ENCYCLOPEDIA OF VITAMIN RESEARCH (2 VOLUME SET)

NUTRITION AND DIET RESEARCH PROGRESS

Additional books in this series can be found on Nova's website
under the Series tab.

Additional E-books in this series can be found on Nova's website
under the E-book tab.

NUTRITION AND DIET RESEARCH PROGRESS

ENCYCLOPEDIA OF VITAMIN RESEARCH (2 VOLUME SET)

JOSHUA T. MAYER

EDITOR

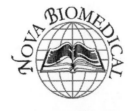

Nova Science Publishers, Inc.

New York

For permission to use material from this book please contact us:
Telephone 631-231-7269; Fax 631-231-8175
Web Site: http://www.novapublishers.com

NOTICE TO THE READER

Additional color graphics may be available in the e-book version of this book.

Library of Congress Cataloging-in-Publication Data

Encyclopedia of vitamin research / editor, Joshua T. Mayer.
    p. ; cm.
 Includes bibliographical references and index.
 ISBN 978-1-61761-928-1 (hardcover : alk. paper)
 1. Vitamins--Encyclopedias. I. Mayer, Joshua T.
 [DNLM: 1. Vitamins. QU 160]
 QP771.E48 2010
 613.2'8603--dc22
                                                                    2010037359

Published by Nova Science Publishers, Inc. † New York

Contents

In: Encyclopedia of Vitamin Research
Editor: Joshua T. Mayer

ISBN 978-1-61761-928-1
© 2011 Nova Science Publishers, Inc.

Chapter 27

Influences of Vitamin D on Prostate Cancer Prevention and Bone Health[*]

Janet Laura Colli
University of Alabama at Birmingham
Birmingham Veteran's Affairs Medical Center, USA

Vitamin D- Commentary/ Short Communication

Prostate cancer is a leading cause of morbidity and mortality among men in North America and northern Europe [1]. Genetics, androgens, dietary and lifestyle factors have been recognized as contributors to risk of prostate cancer [2]. Epidemiological studies suggest associations between environmental factors and prostate cancer risk.

Vitamin D and Prostate Cancer Prevention

Prostate cancer exhibits striking geographical variation, with lower incidences and mortalities in southern latitudes (including China and India), and highest rates occurring in United States, Canada and Scandinavia (countries located in northern hemispheres) [3]. Globally, prostate cancer has higher incidences in countries located in the northern latitudes, and overall has a greater propensity to occur in black and elderly men. These are the same populations most likely to suffer from vitamin D deficiency. Hence it has been hypothesized that low levels of vitamin D (and/or lack of sunlight exposure) may increase the risk of prostate cancer.

---

[*] A version of this chapter was also published in *Vitamin D Biochemistry Nutrition and Roles, edited by William J. Stackhouse* published by Nova Science Publishers, Inc. It was submitted for appropriate modifications in an effort to encourage wider dissemination of research.

Large variations in international prostate cancer incidence and mortality rates suggest that changeable environmental factors exert a role on the etiology of prostate cancer. There are epidemiologic studies which show an inverse relationship between the level of solar altitude and prostate cancer incidence and mortality [3]. Inadequate exposure to sunlight or solar ultraviolet (UV) radiation has been consistently implicated as a risk factor for prostate cancer incidence and mortality in many studies [4]. Further, ecologic analysis of geographic variation in cancer mortality rates suggests that inadequate doses of solar UV radiation cause premature mortality from fifteen different cancers in the United States [5] Exposure to UV radiation leads to the synthesis of vitamin D in humans which has led to the thesis that a vitamin D deficiency may increase the risk of many cancers.

There is evidence the daily requirements for vitamin D increases with age and also are higher in black patients [6]. This is due to evidence suggesting that the skin of older individuals and blacks cannot synthesize vitamin D as effectively as the skin of younger people, and the vitamin D which is produced is less readily absorbed in the intestine [6]. Furthermore, it is important to note that the decrease in serum levels of active Vitamin D lead to an age-related decrease in calcium absorption, which may be as high as 50% [7]. In an affiliate study, prostate cancer was found to occur more frequently in older men in who had documented vitamin D deficiencies. They were able to identify age related declines in enzymes (hydroxylases) responsible for the synthesis of active vitamin D [8]. Further evidence supporting vitamin D as a prostate cancer inhibitor, stems from the study which demonstrated black men to have higher prostate cancer rates compared to white men, while their serum levels of Vitamin D where lower than white men [9]. An additional study reviewing data on Vitamin D and prostate cancer, has shown men in the Orient with diets rich in vitamin D (e.g. derived from fish) have lower incidence of prostate cancer; while those with a high dietary intake of dairy products rich in calcium (which depresses serum levels of vitamin D) are associated with a higher risk of prostate cancer [10]. Prospective, randomized studies have demonstrated that vitamin D suppressed metastatic lesions when administered to patients with advanced prostate cancer [11].

Sources of vitamin D include exposure to sunshine or ultraviolet (UV) irradiation of the skin, dietary intake, and oral supplements. The synthesis of vitamin D in human skin begins with exposure to sunlight (UV) [12]. Vitamin D, obtained by humans from UV exposure or diet, is hydroxylated in the liver to form 25(OH) D (calcidiol), the primary circulating form of the vitamin. Calcidiol is converted to the active hormone 1, 25(OH) 2D (calcitriol) in the kidney and other tissues, including prostate. Calcitriol has been found to hinder prostate cancer cell proliferation and tumor metastasis [13] suggesting protections against both initiation and progression of cancer. Although the biologic evidence for an anti-cancer role of calcitriol is strong for prostate cancer, epidemiological data from prospective studies showed inconsistent associations of pre-diagnostic circulating levels of calcidiol and calcitriol with prostate cancer incidence [13] It has been hypothesized that this lack of correlation may be a result of genetic differences among males. A recent study [14] found that men with the FokI *ff* genotype were more susceptible to prostate cancer if 25(OH) D levels were low. Levels of vitamin D sufficient to prevent cancer in one person may be insufficient in someone with a different genotype and this confounding factor affecting variations has not been taken into consideration in vitamin D studies. This research demonstrated that genetic differences cause some males to become more susceptible to prostate cancer in the presence of low vitamin D levels. Laboratory data suggests that the active metabolite of Vitamin D (1,25-dihydroxy) inhibits growth of prostate cancer cell lines by inducing cell cycle arrest [15], and inhibits the development of prostate cancer in rat models [16].

In summary, many studies have identified mechanisms by which environmental and dietary carcinogens might promote prostate cancer [2]. In addition, investigators have recently characterized several susceptibility loci, somatic mutations, chromosomal rearrangements and genetic alterations (deletions and amplifications) involved in the development and progression of prostate cancer [2].The etiology and progression of prostate cancer is most likely a complex interaction between multiple environmental factors and genetic susceptibility. Since it is difficult to alter ones genetic makeup, prostate cancer prevention and treatment largely depends on our ability to alter environmental and lifestyle factors which lead to molecular changes that cause prostate cancer. Large-scale prevention trials are needed to provide final evidence before making dietary or nutritional recommendations. Future studies, evaluating Vitamin D in prostate cancer prevention need to be performed before we can consider initiating chemoprevention with vitamin D.

Vitamin D and Bone Health in Prostate Cancer

The function of Vitamin D is to enhance the absorption of calcium and phosphate in the intestines to facilitate the mineralization of bone. Vitamin D's action on bone mineralization, and bone readsoption, is indirect through the stimulation of enhanced calcium absorption from the intestinal lumen into the bloodstream. Patients with metastatic or recurrent prostate cancer are frequently placed on androgen deprivation therapy (ADT) for treatment. Evidence that early androgen-deprivation therapy improves survival has led to increased use of androgen deprivation hormone agonists in men with distant metastases and locally advanced nonmetastatic prostate cancer [17].

Osteoporosis is an important complication of androgen-deprivation therapy. Deprivation of androgens has been shown to lead to bone loss in men with prostate cancer by decreasing total bone mineral density. A rapid loss of bone-mineral density occurs within the first 6 to 12 months of androgen-deprivation therapy [18]. Dietary vitamin D supplementation of 400-800IU/d causes a cycle similar to naturally occurring vitamin D: there is an increase in serum 25 (OH) D, a decrease in serum PTH, and a decrease in bone resorption; therefore, decreasing the effect androgen deprivation has on bone mass density [7]. Therefore, patients on androgen deprivation therapy should be placed on Vitamin D and Calcium supplementation to reduce the risk of bone fractures secondary to osteoporosis/osteopenia caused by androgen deprivation therapy.

References

[1]   Jemal A, Murray T, Samuels A, et al. Cancer Statistics, 2003. *Cancer J Clin* 2003; 53: pp 5-26.

[2]   Nelson WG, DeMarzo AM, Isaacs WB, Mechanisms Of Disease – Prostate Cancer. *NEJM*. July 24, 2004, 349; 4, pp 366-381.

[3]   Hanchette CL, Schwartz GG, *Geographic Patterns of Prostate Cancer Mortality. Cancer*. December 15, 1992, Volume 70, No 12, pp 2861-2869.

[4]   Colli JL, Grant WB: Solar ultraviolet B radiation compared with prostate cancer incidence and mortality rates in United States. *Urology* 2008, 71:531–535.

[5]   Grant WB: An estimate of premature cancer mortality in the U.S. due to inadequate doses of solar ultraviolet-B radiation. *Cancer* 2002, 94:1867–1875.

[6]   Russell RM. Vitamin requirements in old age. *Age Nutrition*. 1992; 3:20-23.

[7]   Lips P.Vitamin D deficiency and secondary hyperparathyroidism in the elderly: consequences for bone loss and fractures and therapeutic implications. *Endocr Rev.* 2001; 22:477-501.

[8]   John EM, Schwartz GG, Ingles SA, et al. Sun exposure, vitamin D receptor gene polymorphisms, and risk of advanced prostate cancer. *Cancer Research*. June 15, 2005; 65(12); pp 5470-9.

[9]   Klein E. Opportunities for Prevention of Prostate Cancer: Genetics, Chemoprevention, and Dietary Intervention. *Reviews in Urology.* 2002; 4 (supp 5); pp S18-28.

[10] Peehl DM et al. Pathways mediating the growth-inhibitory actions of vitamin D in prostate cancer. *Journal of Nutrition*, 133: pp 2461S- 2469S.

[11] 11.Schwartz GG, Hall MC, Torti FM, et al. Phase I/II study of 19-nor-1 alpha-25-dihyroxyvitamin D2 (paricalcitol) in advanced, androgen-insensitive prostate cancer. *Clin Cancer Research*. Dec 15, 2005; 11 (24 Pt1): pp 8680-5.

[12] Stein M, Wark JD, Scherer SC. Falls relate to vitamin D and parathyroid hormone in an Australian nursing home and hosteU *Am Geriatr Soc.* 1999; 47:1195-1201.

[13] Giovannucci E: The epidemiology of vitamin D and cancer incidence and mortality: a review (United States). *Cancer Causes Control* 2005, 16: 83–95.

[14] Li H, Stampfer MJ, Hollis JB, et al.: A prospective study of plasma vitamin D metabolites, vitamin D receptor polymorphisms, and prostate cancer. *PLoS Med* 2007, 4:e103.

[15] Peehl DM, Skowronski RJ, Stamey TA, Feldman D, et al. Antiproliferative Effects of 1,25-Didydroxyvitamin D3 on Primary Cultures of Human Prostatic Cells. *Cancer Research*. Feb 1, 1994; 54; pp 805-810.

[16] Carlberg C, Bendik I, Hunziker W, et al. Two Nuclear Signaling Pathways for Vitamin D. *Nature*. Feb 18, 1993; Vol 361, pp 657-660.

[17] The Medical Research Council Prostate Cancer Working Party Investment Group. Immediate versus Deferred Treatment for Advanced Prostatic Cancer: Initial Results of the Medical Research Council Trial, *British Journal of Urology;* 1997; 79, 235-46.

[18] Shahinian V, Kuo Y, Freeman J, Goodwin J, Risk of Fracture after Androgen Deprivation for Prostate Cancer; *NEJM* Volume 352: 154-164, January 13, 2005.

In: Encyclopedia of Vitamin Research
Editor: Joshua T. Mayer

ISBN 978-1-61761-928-1
© 2011 Nova Science Publishers, Inc.

Chapter 28

Effect of Magnesium Deficiency on Vitamin D Metabolism and Action[*]

Robert K. Rude[†1] and Helen E. Gruber[2]

[1]USC Keck School of Medicine and Orthopaedic Hospital, Los Angeles, CA, USA
[2]Department of Orthopaedic Surgery, Carolinas Medical Center, Charlotte, NC, USA

Abstract

Magnesium (Mg) deficiency affects mineral metabolism in a dramatic fashion. Patients with severe Mg deficiency may present with increased neuromuscular hyperexcitablity characterized by paresthesias, muscle cramps and spasm, tetany, and seizures. This is thought to be secondary to profound hypocalcemia and Mg-deficiency induced decreased parathyroid hormone (PTH) secretion and PTH end-organ resistance, although low serum Mg concentrations can produce similar effects without concomitant hypocalcemia. More moderate degrees of Mg deficiency have also been linked to osteoporosis. Serum concentrations of 25(OH)-vitamin D have been observed to be low in patients with severe Mg deficiency and to be resistant to the administration of vitamin D metabolites. Similarly, serum concentrations of 1,25(OH)$_2$-vitamin D are low in Mg deficiency. Experimental Mg depletion in humans and in animal models has resulted in a fall in serum 1,25(OH)$_2$-vitamin D levels. This paper will review the evidence that Mg deficiency in both humans and in animals does adversely affect vitamin D metabolism and/or action.

---

[*] A version of this chapter was also published in *Vitamin D Biochemistry Nutrition and Roles, edited by William J. Stackhouse* published by Nova Science Publishers, Inc. It was submitted for appropriate modifications in an effort to encourage wider dissemination of research.

[†] Corresponding Author: Robert K. Rude, M.D., Orthopaedic Hospital, Endocrinology Research Laboratory, 2400 South Flower Street, Los Angeles, CA 90007, Telephone:213-742-1376, Fax:213-742-1365, Email: rrude60075@aol.com

Introduction

Calcium and the metabolites of vitamin D, 25-hydroxyvitamin D and 1,25-dihydroxyvitmin D, along with parathyroid hormone play an important role in skeletal metabolism as well as other biological processes. Magnesium is also known to modulate the synthesis and action of these hormones and therefore plays an important role in these same processes. Studies have demonstrated that the usual dietary intake or nutritional status of these factors are suboptimal. This chapter will summarize the prevalence of these deficiencies and review the evidence for the role of magnesium deficiency in the action and/or metabolism of vitamin D and its metabolites.

Prevalence of Vitamin D Deficiency and Insufficiency

Vitamin D deficiency is defined as a serum concentration of 25-hydroxyvitamin D of less than 20 ng/ml, and vitamin D insufficiency is defined by a concentration of less that 30 ng/ml. It is estimated that 40-100% of U.S. and European elderly men and women are vitamin D deficient [1]. A recent study of older men in the U.S. demonstrated 26% were vitamin D deficiency and 72% were insufficient in vitamin D [2,3]. The incidence of vitamin D insufficiency appears to be increasing rapidly [4]. This problem also exists in children (1). A recent study in a population aged 1-21 found 9% were vitamin D deficient and 61% were vitamin D insufficient [5]. These data therefore suggest that low vitamin D status may negatively affect skeletal metabolism as well as many other medical problems [1].

Prevalence of Calcium Deficiency

Low dietary calcium (Ca) intake is a recognized risk factor for osteoporosis [6-8]. Low dietary Ca has been reported to predict bone density as well as fracture rate in some studies [8-10]. Dietary Ca intake falls far below the established Adequate Intake (AI) set by the U.S. Food Nutrition Board from adolescence to old age [11]. For example, in females the mean Ca intake at age 14-18 is 753 mg/day (AI = 1300 mg), at age 31-50. 590 mg/day (AI = 1000 mg) and at age 51-70, 510 mg/day (AI = 1200 mg). Ca supplements have been shown to enhance bone mass accumulation in adolescence and retard bone loss in later life [12-15]. Since peak bone mass is an important predictor of osteoporosis in later life, low Ca intake is particularly critical during adolescence when much of the skeleton is formed [14,15]. Ten to twenty percent of adolescent girls have a Ca intake less than 500 mg/day [16]. A recent study reported that pubertal girls only partially adapt to low dietary Ca intake thereby placing them at great risk for inadequate Ca retention [16]. This inability to adapt may be linked to other nutritional deficiencies, as studies that assess multiple nutrient effects on bone suggest that other dietary factors also impact bone mass [17-19]. It is likely that there are substantial detrimental effects on bone when multiple bone-related nutritional deficiencies, such as vitamin D deficiency, are present.

Prevalence of Magnesium Deficiency

Magnesium (Mg), the second most prevalent intracellular cation in the body, plays an important role in enzyme activity, membrane stability and ion transport [20]. Mg exists in macronutrient quantities in bone (0.5-1% bone ash) and dietary Mg deficiency has been implicated as a risk factor for osteoporosis [20-23]. The U.S. Food Nutrition Board established the RDA for Mg for adult males at 420 mg/day and for adult females at 320 mg/day [24]. The usual dietary Mg intake, however, falls below this recommendation.

According to the USDA [25], the mean Mg intake for males is 323 mg/day (81% of the RDA) and the mean intake for females is 228 mg/day (68% of RDA). This deficiency, as with Ca deficiency, is present from adolescence to old age. In females, the mean Mg intake at age 14-18 is 225 mg/day (RDA = 360 mg), at age 31-50, 236 mg/day (RDA = 320 mg), and at age 51-70 , 239 mg/day (RDA = 320mg). This substantial dietary Mg deficit is particularly important in an aging population where gastrointestinal and renal mechanisms for Mg conservation may not be as efficient as in a younger population [26,27]. Ten percent of elderly women in the U.S. consume $\leq$ 136 mg of Mg per day. Morbid conditions associated with body Mg loss (diabetes, alcoholism, malabsorption) and medications (diuretics, cyclosporine, aminiglycosides, cisplatin, amphotericin B) also exacerbate this problem [20].

Effect of Magnesium Deficiency on Parathyroid Hormone Secretion and Action

It is known that Mg deficiency, when severe, will markedly disturb Ca homeostasis, resulting in impaired parathyroid hormone (PTH) secretion and PTH end-organ resistance which lead to hypocalcemia and neuromuscular hyperexcitability (20) Acute changes in the serum Mg concentration in normal subjects modulate PTH secretion (similar to Ca) via the Ca^{2+}-sensing receptor. While acute changes in extracellular Mg concentrations will influence PTH secretion in a manner qualitatively similar to calcium, it is clear that Mg deficiency markedly perturbs mineral homeostasis [28-30].

Hypocalcemia is a prominent manifestation of Mg deficiency in humans [28-30] as well as in most other species [30-32]. In humans, Mg deficiency must become moderate to severe before symptomatic hypocalcemia develops. Mg therapy alone restores serum Ca concentrations to normal [28]. Calcium and/or vitamin D therapy will not correct the hypocalcemia [28, 29].

A major factor resulting in the fall in serum Ca is impaired parathyroid gland function. Determination of serum PTH concentrations in hypocalcemic hypomagnesemic patients has shown that the majority of patients have low or normal serum PTH levels [28,34-36] (Figure 1). Normal serum PTH concentrations are thought to be inappropriately low in the presence of hypocalcemia. Therefore, a state of hypoparathyroidism exists in most hypocalcemic Mg-deficient patients. With Mg therapy, the serum PTH rises to elevated levels within minutes [28]. The serum PTH concentration will gradually fall to normal within several days of therapy with return of the serum calcium concentration to normal [28,33,36].

Some Mg deficient patients, however, have elevated levels of serum PTH [28,36,37] The presence of normal or elevated serum concentrations of PTH in the face of hypocalcemia [28,29,36] suggests that there may also be end organ resistance to PTH action. In one study, PTH administration did not result in elevation in the serum Ca concentration or urinary hydroxyproline excretion in hypocalcemic hypomagnesemic patients [38]. Following Mg repletion, however, a clear response to PTH was observed. PTH has also been shown to have a reduced calcemic effect in Mg-deficient animals [39-41]. In one study of the isolated perfused canine femur, the ability of PTH to simulate an increase in the venous cyclic AMP was impaired during perfusion with low Mg fluid, suggesting skeletal PTH resistance [42].

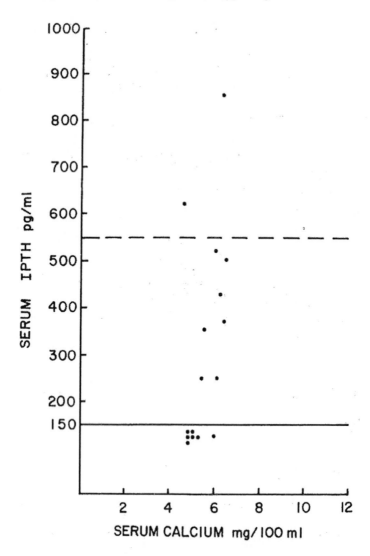

Figure 1. Correlation between the serum PTH concentration with the serum Ca concentration in sixteen hypocalcemic hypomagnesemic patients. The dashed line denotes the upper limit of normal, and the solid line represents the lower level of detection of serum PTH concentration. (Reprinted from reference 28 with permission).

The renal response to PTH has also been assessed by determining the urinary excretion of cyclic AMP and/or phosphate in response to exogenous PTH. Studies in severely Mg-depleted patients demonstrated an impaired response to PTH [28, 29, 38, 43,44]. A decrease in urinary cyclic AMP excretion in response to PTH has also been described in the Mg-deficient dog and rat [40,41].

Effect of Magnesium Deficiency on Vitamin D Metabolism and Action

Mg may also be important in vitamin D metabolism and/or action. Patients with hypoparathyroidism, malabsorption syndromes, and rickets have been reported to be resistant to therapeutic doses of vitamin D until Mg was administered simultaneously [29]. Patients with hypocalcemia and Mg deficiency have also been reported to be resistant to pharmacological doses of vitamin D [45,46], 1α hydroxyvitamin D [47,48] and 1,25-dihydroxyvitamin D [49]. Similarly, an impaired calcemic response to vitamin D has been found in Mg-deficient rats [50], lambs [51], and calves [52].

The exact nature of altered vitamin D metabolism and/or action in Mg deficiency is unclear. Intestinal calcium transport in animal models of Mg deficiency has been found to be reduced in some [53], but not all [54], studies. Calcium malabsorption was associated with low serum levels of 25-hydroxyvitamin D in one study [50], but not in another [54], suggesting that Mg deficiency may impair intestinal Ca absorption by more than one mechanism. Patients with Mg deficiency and hypocalcemia frequently have low serum concentrations of 25-hydroxyvitamin D [55,56], and therefore nutritional vitamin D deficiency may be an important factor in such patients (Figure 2). Therapy with vitamin D, however, results in high serum levels of 25-hydroxyvitamin D without correction of the hypocalcemia [57], suggesting that the vitamin D nutrition is not the major reason. In addition, conversion of radiolabeled vitamin D to 25-hydroxyvitamin D was found to be normal in three Mg-deficient patients [58]. Serum concentrations of 1,25-dihydroxyvitamin D have also been found to be low or low normal in most hypocalcemic Mg-deficient patients (30,55,56, 59) (Figure 2). Mg-deficient diabetic children, when given a low Ca diet, did not exhibit the expected normal rise in serum 1,25-dihydroxyvitamin D or PTH [60]; the response returned to normal, however, following Mg therapy [61].

Recent work has shown that vitamin D insufficient adult women with a blunted response to PTH, had low serum Mg levels [62]. Because PTH is a major trophic for 1,25-dihydroxyvitamin D formation, the low serum PTH concentrations could explain the low 1,25-dihydroxyvitamin D levels. In support of this is the finding that some hypocalcemic Mg-deficient patients treated with Mg have a rise in serum 1,25-dihydroxyvitamin D to high normal or to frankly elevated levels, as shown in Figure 2 [55]. Most patients, however, do not have a significant rise within one week after institution of Mg therapy, despite a rise in serum PTH and normalization of the serum calcium concentration (Fig. 2) [55]. These data suggest that Mg deficiency in humans also impairs the ability of the kidney to synthesize 1,25-dihydroxyvitamin D.

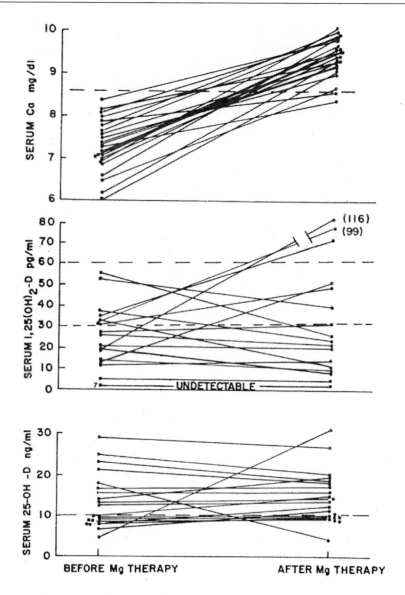

Figure 2. Serum concentrations of Ca, 1,25-dihydroxyvitamin-D and 25-hydroxyvitamin-D in 22 hypocalcemic magnesium-deficient patients before and after 5-8 days of parenteral Mg therapy. The dashed line in the top panel represents the lower normal limit for serum Ca, in the middle panel, the upper and lower limit of normal for serum 1,25-dihydroxyvitamin-D, and in the lower panel, the lower normal limit for 25-hydroxyvitamin D concentrations. (Reprinted from reference 55 with permission).

This is supported by the observation that exogenous administration of 1–34 human PTH to normal subjects after 3 weeks of experimental Mg depletion resulted in a significantly lower rise in serum 1,25-dihydroxyvitamin D concentrations than before institution of the diet (see below) [63]. It appears, therefore, that the renal synthesis of 1,25-dihydroxyvitamin D is sensitive to Mg depletion. While Mg is known to support 25-hydroxy-1α-hydroxylase *in vitro* [64], the exact Mg requirement for this enzymatic process is not known. Reduced bone-specific binding sites for 1,25-dihydroxyvitamin D have also been reported in Mg deficiency [65].

The association of Mg deficiency with impaired vitamin D metabolism and action therefore may be due to several factors, including vitamin D deficiency [55, 56,65,66] and a decrease in PTH secretion [28,33-36], as well as a direct effect of Mg depletion on the ability of the kidney to synthesize 1,25-dihydroxyvitamin D [55,56,63]. Osteoporotic patients with a blunted response to PTH exhibit Mg deficiency [68]. In addition, Mg deficiency may directly impair intestinal Ca absorption [28,53,55]. Skeletal resistance to vitamin D and its metabolites may also play an important role [47,48-50]. It is clear, however, that the restoration of normal serum 1,25-dihydroxyvitamin D concentrations is not required for normalization of the serum calcium level (Figure 2). Most Mg-deficient patients who receive Mg therapy exhibit an immediate rise in PTH, followed by normalization of the serum calcium prior to any change in serum 1,25-dihydroxyvitamin D concentrations [55,56].

Effect of Experimental Magnesium Depletion on Serum Concentrations of 1,25(OH)$_2$-Vitamin D in Humans and Animals

As noted above, Mg deficient patients may have multiple nutritional deficiencies including Ca and vitamin D deficiencies. We therefore conducted experimental human Mg depletion studies by placing 26 normal subjects on a low magnesium diet (12 mg per day) for 21 days. Serum Mg, Ca, PTH and 1,25-dihydroxyvitamin D were determined before and at the conclusion of the dietary period [63]. Magnesium depletion was documented by a fall in serum Mg as well as an increase in the retention of an intravenous infusion of magnesium (Figure 3). There was a significant fall in the serum calcium and 1,25-dihydroxyvitamin D as well (Figure 3). The changes observed in PTH were heterogeneous with 20 of the 26 individuals who exhibited no change (n=8) or a fall in serum PTH (n=12) despite the significant decrease in the serum Ca.

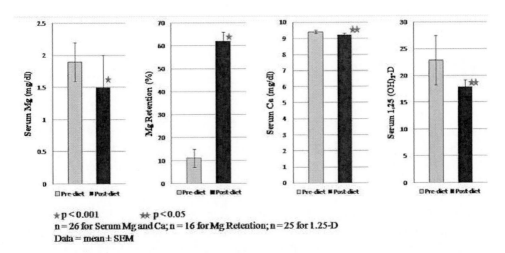

★ p < 0.001   ★★ p < 0.05
n = 26 for Serum Mg and Ca; n = 16 for Mg Retention; n = 25 for 1,25-D
Data = mean ± SEM

Figure 3. Changes in the serum Mg (n = 26), % Mg retention (n = 16), serum Ca (n = 26, and 1,25-dihydroxyvitamin-D (n = 25) in normal human subjects on a low Mg diet for 21 days. (Adapted from reference 63 with permission).

Renal resistance to PTH was assessed in 13 of the study subjects by determining the serum 1,25-dihydroxyvitamin D concentration before and after a 6 hour PTH infusion pre- and post-diet. As noted in Figure 4, there was a significant fall in serum 1,25-dihydroxyvitamin D in the basal level from pre- to post diet. The rise in serum 1,25-dihydroxyvitamin D in response to the PTH infusion post diet was significantly lower than pre-diet suggesting a degree of renal resistance had occurred in response to the low magnesium diet.

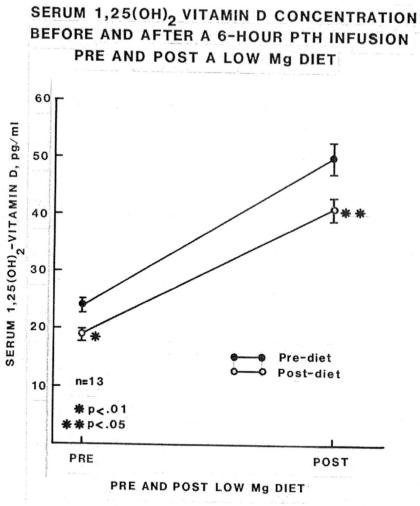

Figure 4. Changes in the serum 1,25-dihydroxyvitamin-D in 13 normal human subjects before and after a low Mg diet for 21 days following a PTH infusion. Data mean ± sem. (Adapted from reference 63 with permission).

The effect of dietary Mg depletion on bone and mineral homeostasis in animals has also been studied, primarily using the rat model. Dietary restriction has usually been severe (0.002 to 0.08 g/Kg diet; normal 0.5 g/Kg diet). A universal observation has been a decrease in growth of both the whole body as well as the skeleton [66-71]. Bone from Mg deficient rats has been described as brittle and fragile [72,73]. Biomechanical testing has directly demonstrated skeletal fragility in both rat and pig [73-75]. Reduction in bone mass compared to control animals occurs in dietary Mg depletion within 6 weeks [71,73-76]. We have also observed a decrease in bone mass and a fall in serum 1,25-dihydroxyvitamin D and PTH in rats on a very low Mg diet (0.002% Mg as percent of total diet) as compared to control (0.063% Mg as percent of total diet) as shown in Figures 5 and 6 [76].

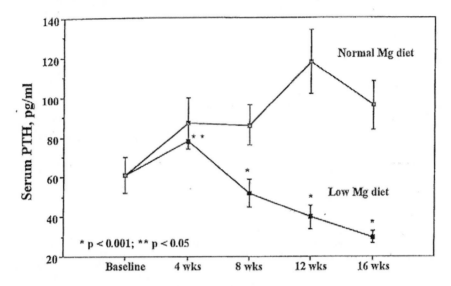

Figure 5. Significant fall in the serum PTH concentration in rats on a very low Mg diet (n = 28) compared to a control diet (n = 34). (Reprinted from reference 76 with permission).

These very low dietary Mg intakes probably do not often occur in the human population. We have, for the first time, studied the effect of less severe dietary Mg restriction on bone metabolism. We employed dietary Mg deprivation in the rat at 10%, 25% and 50% of recommended nutrient (RN) requirement (normal control was 0.05% Mg as percent of total diet) on skeletal metabolism and again found that trabecular bone loss occurred at all these dietary Mg intake levels [77-79]. These dietary intake levels reflect similar levels of dietary Mg inadequacy in segments of our population as discussed above. Data for serum determinations at 6 months in the dietary Mg deprivation group are demonstrated in Table 1. It is noted that the serum Mg was significantly lower in the 10% and 25% NR groups but not in the 50% NR group. The serum Ca tended to be slightly higher in the lower Mg diet groups but slightly lower in the 50% group. This is explained by the fact that Ca and Mg appear to share a common intestinal transport system [80], and, in the absence of intestinal dietary Mg, fractional Ca absorption is increased. A low Ca diet will prevent hypercalcemia in the Mg-deficient rodent [81]. Therefore, at the 50% Mg diet, the changes in serum Ca are similar to humans and other vertebrates. The serum PTH was lower in the 10% and 25% dietary groups, but at the more mild depletion of 50% of NR was elevated. This could be explained by the fact that Mg is acting in a manner similar to Ca by binding to the calcium-sensing receptor at this higher diet Mg intake. Despite these changes, there was a significant fall in serum 1,25-dihydroxyvitamin D in all groups which demonstrates that Mg deficiency reduces this metabolite of vitamin D regardless of the observed changes in serum Mg, Ca, or PTH. These data again suggest that even moderate degrees of Mg depletion adversely affect vitamin D metabolism.

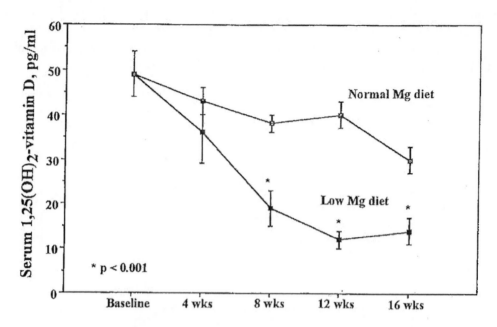

Figure 6. Significant fall in the serum 1,25-dihyroxyvitamin D concentration in rats on a very low Mg diet (n = 28) compared to a control diet (n = 34). (Reprinted from reference 76 with permission).

Table 1. Serum Concentrations of Mg, Ca, PTH, and 1,25(OH)$_2$-Vitamin D in Rats on Low Mg Diets at 10%, 25%, and 50% of Nutritional Requirement (RN) for 6 months.

	10% NR		25% NR		50% NR	
	Control	Low Mg	Control	Low Mg	Control	Low Mg
sMg, mg/dl	1.9 ± 0.2	0.6 ± 0.1*	1.6 ± 0.2	0.9 ± 0.2*	2.0 ± 0.2	1.9 ± 0.3
sCa, mg/dl	8.6 ± 0.5	9.9 ± 0.4*	8.5 ± 0.6	9.2 ± 0.6***	10.1 ± 0.6	$9.6 \pm 0.3^\delta$
sPTH, pg/ml	361 ± 228	141 ± 56**	320 ± 146	$134 \pm 116^\alpha$	381 ± 281	505 ± 302
s1,25D,pg/ml	18.9 ± 16.6	2.9 ± 0.5**	18.0 ± 13	$8.0 \pm 4.0^\beta$	23.5 ± 12.7	10.6 ± 7.1**

Data = mean ± SD. * p<.001; ** p<.01; *** p< .02; α p< .002; β p< .05; δ p<.004
n = 12 for Control and Low Mg in 10%, 25%, and 50% dietary groups.
(adapted from data from ref 77, 78, and 79 with permission)

Conclusion

This review demonstrates that Mg deficiency has a profound effect on vitamin D and PTH metabolism and/or action. This interaction probably plays an important role in skeletal health and the increased risk of osteoporosis observed in Mg deficient humans and animals. Assessment of dietary Mg intake, Mg status, and vitamin D and Ca nutrition should be made in patients with osteoporosis.

References

[1]   Holick, MF. Vitamin D Deficiency. 2007, *N Engl J Med* 357:266-281.

[2]   Orwell, E, Neilson CM, Marshall, LM, Lambert, L, Holton, KF, Hoffman, AR, Barrett-Conner, E, Shikany, JM, Dam, T, and Cauley, JA. Vitamin D deficiency in older men. 2009, *J Clin Endocrinol Metab* 94, 1214-1222.

[3]   Holick, MF. MrOs is D-ficient. 2009, *J Clin Endocrinol Metab* 94, 1092-1093.

[4]   Ginde, AA, Liu, MC, and Camargo, CA. Demographic differences and trends of vitamin D insufficiency in the US population, 1988-2004. 2009, *Arch Intern Med* 169, 626-632.

[5]   Kumar, J, Munter P, Kaskei, FJ, Hailpern, SM, and, Melamed, ML. *Prevalence and associations of 25-hydroxyvitamin D deficiency in US children:* NHANES 2001-2004. 2009, Pediatrics online (doi:10.1542/peds.2009-0051).

[6]   Consensus Development Conference: Prophylaxis and treatment of osteoporosis. 1991, *Am J Med* 90, 107-110.

[7]   *Optimal calcium intake.* 1994, NIH Consensus Statement 12:1-24.

[8]   Heaney, RP. Calcium, dairy products and osteoporosis. 2000, *J Am Coll Nutr* 19, 83s-99s.

[9]   Dawson-Hughes, B, Gallai, GE, Drall, EA, Sadowski, L, Sahyoun N, Tannenbaum, S. A controlled trial of the effect of calcium supplementation on bone density in postmenopausal women. 1990, *N Engl J Med* 323, 878-883.

[10]   Meyer HE. Calcium and osteoporotic fractures. 2004, *Br J Nutr* 91, 505-506.

[11]   *Dietary Reference Intakes for calcium, phosphorus, magnesium, vitamin D, and fluoride.* 1997, National Academy Press, Washington, D.C., 71-145.

[12]   Flynn A. *The role of dietary calcium in bone health.* 2003, Proc Nutr Soc 62, 851-858.

[13]   Cashman KD, Flynn A. Optimal nutrition: calcium, magnesium and phosphorus. 1999, *Proc Nutr Soc* 58, 477-487.

[14]   Bachrach LK. Acquisition of optimal bone mass in childhood and adolescence. 2001, *Trends Endocrinol Metab* 12, 22-28.

[15]   Weaver CM. Calcium and magnesium requirements of children and adolescents and peak bone mass. 2000, *Nutrition* 16, 514-516.

[16]   Abrams SA, Griffin IJ, Hicks PD, Gunn SK. Pubertal girls only partially adapt to low dietary calcium intakes. 2004, *J Bone Miner* Res 19, 759-763.

[17]   Tranquilli AL, Lucino E, Garzetti GG, Romanini C. Calcium, phosphorus and magnesium intakes correlate with bone mineral content in postmenopausal women. 1994, *Gynecol Endocrinol* 8, 55-58.

[18]   New SA, Bolton-Smith C, Grubb DA, Reid DM. Nutritional influences on bone mineral density: A cross-sectional study in premenopausal women. 1997, *Am J Clin Nutr* 65:1831-1839.

[19]   Macdonald HM, New SA, Golden MHN, Campbell MK, Reid DM. Nutritional associations with bone loss during the menopausal transition: evidence of a beneficial effect of calcium, alcohol, and fruit and vegetable nutrients and of a detrimental effect of fatty acids. 2004, *Am Soc Clin Nutr* 79, 155-165.

[20]   Rude RK. Magnesium Deficiency: a heterogeneous cause of disease in humans. 1998, *J Bone Miner Res* 13, 749-758.

[21] Sojka JE, Weaver CM. Magnesium supplementation and osteoporosis. 1995, *Nutr Rev* 53, 71-80.

[22] Cohen L, Kitzes R. 1981, Infrared spectroscopy and magnesium content of bone mineral in osteoporotic women. *Israel J Med Sci* 17, 1123-1125.

[23] Wallach S. Effects of magnesium on skeletal metabolism. 1990, *Magnes Trace Elem* 9, 1-14.

[24] *Dietary Reference Intakes for calcium, phosphorus, magnesium, vitamin D, and fluoride.* 1997, National Academy Press, Washington, D.C., 190-249.

[25] Cleveland LE, Goldman JD, Borrude LG 1994 Data tables: Results from USDA 1994 continuing survey of food intakes by individuals and 1994 diet and health knowledge survey. *Agricultural Research Service,* U.S. Department of Agriculture, Beltsville, MD.

[26] Lowik MRH, van Dokkum W, Kistemaker C, Schaafasma G, Ockhuizen T. Body composition, health status and urinary magnesium excretion among elderly people (Dutch nutrition surveillance system). 1993, *Magnes Res* 63, 223-232.

[27] Martin BJ. The magnesium load test: Experience in elderly subjects. 1990, *Aging* 2, 291-296.

[28] Rude, R. K., Oldham, S. B., and Singer, F. R. Functional hypoparathyroidism and parathyroid hormone end-organ resistance in human magnesium deficiency. 1976, *Clin. Endocrinol.* 5, 209–224.

[29] Rude, R. K. (1994). Magnesium deficiency in parathyroid function. *In "The Parathyroids"* (J. P. Bilezikian, ed.), pp. 829–842. Raven Press, New York.

[30] Rude, R. K., and Shils, M. E. (2006). *Magnesium. In "Modern Nutrition in Health and Disease"* (M. E. Shils, ed.), pp. 223-247. Lippincott Williams and Wilkins, Philadelphia.

[31] Shils, M. E., Magnesium, calcium and parathyroid hormone interactions. 1980, *Ann. N.Y. Acad. Sci.* 355, 165–180.

[32] Anast, C. S., and Forte, L. F. Parathyroid function and magnesium depletion in the rat. 1983, *Endocrinology* 113, 184–189.

[33] Anast, C. S., Mohs, J. M., Kaplan, S. L., and Burns, T. W. Evidence for parathyroid failure in magnesium deficiency. 1972, *Science* 177, 606–608.

[34] Chase, L. R., and Slatopolsky, E. Secretion and metabolic efficacy of parathyroid hormone in patients with severe hypomagnesemia. 1974, J. *Clin. Endocrinol. Metab.* 38, 363–371.

[35] Suh, S. M., Tashjian, A. H., Matsuo, N., Parkinson, D. K., and Fraser, D. Pathogenesis of hypocalcemia in primary hypomagnesemia: Normal end-organ responsiveness to parathyroid hormone, impaired parathyroid gland function. 1973, *J. Clin. Invest.* 52, 153–160.

[36] Rude, R. K., Oldham, S. B., Sharp, C. F., Jr., and Singer, F. R. Parathyroid hormone secretion in magnesium deficiency. 1978, *J. Clin. Endocrinol. Metab.* 47, 800–806.

[37] Allgrove, J., Adami, S., Fraher, L., Reuben, A., and O'Riordan, J. L. H. Hypomagnesaemia: Studies of parathyroid hormone secretion and function. 1984, *Clin. Endocrinol.* 21, 435–449.

[38] Estep, H., Shaw, W. A., Watlington, C., Hobe, R., Holland, W., and Tucker, S. G. Hypocalcemia due to hypomagnesemia and reversible parathyroid hormone unresponsiveness. 1969, *J. Clin. Endocrinol.* 29, 842–848.

[39] MacManus, J., Heaton, F. W., and Lucas, P. W. A decreased response to parathyroid hormone in magnesium deficiency. 1971, *J. Endocrinol.* 49, 253–258.

[40] Levi, J., Massry, S. G., Coburn, J. W., Llach, F., and Kleeman, C. R. Hypocalcemia in magnesium-depleted dogs: Evidence for reduced responsiveness to parathyroid hormone and relative failure of parathyroid gland function. 1974, *Metabolism* 23, 323–335.

[41] Forbes, R. M., and Parker, H. M. Effect of magnesium deficiency on rat bone and kidney sensitivity to parathyroid hormone.1980, *J. Nutr.* 110, 1610–1617.

[42] Freitag, J. J., Martin, K. J., Conrades, M. B., Bellorin-Font, E., Teitelbaum, S., Klahr, S., and Slatopolsky, E. Evidence for skeletal resistance to parathyroid hormone in magnesium deficiency. 1979, *J. Clin. Invest.* 64, 1238–1244.

[43] Medalle, R., and Waterhouse, C. A magnesium-deficient patient presenting with hypocalcemia and hyperphosphatemia. 1973, *Ann. Int. Med.* 79, 76–79.

[44] Mihara, M., Kamikubo, K., Hiramatsu, K., Itaya, S., Ogawa, T., and Sakata, S. Renal refractoriness to phosphaturic action of parathyroid hormone in a patient with hypomagnesemia. 1995, *Intern. Med.* 34, 666-669.

[45] Medalle, R., Waterhouse, C., and Hahn, T. J. Vitamin D resistance in magnesium deficiency. 1976, *Am. J. Clin. Nutr.* 29, 854–858.

[46] Leicht, E., Biro, G., Keck, E., and Langer, H. J. Die hypomagnesiaemie-bedingte hypocalciaemie: funktioneller hypoparathyreoidismus, parathormon-und vitamin D resistenz. 1990, *Klin. Wochenschr.* 68, 678–684.

[47] Ralston, S., Boyle, I. T., Cowan, R. A., Crean, G. P., Jenkins, A., and Thomson, W. S. PTH and vitamin D responses during treatment of hypomagnesaemic hypoparathyroidism. 1983, *Acta Endocrinol.* 103, 535–538.

[48] Selby, P. L., Peacock, M., and Bambach, C. P. Hypomagnesaemia after small bowel resection: Treatment with 1 α-hydroxylated vitamin D metabolites. 1984, *Br. J. Surg.* 71, 334–337.

[49] Graber, M. L., and Schulman, G. Hypomagnesemic hypocalcemia independent of parathyroid hormone. 1986, *Ann. Int. Med.* 104, 804–806.

[50] Lifshitz, F., Harrison, H. C., and Harrison, H. E. Response to vitamin D of magnesium deficient rats.1967, *Proc. Soc. Exp. Biol. Med.* 125, 472–476.

[51] McAleese, D. M., and Forbes, R. M. Experimental production of magnesium deficiency in lambs on a diet containing roughage. 1959, *Nature* 184, 2025–2026.

[52] Smith, R. H. Calcium and magnesium metabolism in calves. 2. Effect of dietary vitamin D and ultraviolet irradiation on milk-fed calves. 1958, *Biochem. J.* 70, 201-205.

[53] Higuchi, J., and Lukert, B. Effects of magnesium depletion on vitamin D metabolism and intestinal calcium transport. 1974, *Clin. Res.* 22, 617.

[54] Coburn, J. W., Reddy, C. R., Brickman, A. S., Hartenbower, D. L., and Friedler, R. M. Vitamin D metabolism in magnesium deficiency. 1975, *Clin. Res.* 23, 3933.

[55] Rude, R. K., Adams, J. S., Ryzen, E., Endres, D. B., Niimi, H., Horst, R. L., Haddad, J. F., and Singer, F. R. Low serum concentrations of 1,25-dihydroxyvitamin D in human magnesium deficiency. 1985, *J. Clin. Endocrinol. Metab.* 61, 933–940.

[56] Fuss, M., Bergmann, P., Bergans, A., Bagon, J., Cogan, E., Pepersack, T., Van Gossum, M., and Corvilain, J. Correction of low circulating levels of 1,25-dihydroxyvitamin D by 25-hydroxyvitamin D during reversal of hypomagnesaemia. 1989, *Clin. Endocrinol.* 31, 31–38.

[57] Medalle, R., Waterhouse, C., and Hahn, T. J. Vitamin D resistance in magnesium deficiency. 1976, *Am. J. Clin. Nutr.* 29, 854–858.

[58] Lukert, B. P. (1980). Effect of magnesium depletion on vitamin D metabolism in man. *In "Magnesium in Health and Disease"* (M. Cantin and M. S. Seelig, eds.), pp. 275–279 Spectrum, New York.

[59] Leicht, E., Schmidt-Gayk, N., Langer, H. J., Sniege, N., and Biro, G. Hypomagnesaemia-induced hypocalcaemia: Concentrations of parathyroid hormone, prolactin and 1,25-dihydroxyvitamin D during magnesium replenishment. 1992, *Magnes. Res.* 5, 33–36.

[60] Saggese, G., Bertelloni, S., Baroncelli, G. I., Federico, G., Calisti, I., and Fusaro, C. (1988). Bone demineralization and impaired mineral metabolism in insulin-dependent diabetes mellitus. *Helv. Paediat. Acta* 43, 405–414.

[61] Saggese, G., Federico, G., Bertelloni, S., Baroncelli, G. I., and Calisti, L. (1991). Hypomagnesemia and the parathyroid hormone-vitamin D endocrine system in children with insulin-dependent diabetes mellitus: Effects of magnesium administration. *J. Pediatr.* 118, 220–225.

[62] Gunnarsson, O, Indridason, OS, Lranzon, L, and Sigurdsson, G. Factors associated with elevater or blunted PTH response in vitamin D insufficient adults. 2008, *J Intern Med.*265, 488-495.

[63] Fatemi, S., Ryzen, E., Flores, J., Endres, D. B., and Rude, R. K. Effect of experimental human magnesium depletion on parathyroid hormone secretion and 1,25-dihydroxyvitamin D metabolism. 1991, *J. Clin. Endocrinol. Metab.* 73, 1067–1072.

[64] Fisco, F., and Traba, M. L. Influence of magnesium on the in vitro synthesis of 24,25-dihydroxyvitamin D3 and 1α,25-dihydroxyvitamin D3. 1992, *Magnes. Res.* 5, 5–14.

[65] Risco, F. and Traba, M.I. Bone specific binding sites for $1,25(OH)-D_3$ in magnesium deficiency. 2004, *J. Physiol. Biochem.* 60, 199-204.

[66] Carpenter, T. O. Disturbances of vitamin D metabolism and action during clinical and experimental magnesium deficiency. 1988, *Magnes. Res.* 1, 131–139.

[67] Leicht, E., and Biro, G. Mechanisms of hypocalcaemia in the clinical form of severe magnesium deficit in the human. 1992, *Magnes. Res.* 5, 37–44.

[68] Sahota, O., Mundey M. K., San, P., Godher, I. M., and Hosking, D. J. Vitamin D insufficiency and the blunted PTH response in established osteoporosis: the role of magnesium deficiency. 2006, *Osteoporos. Int.* 17, 1013-1021.

[69] Kenney, MA, McCoy, H, and Williams, L. Effects of magnesium deficiency on strength, mass and composition of rat femur. 1994, *Calcif Tissue Int* 54:44-49.

[70] Mirra, JM, Alcock, NW, Shils, ME, and Tannenbaum, P. Effects of calcium and magnesium deficiencies on rat skeletal development and parathyroid gland area. 1982, *Magnesium* 1:16-33.

[71] Carpenter, TO, Mackowiak, SJ, Troiano, N, aand Gundberg, CM. Osteocalcin and its message: Relationship to bone histology in magnesium-deprived rats. 1992, *Am J Physiol* 263:E107-E114.

[72] Lai, CC, Singer L, and Armstrong ,WD. Bone composition and phosphatase activity in magnesium deficiency in rats. 1975*J Bone Joint Surg* 57, 516-522.

[73] Kenney, MA, McCoy, H, and Williams, L. Effects of dietary magnesium and nickel on growth and bone characteristics in rats. 1992, *J Am Col Nutr* 11:687-693.

[74] Miller ER, Ullrey DE, Zutaut CL, Baltzer BV, Schmidt DA, Hoefer JA, Luecke RW. Magnesium requirement of the baby pig. *J Nutr* 85:13-20, 1965.

[75] Heroux, O, Peter, D, and Tanner, A. Effect of a chronic suboptimal intake of magnesium on magnesium and calcium content of bone and on bone strength of the rat. 1974, *Can J Physiol Pharmacol* 53:304-310.

[76] Rude, RK, Kirchen ,ME, Gruber, HE, Meyer ,MH, Luck, JS, and Crawford, DL. Magnesium deficiency-induced osteoporosis in the rat: Uncoupling of bone formation and bone resorption. 1999, *Magnes Res* 12:257-267.

[77] Rude, RK, Gruber, HE, Norton, HJ, Wei, LY, Frausto, A, and Mills, BG. Bone loss induced by dietary magnesium reduction to 10% Nutrient Requirement in rats is associated with increase release of substance P and tumor necrosis factor-a. 2004, *J Nutr* 134:79-85.

[78] Rude, RK, Gruber, HE, Norton, HJ, Wei, LY, Frausto, A, and Kilburn ' J. Dietary Magnesium Reduction to 25% of Nutrient Requirement Disrupts Bone and Mineral Metabolism in the Rat. 2005, *Bone* 37: 211-219.

[79] Rude, RK, Gruber, HE, Norton ,HJ, Wei, LY, Frausto, A, and Kilburn, J. Reduction of dietary magnesium by only 50% in the rat disrupts bone and mineral metabolism. 2006, *Osteopor Int* 17: 1022-1032.

[80] Rude RK: *Magnesium Homeostasis*. In: Principles of Bone Biology (3nd edition; Bilezikian JB, Raisz L, Rodan G [editors]). Academic Press, San Diego, CA, pp487– 358-513, 2008.

[81] Rude RK, Gruber HE, Wei LY, Frausto A, Mills BG. 2003. Magnesium deficiency: effect on bone and mineral metabolism in the mouse. *Calcif Tiss Int* 72:32–41.

In: Encyclopedia of Vitamin Research
Editor: Joshua T. Mayer

ISBN 978-1-61761-928-1
© 2011 Nova Science Publishers, Inc.

Chapter 29

Carotenoids in Crops: Roles, Regulation of the Pathway, Breeding to Improve the Content[*]

Marco Fambrini and Claudio Pugliesi[†]

Dipartimento di Biologia delle Piante Agrarie, Sezione di Genetica,
Università di Pisa, Via Matteotti 1B, I-56124 Pisa, Italy

Abstract

The carotenoids are natural phytochemicals important to exploit the nutritional value of fruits and vegetables because they are required as provitamin A, antioxidants and immune system stimulants. At biochemical level, the biosynthetic pathway has been extensively clarified in several organisms and a near complete set of genes encoding enzymes have been identified. Some major crops (i.e. cereals or potato) are characterized by insufficient (or null) carotenoid content and to combat malnutrition, especially in developing countries, food biofortification is a relevant objective. Traditional approaches of breeding have been applied in some vegetables to study the genetic factors implicated in carotenoid accumulation and more recently, several interesting results have been obtained by recombinant DNA techniques. The regulation of carotenoid biosynthesis is only partially known and it deserves particular attention to improve the efficiency of plant breeding. In the introduction of this chapter, we summarize the roles of carotenoids in plants and animals as well as the essential steps of biosynthetic pathway in higher plants. Then, we report basic aspects on regulatory mechanisms of carotenogenesis also including the characterization of some mutants in crop species with altered profile of

---

[*] A version of this chapter was also published in *Beta Carotene: Dietary Sources, Cancer and Cognition,* *edited by Leiv Haugen and Terje Bjornson* published by Nova Science Publishers, Inc. It was submitted for appropriate modifications in an effort to encourage wider dissemination of research.

[†] Corresponding author: Dipartimento di Biologia delle Piante Agrarie, Sezione di Genetica, Università di Pisa, Via Matteotti 1B, I-56124 Pisa, Italy; Tel.: +39(0)502216666; Fax: +39(0)502216661; Email address: cpuglies@agr.unipi.it

carotenoid composition. Finally, with respect to species where traditional and innovative plant breeding have been applied, we review the main results obtained.

Keywords: Antioxidants, biofortification, breeding, carotenoid, pigment mutants, provitamin A, transgenic plants.

Introduction

Carotenoids are yellow, orange and red pigments (>600) present in all major taxa probably appeared for the first time in archaebacteria (Vershinin, 1999). As pointed out by George Britton (1995) carotenoids are not *"another group of pigments"* but *"substances with very special and remarkable properties that no other group of substances possess and that form the basis of their many, varied functions and actions in all kinds of living organisms"*. These peculiar characteristics can be related to their fundamental chemical properties (Britton, 2008). The nature is polyisoprenoid and a key feature is the conjugated system in which π-electrons are delocalized over the entire length. The long sequence of double and single bonds is located in the centre of molecule. Three major processes can modify the basis of the skeleton: cyclization (at the end), modification of hydrogenation level, and addition of oxygen-containing functional groups. If the basic structure contains oxygen function the carotenoid is named xanthophyll. When the oxygen function is absent, the name is carotene. The carotenoids are hydrophobic and usually associated to cell membranes. In alternative, the localization is different if the molecule is associated to proteins (Britton, 1995).

Carotenoids determine the natural color of purple bacteria, or tissues in some species of algae, mussels, crustaceans, fishes, reptiles and birds. The carotenoid-dependent color of vertebrate (i.e. zebra finches, *Taeniopygia guttata*) is a trait awarded in evolution because the ostentation of bright pigments is an ornamental marker of superior immunocompetence (Blount et al., 2003; Blount and McGraw, 2008).

In higher plants, these pigments occur in plastids located in green tissues, flowers and storage organs where guarantee a large spectrum of functions (Bartley and Scolnik, 1995). In leaves their color is masked by chlorophyll but the synthesis in chloroplasts is fundamental to ensure the production of chemical energy from light. From the considerable accumulation of carotenoids in chromoplasts depend the color of flowers and fruits in several species to promote visual attraction. Likewise, carotenoids are frequently used as natural colorants by cosmetic or food manufactures. Fruits and vegetables are common source of carotenoids in human diet. High pigment content has been ascertained in mango (*Mangifera indica* L.), pepper (*Capsicum annuum* L.), melon (*Cucumis melo* L.), apricot (*Prunus armeniaca* L.) and tomato fruits (*Solanum lycopersicum* L.). Among green vegetables, watercress (*Nasturtium officinale* L.), spinach (*Spinacia oleracea* L.), and parsley (*Petroselinum crispum* L.) are particularly enriched in carotenoids (Figure 1) (Müller, 1997; Holden et al., 1999; Fraser and Bramley, 2004). Moreover, carrots (*Daucus carota* L.) are the roots more famous for the high provitamin A content. In general, it is important to emphasize that amongst the characters of horticultural crops with marked value, color is one the most important phenotypic trait because influences consumer's initial perception of product quality. On the other hand, carotenoid pigmentation patterns have profound effects on the apocarotenoid and monoterpene aroma volatiles as demonstrated in tomato and melon (Lewinsohn et al., 2005).

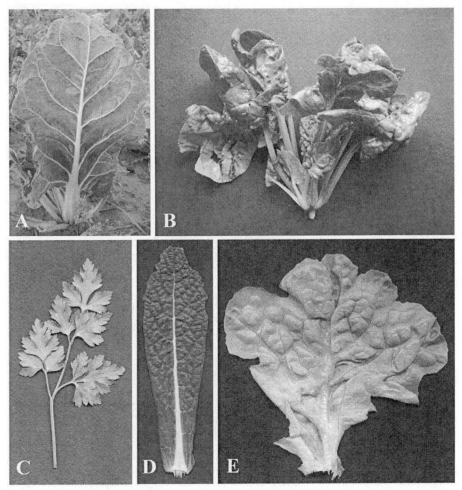

Figure 1. Some green vegetables with significant carotenoid content. A, chard (*Beta vulgaris*); B, spinach (*Spinacia oleracea*); C, parsley (*Petroselinum crispum*); D, kale (*Brassica oleracea* var. *acephala*); E, lettuce (*Lactuca sativa*).

Humans and animals are not able to synthesize carotenoids and after the absorption at the level of mucosal cells, these pigments appear unchanged in the circulation and peripheral tissues while adipose tissue and liver are the common storage depots (Rock, 1997). Moreover, the yellow color of retina depends on ingested carotenoids such as lutein and zeaxanthin (Krinsky et al., 2003).

Carotenoid Biosynthesis in Higher Plants

Carotenoids are tetraterpenoid pigments characterized by a C_{40} backbone with polyene chains that may contain up to 15 conjugated double bonds. Despite the carotenoid biosynthesis takes place in the plastid, all known enzymes in the pathway are nuclear encoded and post-translationally imported into organelle (Cunningham and Gantt, 1998; Sandmann, 2002).

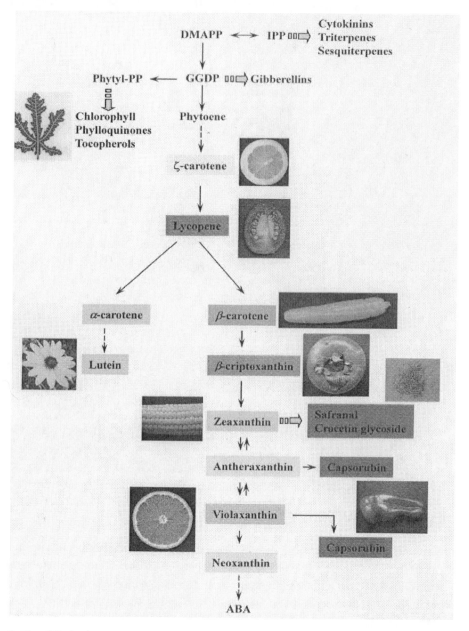

Figure 2. Simplified scheme of carotenoid biosynthesis and related pathways in higher plants. Note, only few steps are indicated and rectangular box color is not representative for the associate carotenoid. Examples of crops characterized by pigment accumulation are showed: *Ficus carica*, leaf abaxial side; *Citrus limon*, transverse hand fruit section; *Solanum lycopersicum* longitudinal hand fruit section; *Daucus carota*, longitudinal hand root section; *Diospyros kaki* fruit (top of view); *Crocus sativus*, dried stlyles; *Helianthus tuberosus*, inflorescence; *Zea mays*, particular of the ear; *Citrus sinensis*, fruit; *Capsicum annuum*, fruit.

In plastids, the carotenoids biosynthesis depends on the non-mevalonate or 2-C-methyl-D-erythritol 4-phosphate (MEP/DOXP) pathway (Lichtenthaler 1999; Rodríquez-Concepción and Boronat 2002; Bouvier et al., 2005b; DellaPenna and Pogson, 2006; Lu and Li, 2008). The first committed step of carotenoid synthesis, the head-to-head condensation of geranylgeranyl diphosphate (GGPP) molecules to produce phytoene, is mediated by the soluble enzyme phytoene synthase (PSY). It is important to note that the C_{20} GGPP is an early precursor not only of carotenoids but also of phylloquinone, chlorophyll, tocopherol and gibberellins (Figure 2; Chappell, 1995). Membrane-localized enzymes carry out subsequent steps of the pathway leading to the coloured carotenoids. The phytoene undergoes four desaturation reactions with the production of lycopene. In this part of the pathway, phytofluene, ζ-carotene and neurosporene are the intermediates. In higher plants, four desaturations are performed by two FAD containing enzymes: the phytoene desaturase (PDS) and the ζ-carotene desaturase (ZDS). The PDS inserts *trans* double bonds at the 11,11' positions, whereas ZDS inserts *cis* double bonds at the 7,7' positions (Giuliano et al., 2002). In the following step, the carotenoid isomerase (CRTISO) enzyme converts pro-lycopene to all-*trans*-lycopene (Isaacson et al., 2002; Park et al., 2002). Lycopene is converted to cyclic carotenoids β-carotene and α-carotene by cyclases such as, lycopene β-cyclase (LCY-b) (Pecker et al., 1996) and lycopene ε-cyclase (LCY-e) (Ronen et al., 1999). Subsequently, substitutions by hydroxyl, oxo, and/or epoxy groups produce xanthophylls with bright orange/yellow colors.

A family of dioxygenases (CCDs) catalyses the cleavage of several carotenoids with the production of apocarotenoids (Bouvier et al., 2005a; Auldridge et al., 2006). Probably, the most known product of carotenoid (neoxanthin) catabolism is the hormone abscisic acid (Nambara and Marion-Poll, 2005) but the spectrum of compounds is wide and includes β-ionone (Schwartz et al., 2003), saffron (Castillo et al., 2005), bixin (Bouvier et al., 2003a) and strigolactones (Akiyama et al., 2005).

Carotenoid Role in Plants

Chloroplasts

The functions of carotenoids in higher plants are influenced where the pigments are synthesized. In chloroplast, the two major roles of carotenoids are related to photosynthesis: light harvesting and protection from photo-oxidation. The carotenoid composition of chloroplasts is usually the following: lutein (45% of the total), β-carotene (25-30%), violaxanthin (10-15%), neoxanthin (10-15%).

A clear demonstration of the pivotal roles of carotenoids in chloroplasts is given by genotypes deficient in carotenoid biosynthesis. For example, in sunflower the *non dormant-1* (*nd-1*) mutant is characterized by an albino and viviparous phenotype (Fambrini et al., 1993). This lethal genotype shows a block in the carotenogenesis after the synthesis of ζ-carotene related to a chromosomal deletion including a region of the *ZDS* locus (Conti et al., 2004). Therefore in the *nd-1* mutant, the absence of end products of the carotenoid pathway determines absence of thylakoids membranes, photobleaching of chlorophyll, no CO_2 uptake and absence of embryo dormancy (Fambrini et al., 1993; Conti et al., 2004).

The conjugated double bonds of carotenoids are responsible of their ability to adsorb photons in the visible wavelengths and this property is very important to increase the spectrum of wavelengths to perform light harvesting (Frank and Cogdell, 1996). The energy transfer from carotenoids to chlorophylls requires a close association. The absorption spectra (primarily from 400 nm to 550 nm) of carotenoids are associated with the transition from the S_0 (ground state) to the second excited state S_2. The latter, converts to S_1 in a few hundred femtoseconds, while the return from S_1 to S_0 occurs in few picoseconds (Ritz et al., 2000). Recently, an additional excited singlet state, S_x has been identified between S_2 and S_1 (Cerullo et al., 2002). Singlet-singlet resonant energy transfer from carotenoid to chlorophyll has been described but the exact mechanisms involved are poorly understood.

Fine-setting of light harvesting efficiency is required because frequently higher plants encounter light intensities that exceed their photosynthetic capacity. Moreover, at the level of photosystem II (PSII), light energy facilitates the generation of a strong oxidant that is capable of oxidizing water molecules and as consequence photooxidative intermediates are inevitable byproducts of photosynthesis (Melis, 1999). Under high light, the light-harvesting system of PSII changed into a state in which energy is dissipated as heat. This process, known as nonphotochemical quenching (NPQ), occurs by the creation of energy quenchers following conformational change in the light-harvesting complexes, which is initiated by the build up of the thylakoid pH gradient and controlled by the xanthophyll cycle. The predominant component of NPQ is referred to as energy-dependent quenching, or qE, and it is rapidly reversible and correlated with zeaxanthin formation. With excess of light, zeaxanthin is formed from violaxanthin via antheraxanthin while the reaction is reversed in the dark (Yamamoto, 1979; Demming-Adams and Adams, 1996). If a mutant is incapable of CO_2 assimilation, the zeaxanthin accumulation can be observed also in low light condition. This case has been effectively verified, for example, in the *xan1* mutant of sunflower with abnormal chloroplast biogenesis (Fambrini et al., 2004).

The non-radiative dissipation is linked to non-photochemical de-excitation of $^1Chl^*$ (singlet excitation of chlorophyll) and this process is normally monitored by a lowering of chlorophyll fluorescence. Although the biological significance of qE is established, the molecular mechanisms involved are unknown. Two different mechanisms have been proposed recently on this topic (Holt et al., 2005; Ruban et al., 2007). Ruban et al. (2007), retain that qE occurs in the peripheral LHCII where the key process is the energy transfer from chlorophyll *a* to a low-lying excited state of a specific carotenoid (lutein 1). The second mechanism, a charge-transfer (CT) mechanism, suggests the existence of energy transfer from the chlorophylls bound to LHCII supercomplex to a chlorophyll-zeaxanthin heterodimer (Holt et al., 2005; Avenson et al., 2008).

The peripheral antenna consists of trimeric complexes composed of LHCII proteins, the major LHC of higher plant antennae; three minor LHCs referred, as CP24, CP26, and CP29 are located between the peripheral LHCII and the reaction center. It is possible that different qE mechanisms are operating in different parts of the PSII antenna (Ahn et al., 2008).

The antenna of photosystem I (PSI) consists of two structurally and functionally parts: the core antenna and the peripheral antenna. Carotenoids of the core antenna are represented by β-carotene molecules while in the peripheral antenna, LHCA proteins bind mainly lutein and violaxanthin.

Molecular genetics of the xanthophyll cycle support the view that carotenoids are involved in the process of $^1Chl^*$ quenching (Baroli and Niyogi, 2000). For example, the *npq1* mutant of *Arabidopsis thaliana* is extremely susceptible to light stress and shows a defect in qE. This phenotype depends on the deficient function of the violaxanthin de-epoxidase that preclude the zeaxanthin accumulation (Niyogi et al., 1998). The characterization of the *lut2* mutant in the same species has demonstrated that the deficient content of lutein is associated to an abnormal induction of NPQ (Pogson et al., 1998).

The protection of carotenoids against photo-oxidative damage is not exhausted in the process of ^{1}Chl* quenching. In fact, carotenoids are also able to quench ^{3}Chl* and ^{1}O$_2$* (Edge et al., 1997; Telfer et al., 1994). In both cases, the end-product is a carotenoid triplet that decays to the ground state by thermal dissipation. Lutein, zeaxanthin and violaxanthin are particularly involved in protection against ^{1}Chl*. On the contrary, neoxanthin is more active in ^{1}O$_2$* quenching (Croce et al., 1999).

Chloroplasts originate from etioplasts from the dark-light transition during photo-morphogenesis (Ellis, 1984). The color of etiolated seedlings is normally yellow due to carotenoids into etioplasts; recently the Pogson's Research Group (Cuttriss et al., 2007) has demonstrated that lutein synthesis is essential to development of lattice-like membranous structure of etioplast, the prolamellar body (PLB).

Other Plastids

With the exception of proplastids, the carotenoids are presents in all types of plastids (chromoplasts, amyloplasts, elaioplasts, leucoplasts and etioplasts) of flowers, fruits, roots, tubers and seeds (Bartley and Scolnik, 1995; Howitt and Pogson, 2006). The biological roles of carotenoids in these different plastids are not completely clear.

In fruits and flowers their role as attractants is evident but other two major functions are important: precursors of scents and antioxidants. In species with pollination mediated by insects the pollen is frequently colored and in many cases, the aspect depends on carotenoid accumulation (Stanley and Linsken, 1974). Carotenoids such as β-carotene, xanthophylls or esterified molecules are present in the adhesive material around pollen grains (pollenkitt) and their origin is the anther tapetum before its final dissolution (Pacini and Hesse, 2005). A structural role of carotenoids in the sporopollenin biosynthesis has been proposed in the past (Brooks and Shaw, 1968) but treatments with inhibitors of carotenegenesis indicate that, also in presence of a deficient accumulation carotenoid synthesis, the structure of sporopollenin is not drastically affected (Wiermann and Gubatz, 1992). Optical attraction of pollinators is probably the main function of carotenoids in pollenkitt but other are suspected such as the protection against ultraviolet radiation, growth stimulation for male cells, or control of the germination process (Stanley and Linsken, 1974). In seeds the carotenoids are precursors of abscisic acid (ABA) and this hormone is fundamental for the induction of dormancy. In fact, only the ABA synthesized *in situ* is important to prevent precocious events of germination. On the other hands, carotenoids protect the seeds from radical oxygen species and this function extends their lifetime. In roots the presence of carotenoids is usually very low and confined into the leucoplasts. In addition to a role linked to ABA production (Li et al., 2008a; Welsch et al., 2008), the presence of carotenoids in roots appears to be related to the production of several types of apocarotenoids with various actions in the rhyzosphera

(Auldridge et al., 2006). Recently, an intriguing role of this pigments as root-derived signal to regulate the level of shoot branching has been also postulated (Leyser, 2008).

Carotenoid Role in Humans

Humans are not able to synthesize carotenoids but have enzymes for their conversion. With respect to health, carotenoids are required both as integer pigment or cleavage products. Xanthophylls such as lutein and zeaxanthin are macular pigments. In the middle of the retina the depression characterized by high number of cone receptors is a yellow area due to carotenoid presence (Bone et al., 1988). Several data suggest the existence of an epidemiological association between ingestion of lutein and zeaxanthin and the risk of age-related macular degeneration (Krinsky et al., 2003). At the basis of this association some biological properties can be evocated: filters for blue-light, modificative compounds of membrane structure, and antioxidants (Krinsky et al., 2003). Epidemiologic studies show that the ingestion of lycopene is correlated with the reduction of risk of some cancers (especially prostate cancers) and cardiovascular diseases (Heber and Lu, 2002; Sesso et al., 2003; Omoni and Aluko, 2005). The positive effects of diets rich in tomato (or derivates) are probably linked to scavenge of singlet oxygen and peroxy radicals as well as the deactivation of excited molecules or DNA chain-breaking agents (Stahl et al., 1997; Nishino et al., 2009). In particular, it is important underline that lycopene lacks provitamin A activity but is one the most potent antioxidants among the dietary carotenoids; moreover, this pigment has a negative effect on HMGCoA reductase that acts in cholesterol synthesis (Fuhrman et al., 1997) and can modulates intercellular signaling at the level of the gap junctions and this latter effect inhibits proliferation of tumor cells (Livny et al., 2002). Another mode of lycopene action is the down regulation of the polypeptide protein hormone insulin-like growth factor 1 (IGF-I). The inhibitory effect of lycopene on IGF signaling has been associated with suppression of IGF stimulated cell cycle progression of serum-starved, synchronized cells (Karas et al., 2000). Several studies suggest that β-carotene might be a natural immunoenhancing agent and this useful function could be related to prevention of oxidative damage, modulation of prostaglandins synthesis and/or modification of the arachidonic acid signaling (Hughes, 2000).

The best studied role of carotenoids in human health is the provitamin A activity of pigments such as β-carotene and β-cryptoxanthin. The key enzyme of the pathway is an intestinal 15-15'-dioxygenase and in mammalian, the first gene that encodes a β-carotene 15-15'-dioxygenase (BCO) has been isolated in mouse (Redmond et al., 2001). The product of the human *Bco* gene is a protein of 547 amino acid residues that catalyzes the conversion of β,β-carotene into two molecules of all-*trans*-retinal (Yan et al., 2001). It important to note that the identification in mammalian of β-carotene 15-15'-dioxygenase has been made on the basis on similarity to plant CCDs. The expression of *Bco* is very high in the retinal pigment epithelium but present also in kidney, intestine, liver, brain, stomach and testis. Moreover, when mutated, the patient develops a retinal degenerative disease (Yan et al., 2001). The *Drosophila melanogaster* genome encodes only one *Bco* gene while in vertebrates *Bco*, *Rpe65* and *Bco2,* have been identified (von Lintig et al., 2005). When *Rpe65* is mutated specific type of blindness affects humans and at biochemical level, the accumulation of all-*trans*-retinyl ester is characteristic. The BCO2 enzyme has β,β-carotene-9',10'-oxygenase activity and the asymmetric oxidative cleavage of β-carotene at the 9',10' double bond determines the formation of β-apo-10'-carotenal and β-ionone (von Lintig et al., 2005). Therefore, in mammalian both centric and excentric cleavage pathways occurred (Giuliano et al., 2003).

Vitamin A (retinol and retinyl esters) is an essential nutrient that is necessary for normal cell growth and differentiation, immunological functions, and vision (Blomhoff et al., 1992; Means and Gudas, 1995; Soprano et al., 2004; Napoli, 2005; Blomhoff and Blomhoff, 2006; Meissburger and Wolfrum, 2008). Retinal is light-sensitive and correspond to the chromophore in photoreceptor cells of the retina (Wald, 1960; Stroeva and Mitashov, 1983). Retinoic acid is the ligand of two classes of nuclear receptors (RARs and RXRs) and the responsive target genes have a wide spectrum of functions in biological processes (Chawla et al., 2001; Sharoni et al., 2004; Wolf, 2008).

Regulation of Carotenogenesis

The mechanisms that influence the accumulation and composition of carotenoids in higher plants and their reciprocal interaction are only partially known (Lu and Li, 2008). In general, basic aspects of control of the carotenoid pathway are the changes in the levels of gene transcription, availability of substrates obtained by MEP pathway, and post-translational mechanisms (Cunningham, 2002). In addition, the precursors of carotenoids are common with many other isoprenoids and this aspect gives more complexity to the regulation. Finally, in some species different genes with tissue-specific expression code key rate-limiting enzyme such as phytoene synthase; therefore the pathway has also elements of redundancy and segregation (Taylor and Ramsay, 2005).

Leaves

In chloroplasts the composition and the relative abundance of carotenoids are generally well preserved because exist a direct link between the carotenogenesis and the assembly of the two photosystems (Frosch and Mohr, 1980). In particular, the fine-tuning of carotenoid accumulation takes place in connection with chlorophyll formation at the level of assembly of carotenoids (i.e. lutein, β-carotene and neoxanthin) into holocomplexes (Oelmüller and Mohr, 1985). The accumulation of large amount of carotenoids in leaves is generally associated with the biosynthesis of chlorophylls; in fact if the accumulation of chlorophylls is excluded by chemical treatments or genetic mutations, the carotenogenesis is also inhibited (Nielsen and Gough, 1974; Corona et al., 1996). The boost expression of the *PDS* promoter when the carotenoid and/or chlorophyll pathway are inhibited by herbicide treatments, suggest that the phytoene desaturation is regulated by end-products (Corona et al., 1996). Tobacco plants with chlorophyll deficiency due to the expression of antisense RNA coding for glutamate 1-semialdehyde aminotransferase showed a strong accumulation of xanthophyll cycle pool in leaves grown under high light condition (Härtel and Grimm, 1998). Moreover, under these conditions, violaxanthin was near completely converted into antheraxanthin and zeaxanthin (Härtel and Grimm, 1998). Recently, Mortain-Bertrand et al. (2008) have demonstrated that when excised tomato plants were incubated in glucose supplemented medium, the accumulation of soluble sugars in young and mature leaves was correlated to a coordinated decrease of chlorophylls and carotenoids. The sugar-dependent reduction of carotenoids biosynthesis was probably mediated through the repression of *1-deoxy-D-xylulose-5-phosphate synthase* (*DXPS*), *PSY2*, *PDS* and *LCY-b* gene expression (Mortain-Bertrand et al., 2008). It is interesting to underline that DXPS controls the synthesis of plastidic isopentenyl pyrosphate (IPP), the general precursor of isoprenoid biosynthesis.

Carotenogenesis and Abiotic Factors

Among the environmental factors that influence the carotenogenesis, light is of primary importance. In cotyledons, the conversion of etioplasts into chloroplasts is a light-dependent process essential to acquire the capacity of CO_2 uptake. Chlorophylls and carotenoids are rapidly synthesized to support the formation of the photosynthetic apparatus. In *Sinapis alba* and *Arabidopsis thaliana* the study of the light-dependent regulation of carotenoid biosynthesis clarified that the major molecular event is the up-regulation of *PSY* expression with a phytochrome-mediated control. The activity of *PSY* promoter of *Arabidopsis thaliana* was observed also in the dark but 24 hours of white light induced a doubling of promoter activity (von Lintig et al., 1997; Welsch et al., 2003). The analysis of *PSY* promoter region showed that *cis*-acting elements involved in the phytochrome response under red light are located between -300 and -196, whereas elements mediating responses to far-red and blue light are positioned in the first 196 bp (Welsch et al., 2003).

Notably, extend of carotenoid synthesis is also associated to favorable conditions for chlorophylls biosynthesis (von Lintig et al., 1997). In the structure of the *PSY* promoter, a TATA box proximal region containing G-box-like elements is involved in light induction and discrimination between different light qualities. A TATA box distal region enables a high basal level of promoter activity (Welsch et al., 2003). Recently, Welsh et al. (2007) have demonstrated that the ATCTA sequence, occurring in tandem in the TATA box distal region, was recognized as the *cis*-acting element for a transcription factor mediating high *PSY* promoter activity. Interestingly, this novel motif is also found in promoter regions of other carotenogenic genes as well as in photosynthesis-related genes; therefore, the *trans*-acting factor could be able to regulate several genes involved in chloroplast biology. AtRAP2.2, a member of the APETALA2 (AP2)/ethylene-responsive element-binding protein transcription factor family, binds to the ATCTA element (Welsch et al., 2007).

The *PSY* promoter activity in *Arabidopsis thaliana* is not influenced by chemicals treatments such as norflurazon (inhibitor of carotenoid biosynthesis) or gabaculine (inhibitor of chlorophyll biosynthesis) suggesting a lack in the regulation by feedback mechanism (Welsch et al., 2003).

A previous point of control has been identified in *Zea mays* where the transformation of etioplast in chloroplast is regulated by increased activity of isopentenyl pyrophosphate isomerase (Albrecht and Sandmann, 1994). The light stimulation of carotenogenesis in *Helianthus annuus* induces a significant increase of transcription of the *HaPSY* and *HaZDS* genes (Fambrini et al., 2004; Salvini et al., 2005). Moreover, the strong increase of carotenoid content in *Nicotiana tabacum* during photomorphogenesis is associated also with the rise of transcription of xanthophylls biosynthetic genes. In particular, the expression profiles of *beta-*

carotene hydroxylase (*CHY-b*) and *zeaxanthin epoxidase* (*ZEP*) are analogous to the expression pattern of a gene encoding a major light-harvesting protein of PSII (Woitsch and Römer, 2003). Using *Daucus carota* as a novel plant model, Stange et al. (2008) have demonstrated that light differentially affects the accumulation of several carotenoid genes in leaves and roots.

The light intensity modifies the chloroplast pigments composition. For example, when *Raphanus sativus* is grown under shade conditions, chloroplasts contain a higher chlorophylls and carotenoids content as compared to sun chloroplasts; moreover, with low light intensities, the content of *β*-carotene, lutein and antheraxanthin is elevated while the xanthophylls to carotene ratio is low. In the same species, the turnover rate of pigments is very strong under high light condition (Grumbach and Lichtenthaler, 1982). The modification of pigment content on the basis of light intensity is associated to change of the chloroplast ultrastructure: sun plastids have few thylakoids and large starch grains while under dim light conditions, chloroplasts have large thylakoid systems with large grana stacks. High light diminishes grana stacking and this ultrastructure modification is linked to reduction of light-harvesting complex II (Anderson et al., 1995). A transcriptional control of pigment modification in plants grown under different light intensities has been described. In *Helianthus annuus*, light-dependent carotenoid accumulation from 5 to 100 PPFD (photosynthetically active photon flux density) is correlated to an increase of mRNA transcript levels of both *HaPSY* and *HaZDS* genes (Salvini et al., 2005; Fambrini et al., 2004).

An interesting regulatory mechanism is the relationship between carotene desaturation and photosynthetic electron transport. In fact, under high light conditions the plastoquinone pool is oxidized and this circumstance is positive to carotene desaturation (Norris et al., 1995).

Light intensity can also influence the carotenogenesis in chromoplasts; for example, during tomato fruit ripening increasing PAR (photosynthetically active radiation) increased the content of lycopene and *β*-carotene (Gautier et al., 2004).

Temperature is another environmental factors that effect carotenoid accumulation. Several study have been conducted in tomato where high temperature induces a strong reduction of lycopene content in fruits (Tomes, 1963; Dumas et al., 2003). The optimal temperature for lycopene accumulation in tomato ranges from 20 to 24 °C (Krumbein et al., 2006). Moreover, the effects of mineral nutrients in the soil on carotenoid content have been analyzed in numerous agronomic trials (Kopsell et al., 2003; Dumas et al. 2003). In tomato fruits, N fertilizers have a negative effect for carotenoid concentration, while K fertilization has the opposite effect. Supply of P fertilizers is generally positive for the level of phytochemicals but the final results is dependent by the interaction with other abiotic factors (Dorais et al., 2008).

A specific interaction of carotenogenesis with abiotic stress has been recently demonstrated in rice where a third *PSY* gene (*OsPSY3*) has been isolated and characterized (Welsch et al., 2008). This gene is not up-regulated by light while a positive regulation has been observed during ABA biosynthesis in roots upon salt and/or drought treatments. In particular, its role is probably related to the compensation of the reduction of the xanthophylls pool caused by the epoxycarotenoid dioxygenases (NCEDs) activity to ensure the ABA biosynthesis stress-induced. Moreover the *OsPSY3* is also induced by ABA treatments suggesting the presence of a positive feedback regulation; some specific traits in the promoter architecture justify the peculiar type of this gene (Welch et al., 2008). Analogously, in maize (*Zea mays* L.) each paralog of the small *PSY* family shows differential gene expression. In particular, the transcription of *PSY3* is an important bottleneck in controlling flux to carotenoid precursors required for the stress-induced ABA accumulation in roots (Li et al., 2008a).

Flowers

Pigments like β,ε-carotenoids, lutein and its derivates are accumulated in chromoplasts and responsible of yellow petals in many flowers (i.e. *Tagetes*, *Gerbera*, and *Chrysanthemum*; Grotewold, 2006). In species with flowers characterized by yellow-orange colors such as *Lilium tigrinum* the carotenoids more prevalent are β-carotene derivates (Figure 3) (Deli et al., 2000).

Marigold *(Tagetes erecta* L.) is a species useful as a source of carotenoids because its petals contain high concentration (up to 20-fold greater than in leaves) of xanthophylls like lutein and its derivates by esterification. Cultivars of marigold flowers range in color from white to dark orange and the intensity is not associated to different products of carotenogenesis but it relates to the level of lutein accumulation. With respect to biosynthesis in leaves, the carotenogenesis in petals is peculiar due to a predominant synthesis of the α-carotene-derived xanthophylls, which contain a β- and ε-cyclic end group (Mohes et al., 2001). The cultivar French Vanilla has white petals, a trait correlated to a very low level of transcripts of several genes (i.e. *PSY, PDS, ZDS, LCY-b, LCY-e*) encoding enzymes of carotenogenesis. On the contrary, at molecular level, the cultivar Golden Lady (yellow petals) is characterized by a reduced accumulation of both *PSY* and *DXPS* transcripts with respect to the Dark Orange Lady (orange petals) variety. It is important to note that at level of leaves all the different cultivars are not distinguishable for carotenoid accumulation or gene expression (Mohes et al., 2001).

In *Chrysanthemum morifolium* the yellow petals depends on accumulation of lutein and its derivates, and it is a recessive trait against white flowers (Langton, 1980; Kishimoto et al., 2004). During petal development of yellow flowers the carotenoid content increases three times and the pigment accumulation is correlated with the up-regulation of several genes for carotenogenic enzymes: *DXPS, PSY, PDS, ZDS, CRTISO, LCY-e* and *CHY-b* (Kishimoto and Ohmiya, 2006). At the very early stage of petal development, the carotenoid content of white type (cultivar Paragon) is similar to that of colored Yellow Paragon but at later stages the level of pigments strongly decreases (Kishimoto and Ohmiya, 2006). The absence of yellow color in the final stage of development is determined by a petal-specific activity of a carotenoid cleavage dioxygenase enzyme (CmCCD4a). Therefore, the white color of Paragon petals is not associated to a deficient carotenoid biosynthesis because the final products are degraded into colorless compounds (Ohmiya et al., 2006).

In Asiatic hybrid lily (*Lilium* spp.) yellow, orange and red flower colours of tepals are very important traits related to carotenoid accumulation. The pigment characterization in different cultivars showed that the major components in yellow tepals of Connecticut King are antheraxanthin, (9Z)-violaxanthin, *cis*-lutein and violaxanthin, while capsanthin was the major pigment accumulated in red tepals of Saija (Yamagishi et al., 2009). Total carotenoid content in Connecticut King was higher than those in Gran Paradiso and Saija. This trait related to a more elevated level of transcriptions of *LhPSY*, *LhPDS*, *LhZDS*, *LhLCYB* and *LhHYB* genes. During tepal development, the amount of carotenoids changed markedly and the authors have demonstrated that at least three regulation systems control accumulation of mRNA encoding carotenoid biosynthetic enzymes in lily tepals. Moreover, to determine the reduced amount of carotenoids in Montreux tepals the Authors suggested that a *CmCCD4-*homologous gene, should act.

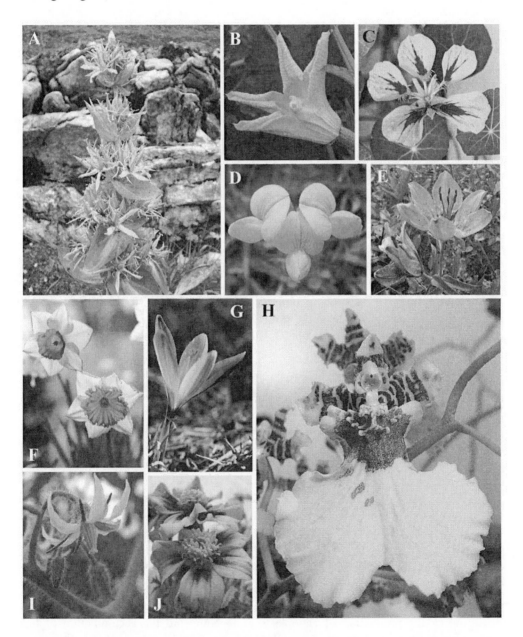

Figure 3. Spontaneous and cultivated species exemplifying carotenoid accumulation in flowers. A, *Gentiana lutea*; B, *Cucurbita pepo*; C, *Tropeolus majus*; D, *Lotus corniculatus*; E, *Lilium bulbiferum*; F, *Narcissus pseudonarcissus*; G, *Crocus biflorus*; H, *Oncidium* Gower Ramsey hybrid; I, *Solanum lycopersicum*; J, *Tagetes*.

The genetic control of carotenoid-dependent color of tomato petals is opposite if compared with that of *Chrysanthemum morifolium*. In fact, in *Solanum lycopersicum* the yellow color is dominant against white flowers (Galpaz et al., 2006). The yellow color of wild type petals is correlated to neoxanthin and violaxanthin accumulation while lutein is present at very low level. Moreover, the concentration of total carotenoids in petals and anthers is 3- to 4-fold higher than in leaves. Petals of white flowers contain about 6-fold lower carotenoids than yellow petals and also the composition differ from that of wild type because only in the mutant β-carotene has been detected (Galpaz et al., 2006). In the recessive *wf* mutant, white flowers are originated by the mutation in a flower-specific β-ring carotene hydroxylase (*CrtR-b2*) gene. In this genotype, the carotenoid biosynthesis is not affected in chloroplasts where the homologous *CrtR-b1* is normally expressed (Galpaz et al., 2006). In spite of the molecular characterization of *wf* mutant, its nearly colorless petals remain an open question. β-ring carotene hydroxylase activity is important to transform β-carotene in xanthophylls and if the enzyme is not active, a strong accumulation of this orange pigment is expected. Nevertheless, the level of β-carotene in the *wf* petals is very low. Some hypotheses have been postulated but Galpaz et al. (2006) retain more probable the presence of a petal-specific enzymatic cleavage because the production of volatiles (e.g. β-ionone and β-cyclocytral) is elevated in the *wf* mutant.

In yellow petals of tomato flower a specific correlation between the chromoplast differentiation and the expression of the *PDS* promoter has been demonstrated (Corona et al., 1996).

Mechanisms of post-transcriptional regulation of carotenogenesis have been also described. For example in daffodil (*Narcissus pseudonarcissus*) petals the activity of PSY and PDS is strictly linked to their association with the chromoplast membranes (Morstadt et al., 2002).

The genetic control of carotenoid-dependent color of petals has been investigated in other species such as *Cucurbita moschata*, *Zinnia angustifolia* and *Helianthus annuus* but molecular characterization of carotenogenesis in chromoplasts of these plants is yet lacking (Fick, 1976; Roe and Bemis, 1977; Boyle and Stimart, 1988; Yue et al., 2008; Fambrini et al., 2009).

In flowers, carotenogenesis is not present only in petals; for example, β-carotene accumulates in nectaries of tobacco. During the development of nectaries up-regulation of genes coding for enzymes involved in carotenogenesis has been detected before the metabolic shift in plastids towards accumulation of sugars. The β-carotene and ascorbate high levels analyzed after the metabolic shift is probably dependent by availability of substrate molecules originated from starch breakdown (Horner et al., 2007).

In the tomato flower buds, the expression of the *PDS* promoter has not been observed but just before the anthesis the action of this promoter was localized throughout the anther connective tissue and in pollen grains (Corona et al., 1996).

The regulation of carotenoids accumulation in tapetum of anthers is completely unknown. A role of plastid-lipid associated proteins (PAPs) has been proposed. PAP genes are expressed during the production of elaioplasts of tapetum and the accumulation of these proteins could be coordinate with the increased level of antioxidants like carotenoids (Ting et al., 1998). In chloroplasts, PAPs on the thylakoid membranes modulate the action of the carotenoids involved in the light reaction of photosynthesis and in photoprotection while in plastids without chlorophyll, the lipid stabilization function is more probable. Each type of PAP could be specialized in the first or second function (Kim et al., 2001a).

In several species, the carotenoids localized in tapetum are important to give pollen color from yellow to orange range. The pigments of pollen grains are of sporophytic origin and mutants with strong reduction of color characterized by a recessive inheritance have been isolated in some species (Qiao et al., 1995; Wakelin et al., 2003; Fambrini et al., 2009). To date, the biochemical analysis of these mutants is only partial and no molecular data have been collected. On the contrary, interesting results have been obtained in species with pollen coats enriched in flavonoids such as *Brassica napus* and *Arabidopsis thaliana*. In addition to genetic lesions on flavonoid biosynthesis the absence of membrane flavonoid transporter is also correlated to pollen grains with substantially reduced levels of flavonoids (Hsieh and Huang, 2007). In particular, the latter result suggests the importance of the delivery mechanisms to guarantee the essential substances of pollen.

Carotenoids in anthers are substrates to ABA biosynthesis and in *Oryza sativa*, the hormone accumulation responds to stress factors such as cold temperature. Recently, Oliver et al. (2007) have demonstrated that *OSZEP1*, *OSNCED2* and *OSNCED3* are expressed in anthers of cold-tolerant rice differently with respect to cold-sensitive rice.

The saffron from style branches of *Crocus sativus* (a triploid sterile species) is a very expensive spice with notable economic value. During the development, the color of stigma changes from white to red with yellow and orange as intermediate phases. The stigma development parallels carotenoid accumulation but the massive accumulation of final products correspond to the red stage (Himeno and Sano, 1987). The chemical nature of this spice is characterized by three major carotenoid derivates (i.e. crocetin glycosides, picrocrocin, and safranal) and for initiate their biosynthesis from zeaxanthin, the zeaxanthin 7,8(7',8')-cleavage dioxygenese (CsZCD), has a key role. The expression of the relative gene (*CsZCD*) is style-specific and positively regulated by water stress (Bouvier et al., 2003b). Moreover, to give a consistent pool of zeaxanthin the simultaneous expression of carotenogenic genes encoding for early steps of the pathway, is also required. In particular, it has been demonstrated a direct correlation between the level of *β-carotene hydroxylase* (*CsBCH*) transcripts and the zeaxanthin accumulation in styles suggesting that the CsBCH enzyme could be the limiting step (Castillo et al., 2005).

Inflorescences

The edible part (curd) of the *Brassica oleracea* (var. *botrytis*) shares characteristics of both the vegetative and reproductive apices (Sadik, 1962). Normally, wild type curd of cauliflower is white with negligible carotenoid content; nevertheless, the interesting *Or* mutation regulates spatial and temporal aspects of carotenogenesis and induced a peculiar orange phenotype (Li et al., 2001). Homozygous genotypes (*Or/Or*) develop a small curd with intense orange color due to massive accumulation of β-carotene in highly ordered sheets within chromoplasts while the heterozygous *Or/or* has normal sized curd but with less intense orange color. The nature of mutation is not liked to up-regulation of carotenogenic genes but to the formation of a deposition sink (Li et al., 2001). The gene *Or* encodes a plastid-associated protein containing a DnaJ Cys-rich domain with a function associated to the conversion of plastids towards chromoplasts; the mutation is caused by the insertion, in the exon 3, of a long terminal repeat retrotransposon (Lu et al., 2006). The mature protein in the mutant is smaller in size than in the wild type and the analysis of its localization indicates a preferential targeting to non-green plastids. In the *Or/Or* genotype, the molecular data suggest that chromoplasts biogenesis is enhanced. The mutant *Or* represents a clear and valuable example of the critical role of the storage structures to provide driving force for carotenoid accumulation also without a significant increase of the transcription of genes encoding enzymes of the carotenoid pathway (Lu et al., 2006).

Tomato Fruits

The tomato is a significant plant model to study carotenoid biosynthesis in fruits (Bramley, 2002). The fruit of tomato is climateric and during ripening several biochemical processes such as hormone synthesis (ethylene), modification of pigments profile, sugar accumulation, textural changes, and production of volatiles compounds are activated (Gillaspy et al., 1993). The ripening process involves the differentiation of chloroplasts in green stage and chromoplasts in ripe red fruits. The plastids are localized (500-1000 per cell) into large vacuolated cells of pericarp. In particular, chromoplasts are cluster arranged and their shape depends on the elongated red lycopene crystals (Pyke and Howells, 2002). Lycopene accumulation is influenced by light and fruit-localized phytochromes regulate the pigment deposit (Alba et al., 2000). During the transition from immature green stage to full red mature stage, a 10-fold increase of the carotenoid content has been detected in the pericarp of the cultivar Rheilands Rhum (Giuliano et al., 1993). In the process of fruit ripening, chromoplasts are derived from chloroplasts with concomitant strong decrease of chlorophyll and accumulation of lycopene in membrane-bound crystals. The ripe fruit has the higher carotenoid content but the maximum level of carotenogenic enzyme activities has been detected in green stage (Fraser et al., 1994). At molecular level, the high carotenoid content observed in the orange stage, is correlated to a relevant enhancement of both *PSY1* and *PDS* expression (Giuliano et al., 1993). PSY1 is the fruit-specific isoform of phytoene synthase and represents the limiting enzyme for carotenoid biosynthesis during tomato fruit ripening (Bartley and Scolnik, 1995). Moreover also the gene *DXPS* showed developmental and organ-specific regulation at transcriptional level because its mRNA accumulation is strictly correlated with carotenoid synthesis during fruit ripening (Lois et al., 2000). On the basis of these data, in the early steps of carotenoid biosynthesis, a putative cross-talk between PSY1 and DXPS activities has been postulated with respect to the fine tuning of carotenoid accumulation in tomato. By contrast, in the later steps of carotenogenesis the drastic reduction of mRNAs level of both lycopene cyclases (*CYC-b* and *LCY-e*) ensures the effective accumulation of lycopene (Pecker et al., 1996; Ronen et al., 1999). These results suggest that a differential regulation of expression of carotenoid biosynthesis genes is the major mechanism that controls lycopene accumulation in tomato fruits.

In *Lycopersicon esculentum* several mutants with altered carotenoid accumulation in fruits have been described. The fruits of the recessive *r* mutant are yellow with only carotenoid traces (7 µg/g *vs.* 65 µg/g of wild type). The carotenogenesis in this genotype is defective in a early step of the biochemical pathway caused by mutation to *PSY1* locus (Fray and Grierson, 1993). On the contrary, the PSY of green tissues (leaf chloroplasts) is not affected and the carotenoid content in the *r* mutant is the same of control plants. *Colourless nonripening* (*Cnr*) is another tomato mutant defective in *PSY1* expression (Thompson et al., 1999). In this mutant the formation of phytoene during fruit ripening is completely abolished (Fraser et al., 2001).

The genetic control of the *B* mutation is partially dominant and the relative *Beta* mutant of tomato develops mature orange fruits where the lycopene content is replaced by *β*-carotene. The *B* gene (*CYC-b*) encodes a fruit- and flower-specific lycopene *β*-cyclase involved in the *β*-carotene production from lycopene. In wild type plants this lycopene *β*-cyclase is expressed only for a short period in chromoplasts of fruits in the breaker stage while in the *Beta* mutant, the *CYC-b* expression is strong and prolonged in time (Ronen et al., 2000). The *old-gold* (*og*) and *old-gold-crimson* (*og^c*) mutants are recessive and characterized by red deep fruits. *B*, *og* and *og^c* are all allelic to the same locus and in the last two genotypes the fruit-specific lycopene *β*-cyclase activity is lost (Ronen et al., 2000).

The mutation *lutescent-2* (*l2*) produces numerous pleiotropic effects, including photobleaching and premature yellowing of leaves, delayed onset of red pigments development in fruit, and reduced level of *β*-carotene and xanthophylls. This mutation could be due to either a structural or a *cis*-acting regulatory mutation in *LCY-b* (Thorup et al., 2000).

Characteristic tangerine-orange fruits have been described for the *tangerine* (*t*) mutant of tomato (Zechmeister et al., 1941; Tomes et al., 1953). The particular fruit color depend on the accumulation of poly-*cis*-isomer of lycopene. In addition, to prolycopene, the mutant fruits accumulate precursors such as phytoene and *ζ*-carotene. In wild type fruits are mainly accumulated *trans*-isomer of lycopene. In the breaker stage of the ripening, the level of *CRTISO* transcripts increased 10-fold in wild type. The CRTISO protein functions in parallel with *ζ*-carotene desaturation, by converting 7,9,9'-tri-*cis*-neurosporene to 9'-*cis*-neurosporene and 7'9'-di-*cis*-lycopene into all-*trans*-lycopene (Isaacson et al., 2004). The genetic lesion of *t* mutants hits the *CRTISO* gene that encodes a carotenoid isomerase required in the desaturation. In the mutant *tangerine^mic*, the elimination of a splicing site generates an incorrect *CRTISO* mRNA. By contrast, in the *tangerine^3183* mutant a deletion of 348 pb in the promoter region of *CRTISO* alters the expression gene profile (Isaacson et al., 2002). In the *CRTISO* mutants (*ccr2* and *tangerine*) accumulation of tetra-*cis*-lycopene characterizes the carotenoid profile of etioplasts and chromoplasts but the pathway proceeds in chloroplasts by photoisomerization of the *cis*-bonds. However, these mutants show a delayed greening, reduced lutein accumulation and chlorosis (Isaacson et al., 2002; Park et al., 2002; Fang et al., 2008). Cazzonelli et al. (2009) cloned the Arabidopsis *CCR1* gene and they demonstrated that a histone methyltransferase is required for the *CRTISO* transcript accumulation. This is a remarkable result because for the first time, an epigenetic mechanism is identified in regulation of carotenoid composition.

The pigment analysis of the *high pigment* (*hp*) mutant showed that both green and ripe fruits accumulated increased level of carotenoids in comparison with the levels observed in the Ailsa Craig parental strain (Bramley, 1997). Therefore, the mutation enhanced the carotenoid content both in chloroplasts and chromoplasts. The evaluation of carotenoids composition in mature fruits has demonstrated that the pattern of individual carotenoids of the *hp* mutant is the same of that of wild type (Bramley, 1997). In tomato *hp* mutants regulatory functions that control plastid development are altered and the phenotype show defects in the photomorphogenic signal transduction. The genes *HP1* and *HP2* encode the tomato orthologes respectively of a *UV-DAMAGED DNA-BINDING PROTEIN 1* (*DDB1*) and *DE-ETIOLATED 1* (*DET1*) from *Arabidopsis thaliana* (Lieberman et al., 2004; Liu et al., 2004; Mustilli et al., 1999). It is interesting to note that in the pericarp of *hp-1* ripe fruits, the chromoplast area per cell is increased with respect to wild type, and the activity of phytoene synthase enzyme was near 2-fold higher. No difference between *hp-1* and wild type has been detected at transcriptional level (Cookson et al., 2003).

Recently, the molecular nature of the *hp-3* mutant has been identified: the *HP3* gene encodes the zeaxanthin epoxidase (ZEP) that converts zeaxanthin to violaxanthin (Galpaz et al., 2008). In the *hp-3* mutant several consequences at phenotypic level have been described: reduction of ABA and xanthophylls pool in leaves, accumulation of zeaxanthin in the fruits, increased plastid numbers. The last effect is probably the causal factor of the increased lycopene content in the fruits (Galpaz et al., 2008).

The tomato mutant *Delta* is characterized by orange fruits due to accumulation of δ-carotene at the expense of lycopene. The phenotype depends on a single dominant gene (*Del*), and the molecular analysis showed that the transcript level of *LCY-e* increases approximately 30-fold during fruit ripening of the mutant (Ronen et al., 1999). The mutation is probably located in the promoter region because *LCY-e* of both *Delta* and wild type are functional after expression in *Escherichia coli* (Ronen et al., 1999).

The dominant *Green-ripe* (*Gr*) and *Never-ripe 2* (*Nr-2*) mutants are characterized by deficient ripening processes with development of fruits unable to accumulate the normal lycopene content. The reduced ripening of these genotypes results from decreased ethylene sensitivity (Barry et al., 2005) and the desaturation of carotenoids during chromoplast differentiation is ethylene-dependent in the carotenogenesis of fruits (Alba et al., 2005).

In the *ghost* mutant, developed under normal light intensity, the immature fruits are small and white while they are yellow/orange at the ripe stage. The yellow/orange pericarp of mature *ghost* fruits is characterized by a drastic reduction of lycopene, low levels of phytofluene, β-carotene and lutein, and a massive accumulation of phytoene (Scolnik, et al., 1987). The white color of immature fruits (green, in wild type) is probably caused by photo-oxidation processes (Barr et al., 2004). The mutation affects the *PLASTID TERMINAL OXIDASE* (*PTOX*) gene encoding an enzyme involved in carotenoid desaturation that has a function equivalent to a quinol:oxygen oxidoreductase (Josse et al., 2000). The presence of lutein and β-carotene in ripe fruits suggest that phytoene desaturation is not completely blocked by the *gh* mutation. The expression analysis of eight different genes (i.e. *PSY1*, *PDS*, *ZDS*, *CRTISO*, *LYC-b*, *BETA*, *LCY-e* and *CHY-b*) has demonstrated a their generalized down regulation in the *gh* fruits before or during the orange stage (Barr et al., 2004).

Citrus Fruits

With respect to tomato, the carotenoid composition of citrus fruits is very different because more than 100 pigments have been isolated. Epoxy and hydroxylated carotenoids are prevalent with respect to linear carotenes but, also genus-specific apocarotenoids have been isolated (Farin et al., 1983; Saunt, 2000). For example, β-cryptoxanthin is the major carotenoid in the flavedo (colored part of the skin) and juice sacs of the mandarin (*Citrus unshiu*) (Ikoma et al., 2001) while mature sweet orange (*Citrus sinensis*) accumulates violaxanthin isomers and in particular 9-*cis*-violaxanthin (Molnár and Szabolcs, 1980). The light yellow color in the flavedo and juice sacs is characteristic of lemon fruit (*Citrus limon*) and the trait is correlated to a small concentration of total xanthophylls with a concomitant and unusual preservation of precursors such as phytoene and ζ-carotene (Yokoyama and Vandercook, 1967; Kato et al., 2004). In general, xanthophylls are the main carotenoids in citrus fruits, and several genes of carotenogenesis must be considered to study the regulatory processes in these crops. The first investigations showed that in Satsuma mandarin, the gene expression of *Citrus limon PSY* (*CitPSY*) increased in the peel and juice sacs with the onset of coloration after the green stage of immature fruit (Kim et al., 2001b), whereas the gene expression of both *CitPDS* and *CitHYb* (β-ring hydroxylase) remained constant once fruit was fully developed (Kim et al., 2001b; Kita et al., 2001). A more complete analysis of carotenogenic genes participating in the xanthophylls synthesis has been conducted in Satsuma mandarin, Valencia orange and Lisbon lemon by Kato et al. (2004). The carotenoid accumulation during fruit maturation was extremely regulated by the coordination among the expression of the carotenoid biosynthetic genes. The carotenogenic pathway changing from β,ε-carotenoids to β,β-carotenoids synthesis was obtained in the flavedos of Satsuma mandarin and Valencia orange by the lost of *CitLCY-e* transcripts and the increase in *CitLCY-b* transcripts during the transition of peel color from green to orange. In the juice sacs, pathway changing was advanced than in flavedo because *CitLCY-e* transcription was not detected even in green fruit. In Satsuma mandarin and Valencia orange during later stages of fruit maturation, a concurrent increase in the expression of genes such as *CitPSY*, *CitPDS*, *CitZDS*, *CitLCY-b*, *CitHY-b*, and *CitZEP* was associated to a massive β,β-xanthophyll accumulation in both the flavedo and juice sacs. In the flavedo of Lisbon lemon and Satsuma mandarin, the accumulation of phytoene was cuncurrent with a decrease of *CitPDS* transcript levels. About the considerable difference in the β,β-xanthophyll compositions of the juice sacs between Satsuma mandarin and Valencia orange Kato et al. (2004) suggested two essential mechanisms: the substrate specificity of CitHY-b and expression balance between upstream synthesis genes (i.e. *CitPSY*, *CitPDS*, *CitZDS*, and *CitLCY-b*) and downstream synthesis genes (i.e. *CitHY-b* and *CitZEP*). In Lisbon lemon, the gene expression of genes required to produce β,β-xanthophylls also increased but at much lower level than those in Satsuma mandarin and Valencia orange. This depleted gene expression may be associated to small concentration of β,β-carotenoids in the flavedo and juice sacs of Lisbon lemon. Notably, the cleavage reaction for ABA synthesis reduces the 9-*cis*-violaxanthin level in Satsuma mandarin and Lisbon lemon juice sacs, whereas the low level of cleavage reaction maintains the predominant 9-*cis*-violaxanthin accumulation in Valencia orange (Kato et al., 2006).

A recent work has been conducted in *Citrus sinensis* in order to evaluate the contribution of carotenoid composition to the color range of the fruit juice sacs in Shamouti (normal orange), Sanguinelli (purple), Cara Cara navel (pink-reddish), and Huang pi Chen (yellowish color) (Fanciullino et al., 2008). Shamouti and Sanguinelli oranges accumulated mainly β,β-xanthophylls as expected in typically colored oranges, whereas Cara Cara navel orange accumulated linear carotenes in addition to *cis*-violaxanthin. Huang pi Chen fruit flesh orange was characterized by a strong reduction of total carotenoid content. The molecular analysis of carotenogenesis revealed in juice sacs an apparent coordination of *DXS* and *PSY* expression and a general increase in mRNA levels of carotenoid biosynthetic genes that correlated with the β,β-xanthophyll accumulation in Shamouti and Sanguinelli oranges. Moreover, the preponderant accumulation of linear carotenes in Cara Cara navel and the very low level of carotenoids in Huang pi Chen oranges were not predominantly due to changes in regulation of carotenoid biosynthetic genes at the transcriptional level (Fanciullino et al., 2008).

In navel orange (*Citrus sinensis*) several mutants with alteration of carotenoid content in the fruits have been described. For example, in the Pinalate mutant, a reduction of the ζ-carotene desaturation determines an abnormal accumulation of linear carotenes (phytoene, phytofluene and ζ-carotene) and a reduction of xanthophylls (Rodrigo et al., 2003). Pinalate displayed a distinctive yellow color. The red color of the mutant Cara Cara is due to accumulation of β-carotene and lycopene while the pink color of the Sarah variety is associated to high level of lycopene only (Lee, 2001; Monselise and Halevy, 1961).

The molecular analysis of the Cara Cara pulp showed the higher expression level of the *DXPS, 1-hydroxy-2-methyl-2-(E)-butenyl-4-diphosphate (HD) synthase (HDS)* and *HD reductase (HDR)* genes of the MEP pathway suggesting that for elevation of early carotenes contents, could be relevant an increased synthesis and channeling of isoprenoid precursors into the carotenoid pathway. Moreover, carotenoid biosynthetic genes downstream ζ-carotene desaturation were also highly expressed in the pulp of Cara Cara demonstrating a positive feedback regulatory mechanism (Alquezar et al., 2008).

The mutant Hong Anliu isolated in sweet orange (*Citrus sinensis*) has a pleiotropic phenotype with peculiar carotenoid accumulation, high sugar, and low acid in the fruits. A very strong lycopene accumulation (until 1000-fold higher than those in comparable wild type fruits) was observed in albedo, segment membranes, and juice sacs. Lycopene biosynthesis in the juice sacs was regulated by co-ordinate expression of carotenoid biosynthetic genes. Conversely, in albedo and segment membranes, the expression of downstream carotenogenic genes seems to be feedback induced by lycopene accumulation. A model proposed that huge amounts of lycopene might be synthesized in the juice sacs and then transported to the segment membrane and the albedo (Liu et al., 2007).

Pepper Fruits

Pepper (*Capsicum* sp.) fruits are characterized by different colors from white to deep red with the addition of green color due to chlorophyll retention. Elevated accumulation of the delphinidin glycoside (anthocyanin) in combination with chlorophyll and accessory carotenoid pigments produced the characteristic black pigmentation observed in no-ripe fruit of selected genotypes while violet immature fruits contained relatively little chlorophyll and carotenoids (Lightbourn et al., 2008). Yellow but above all, red peppers are important edible source of carotenoids and very common food additives for human nutrition. Specific ketocarotenoids such as capsanthin and capsorubin are key components in red pepper, but the carotenoid pathway present in chromoplasts of pepper (fibrillar type) is complex and many other pigments have been isolated (Hornero-Méndez et al., 2000, 2002; Sun et al., 2007). The two common xanthophylls antheraxanthin and violaxanthin are the direct precursors of capsanthin and capsorubin, respectively. The reaction of conversion is catalyzed by the capsanthin-capsorubin synthase (CCS), a fruit-specific bi-functional enzyme (Bouvier et al., 1994).

In immature stage of red pepper, lutein is abundant but during the ripening, its concentration decrease with a gradual increase of β-carotene, β-cryptoxanthin, zeaxanthin and a strong accumulation of capsanthin (Ha et al., 2007). In red colored pepper the total carotenoids at mature stage is higher than that of non-ripe fruit, and the high levels of capsanthin is associated with high transcription of the *CCS* gene. High levels of total carotenoids also required a substantial activity of the *PSY*, *PDS*, and β-*CH* genes. By contrast in non-red types the total carotenoid remains low during ripening (Ha et al., 2007).

The three major genes controlling the ketocarotenoid biosynthesis are: *y*, *c1* and *c2* (Hurtado-Hernandez and Smith, 1985). At the *y* locus the dominat allele y^+ determines the red fruit color while the *y* recessive allele is associated to the yellow morphotype. The *CCS* has been proposed as the candidate gene for the *y* locus present in red fruit while its deletion was hypothesized in the yellow fruit genotypes (Lefebvre et al., 1998; Popovsky and Paran, 2000).

The analysis of a genetic map using RFLP and AFLP markers in the F_2 population of an interspecific cross between *Capsicum annuum* cv TF68 (red fruits) and *Capsicum chinense* cultivar Habanero (orange fruits) has determined that one of the putative candidate genes, *PSY*, cosegregated with fruit color in the F_2 population. Quantitative trait loci (QTL) analysis of the pigment content of F_2 individuals quantified by HPLC also indicated that *PSY* is the locus responsible for the development of fruit color. The *PSY* gene could be the *c2* gene discriminating between red and orange genotypes (Huh et al., 2001). The orange fruits in *Capsicum chinense* cultivar Habanero are related to a drastic reduction in the quantity of capsanthin due to a mutation of *PSY* (Huh et al., 2001). On the contrary, a deletion in the upstream region of *CCS* characterizes orange fruits in the cultivar msGTY-1 of *Capsicum annuum* (Lang et al., 2004). In the *CCS* locus of two varieties of *Capsicum chinense* with yellow ripe fruits, premature stop codon and frame shift mutations have been also detected (Ha et al., 2007).

In pepper chromoplasts the carotenoids are sequestered within the fibrils and the process required a specific protein of 35 kDa (fibrillin) responsible of subplastidial architecture. There is a specific correlation between carotenoid accumulation in chromoplasts and the expression of fibrillin gene (Deruère et al., 1994). Therefore, to allow the enhanced carotenoid storage capacity within chromoplasts, the carotenogenesis must be coordinated to the mechanism of sequestration. Moreover, the transcription of genes that give rise to capsanthin is under positive control of reactive oxygen species (Bouvier et al., 1998).

The ethephon treatment stimulated carotenogenesis in pepper fruit. It was detected that the level of β-carotene increased by more than 30% at the red stage as control (Perucka, 2004).

Apricot Fruits

Apricot fruits (*Prunus armeniaca*) are important dietary sources of provitamin A because the common orange color is caused by a high accumulation of β-carotene (70-80% of the total carotenoids). In the fruits, low concentration of other carotenoids such as precursors (i.e. phytoene, phytofluene, γ-carotene, and lycopene) or xanthophylls (i.e. β-cryptoxanthin, zeaxanthin, and lutein) have been also identified (Curl, 1960; Dragovic-Uzelac et al., 2007). The carotenoid amounts are significantly conditioned by both the genotype and the environment; in particular, the carotenoid content is higher in cultivars grown in Mediterranean region (Dragovic-Uzelac et al., 2007).

Apricot varieties with different skin or flesh color (white, yellow, light orange, orange) have been selected. In these genotypes, carotenoids as well as the provitamin A content are minimum in the white fruits, medium in the yellow fruits and maximum in the orange fruits. The color parameters a^*, b^*, hue angle, and chroma showed good correlations with individual and total carotenoids in both flesh and peel. The best correlation was observed between total carotenoids and a^* value in the case of flesh whereas for the peel the best correlation was between total carotenoids and hue angle (Ruiz et al., 2005).

The expression analysis of early genes of carotenogenesis (*PSY1*, *PDS*, and *ZDS*) showed a systematically higher transcription in white than orange fruits while ethylene production was lower in orange than white fruits (Marty et al., 2005). The regulation of phytoene and phytofluene synthesis was analogous both in white and orange apricots as well as, the ethylene-mediated effect on the up-regulation of *PSY1* and *PDS*. On the contrary, for *ZDS* transcription an ethylene-mediated regulation was not observed. In addition, β-carotene was not accumulated in white fruits despite a higher expression of *ZDS* than orange fruits. A feedback regulation by end-products has been suggested (Marty et al., 2005).

Japanese apricot (*Prunus mume*) is a climateric fruit with large carotenoid accumulation (β,β-carotenoids such as β-carotene, β-cryptoxanthin, zeaxanthin and violaxanthin) during ripening. A key point in carotenoid biosynthesis is the up-regulation, ethylene-mediated, of *Prunus mume PSY* (*PmPSY-1*) gene. This event has positive consequences on transcription of downstream genes of the pathway. Moreover, during the ripening, the metabolic shift from β,ε-carotenoid synthesis to β,β-carotenoid requires a decrease in *PmLCY-e* expression and an increase in *PmLCY-b* expression (Kita et al., 2007).

Peach Fruits

The total carotenoid content of peach fruits (*Prunus persica*) with white flesh is very low but in the cultivars characterized by yellow flesh, 10-fold higher amounts (β-carotene and β-cryptoxanthin) have been detected (Gil et al., 2002). White flesh is dominant to yellow flesh and the symbols *Y* and *y* have been suggested for the two alleles (Connors, 1920; Bailey and French, 1949).

Recently, in the yellow-fleshed cultivar Redhaven and in the white-fleshed mutant *Redhaven Bianca*, Brandi et al. (2008) have analysed the expression levels of several genes involved in the synthesis of isoprenoids and the synthesis/degradation of carotenoids, as well as two genes involved in the ethylene emission at four stages of late fruit ripening (S3, Breaker 1, Breaker 2, S4). The authors have showed a differential temporal regulation of gene expression between the two genotypes, and quantitative and qualitative differences in transcript levels for key genes involved in carotenoid synthesis and degradation. The two genotypes also displayed quantitative and qualitative differences in emission patterns of carotenoid-derived volatiles, with higher levels in genotype with white flesh.

Watermelon and Melon Fruits

The flesh color of watermelon (*Citrullus lanatus* (Thunb.) Matsum & Nakai) depends on the carotenoid accumulation into chromoplasts with specific development (Bangalore et al., 2008), and genotypes characterized by red, orange, salmon yellow, canary yellow, or white have been described. The inheritance of this trait is complex with multiple allelic series at the *Y* locus and epistatic relationship (Poole, 1944; Henderson et al., 1998). Red type (with high lycopene content) is recessive to dominant canary yellow but it is the common trait of many cultivars. A molecular analysis of the mechanisms underlying differences in carotenoid content suggest the hypothesis that in red watermelon a mutation modifies the amino acid sequence of the LCY-b protein resulting in lycopene accumulation (Bang et al., 2007).

Orange mesocarp of melon (*Cucumis melo*) is rich in phytonutrients and provitamin A for human nutrition. Data on the inheritance of carotenoid content in melon are few and not univocal (Monforte et al., 2004; Eduardo et al., 2007) but recently maps of the genetic loci that regulate β-carotene accumulation have been obtained (Cuevas et al., 2008; 2009).

White and pale green varieties have a drastic reduction of β-carotene and β-ionone contents. However, thare are no differences in the transcriptional level of the *Cucumis melo CCD* (*CmCCD1*) gene during the maturation of orange, pale green and white flesh fruits. Therefore, in depigmentated melon fruits the β-ionone is reduced by lack of carotenoid precursors (Ibdah et al., 2006).

Maize Kernels

The carotenoids more abundant in maize grains are xanthophylls (lutein, zeaxanthin and β-cryptoxanthin) while β-carotene represents only the 2% of the total (Kean et al., 2008). The carotenoid accumulation starts 10 days after pollination (DAP) and then, it continues until maturity. A good molecular marker of this process is the *PSY1* expression level at 20 DAP. It is interesting to note that in the maize endosperm, the enzyme PSY1 is specifically localized in amyloplast envelope membranes (Li et al., 2008b).

Numerous mutations affecting maize carotenoid accumulation have been reported (Wurtzel, 2004) and some of these have been analyzed at molecular level. For example, the non-dormancy of the *viviparous-5* mutant (*vp5*) embryos is caused by insertions and/or deletions in the *PDS* locus (Li et al., 1996; Hable et al., 1998). The white *vp5* seedlings dead precociously. In the *pale yellow9* mutant (*y9*) the mutation affects a gene encoding an enzyme required for the *cis*- to *trans*-conversion of the 15-*cis*-bond in 9,15,9'-tri-*cis*-ζ-carotene (Li et al., 2007). The endosperm of the *y9* mutant is depigmentated but the seedlings are viable and developed normal green leaves.

Underground Organs: Carrot Root

Massive accumulation of carotenoids in roots is an unusual phenomenon and the carrot (*Daucus carota*) represents the most distinctive example. The carotenoids are located into crystalline chromoplasts characterized by small crystals of β-carotene. The Raman spectroscopy analysis showed that the accumulation of this pigment in the secondary phloem increased gradually from periderm towards the core, but declined fast in cells close to the vascular cambium (Baranska et al., 2006). The crystalline chromoplasts derive from proplastids without an intermediate chloroplast phase (Ben-Shaul and Klein, 1965).

Several colors of root carrots such as high βC orange, orange, purple, red, yellow, and white, have been selected (Surles et al., 2004). The orange roots present a massive accumulation of β-carotene, low levels of α-carotene and lutein, but are devoid in lycopene, which is accumulated at low level into the high βC orange type. In purple cultivars, in addition to β-carotene, the carotenoid profile is characterized by a relevant content of α-carotene and lutein. Lycopene is the typic carotenoid of the red cultivar while in the yellow carrots the lutein is the main pigment in concomitance with a drastic reduction of both α- and β-carotene. In white carrot the carotenoids are present only in traces (Surles et al., 2004).

Several major genes affecting carotenoid accumulation have been identified. They include dominant alleles such as A (α-carotene accumulation), Io (intense orange xylem), L_1 and L_2 (lycopene accumulation), O (orange xylem) as well as the recessives alleles y (yellow xylem) and rp (reduced pigmentation) (Simon, 2000). The Y, Y_1, and Y_2 loci control differential distribution of α- and β-carotene (xylem/phloem carotene levels) where the mutation Y_2 controls low carotene content of the storage root xylem in high carotene orange backgrounds (Simon, 1996).

The expression level of eight different genes of carotenoid pathway has been recently analyzed in white, yellow, orange, and red carrots (Clotault et al., 2008). Despite the white phenotype, mRNA of all genes were accumulated in the cultivar Blanche demi-longue des Vosges. The control of the absence of carotenoids in white roots is not at transcriptional level but its nature remains yet elusive. In colored roots the correlation between expression level of genes of carotenogenesis and carotenoid accumulation in roots was well defined during the early stages of root development while for the strong pigment accumulation in the late stages the correlation with up-regulation of transcription was less defined. It has been also hypothesized that the elevated transcription of LCY-e is required to obtain the carotenoid profile of yellow roots while the lycopene buildup of red roots could be associate to high expression of $ZDS1$ and/or $ZDS2$ (Clotault et al., 2008). The regulation of carotenoid synthesis on the basis of a control at the transcriptional level was only partially justified in the orange roots (cv. Bolero); therefore, further investigations are required in the future to clarify the differential accumulation of carotenoids in carrot (Clotault et al., 2008).

Underground Organs: Potato Tuber

Commercial tetraploid potato tubers (*Solanum tuberosum* L.), also if with yellow flesh, are characterized by 50-fold lower carotenoid content with respect to the level observed in carrots. Nevertheless, tubers with orange/yellow flesh could be interesting source of xanthophylls for human nutrition considering that potato is one of major horticultural crops with very wide diffusion in the world; therefore, the selection of genotypes with enhanced carotenoid content is an important breeding goal.

The total carotenoid content of potato is influenced by the genotype and the year of cultivation but poor conditioned by fertilizer application (Kotikova et al., 2007).

Orange flesh trait (high zeaxanthin accumulation) is under the genetic control of the O locus that is dominant over both Y (yellow flesh) and y (white flesh) (Bonierbale et al., 1988).

Potato varieties of the Andes such as the diploid in the Groups Phureja and Goniocalyx are the germoplasm with higher carotenoid content (Brown et al., 1993). An interesting trait of the native potato cultivars is the oxygen radical absorbance capacity (ORAC) because is associated to anthocyanin and carotenoids content. The analysis of 38 native potato cultivars of different taxonomic groups from South America demonstrated that total carotenoid content was negatively correlated with total anthocyanins (Brown et al., 2007). Recently, a very interesting clone named Hokkai 93, has been selected from the progeny of open-pollinated Inca-no-mezame (diploid potato variety) seeds. The new variety is a diploid potato characterized by yellowish-orange flesh, very high carotenoid content and chestnut-like nutty flavor. In particular, the total carotenoid content is 40-fold higher compared to a commercial tetraploid potato variety and very rich in zeaxanthin and lutein (Kobayashi et al., 2008).

To date, the analysis of carotenogenesis regulation in potato, at molecular level, is scantily defined. Morris et al. (2004) have conducted a study on carotenoid biosynthesis during tuber development of DB375/1 (*S. phureya*, orange flesh characterized by high zeaxanthin content), Pentland Javelin (*S. tuberosum*, white flesh), and Desiree (*S. tuberosum*, cream/yellow flesh) characterized by a different total carotenoid in mature tubers: 36.3, 1.6 and 4.9 µg/g DW, respectively. Unexpected result has been the higher transcript levels of some genes of the DOXP and carotenogenesis pathways (i.e. *DXPS*, *GGPS* and *ZEP*) in the genotypes with lower carotenoid accumulation. Moreover, the *PSY* expression level was very high in the early stages of DB375/1 tuberization and this result is consistent with the hypothesis that PSY activity is an important point in the control of carotenoid accumulation as demonstrated in other species. The expression profile of genes for carotenogenesis observed in DB375/1 was also specific for the transcript levels of *ε-CYC* and *ZEP*. The significant lutein level accumulated in the DB375/1 tubers was attributed to the large increase in the transcript level of *ε-CYC* compared with Desiree e Pentland Javelin. By contrast, the *ZEP* expression in the DB375/1 was lower than in white flesh tubers. To date, it is not clear why a lowered *ZEP* transcription is associated with a high total carotenoid content of mature tubers. Perhaps, the reduction of zeaxanthin epoxidation restricts the supply of ABA precursors with a positive and concomitant effect of metabolic flux towards the pigment accumulation (Morris et al., 2004).

Recently, the *β-carotene hydroxylase* has been suggested for the identity of the classic Y locus (Brown et al., 2006).

Plant Breeding and Molecular Markers

The increase of the carotenoid content in crops (biofortification) used as food in large groups of people, is considered to be a very effective and sustainable approach to improve human nutrition and health (Nestel et al., 2006; Ortiz-Monasterio et al., 2007; Pfeiffer and McClafferty, 2007). Biofortification provides a praticable mean of reaching undernourished populations in rather remote rural areas, delivering naturally fortified foods to people with limited access to commercially marketed fortified foods (Nestel et al., 2006). In 2003 the Consultative Group on International Agricultural Research (CGIAR) established the

Biofortification Challenge Program, HarvestPlus (http://www.harvestplus.org/) adding food quality to its agricultural production research model (Nestel et al., 2006; Pfeiffer and McClafferty, 2007). The HarvestPlus program include plant breeding at the CGIAR centers and National Agricultural Research and Extension Services (NARES) to develop varieties that combine the best nutritional and agronomic traits in several crops (Pfeiffer and McClafferty, 2007). Because of regulatory and political restrictions on the use of transgenic plants, and because significant advancement can be made also through conventional breeding, 85% of HarvestPlus resources are presently committed in conventional breeding (Nestel et al., 2006). Plant breeding programs are under way for six crops that are largely consumed by the majority of the world's poor in Africa, Asia, and Latin America: rice, maize, cassava (*Manihot esculenta* Crantz), common beans (*Phaseolus vulgaris* L.), common wheat (*Triticum aestivum* L.), and orange-fleshed sweetpotato [*Ipomoea batatas* (L.) Lam.] (Pfeiffer and McClafferty, 2007).

Success in crop improvement through conventional plant breeding strategies depends on the existence of adequate genetic variation for the target traits in the gene pool available to the breeders. When there is sufficient genetic variation, breeders can exploit additive gene effects, transgressive segregation and heterosis to modify carotenoid content. However, to date, only a small portion of genetic diversity for carotenoid has been assayed. It is desirable the screening for carotenoid content in large germplasm collections of different crops. When variation is not available a mutagenic approach may be an option to generate mutants with favorably altered biochemical pathway. Breeding strategies must aim to generate carotenoid-enhanced plant cultivars without compromising tolerance to abiotic and biotic stress, crop productivity, and acceptable end-use quality.

Extensive screening for genetic variation for carotenoid content in crops including tomato (Lincoln and Porter, 1950; Tomes et al., 1954; Tanksley, 1993; Liu et al., 2003), pepper (Hurtado-Hernandez and Smith, 1985; Hornero-Méndez et al., 2000), common wheat (Ortiz-Monasterio et al., 2007), tritordeum (*Tritordeum* Ascherson et Graebner) (Alvarez et al., 1999; Atienza et al., 2007), *Hordeum chilense* (Atienza et al., 2004), maize (Mackinney and Jenkins, 1949; Ortiz-Monasterio et al., 2007), carrot (Buishand and Gabelman, 1979; Simon and Wolff, 1987; Simon, 2000), cassava (Iglesias et al., 1997), *Citrus* spp. (Fanciullino et al., 2006), melon (Monforte et al., 2004) coupled with traditional breeding and selection procedures have resulted in varieties with enhanced levels of total carotenoids and provitamin A (Simon, 1990; 1993; Nestel et al., 2006; Ortiz-Monasterio et al., 2007). Several tests have been also conducted to examine the effect of environment on carotenoid content. An increasing body of evidence suggests that the expression of provitamin A across crops is relatively stable under different growing conditions (Egesel et al., 2003; Menkir and Maziya-Dixon, 2004). Cassava, maize and sweet potato genotypes with high and stable expression across environments were identified, with genotype × environment interactions predominantly of the crossover type (Egesel et al., 2003; Ortiz-Monasterio et al., 2007; Pfeiffer and McClafferty, 2007). These results agree with the findings that provitamin A is controlled by few major genes. Compared to typical carrots, sweet potatoes, and tomatoes, which contains 160, 120, and 7 mg Kg^{-1} (fresh weight) of provitamin A carotenoids, respectively, high carotene genotypes containing 600, >200, and 95 mg Kg^{-1}, respectively, have been realized (Simon, 1990, 1993; Simon et al., 1989; Nestel et al., 2006). Even naturally low-carotene vegetables, as cauliflower (*Brassica oleracea* L) (Dickinson et al.,

1988) and cucumber (*Cucumis sativus* L.) (Simon and Navazio, 1997) have been genetically improved for higher carotenoid content by classical breeding.

Lutein followed by zeaxanthin is the main carotenoids (yellow pigment, YP) found in the seeds of einkorn (*Triticum monococcum* L.) (Hidalgo et al., 2006; Leenhardt et al., 2006); durum wheat (*Triticum durum* L.) (Adom et al., 2003; Leenhardt et al., 2006), common wheat (Adom et al., 2003; Leenhardt et al., 2006; Moore et al., 2005) and tritordeum (Atienza et al., 2007). These two carotenoids show no provitamin A activity. Orange-colored wheat seed, which may have some provitamin A carotenoids, have not been identified (Ortiz-Monasterio et al., 2007). However, the yellow color is a selection criterion for durum wheat breeding worldwide due to its importance in pasta-making (Troccoli et al., 2000). In addition, both lutein and zeaxanthin have important roles in human health in terms of preventing macular degeneration and cataracts. The importance of the carotenoid content have also promoted the search of new sources of variation in related species of wheat such as *Lophopyrum ponticum* (Podp.), and *Hordeum chilense* (Roem. et Schulz) (Alvarez et al., 1994; 1999). *H. chilense* has been used in cross with durum wheat to synthesize the amphidiploid tritordeum that have consistently shown higher carotenoid pigment levels than wheat (Alvarez et al., 1994). The genetic origin of the main component of the difference in carotenoid pigments between wheat and tritordeum has been attributed to two loci for YP content on chromosomes 2H[ch] and 7H[ch] (Alvarez et al., 1998; Atienza et al., 2004; 2007). Carotenoids are stored in specialized carotenoid-sequestering structures within plastids (Vishnevetsky et al. 1999), a feature that suggests the importance of the cytoplasmic genomes for the determination of this trait. It has been observed that in wheat lines, where the native cytoplasm was replaced by donor cytoplasm from *H. chilense* and *Triticum-Aegilops* complex the lutein concentration was significantly increased (Atienza et al., 2008). It is likely that carotenoid accumulation is controlled both by the level of activity of the carotenoid biosynthetic genes and the presence of carotenoid-storing structures (Cookson et al., 2003; Howitt and Pogson, 2006; Atienza et al., 2008).

In maize genetic variation for provitamin A carotenoid concentration is adequate (especially for *β*-carotene and *β*-cryptoxanthin) (Ortiz-Monasterio et al., 2007; Harjes et al., 2008; Vallabhaneni and Wurtzel, 2009). Egesel et al. (2003) reported that general combining ability (GCA) effects, or additive gene action, accounted for 72-87% of the variation for *β*-carotene, *β*-cryptoxanthin, and total carotenoids in a diallel crossing among 10 inbred lines. However, non-additive gene action is important for provitamin A concentrations in some crosses (Egesel et al., 2003) and raises the possibility of exploiting heterosis in breeding for these nutrients (Ortiz-Monasterio et al., 2007). To enhance provitamin A concentration in more than 100 normal and quality protein maize (QPM) lines, an intra-population recurrent selection programme has been initiated at the CYMMIT (Ortiz-Monasterio et al., 2007).

Improvements in carotenoid concentrations using traditional breeding efforts are limited because the high cost associated with analytical laboratory measurements and the time required to quantitatively assessing the carotenoid content in plant organs. The rapid development of molecular tools is expected to speed up the introgression of increased carotenoid concentration from exotic sources into locally adapted elite germoplasm. This is particularly fundamental using wild species that are a considerable resource for extending genetic variation for carotenoid content. Molecular makers offer a tool in which the amount of wild or alien DNA can be monitored during each backcross generation. Selection for these markers could be incorporated into breeding schemes (Molecular Marker-Assisted Selection, MAS), resulting in efficiency gains in terms of faster and greater progress from selection, as well as cost savings relative to current methods. The efficiency of a classical backcross scheme to introgress genes affecting carotenoid concentration from the donor parent into the genomic background of recurrent parent has been improved with the use of molecular marker alleles typical of either parents. Thus, accelerating the recovery of recurrent genome, and reducing the "linkage drag".

Indeed, a large genetic variation for carotenoid content is also available in the wild relatives of crops (Tanksley et al., 1996; Tanksley and McCouch, 1997; Alvarez et al., 1998; Atienza et al., 2004; 2007; Abbo et al., 2005). Near isogenic cultivated lines (NILs) of a given plant species, each containing a small introgressed chromosomal segment from wild relatives of that species have been produced. In these NILs, the wild genes function in a genetic background that is mostly derived from cultivated plants, and hence the agronomic quality of specific wild genes can be assessed. For example, the potential of this approach has been enstablished for improving carotenoid content in tomato. In the NILs of tomato cultivars containing segments derived from *Lycopersicum hyrsutum* (Monforte and Tanksley, 2000), a wild trait locus controls a novel flower and fruit-specific *LCY-b* was identified (Ronen et al., 2000). The manipulation of this gene, which provides an alternative pathway for the synthesis of β-carotene, was conduced to increase β-carotene or lycopene content in fruits (Ronen et al., 2000).

Carotenoid biosynthesis is not fully characterized in many crops because some of the genes encoding certain enzymes still need to be identified. However, the carotenoid biosynthetic pathway is well characterized in several species (i.e., *Arabidopsis*, maize, tomato) and genes encoding major structural enzymes in the pathway have been isolated, mapped, and characterized (Hirschberg, 2001; Thorup et al., 2000; DellaPenna and Pogson, 2006). In addition, the genome of several species, including crops as rice and *Vitis vinifera*, has already been sequenced and expresses sequence tag (EST) databases are available from various tissues of many species. Conserved genes and cDNA sequences from these databases, for which clear functional annotation can be predicted by the current bioinformatic tools, are easily identified and their potential biotechnologies values can be tested. The cloning and sequence information of these genes is useful for PCR-based expression studies and may point toward transgenic approaches to manipulate carotenoid biosynthesis and/or regulation. Moreover, the identification of QTLs associated with key enzymes of the carotenoid biosynthetic pathway, is fundamental to apply marker-assisted selection in breeding for increased carotenoid concentration. Studies in several different plant species have examined the relationship between candidate genes and quantitative variation for carotenoid content. The mapping of QTLs with effects on carotenoid biosynthesis, including QTLs in regions of candidate genes, and to detect molecular markers useful as tags for these traits should enable a better understanding of the genetic control of levels of carotenoids in crops. In addition, if the candidate gene can be validated, then it can be used as an efficient molecular marker to aid in selecting desirable alleles. Since the carotenoid pathway is so highly conserved among flowering plants (Hirschberg, 2001), map positions of these genes in a species could serve as a starting point for comparative mapping studies with other species in genera closely related (Thorup et al., 2000).

PSY and ZDS catalyze rate-limiting steps in the carotenoid biosynthetic pathway and have been found associated with major QTLs controlling carotenoid content in several species

(Thorup et al., 2000; Palaisa et al., 2003; Wong et al., 2004; Gallagher et al., 2004; Pozniak et al., 2007). For example, three functional *PSY* genes (*PSY1*, *PSY2*, and *PSY3*) were identified in maize, but association and QTL mapping studies have shown that only *PSY1* is associated with elevated levels of endosperm carotenoids (Palaisa et al. 2003; Wong et al. 2004; Pozniak et al., 2007; Li et al., 2008b). Four QTLs underlying phenotypic variation in endosperm color were identified on chromosomes 2A, 4B, 6B, and 7B of durum wheat (Pozniak et al., 2007). The *PSY1-1* locus co-segregated with the 7B QTL, demonstrating an association of this gene with phenotypic variation for endosperm color.

In maize, QTLs for lutein, zeaxanthin, β-carotene, β-cryptoxanthin, and total carotenoids also map to region with the candidate gene *viviparous 9* in the chromosome 7 and is associated with *ZDS* (Wong et al., 2004).

Recently, through association analysis, linkage mapping, expression analysis and mutagenesis have been shown that variation at the *LCY-e* locus alters flux down α-carotene versus β-carotene branches of the carotenoid pathway. A maize QTL that showed significant effects for the modification of the ratio of α to β branch carotenoids, and explained 31.7% of the variation for lutein, colocalized with *LCY-e* (Harjes et al., 2008). Notably, this QTL was not significant for total carotenoid, which further support that variation in within *LCY-e* gene underlies this QTL for carotenoid composition (Harjes et al., 2008). As pointed out by Harjes et al. (2008) markers linked to favorable *LCY-e* alleles can now be used to produce maize genotypes with higher provitamin A level.

In *Triticum aestivum*, YP content is mainly provided by the genes located on homoeologous group 7 chromosomes. Parker et al. (1998) found two major QTLs on chromosomes 7A and 3A, explaining 60 and 13% of the phenotypic variance for YP content, respectively. Mares and Campbell (2001) detected two QTLs associated with YP content on chromosomes 7A and 3B in a Sunco/Tasman-derived mapping population. Kuchel et al. (2006) mapped a major QTL for flour yellowness b*, the major criterion to estimate flour color, on chromosome 7B, explaining 48 and 61% of phenotypic variance in different cropping seasons. Zhang et al. (2006) detected a major QTL controlling kernel YP content and flour yellowness b* on chromosome 7A, accounting for 12.9-37.6% of phenotypic variance across the environments. More recently, based on polymorphisms of two haplotypes of *PSY-A1* in cultivars with high and low yellow pigment (YP) content, a STS marker, *YP7A*, was developed by He et al. (2008). Using a recombinant inbred line (RIL) population and a set of Chinese Spring nullisomic-tetrasomic lines and ditelosomic line 7AS, the marker *YP7A* was mapped on chromosome 7AL. *PSY-A1*, co-segregating with the *YP7A* marker, explained 20-28% of the phenotypic variance for YP content across three environments (He et al., 2008). The functional marker *YP7A* was closely related to YP content and, as suggested by He et al. (2008), could be used in breeding programs targeting of YP content for various wheat-based products.

In durum wheat, major QTLs for YP content were found on chromosomes 7A and 7B (Elouafi et al., 2001; Pozniak et al., 2007; Patil et al., 2008). However, QTLs for YP content were also detected on homoeologous group 1 chromosomes (Ma et al., 1999), chromosomes 4A and 5A (Hessler et al., 2002), 2D and 4D (Zhang et al., 2006), 2A, 4B and 6B (Pozniak et al., 2007), and 1A, 3B and 5B (Patil et al., 2008), indicating multigenic control of YP content in durum wheat grain in addition to the major genes on homoeologous group 7 chromosomes.

An extensive genetic variation characterizes the carotenoid content in tomato and pepper, two largely consumed vegetables. Tomato fruit exhibit a wide range of colors, and many mutation (Tanksley, 1993), and QTLs (Fulton et al., 1997; Bernacchi et al., 1998; Liu et al., 2003) affecting fruit color have been characterized and mapped. These results support the strong candidate position of carotenoid genes for qualitative variation in fruit color (Liu et al., 2003). Marker and phenotypic analyses of segregating populations involving crosses of the cultivated tomato with its wild relatives (e.g. *L. pimpinellifolium, L. hirsutum, L. peruvianum, L. parviflorum*) revealed numerous QTLs that modify fruit color (Tanksley et al., 1996; Bernacchi et al., 1998; Fulton et al., 1997; 2000; Chen et al., 1999). Using seventy-five tomato introgression lines (ILs), each containing a single homozygous RFLP-defined chromosome segment from *Lycopersicon pennellii*, a candidate gene approach has been useful for the identification of sequences that regulates major fruit color loci (i.e. *r*, *B* and *Del*), but not for quantitative variation of red color (Liu et al., 2003). Notably, as showed in a previous section of this chapter, other genes (i.e, *HP2* and *NR*) not directly involved in carotenoid pathway, can dramatically modify the carotenoid content of the tomato fruit. Deployment of color intensifier mutants *crimson* (og^c) and *hp* in combination with ripening mutants may represent a viable alternative for the development of tomato cultivars with both improved shelf life and normal fruit color development (Robinson and Tomes, 1968; Tigchelaar et al., 1978; de Araújo et al., 2002; Vrebalov et al., 2002).

All carotenoid pigments presents in the pepper are C_{40} isoprenoid, containing nine conjugated double bonds in the central polyenic chain, which can be classified in two isochromic families: red (R) and yellow (Y) (Hornero-Méndez et al., 2000). Notably, the R fractions contains the pigments exclusive to the *Capsicum* genus (capsanthin, capsanthin-5,6-epoxide, and capsorubin), and the Y fractions contains the rest of the pigments (zeaxanthin, violaxanthin, antheraxanthin, β-cryptoxanthin, β-carotene and cucubitaxanthin A), which act as precursor of the former (Hornero-Méndez et al., 2000). Ten structural genes of carotenoid biosynthetic pathway have been localized on a (*Capsicum annuum* × *C. chinense*)F_2 genetic map anchored in tomato (Thorup et al., 2000). One of three QTLs determining pepper fruit color cosegregated with *PSY*. In addition, it has been suggested that *PSY* may be responsible for the *c2* gene discriminating between red and orange cultivars (Huh et al., 2001). The *CCS* locus, shown to cosegregate with *y* (Popovsky and Paran, 2000), another pepper fruit color locus mapped to chromosome 6 (Thorup et al., 2000). A QTL affecting the intensity of mature red color was detected in this region that also correspond to the position of the *B* locus for hyperaccumulation of β-carotene in tomato fruits (Ronen et al., 2000).

Carrot (*Daucus carota* L.) is one of the most consumed plant food in the world in all seasons, and is the major single source of provitamin A, providing 14% to 17% of total vitamin A consumption (Simon, 2000). The root of carrot contains carotenoids that accounts for their orange, yellow and red color (Buishand and Gabelman, 1979; Simon et al., 1989; Surles et al., 2004). The inheritance of root color variation has been extensively studied (Simon, 2000). Broad sense heritabilities and gene numbers estimation provided evidence for continuous inheritance of α-carotene, β-carotene and total carotenoids in the orange × dark orange cross and discrete inheritance for β-carotene and total carotenoids in the orange × white cross (Santos and Simon, 2006). A collection of naturally occurring single-locus mutations of master genes (e.g. *A*, *Io*, *L$_1$* and *L$_2$*, *O*, *Y*, *Y$_1$* and *Y$_2$*) controlling carotenoid accumulation in carrot roots is also available (Gabelman and Peters, 1979; Simon, 1996).

Initially, six AFLP fragments linked to the Y_2 locus, which controls carotene content of the storage root xylem in high carotene orange backgrounds (Simon, 1996), were identified through a combination of F_2 mapping and bulked segregant analysis (Bradeen and Simon, 1998). Moreover, Santos and Simon (2002) observed numerous QTLs for major component carotenoid pigments using single marker analysis. More recently, twenty-two putative genes coding for carotenoid biosynthesis enzymes were placed on a carrot genetic linkage map developed from a cross orange-rooted × white-rooted carrot (Just et al., 2007). The carotenoid genes were distributed in eight of the nine linkage groups in the carrot genome and two genes co-localized with a genomic region spanning one of the most significant QTLs for carotenoid accumulation (Santos and Simon, 2002).

The seeds of chickpea (*Cicer arietinum* L.) contain carotenoids such as *β*-carotene, cryptoxanthin, lutein and zeaxanthin in amounts above the engineered *β*-carotene-containing "Golden Rice" level. Thus, in countries where chickpea is a dominant staple food, and fruits and other vegetables are scarce or expensive, chickpea would therefore be a much superior source of dietary carotenoids than "Golden Rice"(Abbo et al., 2005). High hereditability values, detected for lutein and *β*-carotene in segregating progeny from a cross between an Israeli cultivar and wild *Cicer reticulatum* Ladiz, suggest that only a few genes were involved in controlling the content of these two carotenoids (Abbo et al., 2005). Four QTLs for *β*-carotene level and a single QTL for lutein concentration were detected. If these QTLs represent genes coding for enzymes involved in the biosynthetic pathway or regulating factors controlling their quantity in seeds is unknown (Abbo et al., 2005).

Several genes control the flesh and epidermis color of typically orange-fleshed cucurbit fruit (Robinson et al., 1976). In *Cucumis melo*, orange flesh color is dominant to both white flesh (*wf*) and green flesh (*gf*). In watermelon, red flesh is dominant to one gene for yellow flesh (*yf*) but recessive to another flesh gene and to white flesh (*Wf*) (Robinson et al., 1976; Simon, 1992).

Although some varieties of melon are source of *β*-carotene with more than 80% of the carotenoids being produced in the fruit, mapping of carotenoid genes in this specie has not been documented, and enhanced high carotene germplasm is not publicly available (Cuevas et al., 2008). Monforte et al. (2004) evaluated the inheritance of orange mesocarp color using F_2 populations and double haploid lines of melon, and hypothesized that three putative loci control the orange color in melon. However, this hypothesis was not confirmed by comparative analysis of nearly isogenic lines differing in fruit color variation (Eduardo et al., 2007). More recently, Cuevas et al. (2008) detected eight QTLs distributed across four linkage group of melon, which explained a significant portion of the associated phenotypic variation for quantity of *β*-carotene (QbC). Although QTL map positions were not uniformly associated with putative carotenoid genes, one QTL was located 10 cM from a *β*-carotene hydroxylase gene (Cuevas et al., 2008).

Some linkage maps have been constructed for watermelon. One linkage map constructed with RAPDs, isozymes and RFLPs spanning 524 cM revealed the loci for rind color and flesh color (Hashizume et al. 1996). Another one, covering 354 cM and based on isozymes and seed protein, revealed the loci for flesh color (Navot and Zamir, 1986; Navot et al., 1990). However, these linkage maps covered only a small part of the genome. More recently, using F_2 populations derived from a cross between a cultivated watermelon and an African wild form, Hashizume and coworker (2003) mapped 554 loci to 11 linkage groups that extended for 2,384 centimorgans (cM). In addition another linkage map with a total length of 1,729 cM was constructed in a BC_1 population using genetic markers found to segregate in the F_2 population (Hashizume et al., 2003). A QTL analysis based on the data of the BC_1 population also allowed the localization of a QTL for flesh color that explained 55.2% and 35.8% of the phenotypic variance for yellow and red, respectively. Another QTL was detected for the red value of the flesh, accounting for 35.5% of the phenotypic variance (Hashizume et al., 2003).

Molecular markers and high-throughput genome sequencing efforts have increased knowledge on genetic diversity for carotenoid content in the germplasm pool for the above mentioned crops. High-resolution genetic maps and genetic linkage between markers and carotenoid variation are expected to speed up the constitution of biofortificated genotypes. The carotenoid content is also expected to be increased in other crop cultivars breed for developing countries and, in the HarvestPlus program, prebreeding feasibility studies are being undertaken on barley (*Hordeum vulgare* L.), millet (*Panicum miliaceum* L.), sorghum [*Sorghum bicolor* (L.) Moench], potato, bananas/plantains (*Musa acuminata* x *M. balbisiana* Colla), cowpea [*Vigna unguiculata* (L.) Walp.], groundnut [*Vigna subterranea* (L.) Verdc.], yam (*Dioscorea* spp.), lentil (*Lens culinaris* Medik.) and pigeon pea [*Cajanus cajan* (L.) Millsp. syn. *Cajanus indicus* Spreng.] (Pfeiffer and McClafferty, 2007). At the same time, it will be necessary to determine in improved crop varieties for high concentrations of total carotenoids the proportion of carotenoids with provitamin A activity and their bioavailability and stability during processing and storage before such varieties are promoted for production and consumption. In addition, despite the controversy surrounding genetically modified plants, it is likely that in some species, for example rice where β-carotene has not been identified in the endosperm of any variety, the transgenic approach may be the only option to modify the carotenoid content.

Transformation Strategies to Improve the Carotenoid Content and Composition

A large number of studies have been conducted in several crops to improve the carotenoid content (and/or composition) using the recombinant DNA techniques and, on this subject, many excellent reviews are available (DellaPenna, 1999; Fraser and Bramley, 2004; Taylor and Ramsay, 2005; Sandmann et al., 2006; Botella-Pavía et al., 2006; Giuliano et al., 2008; Lu and Li, 2008; Mayer et al., 2008; Newell-McGloughlin, 2008; Zhou et al., 2008; Fraser et al., 2009). The results obtained are promising in basic crops such as tomato, rice, potato, and, more recently in maize but the fundamental obstacle remains the reserve of consumer to accept GM crops.

Here, we focalize the attention only on the most interesting approaches used to obtain transgenic plants with enhanced nutritional value.

Obviously, a major strategy is the overexpression of carotenogenic genes encoding enzymes with highest flux control coefficient (rate-limiting). In this context, a candidate gene frequently used is the *PSY* under the control of a constitutive promoter. For example, Fraser et al. (2007) have been conducted in tomato a deep characterization of transgenic plants for the overexpression of *PSY-1*. However, some problems have been observed in the transgenic plants. In addition to increased levels of β-carotene (up to 1.5-fold in the 60% of plants), the population of primary transgenic plants showed also dwarfism, leaf chlorosis, and yellow fruits with decreased pigment content. The origin of undesirable traits could be related to metabolite interaction between pathways, because carotenoid biosynthesis is included into the wide terpenoid metabolism of plastid. The overproduction of one key enzyme in the early step of carotenogenesis can induce deleterious consequences in other branches such as chlorophyll or gibberellin biosynthesis (i.e. through depletion of the endogenous precursors of geranylgeranyl pyrophosphate) (Sandmann et al., 2006). A pleiotropic effect of *PSY* overexpression has been observed also in *Arabidopsis thaliana* seeds where the increased level of carotenoids is coupled to enhancement of ABA-dependent embryo dormancy (Lindgren et a., 2003). In this case, the metabolite interaction is within the same pathway because the abscisic acid is a product of xanthophylls cleavage.

Deleterious consequences on isoprenoid metabolism in tomato were not observed after the use of *PSY* gene from the bacterium *Erwinia uredovora* (*crtB*) under the control of a fruit-specific promoter (Fraser et al., 2002). In this case, the carotenoid accumulation in fruit (up to 4-fold) was not related to alteration of tocopherols, plastoquinone and ubiquinone. The same strategy has produced interesting results also in canola and potato using the *crtB* gene with a tissue-specific promoter (Shewmaker et al., 1999; Ducreux et al., 2005). The synthetic modification of *PSY* sequence is an alternative approach to overcome the detrimental effects on phenotype of transgene overexpression (Schuch et al., US patent wo97/ 1996:46690).

Genetic engineering with two or more genes represents another strategy. For example, in the famous "Golden Rice" selected to alleviate the pro-vitamin A deficiency in developing countries was first inserted *PSY* from daffodil in combination with the carotene desaturase from *Erwinia uredovora* (*crtI*) (Ye et al., 2000) and then improved through a change of the *PSY* origin: from daffodil to maize (Golden Rice II; Paine et al., 2005). The analysis of carotenoid biosynthesis in wild type endosperm of rice demonstrated that mRNA of *PSY* was virtually absent while the expression of *PDS*, *ZDS*, *CRTISO*, *LCY* and, *CHY-b*, were showed. Therefore the action of a *PSY* transgene under a constitutive promoter is of crucial importance whereas the need of *crtI* probably depends on an insufficient activity of PDS and/or ZDS in the rice endosperm (Schaub et al., 2005). The reason for the differing efficiency of the *PSY* from various sources is unclear. Perhaps the organellar environment (endosperm amyloplasts) in rice provides optimal setting for PSY enzyme from maize (Paine et al., 2005).

The concomitant overexpression of two genes was also utilized in tomato. This strategy has permitted the xanthophylls enrichment (β-carotene, β-cryptoxanthin and zeaxanthin) of ripe fruit through the overexpression of *LCY-b* and *CHY-b* genes under the control of the fruit-specific *PDS* promoter (Dharmapuri et al., 2002).

Two different bacterial genes (*crtB* and *crtI*) under the control of a modified γ-zein promoter have been also utilized to increase the provitamin A content of maize kernel (Aluru et al., 2008). A strong carotenoid increment (up to 34-fold) and a preferential β-carotene synthesis were obtained. The carotenoid content was extremely variable in T_1 maize transformants as observed for Golden Rice II (Paine et al., 2005; Aluru et al., 2008); nevertheless, high β-carotene trait is heritable and maintained through generations.

Recently, the combinatorial nuclear transformation to obtain multiplex-transgenic plants has been applied in maize to create metabolically diverse transgenic libraries. Immature zygotic embryos of South African the elite white maize variety M37W have been transformed by biolistic method using *PSY*, *PDS*, *LCY-b*, *CHY-b* and *β-carotene ketolase* genes from 5 different organisms. Each gene was driven by a different endosperm-specific promoter (Zhu et al., 2008).

A different strategy is the use of antisense constructs. For example, the down-regulation of *LCY-b* has been applied with success in tomato in order to increase the lycopene content of ripe fruits (Rosati et al., 2000). Silencing strategies to modify the carotenoid biosynthesis in plants need a tissue-specific control to exclude deleterious effects at chloroplast level. In the example above cited the silencing of *LCY-b* gene was induced in a fruit-specific fashion (Rosati et al., 2000). In potato, a key target to increase the provitamin A content is the silencing of *CHY-b*. Van Eck et al. (2007) introduced RNAi construct under a tuber-specific granule-bound starch synthetase promoter to block the activity of β-carotene hydroxylase that converts β-carotene to zeaxanthin. Diretto et al. (2007) silenced *CHY-b-1* and *-2* by constructs in antisense orientation under the tuber-specific patatin B33 promoter. In the trasformants, a significant increase of the β-carotene content (up to 38-fold) and a concomitant zeaxanthin decrease was observed (Diretto et al., 2007).

The enhancement of carotenoid content in edible crops is not necessarily linked to direct modification of expression of genes encoding enzymes for the carotenogenic pathway. In fact, an alternative strategy is the transformation with genes that are involved in light signal trasduction, photoreceptors, chloroplast biogenesis, and carotenoid-sequestration. The remarkable selection of tomato transformants characterized by the enhancement of both carotenoid and flavonoid content has been obtained through the fruit-specific suppression of the photomorphogenesis regulatory gene *DET1* (Davuluri et al., 2005). It is interesting to note that constitutive silencing of the *DET1* gene determined a phenocopy of the *hp2* mutant because the transformants showed deleterious phenotypic effects such as bushiness and dwarfing. Therefore, the choice of a fruit-specific promoter has been decisive to improve fruit quality without negative effects on plant vigor. The increase of the fruit antioxidant content (up to 1.7 and 2.9-fold of carotenoids and flavonoids content, respectively) has been obtained in tomato also with the overexpression of the *CRY-2* gene encoding the blue light photoreceptor cryptochrome 2 (Giliberto et al., 2005). However, the use of a constitutive promoter realized transgenic plants with a dwarf phenotype, outgrowth of axillary meristems, dark green leaves, anthocyanic veins and a longer vegetative phase.

The enhancement of sink strength to drive the accumulation of carotenoids in edible crops is a new and promising strategy that has been elaborated on the basis of the molecular characterization of the cauliflower *Or* mutant (Lu et al., 2006; Zhou et al., 2008). Recently, Lopez et al. (2008) have demonstrated that the ectopic and tuber-specific expression of the *Or* gene in potato induces the concomitant carotenoid accumulation (up to 6-fold) and chromoplasts development.

In order to modify the sink strength in tomato a particular strategy has been made by Simkin et al. (2007) through the ectopic expression of the pepper gene encoding the protein fibrillin. In this work transgenic tomato plants increased the fruit carotenoid content (up to 2-fold) without the development of fibrils in chromoplasts; on the contrary, the transformants showed an unusual type of transient plastids characterized by the retention of thylakoid structures.

The interesting option of engineering the carotenoid biosynthesis pathway of tomato fruits via plastid transformation has been successfully applied using the *LCY-b* gene from *Erwinia*. The methods required an efficient *in vitro* regeneration system from leaf explants and a particle gun approach. Transplastomic tomato plants harboring microbial carotenoid biosynthesis transgene showed a 4-fold enhanced pro-vitamin A content in the fruits. This strategy offers some advantages: absence of epigenetic gene inactivation by co-suppression, the possibility of transformation with multiple transgenes and the reduction of the risk of transgene dispersion in the environment (Wurbs et al., 2007). More recently, Apel and Bock (2009) have introduced the lycopene β-cyclase gene from *Narcissus pseudonarcissus* into the tomato plastid genome with significative modification of carotenoid profile both in leaves and fruits.

Conclusion

Carotenoid content and composition of edible crops depends on the regulation of biosynthesis, degradation and sequestration mechanisms. All of these aspects deserve specific attention and further data are necessary in the future to improve the selection efficiency of crops with better nutrient properties. In particular, about the regulation of carotenogenesis, only a few is known on the nature of promoter sequences of genes encoding enzymes while even less we know about transcription factors and their binding partners. The modification of carotenoid profile is influenced also by plastid development; therefore the identification of genetic factors correlated to the process of transformation from chloroplast to chromoplasts is useful. On the same time, the production of specific metabolic sink can be crucial to preclude the pigment degradation and to allow massive accumulation. Therefore, the identification of genetic control of this phenomenon has obvious value.

As demonstrated in tomato and cauliflower, the isolation and molecular characterization of mutants with altered carotenoid composition represents a very informative strategy to identify regulatory genes. In addition, for the main crops with carotenoids in the edible organs the mapping of main QTLs has direct and immediate application for the breeding while the modern techniques of transcriptome analysis will provide basic details on carotenogenic regulation.

References

Abbo, S., Molina, C., Jungmann, R., Grusak, M. A., Berkovitch, Z., Reifen, R., Kahl, G., Winter, P. & Reifen, R. (2005). Quantitative trait loci governing carotenoid concentration and weight in seeds of chickpea (*Cicer arietinum* L.). *Theoretical and Applied Genetics*, *111*, 185-195.

Adom, K. K., Sorrells, M. E. & Liu, R. H. (2003). Phytochemical profiles and antioxidant activity of wheat varieties. *Journal of Agricultural and Food Chemistry*, *51*, 7825-7834.

Ahn, T. K., Avenson, T. J., Ballottari, M., Cheng, Y. C., Niyogi, K. K., Bassi, R. & Fleming, G. R. (2008). Architecture of a charge-transfer state regulating light harvesting in plant antenna protein. *Science*, *320*, 794-797.

Akiyama, K., Matsuzaki, K. & Hayashi, H. (2005). Plant sesquiterpenes induce hyphal branching in arbuscular mycorrhizal fungi. *Nature*, *435*, 824-827.

Alba, R., Cordonnier-Pratt, M. M. & Pratt, L. H. (2000). Fruit-localized phytochromes regulate lycopene accumulation independently of ethylene production in tomato. *Plant Physiology*, *123*, 363-370.

Alba, R., Payton, P., Fei, Z., McQhuinn, R., Debbie, P., Martin, G. B., Tanksley, S. D. & Giovannoni, J. J. (2005). Transcriptome and selected metabolite analysis revealed multiple points of ethylene control during tomato fruit development. *The Plant Cell*, *17*, 2954-2965.

Albrecht, M. & Sandmann, G. (1994). Light-stimulated carotenoid biosynthesis during transformation of maize etioplasts is regulated by increases activity of isopentenyl pyrophosphate isomerase. *Plant Physiology*, *105*, 529-534.

Alquezar, B., Rodrigo, M. J. & Zacarías, L. (2008). Regulation of carotenoid biosynthesis during fruit maturation in the red-fleshed orange mutant Cara Cara. *Phytochemistry*, *69*, 1997-2007.

Aluru, M., Xu, Y., Guo, R., Wang, Z., Li, S., White, S., Wang, K. & Rodermel, S. (2008). Generation of transgenic maize with enhanced provitamin A content. *Journal of Experimental Botany*, *59*, 3551-3562.

Alvarez, J. B., Martín, L. M. & Martín, A. (1998). Chromosomal localization of genes for carotenoid pigments using addition lines of *Hordeum chilense* in wheat. *Plant Breeding*, *117*, 287-289.

Alvarez, J. B., Martín, L. M. & Martín, A. (1999). Genetic variation for carotenoid pigment content in the amphidiploid *Hordem chilense* × *Triticum turgidum* conv. *durum*. *Plant Breeding*, *118*, 187-189.

Alvarez, J. B., Urbano, J. M. & Martín, L. M. (1994). Effect on flour quality from inclusion of the *Hordeum chilense* genome into the genetic background of wheat. *Cereal Chemistry*, *71*, 517-519.

Anderson, J. M., Chow, W. S. & Park, Y. I. (1995). The grand design of photosynthesis: acclimation of the photosynthetic apparatus to environmental cues. *Photosynthesis Research*, *46*, 129-139.

Apel, W. & Bock, R. (2009). Enhancement of carotenoid biosynthesis in transplastomic tomatoes by induced lycopene-to-provitamin A conversion. *Plant Physiology*, doi: 10.1104/pp.109.140533

Atienza, S. G., Ballesteros, J., Martín, A. & Hornero-Méndez, D. (2007). Genetic variability of carotenoid concentration and degree of esterification among tritordeum (*Tritordeum* Ascherson et Graebner) and durum wheat accessions. *Journal of Agricultural and Food Chemistry*, *55*, 4244-4251.

Atienza, S. G., Martín, A., Pecchioni, N., Plantani, C. & Cattivelli, L. (2008). The nuclear-cytoplasmic interaction controls carotenoid content in wheat. *Euphytica*, *159*, 325-331.

Atienza, S. G., Ramírez, M. C., Hernández, P. & Martín, A. (2004). Chromosomal location of genes for carotenoid pigments in *Hordeum chilense*. *Plant Breeding*, *123*, 303-304.

Auldridge, M. E., McCarty, D. R. & Klee, H. J. (2006). Plant carotenoid cleavage oxygenases and their apocarotenoid products. *Current Opinion in Plant Biology*, *9*, 315-321.

Avenson, T. J., Ahn, T. K., Zigmantas, D., Niyogi, K. K., Li, Z., Ballottari, M., Bassi, R. & Fleming, G. R. (2008). Zeaxanthin radical cation formation in minor light-harvesting complexes of higher plant antenna. *Journal of Biological Chemistry*, *283*, 3550-3558.

Bailey, J. S. & French, A. P. (1949). The inheritance of certain fruit and foliage characters in the peach. *Massachusetts Agricultural Experiment Bulletin, No. 452.*

Bang, H., Kim, S., Leskovar, D. & King, S. (2007). Development of a codominant CAPS marker for allelic selection between canary yellow and red watermelon based on SNP in lycopene β-cyclase (*LCYB*) gene. *Molecular Breeding, 20*, 63-72.

Bangalore, D. V., McGlynn, W. G. & Scott, D. D. (2008). Effects of fruit maturity on watermelon ultrastructure and intercellular lycopene distribution. *Journal of Food Science, 73*, S222-S228.

Baranska, M., Baranski, R., Schultz, H. & Nothnagel, T. (2006). Tissue-specific accumulation of carotenoids in carrot roots. *Planta, 224*, 1028-1037.

Bartley, G. E. & Scolnik, P. A. (1995). Plant carotenoids: pigments for photoprotection, visual attraction, and human health. *The Plant Cell, 7*, 1027-1038.

Baroli, I. & Niyogi, K. K. (2000). Molecular genetics of xanthophylls-dependent photoprotection in green algae and plants. *Philosophical Transactions of the Royal Society B, Biological Sciences, 355*, 1385-1394.

Barr, J., White, W. S., Chen, L., Bae, H. & Rodermel, S. (2004). The GHOST terminal oxidase regulates developmental programming in tomato fruit. *Plant, Cell & Environment, 27*, 840-852.

Barry, C. S., McQuinn, R. P., Thompson, A. J., Seymour, G. B., Grierson, D. & Giovannoni, J. J. (2005). Ethylene insensitivity conferred by the *Green-ripe* and *Never-ripe 2* ripening mutants of tomato. *Plant Physiology, 138*, 267-275.

Ben-Shaul, Y. & Klein, S. (1965). Development and structure of carotene bodies in carrot roots. *Botanical Gazette, 126*, 79-85.

Bernacchi, D., Beck-Bunn, T., Eshed, Y., Lopez, J., Petiard, V., Uhlig, J., Zamir, D. & Tanksley, S. (1998). Advanced backcross QTL analysis in tomato. I. Identification of QTL for traits of agronomic importance from *Lycopersicon hirsutum*. *Theoretical and Applied Genetics, 97*, 381-397.

Blomhoff, R. & Blomhoff, H. K. (2006). Overview of retinoid metabolism and function. *Journal of Neurobiology, 66*, 606-630.

Blomhoff, R., Green, M. H. & Norum, K. R. (1992). VITAMIN A: Physiological and biochemical processing. *Annual Review of Nutrition, 12*, 37-57.

Blount, J. D. & McGraw K. J. (2008). Signal functions of carotenoid colouration. In: G. Britton, S. Liaan-Jensen & H. Pfander, (Eds.). *Carotenoids* (Vol. *4* Natural Functions, pp. 213-236). Basel: Birkhäuser Ltd.

Blount, J. D., Metcalfe, N. B., Birkhead, T. R. & Surai, P. F. (2003). Carotenoid modulation of immune function and sexual attractiveness in zebra finches. *Science, 300*, 125-127.

Bone, R. A., Landrum, J. T., Fernandez, L. & Tarsis, S. L. (1988). Analysis of the macular pigment by HPLC: retinal distribution and age study. *Investigative Ophthalmology & Visual Science, 29*, 843-849.

Bonierbale, M. W., Plaisted, R. L. & Tanksley, S. D. (1988). RFLP maps based on a common set clones reveal modes of chromosomal evolution in potato and tomato. *Genetics, 120*, 1095-1103.

Botella-Pavía, P. & Rodríguez-Concepción, M. (2006). Carotenoid biotechnology in plants for nutritionally improved foods. *Physiologia Plantarum, 126*, 369-381.

Bouvier, F., Backhaus, R. A. & Camara, B. (1998). Induction and control of chromoplasts-specific carotenoid genes by oxidative stress. *Journal of Biological Chemistry, 273*, 30651-30659.

Bouvier, F., Dogbo, O. & Camara, B. (2003a). Biosynthesis of the food and cosmetic plant pigment bixin (annatto). *Science, 300*, 2089-2091.

Bouvier, F., Hungueney, P., d'Harlingue, A., Kuntz, M. & Camara, B. (1994). Xanthophyll biosynthesis in chromoplasts: isolation and molecular cloning of an enzyme catalyzing the conversion of 5,6-epoxycarotenoid into ketocarotenoid. *The Plant Journal, 6*, 45-54.

Bouvier, F., Isner, J. C., Dogbo, O. & Camara, B. (2005a). Oxidative tailoring of carotenoids: a prospect towards novel functions in plants. *Trends in Plant Science, 10*, 187-194.

Bouvier, F., Rahier, A. & Camara, B. (2005b). Biogenesis, molecular regulation and function of plant isoprenoids. *Progress in Lipid Research, 44*, 357-429.

Bouvier, F., Suire, C., Mutterer, J. & Camara, B. (2003b). Oxidative remodeling of chromoplast carotenoids: identification of the carotenoid dioxygenase *CsCCD* and *CsZCD* genes involved in Crocus secondary metabolite biogenesis. *The Plant Cell, 15*, 47-62.

Boyle, T. H. & Stimart, D. P. (1988). Inheritance of ray floret color in *Zinnia angustifolia* HBK and *Z. elegans* Jacq. *The Journal of Heredity, 79*, 289-293.

Bradeen, J. M. & Simon, P. W. (1998). Conversion of an AFLP fragment linked to the carrot Y_2 locus to a simple, codominant, PCR-based marker form. *Theoretical and Applied Genetics, 97*, 960-967.

Bramley, P. (1997). The regulation of genetic manipulation of carotenoid biosynthesis in tomato fruit. *Pure and Applied Chemistry, 69*, 2159-2162.

Brandi, F., Bar, E., Mourgues, F., Liverani, A., Giuliano, G., Lewinsohn, E. & Rosati, C. (2008). Regulation of carotenoid gene expression and volatile compound emission in white- and yellow-fleshed peach genotypes. *Proceedings of the 52nd Italian Society of Agricultural Genetics Annual Congress* Padova, Italy – 14/17 September, 2008; ISBN 978-88-900622-8-5.

Britton, G. (1995). Structure and properties of carotenoids in relation to function. *The FASEB Journal, 9*, 1551-1558.

Britton, G. (2008). Functions of intact carotenoids. In: G. Britton, S. Liaan-Jensen & H. Pfander, (Eds.). *Carotenoids* (Vol. *4* Natural Functions, pp. 189-212). Basel: Birkhäuser Ltd.

Brooks, J. & Shaw, G. (1968). Chemical structure of the exine of pollen walls a new function for carotenoids in nature. *Nature, 219*, 523-524.

Brown, C. R., Culley, D., Bonierbale, M. & Amorós, W. (2007). Anthocyanin, carotenoid content, and antioxidant values in native South American potato cultivars. *HortScience, 42*, 1733-1736.

Brown, C. R., Edwards, C. G., Yang, C. P. & Dean, B. B. (1993). Orange flesh trait in potato: inheritance and carotenoid content. *Journal of the American Society of Horticultural Science, 118*, 145-150.

Brown, C. R., Kim, T. S., Ganga, Z., Haynes, K., De Jong, D., Jahn, M., Paran, I., De Jong, W. (2006). Segregation of total carotenoid in high level potato germplasm and its relationship to beta-carotene hydroxylase polymorphism. *American Journal of Potato Research, 83*, 365-372.

Buishand, J. G. & Gabelman, W. H. (1979). Investigations on the inheritance of color and carotenoid content in phloem and xylem of carrot roots (*Daucus carota* L.). *Euphytica, 28*, 611-632.

Castillo, R., Fernández, J. A. & Gómez-Gómez, L. (2005). Implications of carotenoid biosynthetic genes in apocarotenoid formation during the stigma development of *Crocus sativus* and its closer derivates. *Plant Physiology*, *139*, 674-689.

Cazzonelli, C. I., Cuttriss, A. J., Cossetto S. B., Pye, W., Crisp, P., Whelan, J., Finnegan, E. J., Turnbull, C. & Pogson, B. J. (2009). Regulation of carotenoid composition and shoot branching in Arabidopsis by chromatin modyfying histone methyltransferase, SDG8. *The Plant Cell*, *21*, 39-53.

Cerullo, G., Polli, D., Lanzani, G., De Silvestri, S., Hashimoto, H. & Cogdell, R. J. (2002). Photosynthetic light harvesting by carotenoids: detection of an intermediate excited state. *Science*, *298*, 2395-2398.

Chappell, J. (1995). Biochemistry and molecular biology of the isoprenoid biosynthetic pathway in plants. *Annual Review of Plant Physiology and Plant Molecular Biology*, *46*, 521-547.

Chawla, A., Repa, J. J., Evans, R. M. & Mangelsdorf, D. J. (2001). Nuclear receptors and lipid physiology: opening the X files. *Science*, *294*, 1866-1870.

Chen, F. Q., Foolad, M. R., Hyman, J., St. Clair, D. A. & Beelaman, R. B. (1999). Mapping of QTLs for lycopene and other fruit traits in a *Lycopersicon esculentum* × *L. pimpinellifolium* cross and comparison of QTLs across tomato species. *Molecular Breeding*, *5*, 283-299.

Clotault, J., Peltier, D., Berruyer, R., Thomas, M., Briard, M. & Geoffriau, E. (2008). Expression of carotenoid biosynthesis during carrot root development. *Journal of Experimental Botany*, *59*, 3563-3573.

Connors, C. H. (1920). Some notes on the inheritance of unit characters in the peach. *Proceedings of the American Society for Horticultural Science*, *16*, 24-36.

Conti, A., Pancaldi, S., Fambrini, M., Michelotti, V., Bonora, A., Salvini, M. & Pugliesi, C. (2004). A deficiency at the gene coding for ζ-carotene desaturase characterizes the sunflower *non dormant-1* mutant. *Plant & Cell Physiology*, *45*, 445-455.

Cookson, P. J., Kiano, J. W., Shipton, C. A., Fraser, P. D., Romer, S., Schuch, W., Bramley, P. M. & Pyke, K. A. (2003). Increases in cell elongation, plastid compartment size and phytoene synthase activity underlie the phenotype of the *high pigment-1* mutant of tomato. *Planta*, *217*, 896-903.

Corona, V., Aracri, B., Kosturkova, G., Bartley, G. E., Pitto, L., Giorgetti, L., Scolnik, P. A. & Giuliano, G. (1996). Regulation of a carotenoid biosynthesis gene promoter during plant development. *The Plant Journal*, *9*, 505-512.

Croce, R., Weiss, S. & Bassi, R. (1999). Carotenoid-binding sites of the major light-harvesting complex II of higher plants. *Journal of Biological Chemistry*, *274*, 29613-29623.

Cuevas, H. E., Staub, J. E., Simon, P. W. & Zalapa, J. E. (2009). A consensus linkage map identifies genomic regions controlling fruit maturity and beta-carotene-associated flesh color in melo (*Cucumis melo* L.). *Theoretical and Applied Genetics*, doi: 10.1007/s00122-009-1085-3.

Cuevas, H. E., Staub, J. E., Simon, P. W., Zalapa, J. E. & Mc Creight, J. E. (2008). Mapping of genetic loci that regulate quantity of beta-carotene in fruit of US Wester Shipping melon (*Cucumis melo* L.). *Theoretical and Applied Genetics*, *117*, 1345-1359.

Cunningham, Jr. F. X. & Gantt, E. (1998). Genes and enzymes of carotenoid biosynthesis in plants. *Annual Review of Plant Physiology and Plant Molecular Biology*, *49*, 557-583.

Cunningham, Jr F. X. (2002). Regulation of carotenoid synthesis and accumulation in plants. *Pure and Applied Chemistry*, *74*, 1409-1417.

Curl, A. L. (1960). The carotenoids of apricots. *Journal of Food Science*, *25*, 190-196.

Cuttriss, A. J., Chubb, A. C., Alawady, A., Grimm, B. & Pogson, B. J. (2007). Regulation of lutein biosynthesis and prolamellar body formation in *Arabidopsis*. *Functional Plant Biology*, *34*, 663-672.

Davuluri, G. R., van Tuinen, A., Fraser, P. D., Manfredonia, A., Newman, R., Burgess, D., Brummell, D. A., King, S. R., Palys, J., Uhlig, J., Bramley, P. M., Pennings, H. M. J. & Bowler, C. (2005). Fruit-specific RNAi-mediated suppression of *DET1* enhances carotenoid and flavonoid content in tomato. *Nature Biotechnology*, *23*, 890-895.

de Araújo, M. L., Maluf, W. R., Gomes, L. A. A. & Oliveira, A. C. B. (2002). Intra and interlocus interactions between *alcobaça* (*alc*), *crimson* (*og^c*), and *high pigment* (*hp*) loci in tomato *Lycopersicum esculentum* Mill. *Euphytica*, *125*, 215-226.

Deli, J., Molnar, P., Pfander, H. & Tóth, G. (2000). Isolation of capsanthin 5,6-epoxide from *Lilium tigrinum*. *Acta Botanica Hungarica*, *42*, 105-110.

DellaPenna, D. & Pogson, B. J. (2006). Vitamin synthesis in plants: tocopherols and carotenoids. *Annual Review of Plant Biology*, *57*, 711-738.

DellaPenna, D. (1999). Nutritional Genomics: Manipulating plant micronutrients to improve human health. *Science*, *285*, 375-379.

Demmig-Adams, B. & Adams III, W. W. (1996). The role of xanthophyll cycle carotenoids in the protection of photosynthesis. *Trends in Plant Science*, *1*, 21-26.

Deruère, J., Römer, S., d'Harlingue, A., Backhaus, R. A., Kuntz, M. & Camara, B. (1994). Fibril assembly and carotenoid overaccumulation: a model for superamolecular lipoprotein structures. *The Plant Cell*, *6*, 119-133.

Dharmapuri, S., Rosati, C., Pallara, P., Aquilani, R., Bouvier, F., Camara, B. & Giuliano, G. (2002). Metabolic engineering of xanthophyll content in tomato fruits. *FEBS Letters*, *519*, 30-34.

Diretto, G., Welsch, R., Tavazza, R., Mourgues, F., Pizzichini, D., Beyer, P. & Giuliano, G. (2007). Silencing of beta-carotene hydroxylase increases total carotenoid and beta-carotene content. *BMC Plant Biology 7*, *11*, doi:10.1186/1471-2229/7/11.

Dorais, M., Ehret, D. L. & Papadopoulos, A. P. (2008). Tomato (*Solanum lycopersicum*) health components from the seed to the consumer. *Phytochemistry Reviews*, *7*, 231-250.

Dragovic-Uzelac, V., Levaj, B., Mrkic, V., Bursac, D., & Boras, M. (2007). The content of polyphenols and carotenoids in three apricot cultivars depending on stage of maturity and geographical region. *Food Chemistry*, *102*, 966-975.

Ducreux, L. J., Morris, W. L., Hedley, P. E., Shepherd, T., Davies, H. V., Millam, S. & Taylor, M. A. (2005). Metabolic engineering of high carotenoid potato tubers containing enhanced levels of β-carotene and lutein. *Journal of Experimental Botany*, *56*, 81-89.

Dumas, Y., Dadomo, M., Di Lucca, G. & Grolier, P. (2003). Effects of environmental factors and agricultural techniques on antioxidant content of tomatoes. *Journal of the Science of Food and Agriculture*, *83*, 369-382.

Edge, R., McGarvey, D. J. & Truscott, T. G. (1997). The carotenoids as anti-oxidants: a review. *Journal of Photochemistry and Photobiology B: Biology*, *41*, 189-200.

Eduardo, I., Arus, P. & Monforte, A. J. (2007). Estimating the genetic architecture of fruit quality traits in melon using a genomic library of near isogenic lines. *Journal of the American Society for Horticultural Science*, *132*, 80-89.

Egesel, C. O., Wong, J. C., Lambert, R. J. & Rocheford, T. R. (2003). Combining ability of maize inbreds for carotenoids and tocopherols. *Crop Science*, *43*, 818-823.

Ellis, R. J. (1984). Chloroplast biogenesis. Cambridge, UK: Cambridge University Press.

Elouafi, I., Nachit, M. M. & Martin, L. M. (2001). Identification of a microsatellite on chromosome 7B showing a strong linkage with yellow pigment in durum wheat (*Triticum turgidum* L. var. *durum*). *Hereditas*, *135*, 255-261.

Fambrini, M., Castagna, A., Dalla Vecchia, F., Degl'Innocenti, E., Ranieri, A., Vernieri, P., Pardossi, A., Guidi, L., Rascio, N. & Pugliesi, C. (2004). Characterization of a pigment-deficient mutant of sunflower (*Helianthus annuus* L.) with abnormal chloroplast biogenesis, reduced PS II activity and low endogenous level of abscisic acid. *Plant Science*, *167*, 79-89.

Fambrini, M., Michelotti V. & Pugliesi, C. (2009). Orange, yellow and white-cream: inheritance of carotenoid-based color in sunflower pollen. *Plant Biology*, doi: 10.1111/j.1438-8677.2009.00205.x.

Fambrini, M., Pugliesi, C., Vernieri, P., Giuliano, G. & Baroncelli, S. (1993). Characterization of a sunflower (*Helianthus annuus* L.) mutant deficient in carotenoid synthesis and abscisic-acid content induced by in vitro tissue culture. *Theoretical and Applied Genetics*, *87*, 65-69.

Fambrini, M., Salvini, M., Conti, A., Michelotti, V. & Pugliesi, C. (2004). Expression of the ζ-carotene desaturase gene in sunflower. *Plant Biosystems*, *138*, 203-206.

Fanciullino, A.- L., Cercós, M., Dhuique-Mayer, C., Froelicher, Y., Talón, M., Ollitrault, P. & Morillon R. (2008). Changes in carotenoid content and biosynthetic gene expression in juice sacs of four orange varieties (*Citrus sinensis*) differing in flesh friut color. *Journal of Agricultural and Food Chemistry*, *56*, 3628-3638.

Fanciullino, A.- L., Dhuique-Mayer, C., Luro, F., Casanova, J., Morillon, R. & Ollitrault, P. (2006). Carotenoid diversity in cultivated citrus is highly influenced by genetic factors. *Journal of Agricultural and Food Chemistry*, *54*, 4397-4406.

Fang, J., Chai, C., Qian, Q., Li, C., Tang J., Sun L., Huang, Z., Guo, X., Sun, C., Liu, M., Zhang, Y., Lu, Q., Wang, Y., Lu, C., Han, B., Chen, F., Cheng, Z. & Chu, C. (2008). Mutations of genes in synthesis of the carotenoid precursors of ABA lead to pre-harvest sprouting and photo-oxidation in rice. *The Plant Journal*, *54*, 177-189.

Farin, D., Ikan, R. & Gross, J. (1983). The carotenoid pigments in the juice and flavedo of mandarin hybrid (*Citrus reticulata* cv. Michal) during ripening. *Phytochemistry*, *22*, 403-408.

Fick, G. N. (1976). Genetics of floral color and morphology in sunflower. *The Journal of Heredity*, *67*, 227-230.

Frank, H. A. & Cogdell, R. J. (1996). Carotenoids in photosynthesis. *Photochemistry and Photobiology*, *63*, 257-264.

Fraser, P. D. & Bramley, P. M. (2004). The biosynthesis and nutritional uses of carotenoids. *Progress in Lipid Research*, *43*, 228-265.

Fraser, P. D., Bramley, P. & Seymour, G. B. (2001). Effect of *Cnr* mutation on carotenoid formation during tomato fruit ripening. *Phytochemistry*, *58*, 75-79.

Fraser, P. D., Enfissi, E. A. M. & Bramley, P. (2009). Genetic engineering of carotenoid formation in tomato fruit and the potential application of systems and synthetic biology approaches. *Archives of Biochemistry and Biophysics*, *483*, 196-204.

Fraser, P. D., Enfissi, E. A. M., Halket, J. M., Truesdale, M. R., Yu, D., Gerrish, C. & Bramley, P. M. (2007). Manipulation of phytoene levels in tomato fruit: effects on isoprenoids, plastids, and intermediary metabolism. *The Plant Cell, 19*, 3194-3211.

Fraser, P. D., Römer, S., Shipton, C. A., Mills, P. B., Kiano, J. W., Misawa, N., Drake, R. G., Schuch, W. & Bramley, P. M. (2002). Evaluation of transgenic tomato plants expressing an additional phytoene synthase in a fruit-specific manner. *Proceedings of the National Academy of Sciences of the USA, 99*, 1092-1097.

Fraser, P. D., Truesdale, M. R., Bird, C. R., Schuch, W. & Bramley, P. M. (1994). Carotenoid biosynthesis during tomato fruit development. *Plant Physiology, 105*, 405-413.

Fray, R. G. & Grierson, D. (1993). Identification and genetic analysis of normal and mutant phytoene synthase genes of tomato by sequencing, complementation and co-suppression. *Plant Molecular Biology, 22*, 589-602.

Frosch, S. & Mohr, H. (1980). Analysis of light-controlled accumulation of carotenoids in mustard (*Sinapis alba* L.). *Planta, 148*, 279-286.

Fulton, T. M., Beck-Bunn, T., Emmatty, D., Eshed, Y., Lopez, J., Uhlig, J., Zamir, D. & Tanksley, S. D. (1997). QTL analysis of an advanced backcross of *Lycopersicon peruvianum* to the cultivated tomato and comparison of QTLs found in other wild species. *Theoretical and Applied Genetics, 95*, 881-894.

Fulton, T. M., Grandillo, S., Beck-Bunn, T., Fridman, E., Frampton, A., Lopez, J., Petiard, V., Uhlig, J., Zamir, D. & Tanksley, S. D. (2000). Advanced backcross analysis of *Lycopersicon esculentum* × *L. parviflorum* cross. *Theoretical and Applied Genetics, 100*, 1025-1042.

Fuhrman, B., Elis, A. & Aviram, M. (1997). Hypocholesterolemic effect of lycopene and β-carotene is related to suppression of cholesterol synthesis and augmentation of LDL receptor activity in macrophages. *Biochemical and Biophysical Research Communications, 233*, 658-662.

Gabelman, W. H. & Peters, S. (1979). Genetical and plant breeding possibilities for improving the quality of vegetables. *Acta Horticulturae, 93*, 243-259.

Gallagher, C. E., Matthews, P. D., Li, F. & Wurtzel, E. T. (2004). Gene duplication in the carotenoid biosynthetic pathway preceded evolution of the grasses. *Plant Physiology, 135*, 1776-1783.

Galpaz, N., Ronen, G., Khalfa, Z., Zamir, D. & Hirschberg, J. (2006). A chromoplast-specific carotenoid biosynthesis pathway is revealed by cloning of the tomato *white-flower* locus. *The Plant Cell, 18*, 1947-1960.

Galpaz, N., Wang, Q., Menda, N., Zamir, D. & Hirschberg, J. (2008). Abscisic acid deficiency in the tomato *high-pigment 3* leading to increased plastid number and higher fruit lycopene content. *The Plant Journal, 53*, 717-730.

Gautier, H., Rocci, A., Buret, M., Grasselly, D., Dumas, Y. & Causse, M. (2004). Effect of photoselective filters on the physical and chemical traits of vine-ripened tomato fruits. *Canadian Journal of Plant Science, 85*, 1009-1016.

Gil, M. I., Tomás-Barberán, F. A., Hess-Pierce, B. & Kader, A. A. (2002). Antioxidant capacities, phenolic compounds, carotenoids, and vitamin C contents of nectarine, peach, and plum cultivars from California. *Journal of Agricultural and Food Chemistry, 50*, 4976-4982.

Giliberto, L., Perrotta, G., Pallara, P., Weller, J. L., Fraser, P. D., Bramley, P. M., Fiore, A., Tavazza, M. & Giuliano, G. (2005). Manipulation of the blue light photoreceptor cryptochrome 2 in tomato affects vegetative development, flowering time, and fruit antioxidant content. *Plant Physiology, 137,* 199-208.

Gillaspy, G., Ben-David, H. & Gruissem, W. (1993). Fruits: a developmental perspective. *The Plant Cell, 5,* 1439-1451.

Giuliano, G., Al-Babili, S. & von Lintig, J. (2003). Carotenoid oxygenases: cleave it or leave it. *Trends in Plant Science, 8,* 145-149.

Giuliano, G., Giliberto, L. & Rosati, C. (2002). Carotenoid isomerase: a tale of light and isomers. *Trends in Plant Science, 7,* 427-429.

Giuliano, G., Tavazza, R., Diretto, G., Beyer, P. & Taylor, M. A. (2008). Metabolic engineering of carotenoid biosynthesis in plants. *Trends in Biotechnology, 26,* 139-145.

Grotewold, E. (2006). The genetics and biochemistry of floral pigments. *Annual Review of Plant Biology, 57,* 761-780.

Grumbach, K. H. & Lichtenthaler, H. K. (1982). Chloroplast pigments and their biosynthesis in relation to light intensity. *Photochemistry and Photobiology, 35,* 209-212.

Ha, S. H., Kim, J. B., Park, J. S., Lee, S. W. & Cho, K. J. (2007). A comparison of carotenoid accumulation in *Capsicum* varieties that show different ripening colours: deletion of the capsanthin-capsorubin synthase is not a prerequisite for the formation of a yellow pepper. *Journal of Experimental Botany, 58,* 3153-3144.

Hable, W. E., Oishi, K. K. & Schumaker, K. S. (1998). *Viviparous-5* encodes phytoene desaturase, an enzyme essential for abscisic acid (ABA) accumulation and seed development in maize. *Molecular and General Genetics, 257,* 167-176.

Harjes, C. E., Rocheford, T. R., Bai, L., Brutnell, T. P., Bermundez Kandianis, C., Sowinski, S. G., Stapleton, A. E., Vallabhanemi, R., Williams, M., Wurtzel, E. T., Yan, J. & Buckler, E. S. (2008). Natural genetic variation in *lycopene epsilon cyclase* tapped for maize biofortification. *Science, 319,* 330-333.

Härtel, H. & Grimm, B. (1998). Consequences of chlorophyll deficiency for leaf carotenoid composition in tobacco synthesizing glutamate 1-semialdehyde aminotransferase antisense RNA: dependency on development age and growth light. *Journal of Experimental Botany, 49,* 535-546.

Hashizume, T., Shimamoto, I. & Hirai, M. (2003). Construction of a linkage map and QTL analysis of horticultural traits for watermelon [*Citrullus lanatus* (THUNB.) MATSUM & NAKAI] using RAPD, RFLP and ISSR markers. *Theoretical and Applied Genetics, 106,* 779-785.

Hashizume, T., Shimamoto, I., Harushima, Y., Yui, M., Sato, T., Imai, T. & Hirai, M. (1996). Construction of a linkage map for watermelon (*Citrullus lanatus*) using random amplified polymorphic DNA (RAPD). *Euphytica, 90,* 265-273.

He, H. Y., Zhang, Y. L., He, Z. H., Wu, Y. P., Xiao, Y. G., Ma, C. X. & Xia, X. C. (2008). Characterization of phytoene synthase 1 gene (*Psy1*) located on common wheat chromosome 7A and development of a functional marker. *Theoretical and Applied Genetics, 116,* 213-221.

Heber, D. & Lu, Q. Y. (2002). Overview of mechanisms of action of lycopene. *Experimental Biology and Medicine, 227,* 920-923.

Henderson, W. R., Scott, G. H. & Wehner, T. C. (1998). Interaction of flesh color genes in watermelon. *The Journal of Heredity, 89,* 50-53.

Hessler, T. G., Thomson, M. J., Benscher, D., Nachit, M. M., Sorrells, M. E. (2002). Association of a lipoxygenase locus, *Lpx-B1*, with variation in lipoxygenase activity in durum wheat seeds. *Crop Science*, *42*, 1695-1700.

Hidalgo, A., Brandolini, A., Pompei, C. & Piscozzi, R. (2006). Carotenoids and tocols of einkorn wheat (*Triticum monococcum* ssp *monococcum* L.). *Journal of Cereal Science*, *44*, 182-193.

Himeno, H. & Sano K. (1987). Synthesis of crocin, picrocrocin and safranal by saffron stigma-like structures proliferated *in vitro*. *Agricultural and Biological Chemistry*, 51, 2395-2400.

Hirschberg, J. (2001). Carotenoid biosynthesis in flowering plants. *Current Opinion in Plant Biology*, *4*, 210-218.

Holden, J. M., Eldridge, A. L., Beecher, G. R., Buzzard, I. M., Bhagwat, S., Davis, C. S., Douglass, L. W., Gebhardt, S., Haytowitz, D. & Schakel, S. (1999). Carotenoid content of U.S. foods: an update of the database. *Journal of Food Composition and Analysis*, *12*, 169-196.

Holt, N. E., Zigmantas, D., Valkunas, L., Li, X.- P., Niyogi, K. K. & Fleming, G. R. (2005). Carotenoid cation formation and regulation of photosynthetic light harvesting. *Science*, *307*, 433-436.

Horner, H. T., Healy, R. A., Ren, G., Fritz, D., Klyne, A., Seames, C. & Thornburg, R. W. (2007). Amyloplast to chromoplast conversion in developing ornamental tobacco floral nectaries provides sugar for nectar and antioxidants for protection. *American Journal of Botany*, *94*, 12-24.

Hornero-Méndez, D., Costa-García, J. & Mínguez-Mosquera, M. I. (2002). Characterization of carotenoid high-producing *Capsicum annuum* cultivars selected for paprika production. *Journal of Agriculture and Food Chemistry*, *50*, 5711-5716.

Hornero-Méndez, D., Gómez-Landrón de Guevara, R. & Mínguez-Mosquera, M. I. (2000). Carotenoid biosynthesis changes in five red pepper (*Capsicum annuum* L.) cultivars during ripening. Cultivar selection for breeding. *Journal of Agricultural and Food Chemistry*, *48*, 3857-3864.

Howitt, C. A. & Pogson, B. J. (2006). Carotenoid accumulation and function in seeds and non-green tissues. *Plant, Cell & Environment*, *29*, 435-445.

Hsieh, K. & Huang, A. H. C. (2007). Tapetosomes in *Brassica* tapetum accumulate endoplasmic reticulum-derived flavonoids and alkanes for delivery to pollen surface. *The Plant Cell*, *19*, 582-596.

Hughes, D. A. (2000). Dietary antioxidants and human immune function. *Nutrition Bulletin*, *25*, 35-41.

Huh, J. H., Kang, B. C., Nahm, S. H., Kim, S., Ha, K. S., Lee, M. H. & Kim, B. D. (2001). A candidate gene approach identified phytoene synthase as the locus for mature fruit color in red pepper (*Capsicum* spp.). *Theoretical and Applied Genetics*, *102*, 524-530.

Hurtado-Hernandez, H. & Smith, P. (1985). Inheritance of mature fruit color in *Capsicum annuum* L. *The Journal of Heredity*, *76*, 211-213.

Ibdah, M., Azulay, Y., Portnoy, V., Wasserman, B., Bar, E., Meir, A., Burger, Y., Hirschberg, J., Schaffer, A. A., Katzir, N., Tadmor, Y. & Lewinsohn, E. (2006). Functional characterization of *CmCCD1*, a carotenoid cleavage dioxygenase from melon. *Phytochemistry*, *67*, 1579-1589.

Iglesias, C., Mayer, J., Chavez, L. & Calle, F. (1997). Genetic potential and stability of carotene content in cassava roots. *Euphytica*, *94*, 367-373.

Ikoma, Y., Komatsu, A., Kita, M., Ogawa, K., Omura, M., Yano, M. & Moriguchi, T. (2001). Expression of a phytoene synthase gene and characteristic carotenoid accumulation during citrus fruit development. *Physiologia Plantarum*, *111*, 232-238.

Isaacson, T., Ohad, I., Beyer, P. & Hirschberg, J. (2004). Analysis in vitro of the enzyme CRTISO establishes a poly-cis-carotenoid biosynthesis pathway in plants. *Plant Physiology*, *136*, 4246-4255.

Isaacson, T., Ronen, G., Zamir, D. & Hirschberg, J. (2002). Cloning of *tangerine* from tomato reveals a carotenoid isomerase essential for production of carotene and xanthophylls in plants. *The Plant Cell*, *14*, 333-342.

Jensen, P. E., Bassi, R., Boekema, E. J., Dekker, J. P., Jansson, S., Leister, D., Robinson, C. & Scheller, H. V. (2007). Structure, function and regulation of plant photosystem I. *Biochimica et Biophysica Acta – Bioenergetics*, *1767*, 335-352.

Josse, E. M., Simkin, A. J., Gaffé, J., Labouré, A. M., Kuntz, M. & Carol, P. (2000). A plastid terminal oxidase associated with carotenoid desaturation during chromoplast differentation. *Plant Physiology*, *123*, 1427-1436.

Just, B. J, Santos, C. A. F., Fonseca, M. E. N., Boiteux, L. S., Oloizia, B. B. & Simon, P. W. (2007). Carotenoid biosynthesis structural genes in carrot (*Daucus carota*): isolation, sequence-characterization, single nucleotide polymorphism (SNP) markers and genome mapping. *Theoretical and Applied Genetics*, *114*, 693-704.

Karas, M., Amir, H., Fishman, D., Danilenko, M., Segal, S., Nahum, A., Koifmann, A., Giat, Y., Levy, J. & Sharoni, Y. (2000). Lycopene interferes with cell cycle progression and insulin-like growth factor I signaling in mammary cancer cells. *Nutrition and Cancer*, *36*, 101-111.

Kato, M., Ikoma, Y., Matsumoto, H., Sugiura, M., Hyodo, H. & Yano, M. (2004). Accumulation of carotenoids and expression of carotenoid biosynthetic genes during maturation in citrus fruit. *Plant Physiology*, *134*, 824-837.

Kato, M., Matsumoto, H., Ikoma, Y., Okuda, H. & Yano, M. (2006). The role of carotenoid cleavage dioxygenases in the regulation of carotenoid profiles during maturation in citrus fruit. *Journal of Experimental Botany*, *57*, 2153-2164.

Kean, E. G., Hamaker, B. R. & Ferruzzi, M. G. (2008). Carotenoid bioaccessibility from whole grain and degermed maize meal products. *Journal of Agricultural and Food Chemistry*, *56*, 9918-9926.

Khachik, F., Steck, A. & Pfander, H. (1999). Isolation and structural elucidation of (13Z, 13'Z, 3R, 3'R, 6'R)-lutein from marigold flowers, kale, and human plasma. *Journal of Agricultural and Food Chemistry*, *47*, 455-461.

Kim, H. U., Wu, S. S. H., Ratnayake, C. & Huang, A. H. C. (2001a). *Brassica rapa* has three genes that encode proteins associated with different neutral lipids in plastids of specific tissues. *Plant Physiology*, *126*, 330-341.

Kim, I. J., Ko, K. C., Kim, C. S. & Chung, W. I. (2001b). Isolation and characterization of cDNAs encoding β-carotene hydroxylase in *Citrus*. *Plant Science*, *161*, 1005-1010.

Kishimoto, S., Maoka, T., Nakayama, M. & Ohmiya, A. (2004). Carotenoid composition in petals of chrysanthemum (*Dendranthema grandiflorum* (ramat.) Kitamura). *Phytochemistry*, *65*, 2781-2787.

Kishimoto, S. & Ohmiya, A. (2006). Regulation of carotenoid biosynthesis in petals and leaves of chrysanthemum (*Chrysanthemum morifolium*). *Physiologia Plantarum*, *128*, 436-447.

Kita, M., Kato, M., Ban, Y., Honda, C., Yaegaki, H., Ikoma, Y. & Moriguchi, T. (2007). Carotenoid accumulation in Japanese apricot (*Prunus mume* Siebold & Zucc.): molecular analysis of carotenogenic gene expression and ethylene regulation. *Journal of Agriculture and Food Chemistry*, *55*, 3414-3420.

Kita, M., Komatsu, A., Omura, M., Yano, M., Ikoma, Y. & Moriguchi, T. (2001). Cloning and expression of CitPDS1, a gene encoding phytoene desaturase in *Citrus*. *Bioscience, Biotechnology, and Biochemistry*, *65*, 1424-1428.

Kobayashi, A., Ohara-Takada, A., Tsuda S., Matsuura-Endo, C., Takada, N., Umemura, Y., Nakao, T., Yoshida, T., Hayashi, K. & Mori, M. (2008). Breeding of potato variety "Inca-no-hitomi" with a very high carotenoid content. *Breeding Science*, *58*, 77-82.

Kopsell, D. E., Kopsell, D. A., Randle, W. M., Coolong, T. W., Sams, C. E. & Curran-Celentano, J. (2003). Kale carotenoids remain stable while flavor compounds respond to changes in sulfur fertility. *Journal of Agricultural and Food Chemistry*, *51*, 5319-5325.

Kotiková, Z., Hejtmánková, A., Lachman, J., Hamouz, K., Trnková, E. & Dvořák, P. (2007). Effect of selected factors on total carotenoid content in potato tubers (*Solanum tuberosum* L.). *Plant, Soil and Environment*, *53*, 355-360.

Krinsky, N. I., Landrum, J. T. & Bone, R. A. (2003). Biologic mechanisms of the protective role of lutein and zeaxanthin in the eye. *Annual Review of Nutrition*, *23*, 171-201.

Krumbein, A., Schwarz, D. & Klaring, H. P. (2006). Effects of environmental factors on carotenoid content in tomato (*Lycopersicon esculentum* (L.) Mill.) grown in a greenhouse. *Journal of Applied Botany and Food Quality*, *80*, 160-164.

Kuchel, H., Langridge, P., Mosionek, L., Williams, K. & Jefferies, S. P. (2006). The genetic control of milling yield, dough rheology and baking quality of wheat. *Theoretical and Applied Genetics*, *112*, 1487-1495.

Laferriere, L. & Gabelman, W. H. (1968). Inheritance of color, total carotenoids, alpha-carotene, and beta-carotene in carrots, *Daucus carota* L. *Proceedings of the American Society for Horticultural Science*, *93*, 408-411.

Lang, Y.-Q., Yanagawa, S., Sasanuma, T. & Sasakuma, T. (2004). Orange fruit color in *Capsicum* due to deletion of capsanthin-capsorubin synthase gene. *Breeding Science*, *54*, 33-39.

Langton, F. A. (1980). Chemical structure and carotenoid inheritance in *Chrysanthemum morifolium* (Ramat.). *Euphytica*, *29*, 807-812.

Lee, H. S. (2001). Characterization of carotenoids in juice of red Navel orange (Cara Cara). *Journal of Agriculture and Food Chemistry*, *49*, 2563-2568.

Leenhardt, F., Lyan, B., Rock, E., Boussard, A., Potus, J., Chanliaud, E. & Remesy, C. (2006). Genetic variability of carotenoid concentration, and lipoxygenase and peroxidase activities among cultivated wheat species and bread wheat varieties. *European Journal of Agronomy*, *25*, 170-176.

Lefebvre, V., Kuntz, M., Camara, B. & Palloix, A. (1998). The capsanthin-capsorubin synthase gene: a candidate gene for the *y* locus controlling the red fruit colour in pepper. *Plant Molecular Biology*, *36*, 785-789.

Lewinsohn, E., Sitrit, Y., Bar, E. Azulay, Y., Ibdah, M., Meir, A., Yosef, E., Zamir, D. & Tadmor, Y. (2005). Not just color - carotenoid degradation as a link between color and aroma in tomato and watermelon fruit. *Trends in Food Science & Technology*, *16*, 407-415.

Leyser, O. (2008). Strigolactones and shoot branching: a new trick for a young dog. *Developmental Cell*, *15*, 337-338.

Li, F., Maurillo, C., Wurtzel, E. T. (2007). Maize *Y9* encodes a product essential for 15-cis-ζ-carotene isomerization. *Plant Physiology*, *144*, 1181-1189.

Li, F., Vallabhanemi, R., Yu, J., Rocheford, T. & Wurtzel, E. T. (2008a). The maize phytoene synthase gene family: overlapping roles for carotenogenesis in endosperm, photomorphogenesis and thermal stress tolerance. *Plant Physiology*, *147*, 1334-1346.

Li, F., Vallabhaneni, R. & Wurtzel, E. T. (2008b). *PSY3*, a new member of the phytoene synthase gene family conserved in the Poaceae and regulator of abiotic stress-induced root carotenogenesis. *Plant Physiology*, *146*, 1333-1345.

Li, L., Paolillo, D. J., Parthasarathy, M. V., DiMuzio, E. M. & Garvin, D. F. (2001). A novel gene mutation that confers abnormal patterns of β-carotene accumulation in cauliflower (*Brassica oleracea* var. *botrytis*). *The Plant Journal*, *26*, 59-67.

Li, Z. H., Matthews, P. D., Burr, B. & Wurztel, E. T. (1996). Cloning and characterization of a maize cDNA encoding phytoene desaturase, an enzyme of the carotenoid biosynthestic pathway. *Plant Molecular Biology*, *30*, 269-279.

Lichtenthaler, H. K. (1999). The 1-deoxy-D-xylulose-5-phosphate pathway of isoprenoid biosynthesis in plants. *Annual Review of Plant Physiology and Plant Molecular Biology*, *50*, 47-65.

Lieberman, M., Segev, O., Gilboa, N., Lalazar, A. & Levin, I. (2004). The tomato homolog of the gene encoding UV-damaged DNA binding protein 1 (DDB1) underline as the gene that causes the *high pigment-1* mutant phenotype. *Theoretical and Applied Genetics*, *108*, 1574-1581.

Lightbourn, G. J., Griesbach, R. J., Novotny, J. A., Clevidence, B. A., Rao, D. D. & Stommel, J. R. (2008). Combination of anthocyanin and carotenoid combinations on a foliage and immature fruit color of *Capsicum annuum* L. *The Journal of Heredity*, *99*, 105-111.

Lincoln, E. R. & Porter, J. W. (1950). Inheritance of beta carotene in tomatoes. *Genetics*, *35*, 206-211.

Lindgren, L. O., Stalberg, K. G. & Höglund, A. S. (2003). Seed-specific overexpression of an endogenous *Arabidopsis* phytoene synthase gene results in delayed germination and increased levels of carotenoids, chlorophyll, abscisic acid. *Plant Physiology*, *132*, 779-785.

Liu, Q., Xu, J., Liu, Y., Zhao, X., Deng, X., Guo, L. & Gu, J. (2007). A novel bud mutation that confers abnormal patterns of lycopene accumulation in sweet orange fruit (*Citrus sinensis* L. Osbeck). *Journal of Experimental Botany*, *58*, 4161-4171.

Liu, Y., Roof, S., Ye, Z., Barry, C., van Tuinen, A., Vrebalov, J., Bowler, C. & Giovannoni, J. (2004). Manipulation of light signal transduction as a means of modifying fruit nutritional quality in tomato. *Proceedings of the National Academy of Sciences of the USA*, *101*, 9897-9902.

Liu, Y-S., Gur, A., Causse, M., Damidaux, R., Buret, M., Hirschberg, J. & Zamir, D. (2003). There is more to tomato fruit colour than candidate carotenoid genes. *Plant Biotechnology Journal*, *1*, 195-207.

Livny, O., Kaplan, I., Reifen, R., Polak-Charcon, S., Madar, Z. & Schwartz, B. (2002). Lycopene inhibits proliferation and enhances gap-junctional communication of KB-1 human oral tumor cells. *Journal of Nutrition*, *132*, 3754-3759.

Lois, L. M., Rodríguez-Concepción, M., Gallego, F., Campos, N. & Boronat, A. (2000). Carotenoid biosynthesis during tomato fruit development: regulatory role of 1-deoxy-D-xylulose 5-phosphate synthase. *The Plant Journal*, *22*, 503-513.

Lopez, A. B., Van Eck, J., Conlin, B. J., Paolillo, D. J., O'Neill, J. & Li, L. (2008). Effect of the cauliflower *Or* transgene on carotenoid accumulation and chromoplast formation in transgenic potato tubers. *Journal of Experimental Botany*, *59*, 213-223.

Lu, S. & Li, L. (2008). Carotenoid metabolism: biosynthesis, regulation and beyond. *Journal of Integrative Plant Biology*, *50*, 778-785.

Ma, W., Daggard, G., Sutherland, M. & Brennan, P. (1999). Molecular markers for quality attributes in wheat. In: P. Williamson, P. Banks, I. Haak, J. Thompson & A. Campbell (Eds.). *Proceedings of the Ninth Assembly of the Wheat Breeding Society of Australia, Toowoomba*, Vol. *1*. pp 115-117.

Mackinney, G. & Jenkins, J. A. (1949). Inheritance of carotenoid differences in *Lycopersicum esculentum* strains. *Proceedings of the National Academy of Sciences of the USA*, *35*, 284-291.

Mares, D. J., Campbell, A. W. (2001). Mapping components of four and noodle colour in Australian wheat. *Australian Journal of Agricultural Research*, *52*, 1297-1309.

Marty, I., Bureau, S., Sarkissian, G., Gouble, B., Audergon, J. M. & Albagnac, G. (2005). Ethylene regulation of carotenoid accumulation and carotenogenic gene expression in colour-contrasted apricot varieties (*Prunus armeniaca*). *Journal of Experimental Botany*, *56*, 1877-1886.

Mayer, J. E., Pfeiffer, W. H. & Beyer, P. (2008). Biofortified crops to alleviate micronutrient malnutrition. *Current Opinion in Plant Biology*, *11*, 166-170.

Means, A. L. & Gudas, L. J. (1995). The roles of retinoids in vertebrate development. *Annual Review of Biochemistry*, *64*, 201-233.

Meissburger, B. & Wolfrum, C. (2008). The role of retinoids and their receptors in metabolic disorders. *European Journal of Lipid Science and Technology*, *110*, 191-205.

Melis, A. (1999). Photosystem-II damage and repair cycle in chloroplasts: what modulates the rate of photodamage *in vivo*? *Trends in Plant Science*, *4*, 130-135.

Menkir, A. & Maziya-Dixon, B. (2004). Influence of genotype and environment on β-carotene content of tropical yellow-endosperm maize genotypes. *Maydica*, *49*, 313-318.

Moehs, C. P., Tian, L., Osteryoung, K. W. & DellaPenna, D. (2001). Analysis of carotenoid biosynthetic gene expression during marigold petal development. *Plant Molecular Biology*, *45*, 281-293.

Molnár, P. & Szabolcs, J. (1980). β-Citraurin epoxide, a new carotenoid from Valencia orange peel. *Phytochemistry*, *19*, 633-637.

Monforte, A. J. & Tanksley, S. D. (2000). Development of a set of near isogenic and backcross recombinant inbred lines containing most of the *Lycopersicon hirsutum* genome in a *L. esculentum* genetic background: A tool for gene mapping and gene discovery. *Genome*, *43*, 803-813.

Monforte, A. J., Oliver, M., Gonzalo, M. J., Alvarez, J. M., Dolcet-Sanjuan, R. & Arus, P. (2004). Identification of quantitative trait loci involved in fruit quality traits in melon (*Cucumis melo* L.). *Theoretical and Applied Genetics*, *108*, 750-758.

Monselise, S. P. & Halevy, A. H. (1961). Detection of lycopene in pink orange fruit. *Science*, *129*, 639-640.

Moore, J., Hao, Z. G., Zhou, K. Q., Luther, M., Costa, J. & Yu, L. L. (2005). Carotenoid, tocopherol, phenolic acid, and antioxidant properties of Maryland-grown soft wheat. *Journal of Agricultural Food Chemistry*, *53*, 6649-6657.

Morris, W. L., Ducreux, L., Griffiths, D. W., Stewart, D., Davies, H. V. & Taylor, M. A. (2004). Carotenogenesis during tuber development and storage in potato. *Journal of Experimental Botany*, *55*, 1-8.

Morstadt, L., Graber, P., de Pascalis, L., Kleinig, H., Speth, V. & Beyer, P. (2002). Chemiosmotic ATP synthesis in photosynthetically inactive chromoplasts from *Narcissus pseudonarcissus* L. linked to a redox pathway potentially also involved in carotene desaturation. *Planta*, *215*, 134-140.

Mortain-Bertrand, A., Stammitti, L., Telef, N., Colardelle, P., Brouquisse, R., Rolin, D. & Gallusci, P. (2008). Effects of exogenous glucose on carotenoid accumulation in tomato leaves. *Physiologia Plantarum*, *134*, 246-256.

Müller, H. (1997). Determination of the carotenoid content in selected vegetables and fruit by HPLC and photodiode array detection. *Zeitschrift für Lebensmitteluntersuchung und -Forschung A*, *204*, 88-94.

Mustilli, A. C., Fenzi, F., Ciliento, R., Alfano, F. & Bowler, C. (1999). Phenotype of the tomato *high pigment-2* mutant is caused by a mutation in the tomato homolog of *DEETIOLATED1*. *The Plant Cell*, *11*, 145-158.

Nambara, E. & Marion-Poll, A. (2005). Abscisic acid biosynthesis and catabolism. *Annual Review of Plant Biology*, *56*, 165-185.

Napoli, J. L. (2005). Vitamin A: biochemistry and physiological role. In: B. Caballero, L. Allen & A. Prentice, (Eds.) *Encyclopedia of Human Nutrition* (2nd edition, pp. 339-347). Amsterdam: Elsevier Ltd.

Navot, N. & Zamir, D. (1986). Linkage relationships of 19 protein coding genes in watermelon. *Theoretical and Applied Genetics*, *72*, 274-278.

Navot, N., Sarfatti, M. & Zamir, D. (1990). Linkage relationships of genes affecting bitterness and flesh color in watermelon. *The Journal of Heredity*, *81*, 162-165.

Nestel, P., Bouis, H. E., Meenakshi, J. V. & Pfeiffer, W. (2006). Biofortification of stable food crops. *The Journal of Nutrition*, *136*, 1064-1067.

Newell-McGloughlin, M. (2008). Nutritionally improved agricultural crops. *Plant Physiology*, *147*, 939-953.

Nielsen, O. F. & Gough, S. (1974). Macromolecular physiology of plastids XI. Carotenes in etiolated *tigrina* and *xantha* mutants of barley. *Physiologia Plantarum*, *30*, 246-251.

Nishino, H., Murakoshi, M., Tokuda, H. & Satomi, Y. (2009). Cancer prevention by carotenoids. *Archives of Biochemistry and Biophysics*, *43*, 165-168.

Niyogi, K. K., Grossman, A. R. & Bjorkman, O. (1998). *Arabidopsis* mutants define a central role for the xanthophyll cycle in the regulation of photosynthetic energy conversion. *The Plant Cell*, *10*, 1121-1134.

Norris, S. R., Barrette, T. R. & DellaPenna, D. (1995). Genetic dissection of carotenoid synthesis in arabidopsis defines plastoquinone as an essential component of phytoene desaturation. *The Plant Cell*, *7*, 2139-2149.

Oelmüller, R. & Mohr, H. (1985). Carotenoid composition in milo (*Sorghum vulgare*) shoots as affected by phytochrome and chlorophyll. *Planta*, *164*, 390-395.

Ohmiya, A., Kishimoto, S., Aida, R., Yoshioka, S. & Sumitomo, K. (2006). Carotenoid cleavage dioxygenase (CmCCD4a) contributes to white color formation in chrysantemum petals. *Plant Physiology*, *142*, 1193-1201.

Oliver, S. N., Dennis, E. S. & Dolferus, R. (2007). ABA regulates apoplastic sugar transport and is a potential signal for cold-induced pollen sterility in rice. *Plant & Cell Physiology*, *48*, 1319-1330.

Omoni, A. O. & Aluko, R. E. (2005). The anti-carcinogenic and anti-atherogenic effects of lycopene: a review. *Trends in Food Science & Technology*, *16*, 344-350.

Ortiz-Monasterio, J. I., Palacios-Rojas, N., Meng, E., Pixley, K., Trethowan, R. & Peña, R. J. (2007). Enhancing the mineral and vitamin content of wheat and maize through plant breeding. *Journal of Cereal Science*, *46*, 293-307.

Pacini, E. & Hesse, M. (2005). Pollenkitt – its composition, forms and functions. *Flora*, *200*, 399-415.

Paine, A. J., Shipton, C. A., Chaggar, S., Howells, R. M., Kennedy, M. J., Vernon, G., Wright, S. Y., Hinchliffe, Adams J. L., Silverstone, A. L. & Drake, R. (2005). Improving the nutritional value of Golden Rice through increased pro-vitamin A content. *Nature Biotechnology*, *23*, 482-487.

Palaisa, K. A., Morgante, M., Williams, M. & Rafalski, A. (2003). Contrasting effects of selection on sequence diversity and linkage disequilibrium at two phytoene synthase loci. *The Plant Cell*, *15*, 1795-1806.

Park, H., Kreunen, S. S., Cuttriss, A. J., DellaPenna, D. & Pogson, B. J. (2002). Identification of the carotenoid isomerase provides insight into carotenoid biosynthesis, prolamellar body formation, and photomorphogenesis. *The Plant Cell*, *14*, 321-332.

Parker, G. D., Chalmers, K. J., Rathjen, A. J. & Langridge, P. (1998). Mapping loci associated with flour colour in wheat (*Triticum aestivum* L.). *Theoretical and Applied Genetics*, *97*, 238-245.

Parker, G. D. & Langridge, P. (2000). Development of a STS marker linked to a major locus controlling four colour in wheat (*Triticum aestivum* L.). *Molecular Breeding*, *6*, 169-174.

Patil, M. R., Oak, M. D., Tamhankar, S. A., Sourdille, P. & Rao, V. S. (2008). Mapping and validation of a major QTL for yellow pigment content on 7AL in durum wheat (*Triticum turgidum* L. spp. *durum*). *Molecular Breeding*, *21*, 485-496.

Pecker, I., Gabbay, R., Cunningham, F. X. Jr. & Hirschberg, J. (1996). Cloning and characterization of the cDNA for lycopene β-cyclase from tomato reveals decrease in its expression during fruit ripening. *Plant Molecular Biology*, *30*, 807-819.

Perucka, I. (2004). Changes of carotenoid contents during ripening of pepper fruits and ethephon treatment. *Acta Scientiarum Polonorum*, *3*, 85-92.

Pfeiffer, W. & McClafferty, B. (2007). HarvestPlus: breeding crops for better nutrition. *Crop Science*, *47*(S3), S88-S105.

Pogson, B. J., Niyogi, K. K., Bjorkman, O. & DellaPenna, D. (1998). Altered xanthophylls compositions adversely affect chlorophyll accumulation and non photochemical quenching in *Arabidopsis* mutants. *Proceedings of the National Academy of Sciences of the USA*, *95*, 13324-13329.

Poole, C. F. (1944). Genetics of cultivated cucurbits. *The Journal of Heredity*, *35*, 122-128.

Popovsky, S. & Paran, I. (2000). Molecular analysis of the *Y* locus in pepper: its relation to capsanthin-capsorubin synthase and to fruit color. *Theoretical and Applied Genetics*, *101*, 86-89.

Pozniak, C. J., Knox, R. E., Clarke, F. R., Clarke, J. M. (2007). Identification of QTL and association of a phytoene synthase gene with endosperm colour in durum wheat. *Theoretical and Applied Genetics*, *114*, 525-537.

Pyke, K. A. & Howells, C. A. (2002). Plastid and stromule morphogenesis in tomato. *Annals of Botany*, *90*, 559-566.

Qiao, C. G., Li, S. Q., Li, M. N. & Shan, L. M. (1995). A study of the inheritance of the characters of white pollen in sunflower (*Helianthus annuus* L.). *Oil Crops of China*, *17*, 10-12.

Redmond, T. M., Gentleman, S., Duncan, T., Yu, S., Wiggert, B., Gantt, E. & Cunningham, Jr. F. X. (2001). Identification, expression, and substrate specifity of a mammalian *β*-carotene 15,15'-dioxygenase. *Journal of Biological Chemistry*, *276*, 6560-6565.

Ritz, T., Damjanovic, A., Schulten, K., Zhang, J. R. & Koyama, Y. (2000). Efficient light harvesting through carotenoids. *Photosynthesis Research*, *66*, 125-144.

Robinson, R. W., Munger, H. M., Whitaker, T. W. & Bohn, G. W. (1976). Genes of the cucurbitaceae. *HortScience*, *11*, 554-568.

Robinson, R. W. & Tomes, M. L. (1968). Ripening inhibitor: a gene with multiple effects on ripening. *Report of the Tomato Genetics Cooperative*, *18*, 36-37.

Rock, C. L. (1997). Carotenoids: biology and treatment. *Pharmacology & Therapeutics*, *75*, 185-197.

Rodrigo, M. J., Marcos, J. F., Alférez, F., Mallent, D. & Zacarías, L. (2003). Characterization of Pinalate, a novel *Citrus sinensis* mutant with a fruit-specific alteration that results in yellow pigmentation and decreased ABA content. *Journal of Experimental Botany*, *54*, 727-738.

Rodríquez-Concepción, M. & Boronat, A. (2002). Elucidation of the methylerythritol phosphate pathway for isoprenoid biosynthesis in bacteria and plastids. A metabolic milestone achieved through genomics. *Plant Physiology*, *130*, 1079-1089.

Roe, N. E. & Bemis, W. P. (1977). Corolla color in *Cucurbita*. *The Journal of Heredity*, *68*, 193-194.

Ronen, G., Carmel-Goren, L., Zamir, D. & Hirschberg, J. (2000). An alternative pathway to *β*-carotene formation in plant chromoplasts discovered by map-based cloning of *Beta* and *old-gold* color mutations in tomato. *Proceedings of the National Academy of Sciences of the USA*, *97*, 11102-11107.

Ronen, G., Cohen, M., Zamir, D. & Hirschberg, J. (1999). Regulation of carotenoid biosynthesis during tomato fruit development: Expression of the gene for lycopene epsilon-cyclase is down-regulated during ripening and is elevated in the mutant *Delta*. *The Plant Journal*, *17*, 341-351.

Rosati, C., Aquilani, R., Dharmapuri, S., Pallara, P., Marusic, C., Tavazza, R., Bouvier, F., Camara, B. & Giuliano, G. (2000). Metabolic engineering of beta-carotene and lycopene content in tomato fruit. *The Plant Journal*, *24*, 413-419.

Ruban, A. V., Berera, R., Ilioaia, C., van Stokkum, I. H. M., Kennis, J. T. M., Pascal, A. A., van Amerongen, H., Robert, B., Horton, P. & van Grondelle, R. (2007). Identification of a mechanism of photoprotective energy dissipation in higher plants. *Nature, 450,* 575-578.

Ruiz, D., Egea, J., Toms-Barbern, F. A. & Gil, M. I. (2005). Carotenoids from new apricot (*Prunus armeniaca* L.) varieties and their relationship with flesh and skin color. *Journal of Agricultural and Food Chemistry, 53,* 6368-6374.

Sadik, S. (1962). Morphology of the curd of cauliflower. *American Journal of Botany, 49,* 290-297.

Salvini, M., Bernini, A., Fambrini, M. & Pugliesi, C. (2005). cDNA cloning and expression of the phytoene synthase gene in sunflower. *Journal of Plant Physiology, 162,* 479-484.

Sandmann, G. (2002). Molecular evolution of carotenoid biosynthesis from bacteria to plants. *Physiologia Plantarum, 116,* 431-440.

Sandmann, G., Römer, S. & Fraser, P. D. (2006). Understanding carotenoid metabolism as a necessity for genetic engineering of crop plants. *Metabolic Engineering, 8,* 291-302.

Santos, C. A. F. & Simon, P. W. (2002). QTL analyses reveal clustered loci for accumulation of major provitamin A carotenes and lycopene in carrot roots. *Molecular Genetics and Genomics, 268,* 122-129.

Santos, C. A. F. & Simon, P. W. (2006). Hereditability and minimum gene number estimates of carrot carotenoids. *Euphytica, 151,* 79-86.

Saunt, J. (2000). *Citrus Varieties of the World.* (pp. 16-17). Norwich NR5 *950,* England: Sinclair International Limited, Jarrold Way Bowthnope.

Schaub, P., Al-Babili, S., Drake, R. & Beyer, P. (2005). Why is golden rice golden (yellow) instead of red? *Plant Physiology, 138,* 441-450.

Schwartz, S. H., Qin, X. & Zeevaart, J. A. (2003). Characterization of a novel carotenoid cleavage dioxygenases from plant. *Journal of Biological Chemistry, 276,* 25208-25211.

Scolnik, P. A., Hinton, P., Greenblatt, I. M., Giuliano, G., Delanoy, M. R., Spector, D. L. & Pollock, D. (1987). Somatic instability of carotenoid biosynthesis in the tomato ghost mutant and its effect on plastid development. *Planta, 171,* 11-18.

Sesso, H. D., Liu, S., Graziano, M. & Buring, J. E. (2003). Dietary lycopene, tomato-based food products and cardiovascular disease in women. *Journal of Nutrition, 133,* 2336-2341.

Sharoni, Y., Danilenko, M., Dubi, N., Ben-Dor, A. & Levy, J. (2004). Carotenoids and transcription. *Archives of Biochemistry and Biophysics, 430,* 89-96.

Shewmaker, C. K., Sheehy, J. A., Daley, M., Colburn, S. & Ke, D. Y. (1999). Seed-specific overexpression of phytoene synthase: increase in carotenoids and other metabolic effects. *The Plant Journal, 20,* 401-412.

Simkin, A. J., Gaffé, J., Alcaraz, J. P., Carde, J. P., Bramley, P. M., Fraser, P. D. & Kuntz, M. (2007). Fibrillin influence plastid ultrastructure and pigment content in tomato fruit. *Phytochemistry, 68,* 1545-1556.

Simon, P. W. (1990). Carrots and other horticultural crops as a source of provitamin A carotenes. *HortScience, 24,* 174-175.

Simon, P. W. (1992). Genetic improvement of vegetable carotene content. In: D. D. Bills & S.-D. Kung (Eds.). *Biotechnology and Nutrition, Prooceedings of the Third International Symposium* (pp. 291-300). Boston, MA: Butterworth-Heinemann.

Simon, P. W. (1993). Breeding carrot, cucumber, onion and garlic for improved quality and nutritional value. *Horticultura Brasileira, 11*, 171-173.

Simon, P. W. (1996). Inheritance and expression of purple and yellow storage root color in carrot. *The Journal of Heredity, 87*, 63-66.

Simon, P.W. (2000). Domestication, historical development, and modern breeding of carrot. *Plant Breeding Review, 19*, 157-190.

Simon, P. W. & Navazio, J. P. (1997). Early orange mass 400, early orange mass 402, and late orange mass 404: high carotene cucumber germplasm. *HortScience, 32*, 144-145.

Simon, P. W. & Wolff, X. Y. (1987). Carotenes in typical and dark orange carrots. *Journal of Agricultural and Food Chemistry, 35*, 1017-1022.

Simon, P. W., Wolff, X. Y., Peterson, C. E., Kammerlohr, D. S., Rubatzky, V. E., Strandberg, J. O., Bassett, M. J. & White, J. M. (1989). High carotene mass carrot population. *HortScience, 24*, 174-175.

Soprano, D. R., Qin, P. & Soprano, K. J. (2004). Retinoic acid receptors and cancer. *Annual Review of Nutrition, 24*, 210-221.

Stahl, W., Nicolai, S., Briviba, K., Hanusch, M., Broszeit, G., Peters, M., Martin, H. D. & Sies, H. (1997). Biological activities of natural and synthetic carotenoids: Induction of gap junctional communication and singlet oxygen quenching. *Carcinogenesis, 18*, 89-92.

Stange, C., Fuentes P., Handford M. & Pizarro L. (2008). *Daucus carota* as a novel model to evaluate the effect of light on carotenogenic gene expression. *Biological Research, 41*, 289-301.

Stanley, R. G. & Linskens, H. F. (1974). Pollen pigments. In: *Pollen Biology Biochemistry Management* (1st edition, pp. 223-246). Berlin, Heidelberg, New York: Springer-Verlag.

Stroeva, O. G. & Mitashov, V. I. (1983). Retinal pigment epithelium: proliferation and differentiation during development and regeneration. *International Review of Cytology, 83*, 221-293.

Sun, T., Xu, Z., Wu, C. T., Janes, M., Prinyawiwatkul, W. & No, H. K. (2007). Antioxidant activities of different colored sweet bell peppers. *Journal of Food Science, 72*, S98-S102.

Surles, R. L., Weng, N., Simon, P. W. & Tanumihardjo, S. A. (2004). Carotenoid profiles and consumer sensory evaluation of specially carrots (*Daucus carota* L.) of various colors. *Journal of Agricultural and Food Chemistry, 52*, 3417-3421.

Tanksley, S. D. (1993). Linkage map of tomato (*Lycopersicon esculentum*) (2N = 24). In: S. J. O'Brien (Ed.), *Genetic Maps: Locus Maps of Complex Genomes* (6th edition, pp. 639-660). Cold Spring Harbor, NY: Cold Spring Harbor Laboratory Press.

Tanksley, S. D., Grandillo, S., Fulton, T. M., Zamir, D., Eshed, Y., Petiard, V., Lopez, J. & Beck-Bunn, T. (1996). Advanced back cross QTL analysis in a cross between an elite processing line of tomato and its wild relative *L. pimpinellifolium. Theoretical and Applied Genetics, 92*, 213-224.

Tanksley, S. D. & McCouch, S. R. (1997). Seed banks and molecular maps: unlocking genetic potential from the wild. *Science, 277*, 1063-1066.

Taylor, M. & Ramsay, G. (2005). Carotenoid biosynthesis in plant storage organs: recent advances and prospects for improving plant food quality. *Physiologia Plantarum, 124*, 143-151.

Telfer, A., Dhami, S., Bishop, S., Phillips, D. & Barber, J. (1994). *β*-carotene quenches singlet oxygen formed by isolated photosystem II reaction centers. *Biochemistry, 33*, 14469-14474.

Thompson, A. J., Tor, M., Barry, C. S., Vrebalov, J., Orfila, C., Jarvis, M. C., Giovannoni, J. J., Grierson, D. & Seymour, G. B. (1999). Molecular genetic characterization of a novel pleiotropic tomato-ripening mutant. *Plant Physiology, 120*, 383-390.

Thorup, T. A., Tanyolac, B., Livingstone, K. D., Popovsky, S., Paran, I., Jahn, M. (2000). Candidate gene analysis of organ pigmentation loci in the Solanaceae. *Proceedings of the National Academy of Sciences of the USA, 97*, 11192-11197.

Tigchelaar, E. C., McGlasson, W. B. & Buescher, R. W. (1978). Genetic regulation of tomato fruit ripening. *HortScience, 13*, 508-513.

Ting, J. T. L., Wu, S. S. H., Ratnayake, C. & Huang, A. H. C. (1998). Constituents of the tapetosomes and elaioplasts in *Brassica campestris* and their degradation and retention during microsporogenesis. *The Plant Journal, 16*, 541-551.

Tomes, M. L. (1963). Temperature inhibition of carotene synthesis in tomato. *Botanical Gazette, 124*, 180-185.

Tomes, M. L., Quackenbush, F. W. & McQuistan, M. (1954). Modification and dominance of the gene governing formation of high concentration of *beta*-carotene in the tomato. *Genetics, 39*, 810-817.

Tomes, M. L., Quackenbush, F. W., Nelson, O. E. & North, B. (1953). The inheritance of carotenoid pigment system in the tomato. *Genetics, 38*, 117-127.

Troccoli, A., Borrelli, G. M., De Vita, P., Fares, C. & Di Fonzo, N. (2000). Durum wheat quality: a multidisciplinary concept. *Journal of Cereal Science, 32*, 99-113.

Vallabhaneni R. & Wurzel E. T. (2009). Timing and biosynthetic potential for carotenoid accumulation in genetically diverse germplasm of maize. *Plant Physiology, 150*, 562-572.

Van Eck, J., Conlin, B., Garvin, D. F., Mason, H., Navarre, D. A. & Brown, C. R. (2007). Enhancing beta-carotene content in potato by RNAi-mediated silencing of the beta-carotene hydroxylase gene. *American Journal of Potato Research, 84*, 331-342.

Vershinin, A. (1999). Biological function of carotenoids – diversity and evolution. *BioFactors, 10*, 99-104.

Vishnevetsky, M., Ovadis, M. & Vainstein, A. (1999). Carotenoid sequestration in plants: the role of carotenoid-associated proteins. *Trends in Plant Science, 4*, 232-235.

von Lintig, J., Hessel, S., Isken, A., Kiefer, C., Lampert, J. M., Voolstra, O. & Vogt, K. (2005). Towards a better understanding of carotenoid metabolism in animals. *Biochimica et Biophysica Acta, 1740*, 122-131.

von Lintig, J., Welsch, R., Bonk, M., Giuliano, G., Batschauer, A. & Kleinig, H. (1997). Light-dependent regulation of carotenoid biosynthesis occurs at the level of phytoene synthase expression and is mediated by phytochrome in *Sinapis alba* and *Arabidopsis thaliana* seedlings. *The Plant Journal, 12*, 625-634.

Vrebalov, J., Ruezinsky, D., Padmanabhan, V., White, R., Medrano, D., Drake, R., Schuch, W. & Giovannoni, J. (2002). A MADS-box gene necessary for fruit ripening at the tomato *ripening-inhibitor* (*rin*) locus. *Science, 12*, 343-346.

Wakelin, A. M., Lister, C. E. & Conner, A. J. (2003). Inheritance and biochemistry of pollen pigmentation in california poppy (*Eschscholzia californica* Cham.). *International Journal of Plant Science, 164*, 867-875.

Wald, G. (1960). The molecular basis of visual excitation. *Nature, 219*, 800-807.

Welsch, R., Maass D., Voegel, T., DellaPenna, D. & Beyer, P. (2007). Transcription factor RAP2.2 and its interacting partner SINAT2: stable elements in the carotenogenesis of Arabidopsis leaves. *Plant Physiology, 145*, 1073-1085.

Welsch, R., Medina, J., Giuliano, G., Beyer, P. & von Lintig, J. (2003). Structural and functional characterization of the phytoene synthase promoter from *Arabidopsis thaliana*. *Planta, 216*, 523-534.

Welsch, R., Wüst, F., Bär, C., Al-Babili, S. & Beyer, P. (2008). A third phytoene synthase is devoted to abiotic stress-induced abscisic acid formation in rice and defines functional diversification of phytoene synthase genes. *Plant Physiology, 147*, 367-380.

Wiermann, R. & Gubatz, S. (1992). Pollen wall and sporopollenin. *International Review of Cytology, 140*, 35-72.

Woitsch, S. & Römer, S. (2003). Expression of xanthophylls biosynthetic genes during light-dependent chloroplast differentation. *Plant Physiology, 132*, 1508-1517.

Wolf, G. (2008). Retinoic acid as cause of cell proliferation or cell growth inhibition depending on activation of one of two different nuclear receptors. *Nutrition Reviews, 66*, 55-59.

Wong, J. C., Lambert, R. J., Wurtzel, E. T. & Rocheford, T. R. (2004). QTL and candidate genes phytoene synthase and ζ-carotene desaturase associated with the accumulation of carotenoids in maize. *Theoretical and Applied Genetics, 108*, 349-359.

Wurbs, D., Ruf, S. & Bock, R. (2007). Contained metabolic engineering in tomatoes by expression of carotenoid biosynthesis genes from the plastid genomes. *The Plant Journal 49*, 276-288.

Wurtzel, E. T. (2004). Genomics, genetics, and biochemistry of maize carotenoid biosynthesis. In: J. Romero, (Ed.). *Recent Advances in Phytochemistry*, (Vol. *38*, pp. 85-110). New York, NY: Elsevier Ltd.

Yamagishi, M., Kishimoto, S. & Nakayama, M. (2009). Carotenoid composition and changes in expression of carotenoid biosynthetic genes in tepals of Asiatic hybrid lily. *Plant Breeding*, doi:10.1111/j.1439-0523.2009.01656.x.

Yamamoto, H. (1979). Biochemistry of the violaxanthin cycle in higher plants. *Pure and Applied Chemistry, 51*, 639-648.

Yan, W., Jang, G.-F., Haeseleer, F., Esumi, N., Chang, J., Kerrigan, M., Campochiaro, M., Campochiaro, P., Palczewski, K. & Zack, D. J. (2001). Cloning and characterization of a human β,β-carotene-dioxygenase that is highly expressed in the retinal pigment epithelium. *Genomics, 72*, 193-202.

Ye, X., Al-Babili, S., Klöti, A., Zhang, J., Lucca, P., Beyer, P. & Potrykus, I. (2000). Engineering the provitamin A (β-carotene) biosynthetic pathway into (carotenoid-free) rice endosperm. *Science, 287*, 303-305.

Yokoyama, H. & Vandercook, C. E. (1967). Citrus carotenoids. I. Comparison of carotenoids of mature-green and yellow lemons. *Journal of Food Science, 32*, 42-48.

Yue, B., Vick, B. A., Yuan, W. & Hu, J. (2008). Mapping one of the 2 genes controlling ray flower color in sunflower (*Helianthus annuus* L.). *The Journal of Heredity, 99*, 564-567.

Zechmeister, L., LeRosen, A. L., Went, F. W. & Pauling, L. (1941). Prolycopene, a naturally occurring stereoisomer of lycopene. *Proceedings of the National Academy of Sciences of the USA, 27*, 468-474.

Zhang, L. P., Yan, J., Xia, X. C., He, Z. H. & Sutherland, M. W. (2006). QTL mapping for kernel yellow pigment content in common wheat. *Acta Agronomica Sinica*, *32*, 41-45.

Zhou X., Van Eck, J. & Li, L. (2008). Use of the cauliflower *Or* gene for improving crop nutritional quality. *Biotechnology Annual Review*, *14*, 171-190.

Zhu, C., Naqvi, S., Breitenbach, J., Sandmann, G., Christou, P. & Capell, T. (2008). Combinatorial genetic transformation generates a library of metabolic phenotypes for the carotenoid pathway in maize. *Proceedings of the National Academy of Sciences of the USA*, *105*, 18232-18237.

In: Encyclopedia of Vitamin Research
Editor: Joshua T. Mayer

Chapter 30

Evaluating the Effectiveness of Beta-Carotene-Rich Food Interventions for Improving Vitamin A Status[*]

Betty J. Burri and Tami Turner
Western Human Nutrition Research Center, ARS, USDA,
430 West Health Sciences Drive, Davis, CA 95616, USA

Abstract

Despite years of interventions with vitamin A (VA) supplement programs, VA deficiency remains a leading cause of morbidity and blindness in Southern Asia and Africa. Although high dose VA supplements can be a very effective means of preventing VA deficiency, they have several drawbacks: VA capsules can cause toxicity symptoms, and capsule distribution programs are difficult to sustain and have incomplete coverage. Beta-carotene forms VA, and beta-carotene-rich crops are the major source of VA in much of the world, including all areas where VA deficiency is common. For this reason, growing beta-carotene-rich crops to improve VA status has obvious attractions. Several small scale studies and projects have successfully used beta-carotene-rich crops to improve or at least maintain VA status in areas where VA deficiency is common. The results of these small scale programs will be evaluated, and we will use results from these studies to estimate the potential exposure to VA that is likely from food-based interventions. We will evaluate the potential effectiveness of beta-carotene rich crops such as Golden Rice, red palm oil, and mangoes in VA deficiency prevention.

---

[*] A version of this chapter was also published in *Beta Carotene: Dietary Sources, Cancer and Cognition, edited by Leiv Haugen and Terje Bjornson* published by Nova Science Publishers, Inc. It was submitted for appropriate modifications in an effort to encourage wider dissemination of research.

Introduction

Vitamin A is an essential nutrient, required for normal eyesight, growth and development (World Health Organization 2004). Recent estimates suggest that vitamin A deficiency (VAD) is directly responsible for 600,000 deaths per year (Black et al 2008). Coupled with other nutrient deficiencies (such as iron, zinc, and energy) VAD was responsible for about 35% of child deaths and 11% of the total global disease burden (Black et al 2008). VAD is most common in Sub-Saharan Africa and Southern Asia, where small children (aged approximately 2 to 5 years of age) and pregnant women are at highest risk for morbidity and mortality associated with VAD (World Health Organization 2007).

The amount of VA required in the diet varies with age, sex, and pregnancy, as could be expected. Although different nations have somewhat different estimates of the amount of VA required for maintaining human health, most estimates are similar to those derived for the United States population (Table 1; Food and Nutrition Board 2004)

VA supplementation can prevent xeropthalmia, the leading cause of preventable blindness in the world (Sommer and West 1996), and has been associated with significant reductions in infant and maternal mortality in areas where VAD is common (West et al 1999). VAD is generally treated by providing a high-dose oral supplement of VA twice a year (Sommer and West 1999). Currently these VA supplementation programs operate in approximately 43 countries (World Health Organization 2007; Figure 1). In principle, VA supplementation programs using high dose VA capsules are an inexpensive and cost-effective nutrient intervention that can be combined with childhood immunizations and other nutrient interventions. In practice, however, results for VA supplement programs are mixed. These intervention programs have been difficult to sustain and their coverage is often inadequate. For example, although India has supported national VA supplementation programs for over 30 years, they have attained less than 25% coverage of the population (Stein et al 2006, supplemental material), a rate that has not improved for many years. Furthermore, these VA capsule supplementation programs have been associated with price-gouging by manufacturers and have possibly led to inadvertent overdosing, which resulted in much unwelcome publicity for India's public health program (Mudur 2001; West and Sommer 2002).

Growing fruits and vegetables that are rich in beta-carotene, the most abundant precursor of VA, is an attractive alternative or complement to providing VA supplements (Strobel et al 2007). Fruits and vegetables can provide a variety of nutrients in addition to VA, and might also provide income to small farmers and shop keepers whose families are at risk for nutrient deficiencies. Theoretically, long-term sustainability of food-based programs might be easier to achieve then it has been for supplement programs, because fruit and vegetable seeds can be harvested and shared at a local level instead of being provided by a national program. Indeed, studies show that greater household expenditures on fruits and vegetables can improve VA status and health. For example, increased expenditures on fruits and vegetables (but not on animal-based foods) were associated with decreased risks of child mortality in Indonesia (Campbell et al 2008).

There is essentially no data on the outcome and sustainability of national dietary interventions to improve VA status through increasing fruit and vegetable consumption. However, several small scale interventions have successfully used fruit and vegetable crops to increase VA status (Ruel 2001; Leitz et al 2001; Haskell et al 2005, Low et al 2007). Many of these interventions have used a mixture of foods containing VA and beta-carotene (Haskell et al 2005), but several have successfully used a single type of food, such as red palm oil, mangos, and sweet potatoes to increase VA status. We will review these studies, then use their results along with agricultural data to evaluate their potential to decrease VAD on a larger scale. Additionally, we will review the potential and problems associated with Golden Rice.

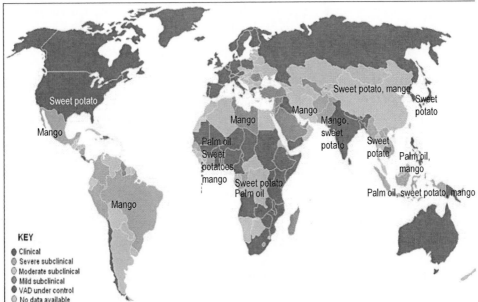

Figure 1. Worldwide distribution of VAD. Severity noted by color.

Table 1. Vitamin A RDI by life stage.

Life Stage/Group	DRI VITAMIN A µg/day
Infants 0-6mo	400 (AI)
Infants 7-12mo	500 (AI)
Children 1-3 y	300
Children 4-8y	400
Children 9-13y	600
Adult males 14+y	900
Adult Females 14+y except pregnant/lactating	700
Pregnant (14-18y) / (19+)	750 / 770
Lactating (14-18y) / (19+)	1,200 / 1,300

Ref. Food and Nutrition Board 2004.

Materials and Methods

Data was collected from library and internet searches conducted in Fall 2008. The search engines used were PubMed, Agricola, and Google. Keywords were 'golden rice', 'mango', 'sweet potato', and 'palm oil' coupled with 'vitamin A, carote* or retino*'. An attempt to evaluate the quality and consistency of the literature was made, with preference given to data published in recent (2004 or later) peer-reviewed journals. However, peer reviewed journals seldom publish nutrition survey data or food composition and production data. Therefore, most data was collected from National (US) data or international (United Nations) sources. In these cases, preference was given to data published by the World Health Organization, the United Nations Food and Agriculture Organization, and the United States Department of Agriculture. However, this data was supplemented with data from major non-governmental agencies known to have major interests and activities in VAD or agriculture, such as HarvestPlus and Greenpeace.

Estimates of the conversion ratio of beta-carotene to VA, and of beta-carotene-rich foods to VA, have changed over the years and remain controversial (Food and Nutrition Board 2004; Matsuda-Inoguchi et al 2006). A major reason for this is that a variety of factors influence beta-carotene absorption and conversion, and these factors can be difficult to control (Ahmed et al 2002).

Although recent studies of the absorption of beta-carotene from foods have led to proposals to decrease the conversion ratio of beta-carotene to VA, and these proposals are supported by substantial evidence, there is as yet insufficient evidence to change them. Therefore, we use the 12:1 conversion ratio for beta-carotene in plant foods proposed by the Food and Nutrition Board (2004). This results in an underestimate of the VA provided from red palm oil, and probably overestimates the amount of VA that could be derived from Golden rice.

Potential impact of any dietary intervention can be estimated by using the disability-adjusted life year (DALY) method (Stein 2006, supplemental material). The DALY method defines the number of DALY lost to VAD each year as:

$$\text{DALY} = \sum jTjMj\left(\frac{1-e^{-rLj}}{r}\right) + \sum i\sum jTjIijDij\left(\frac{1-e^{-rd_{ij}}}{r}\right)$$

When Tj is the number of people in the target group (j), Mj is the mortality associated with VAD in that group, Lj is their average remaining life expectancy, Iij is the incidence of a disease (i) in the target group, Dij is the disability weight for disease i in the group, and r is a standard set at 3% which is the 'discount rate' for future life years.

However, many of the factors used in the DALY equation are determined by the characteristics of VAD itself, not the interventions to prevent VAD. If we make the admittedly simplistic assumption that when a food-based intervention to prevent VAD is begun, it changes the number of people with VAD but not the fundamental characteristics of VAD (i.e., its mortality rate, its disability weight, and the age at which VAD appears), then this diminishes the complexity of the DALY equation. Essentially, if one also assumes that diseases of interest are similar in VAD deficient countries (e.g., that VAD causes xeropthalmia and increases the risk of death in each country), then the impact of a food based intervention on DALY caused by VAD can be estimated by its coverage; it depends mainly on the change in the number of people at risk for VAD in that country. Thus, the likely impact of a food-based intervention on VAD can be estimated by its probable coverage, which can in turn be estimated by the percentage of people at risk in the population, and the local cost, availability, and beta-carotene content of the food used in the intervention.

Therefore, we evaluated potential food based interventions by: 1) calculating the amount of food needed to supply the VA requirements for children, women, and men; 2) identifying the countries that were major producers of each food, their production volume, and emerging issues that might influence their ability to increase production; and 3) calculating whether production of beta-carotene rich foods could meets VA demand.

Results

Major Single-food-based Intervention Strategies

Many food based interventions to decrease VAD use a mixed approach, relying on gardening projects or mixed fruit and vegetable interventions (Ruel 2001, Haskell et al 2004). However, a review of the literature shows that currently three food-based interventions to prevent VAD have been tested in several populations. The beta-carotene-rich foods used in these interventions are red palm oil, orange-fleshed sweet potatoes, and mangoes. All of these beta-carotene rich foods have successfully raised beta-carotene concentrations and improved VA status in small scale studies (Goudo et al 2007, Stapleton 2008, van Jaarlsveld et al 2005, Ruel 2001, Leitz et al 2001, Low et al 2007, van Stuijvenberg et al 2001, Mahapatra and Manorama 1997, Haskell et al 2004). In addition, Golden rice, bioengineered rice with high beta-carotene content, has been in the testing and development stage for many years (Anderson et al 2004, Potrykus 2001). The estimated amount of VA in these fruits and vegetables are shown in Table 2. Note that the beta-carotene content and estimated amounts of VA derived from these foods vary considerably. All food based interventions use natural products that are not as uniform as the VA supplement capsules they intend to replace. Beta-carotene content in these fruits and vegetables varies with variety, climate, growing and harvesting conditions, and cooking (Diedhiou et al 2007, Gomez-Lim 1993, Veda et al 2007, United States Department of Agriculture 2008). Since these interventions are meant to become a component of average diets, some of the variability that occurs in fruits and vegetables would be averaged out over time. However, careful selection of cultivars to introduce higher yields and higher carotenoid content could increase the estimated amount of VA provided by these interventions considerably (Veda et al 2007).

Table 2. Estimated amount of VA in 100g of common intervention foods.

Food	Estimated VA RAE/100g
Mango (edible portion) [a,b]	50 [a], 46 − 268 [b]
Sweet potato (assumed orange; canned, boiled ,or baked) [a]	435, 787, 961
Golden rice (Dry; in various gmo varieties) [c]	73-308*
Red palm oil (*E. tenera,* common commercial) [d]	4,166 - 25,000†

*880-3700µg total carotenoids in 100g dry rice from newer varieties
†up to 50,000 µg total carotenoids for some low-yield (and lesser used) varieties
[a] United States Department of Agriculture, Agricultural Research Service, National Nutrient Database for Standard Reference, Release 21. 2008.
[b] Veda et al 2007. [c] Paine et al 2008. [d] Rodriquez-Amaya 1996, Caritino 2005.

Table 3. Estimated g/day and servings/day needed to meet DRI at different life stages.

Life Stage	Estimated grams/day of food needed to meet RDA or AI*		Estimated serving(s)/day needed to meet DRI†
Infants (0-12 mo)	Assumed mainly breast-fed		See values under Children (4-8y)
Children (1-3y)	Mango	112	0.7 cups (3/4 cup)
	Sweet potato	69 (canned) 31 (baked) 36 (boiled)	0.1 - 0.3 cup
	Golden rice 2	97 (dry)	0.5 cups (dry)
	Red palm oil	4 – 5	0.3 Tbsp (or 1 tsp)
Children (4-8y)	Mango	149	0.9 cup
	Sweet potato	92 (canned) 41 (baked) 48 (boiled)	0.1- 0.4 cups
	Golden rice 2	130 (dry)	0.7 cups (dry)
	Red Palm oil	5 – 6	0.4 - 0.5 Tbsp
Adult males (14+y)	Mango	336	2 cups
	Sweet potato	207 (canned) 93 (baked) 117 (boiled)	0.3 – 0.8 cup
	Golden rice 2	292 (dry)	1.6 cups (dry)
	Red Palm oil	12-14	0.8 - 1 Tbsp
Adult Females (Not pregnant/ lactating 14y+)	Mango	261	1.5 cups
	Sweet potato	161(canned) 72 (baked) 91 (boiled)	0.2 - 0.7 cups
	Golden Rice 2	227 (dry)	1.2 cups (dry)
	Red Palm Oil	9 – 11	0.6-0.8 Tbsp
Pregnant Females (14+)	Mango	282	1.7 cups
	Sweet potato	174(canned) 78 (baked) 98 (boiled)	0.2 - 0.8 cups
	Golden rice 2	244 (dry)	1.3 cups (dry)
	Red Palm Oil	10 – 12	0.7-0.9 Tbsp
Lactating Females (14+)	Mang	464	2.2 cups
	Sweet potato	286 (canned) 162 (boiled) 128 (baked)	0.5 – 1.1 cups
	Golden rice	390 (dry)	2 cups (dry)
	Red Palm Oil	16-21	1.1-1.5 Tbsp

*Assumes high and comparable bioavailability of beta-carotene, conversion ratio of beta-carotene to VA set at 12:1. †Estimated serving amounts gathered by data from USDA Nutrient Database for Standard Reference, Release 21, 2008

Table 3 compares the amounts of beta-carotene-rich food needed to maintain VA status in people at various life stages. As can be seen, only small amounts of red palm oil or orange-fleshed sweet potato are necessary at any life stage. Average mangos (46 – 40 RAE per 100 gm edible portion) would not be a practical method for achieving VA sufficiency, since a 1-3 yr old child would have to consume about 6 cups of mangos (3 mangos) per day to maintain VA status. Therefore, we have used the high RAE *Mangifera indica Badami;* Veda et al 2007*)* in our calculations. Even for this high VA cultivar, mangos would have to become a significant part of the diet if it were to be the sole source of VA in the diet.

Red palm oil (*Arecaceae Elaeis*)

Red palm oil has perhaps the most potential for ameliorating or preventing VAD because of its high concentration and high bioavailability of beta-carotene (Tables 2 and 3). Its red color comes from its high content of beta-carotene, although when it is boiled for a few minutes it becomes colorless because the carotenoids are destroyed. Palm oil is a very common vegetable oil with unusually high saturated fat content, derived from the fruit of the *Arecaceae Elaeis* oil palm. It is perhaps the most widely produced edible oil in the world (FAOPRODSTAT Crops 2007), and is used for making fatty foods and snacks as well as cooking oil. In its unprocessed form it is used extensively for cooking in Africa. However, in most applications it is processed, and the red color and carotenoid content are removed Hussein et al 2001). Therefore, this oil is listed as having no VA content in the United States (United States Department of Agriculture 2008).

Red palm oil is extensively grown in Southern Asia, particularly in Malaysia and Indonesia, and also in West Africa and Columbia. In West Africa, oil palms are grown by small farmers, and local populations obtain significant amounts of VA from this food (Buerkle 2003). Several small scale interventions have successfully used red palm oil, or red palm oil baked into biscuits, to increase VA status in African pregnant women (Mahapatra and Manorama 1997; Radhika et al 2003; and to a lesser extent Lietz et al 2001) and African school children (van Stuijvenberg et al 2001). The United Nations Food and Agriculture program and other non-governmental organizations (NGOs) are encouraging small farmers across Africa to grow palm oil, because the crop offers opportunities to improve both nutrition and incomes (Buerkel 2003; Nestel and Naluboal 2003).

Malaysia and Indonesia account for roughly 90% of both global production and global trade in palm oil (Table 4), with Columbia and several West African countries also producing much of the remainder. However, in Malaysia, Indonesia and Columbia most palm oil is not used as a food or cooking oil. Instead, it is used in soaps and personal care products, and more recently for biofuel. In fact, its major use world-wide is now in biofuel production.

The use of red palm oil as a biofuel is controversial, with important environmental groups claiming that the damage caused by its production for biofuel is more destructive to the environment than the benefits gained by using biofuel (Greenpeace 2007, Friends of the Earth International 2008, but see Basiron 2008). Specifically, its production is blamed for deforestation, the loss of peat beds, and is estimated to contribute as much as 4% to global warming. Furthermore, the burgeoning market in biofuel has apparently led to price increases for grains and oils that are a problem for low income populations (Rosen and Shapouri 2008; FAOSTAT 2008). In addition, the use of palm oil as biofuel has been criticized as potentially leading to more dependence on export markets and concerns regarding the social and environmental sustainability of production expansion. Recently, this controversy appears to be resulting in some efforts to decrease the environmental impact of palm oil growth and production (Young 2008, Crowley 2008).

Table 4. Palm fruit oil – Area harvested, yield, and production, 2007. Major producers, plus United States. FAO ProdSTAT Crops 2007.

Country	Area Harvested Hectares	Country	Yield Hg/ha	Country	Production Metric Tons
Indonesia	4,580,000	Cameroon	224,138	Indonesia	78,000,000
Malaysia	3,790,000	Malaysia	205,013	Malaysia	77,700,000
Nigeria	3,150,000	Indonesia	170,306	Nigeria	8,500,000
Ghana	300,000	China	138,541	Ghana	1,900,000
Congo, Dem. Republic	170,000	Brazil	103,509	Cameroon	1,300,000
Cameroon	58,000	Congo, Dem. Republic	64,705	Congo, Dem. Republic	1,100,000
Brazil	57,000	Ghana	63,333	China	665,000
China	48,000	Nigeria	26,984	Brazil	590,000
U.S.	No data	U.S.	No data	U.S.	No data

Orange-Fleshed Sweet Potatoes (*Ipomoea batatas*)

Sweet potatoes (*Ipomoea batatas*) are an important root vegetable, a staple crop in some regions. Per-capita production is greatest in countries where sweet potatoes are a staple food, such as the Solomon Islands (160 kg/person/year), Burundi (130 kg/person/year), and Uganda (100 kg/person/year). There are many varieties of sweet potato, some of which are white and which contain very little pro-VA (Stapleton 2008). However, orange-fleshed sweet potatoes (OFSP) are a rich source of carotenoids and have been used successfully to improve VA status in several populations (Haskell et al 2004, Low et al 2007; van Jaarsveld 2005). The major sweet potato producers are shown in Table 5.

Since white-fleshed sweet potatoes are produced and eaten by the people of many countries with low VA status, it is probable that increasing the VA content of these potatoes could help prevent VAD (Low et al 2007). Projects to increase the availability of OFSP have been implemented especially in Africa. For example, The International Potato Center (CIP) has developed about 40 new OFSP varieties with resistance to viruses. The VA Partnership for Africa (VITAA) is promoting the increased production and use of OFSP in partnership with more than 70 agencies from the health, nutrition, and agricultural sectors in ten countries in sub-Saharan Africa (Mwaniki 2007).

China produces that most sweet potatoes (by far) in the world; Nigeria, Uganda, Indonesia, and Vietnam follow (Table 5). Israel, although not a large producer of sweet potatoes, has had the highest yields for the last 7 years, with results that suggest that better breeding, cultivating and storage practices could increase OFSP yields and VA availability for major producers in Africa who adopt their practices.

Table 5. Major Sweet Potato Producers – Area Harvested, Production, and Yield, 2007. FAO ProdSTAT Crops 2007.

Country	Area Harvested Hectares	Country	Yield hg/ha	Country	Production Metric Tons
China	4,761,003	Israel	358,209	China	102,240,110
Nigeria	1,030,000	Egypt	295,455	Nigeria	3,490,000
Uganda	578,000	Japan	243,902	Uganda	2,602,000
Tanzania	505,000	China	214,744	Indonesia	1,829,042
Viet Nam	180,000	U.S.	212,127	Viet Nam	1,450,000
Indonesia	173,179	Indonesia	105,616	Japan	1,000,000
Rwanda	158,000	India	89,908	India	980,000
Burundi	125,000	Viet Nam	80,555	Tanzania	960,000
U.S.	39,456	Burundi	66,800	U.S.	836,970

OFSP grow well in many soils and farming conditions and have few natural enemies so pesticides are rarely needed. Properly cured sweet potatoes can be kept for up to a year under certain controlled conditions (Ray and Ravi 2005) As with red palm oil, however, most OFSP are not used for human food. Instead, approximately 60% is used animal food, mainly as pig feed (in China) or chicken feed (in Africa; FAOSTAT 2007). Furthermore, and similar to the case of red palm oil, China is starting to focus on using sweet potatoes as biofuel (Biopact Team 2007).

Mangoes (*Mangifera indica*)

Mangoes are fruit tree grown in frost-free climates, mainly tropical, with over 1,000 cultivars. Although their perishability, short season, and relatively low beta-carotene content would at first seem to make them unlikely candidates for VA interventions, they have been used successfully and are popular because they are sweet and acceptable to children. Also, unlike orange fleshed sweet potatoes and especially red palm oil, they as yet are used mainly for human food. India produces 50% of world's supply (Sauco 2004; United States Department of Agriculture 2005; Table 6). Unfortunately, because of their short shelf life and growing season, many mango farmers receive a low price for their produce, and India accounts for less than one percent of the global mango trade because Indian farmers have little access to foreign markets.

Mangos have been tested in several intervention studies, presumably because they are a most popular fruit enjoyed by children in tropical countries (Goudo et al 2007; Nana et al 2006). However, mangos contain far less beta-carotene then red palm oil or sweet potatoes (Tables 2 and 3). Mango production suffers from fruit rotting due to post-harvest diseases during ripening, which reduce fruit quality and cause severe losses. Furthermore, mangos are relatively expensive, with high import/export costs, short ripening seasons, and susceptibility to chilling injury (Gomez-Lim 1993, Diedhiou et al 2007). These considerations make mangos a poor choice for nutrient interventions, although they have great potential as nutritious snacks.

Table 6. Mango Producers - Area Harvested, Yield, and Total Production in 2007 (includes mangosteens and guavas). Major producers, plus United States. FAO ProdSTAT Crops 2007.

Country	Area harvested hectares	Country	Yield hg/ha	Country	Production Metric Tons
India	2,143,000	Brazil	172,160	India	13,501,000
China	445,000	Pakistan	104,651	China	3,752,000
Thailand	285,000	Egypt	103,226	Pakistan	2,250,000
Indonesia	266,000	Mexico	102,500	Mexico	2,050,000
Pakistan	215,000	China	84,314	Thailand	1,800,000
Mexico	200,000	Thailand	63,157	Indonesia	1,620,000
Philippines	181,000	India	63,000	Brazil	1,546,000
Nigeria	126,500	Indonesia	60,902	Philippines	975,000
U.S.	675	U.S.	43,703	U.S.	2,950

Golden rice (*Oryza sativa*)

Golden rice was the first example of a genetically engineered plant developed as a fortified food (Potkyrus 2001, Anderson et al 2004). Golden rice is produced through genetic engineering to form beta-carotene in the edible parts of rice. Originally it produced relatively small amounts of beta-carotene, but was re-engineered in 2005 to form a new variety (Golden Rice 2, GR2) that produces about 23X more beta-carotene than the original variety (Paine et al 2005). A simplified diagram showing the genes that are transformed in Golden rice is given in Figure 2.

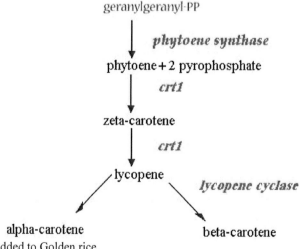

Figure 2. The genes added to Golden rice.

Golden rice was meant to replace rice in areas where there is a shortage of dietary VA, since polished white rice contains essentially no VA. Golden rice was developed for humanitarian purposes as a nutritional intervention and its inventors spearheaded considerable efforts to have golden rice distributed without need to pay royalties to subsistence farmers earning less than $10,000 per year (Potkyrus 2001). There is no fee for the use of Golden rice by these small farmers, and farmers are permitted to keep and replant seed. Initially, Golden rice was touted as having great potential to prevent VAD (Dawe et al 2002; Stein et al 2006). Golden rice was created by introducing two beta-carotene biosynthesis genes (Figure 2).

Golden Rice 1

psy (phytoene synthase) from daffodil (*Narcissus pseudonarcissus*)
crt1 from the soil bacterium *Erwinia uredovora*

Golden Rice 2

psy (phytoene synthase) from maize (*Zea mays*)

Even so, it met strong opposition from environmental and anti-globalization activists and is not now available for human consumption. In particular, Greenpeace opposes the introduction of any genetically modified organisms (GMOs), and has led a very successful campaign against Golden rice in the belief that it is a Trojan horse that will open the door to more widespread use of GMOs (Greenpeace 2005).

Table 7. Major Rice Producers, Area Harvested, Yield, and Total Production in 2007. Major producers, plus United States. FAO ProdSTAT Crops 2007.

Country	Area Harvested Hectares	Country	Yield hg/ha	Country	Production Metric Tons
India	44,000,000	Egypt	99,721	China	187,040,000
China	29,495,000	U.S.	80,538	India	141,134,000
Indonesia	12,165,607	China	63,414	Bangladesh	43,504,000
Bangladesh	11,200,000	Korea, Republic of	62,731	Viet Nam	35,566,800
Thailand	10,360,000	Viet Nam	48,688	Thailand	27,879,000
Viet Nam	7,305,000	Indonesia	46,893	Philippines	16,000,000
Philippines	4,250,000	Bangladesh	38,842	Brazil	11,079,849
Nigeria	3,000,000	Brazil	38,190	U.S.	8,956,450
U.S.	1,112,076	Korea, Dem. People's Republic	37,652	Pakistan	8,300,000

Further arguments against Golden rice were that by focusing on a narrow problem (VA deficiency), Golden rice advocates were obscuring the larger issue of a lack of widespread inexpensive diverse and nutritionally adequate sources of food, and that the introduction of monocultures such as Golden rice have actually increased malnutrition among the poor.

Finally, environmental organizations worried about the possible spread of the genetic engineered substitutions to native rice and other grains, since this migration can occur in wild-type varieties (Chen et al 2004).

Table 7 shows rice production. As can be clearly seen, rice is a widely grown, immensely popular staple crop that is prevalent in areas with VAD. If Golden rice ever replaced a significant fraction of white rice in the diet, then it has the potential for improving VA status for millions of people. At present, however, its potential impact, if any, is still years away, and many prominent NGOs and governmental agencies are developing programs that do not rely on GMOs. Research on Golden rice continues: it has been bred with local rice cultivars in the Philiprpines, Taiwan and with the American rice variety *Cocodrie*. The first field trials of these Golden rice cultivars were conducted by Louisiana State University Agricultural Center (Datta et al 2007). However, several important initiatives (such as Harvest Plus) that attempt to prevent VAD have chosen to avoid GMOs, focusing instead on conventional crops (Enserink 2008).

Best Food Sources of Beta-carotene, based on Production Estimates

We evaluated red palm oil, orange-fleshed sweet potatoes, mangos, and Golden rice for their potential to provide VA, using data from Tables 3 to 7. First, we estimated the production of each beta-carotene rich food required to supply VA requirement to one average person at risk for VAD as roughly 100 kg mangos, 40 kg orange-fleshed sweet potato, 2 kg red palm oil, and 75 kg Golden rice. Assuming that 1 billion people are at risk for VAD that means that 100 million metric tons of mangos, 40 million metric tons of orange-fleshed sweet potato, 2 million metric tons of red palm oil, and 75 million metric tons of Golden rice would have to be produced and distributed per year.

Thus, the amount of red palm oil needed per person is small and supplies of palm oil are ample, if palm oil were prepared so that it retained VA, or if the VA now removed from palm oil during production were extracted and used for human consumption. On the other hand, it is difficult to construct a scenario where mangos could realistically be the major source of VA for the world's population. The amounts of mango required per person is very high and production rather low.

Orange fleshed sweet potatoes probably could not supply VA requirements now, since much of the sweet potatoes currently produced are not orange and contain little VA. Furthermore, a significant percentage of world-wide production would have to be used to provide VA for 1 billion people, instead of food for pigs and chickens or biofuel. However, higher yielding varieties of OFSP with greater VA content are being developed and used. OFSP have potential for being a major source of VA in the future, especially in Africa. Finally, Golden rice might also be able to supply enough VA, but only if it a significant percentage of the population at risk for VAD adopted it and substituted it for white rice in their diets: it would have to become about 14% of the world's rice production at its current concentration of beta-carotene. Since Golden rice is engineered, however, it is quite possible that higher yields of beta-carotene are obtainable—and it is unlikely that Golden rice would be diverted for fuel.

Data on Current Impact of Food-based Interventions

Obviously, it would be interesting to determine if any country has been successful in improving VA status though food-based interventions on a large scale. Unfortunately, few countries with VAD have attempted to survey and document changes in the percentage of people with VAD or to estimate VA status on a national level (World Health Organization 2007) over time. Even fewer have documented VAD using adequate sample sizes and consistent methods. For example, there is little recent national data for Indonesia and Malaysia, two countries with VA supplementation programs which have seen a surge in the production and export of red palm oil. Furthermore, there is very little data linking changes in dietary intakes, especially of individual beta-carotene rich foods that might be useful in food-based interventions to increase VA status.

Bangladesh is a rare exception: they have published national surveys regularly since 1990, and more erratically since 1975. Furthermore, they have used at least one common measure (the presence of current xeropthalmia) consistently as a measure of VAD. Their records show that VAD persists in Bangladesh, but that efforts to monitor and eradicate it have had some success, with a substantial decline between 1995 and 2006. The decline even in this impoverished nation is heartening, and shows that VAD can be reduced when resources and education are used appropriately. However, this decline could not be linked to dietary interventions with red palm oil, orange-fleshed sweet potatoes, or mangos, although information about successful small-scale interventions may have increased dietary intakes of these foods.

The data also suggests that VA status has improved substantially in both Indonesia and Malaysia over the last 40 years, with both countries improving from having severe risks for marginal deficiency (estimated through serum retinol concentrations or corneal lesions) to mild risks (World Health Organization 2007; Khor 2005; Pangaribuan et al 2003, Sitorus et al 2007). However, these improvements are attributed to vitamin supplement capsule distribution programs as well as to general economic development. Thus no evidence that their mass production of red palm oil has directly resulted in improved VA status exists.

WHO data for India are sparse, and show no effect of mango production, which is understandable given the short growing season and short shelf-life of this intervention. However, in the case of India much more relevant data are referenced in Stein (Stein et al 2006) supplemental materials. Again, this data has shown a substantial reduction of VAD over the past 30 years despite the poor coverage of its supplementation programs, but there is insufficient data to link it to any crop-based intervention. Indeed, data from India suggest that implementing any intervention to diminish VAD may be very difficult, since its long-term VA supplementation program has still reached only a fraction of the children that are at risk for VAD (Stein et al 2006).

Although several promising food-based intervention programs have begun in Africa, there is again no data suggesting that these programs have had an impact on a national level. Furthermore, VAD in Africa has not received much long-term attention and study. Thus, there is currently no data suggesting that any food-based intervention has increase VA status on a national or international level, but there is substantial data suggesting that improving diets or economic status has decreased VAD in several Asian countries.

Discussion

VAD is a serious health problem for much of the developing world, especially in Southern Asia and Sub-Saharan Africa (Figure 1). It is a leading cause of blindness, morbidity, and mortality especially to small children and pregnant and lactating women and is responsible for millions of DALYs lost to those countries (Stein et al 2006). Although VAD is usually prevented by distributing high-dose supplement capsules of purified VA, it could be prevented in most people by increasing the availability and consumption of fruits and vegetables rich in pro-VA. Indeed, small scale interventions using fruits and vegetables that are rich sources of pro-VA carotenoids (especially beta-carotene, but also alpha-carotene and beta-cryptoxanthin) have successfully increased VA in several populations in African and Southern Asia. However, translating these small-scale interventions to national and international programs will require planning, work, and a good appreciation of the economic and environmental issues involved in growing and distributing large quantities of crops for food-based interventions.

In comparing Golden rice, mangoes, sweet potatoes, and palm oil as potential food sources for VA, we used a combination of agricultural, population, and consumption factors to evaluate their potential as a VA source. Although each country with VAD has unique environmental circumstances and nutritional needs, it appears that red palm oil could be the best individual food source for beta-carotene, and thus VA in most countries if it were produced to retain its VA and a fraction of it was used for nutrient interventions instead of biofuel. Red palm oil is a highly available source of pro-VA carotenoids and has been successful in alleviating VAD in small scale interventions, and clearly palm oil is produced in large amounts in several countries with VAD. Although mangoes are grown in abundance in many tropical areas and are well-liked by most children, they cannot be recommended as a sole source of VA for most of the world. A possible exception is India, which is the largest world producer of mangoes.

Orange-fleshed sweet potatoes and Golden rice have potential as food sources of VA. China, Nigeria, and most countries in East and Southern Africa grow sweet potatoes, though not always in good yield. Overall, increasing yields and beta-carotene content in sweet potatoes would benefit most African and many South Asian countries and is well worth exploring. Golden rice also has potential, if it is successfully released.

However, environmental issues associated with Golden rice, palm oil, and even sweet potatoes serve as a reminder that producing large quantities of a single crop, even for nutritional and humanitarian purposes, is not a trivial undertaking. Such production impacts a variety of societal, social, economic, and health factors. Clearly, more research is needed to understand the potential impact of these interventions so that their benefits can be maximized and their negative impacts minimized.

References

Ahmed, F; Azim, A; Akhtarzzaman, M. VA deficiency in poor, urban, lactating women in Bangladesh: factors influencing VA status. *Public Health Nutrition,* 2002, 6, 447-452.

Anderson, K; Jackson, LA; Pohl Nielsen, C. Genetically modified rice adoption: implications for welfare and poverty alleviation. Policy Research Working Paper no. 3380. Washington DC. World Bank. 2004.

Basiron, TSD. Response to Friends of the Earth (FoE) report on Malaysian palm oil. Available from: URL: http://www.mpoc.org.my/envo_111108_01.asp. Accessed 2008/10/10.

Biopact Team. China mulls switch to non-food crops for biofuel. Available from: URL: http://biopact.com/2007/06/china-mulls-switch-to-non-food-crops.html. Accessed 2008/12/01.

Black, RE; Allen, RH; Bhutta, ZA; Caulfield, LE; de Onis, M; Ezatti, M; Mathers, C; Rivera, J. Maternal and child undernutrition: global and regional exposures and health consequences. *The Lancet,* 2008, 371, 243-260

Buerkel, T. Hybrid oil palms bear fruit in western Kenya: FAO project improves incomes and diets, and may reduce imports of food oil. Available from URL: http://www.fao.org/english/newsroom/field/2003/1103_oilpalm.htm. Accessed 2008/12/10.

Campbell. AA; Thorne-Lyman, A; Sun, K; de Pee, S; Kraemer, K; Moench-Pfanner, R; S Mayang; Akhter, N; Bloem, MW; Semba, RD. Greater household expenditures on fruits and vegetables but not animal source foods are associated with decreased risk of under-five child mortality among families in rural Indonesia. *Journal of Nutrition,* 2008, 138, 2244-2249.

Caritino. Caritino from nature to you. 2006. URL: http://www.carotino.com/21.html Accessed 2008/10/15.

Chen, LJ; Lee, DS; Song, ZP; Suh, HS; Lu, BR. Gene flow from cultivated rice (*Oryza sativa*) to its weedy and wild relatives. *Annals of Botany,* 2004, 93, 67-73.

Crowley, L. Unilever commits to sustainable palm oil. 2008. Available from: URL: http://www.foodnavigator.com/Financial-Industry/Unilever-commits-to-sustainable-palm-oil-05/02/2008. Accessed 2008/10/27.

Datta, SK; Datta, K; Parkhi, V; Rai, M; Baisakh, N; Sahoo, G; Rehana, S; Bandyopadhyay, A; Alamgir; Ali, S; Abrigo, E; Oliva, N; Torrizo, L. Golden rice: introgression, breeding, and field evaluation. *Euphytica,* 2007, 154, 271-278.

Dawe, D; Robertson, R; Unnevehr, L. Golden rice: what role could it play in alleviation of Vitamin A deficiency?, *Food Policy,* 2002, 27, 541-560.

Diedhiou, PM; Drame, A; Samb, PI. Alteration of post harvest diseases of mango *Mangifera indica* through production practices and climatic factors, *African Journal of Biotechnology,* 2007, 6, 1087-1097.

Enserink, M. Tough lessons from golden rice. *Science,* 2008, 320, 468-471.

Food and Agriculture Organization of the United Nations, FAOSTAT Production, ProdSTAT, Crops, 2007 Data. URL: http://faostat.fao.org/site/567/default.aspx#ancor. Accessed 2008/11/24.

Food and Agriculture Organization of the United Nations, FAOSTAT, Consumption, Crops Primary Equivalent, FAO, 2008. URL: http://faostat.fao.org/site/535/default.aspx#ancor. Accessed 2008/11/22.

Food and Agriculture Organization of the United Nations, FAOTradeSTAT, Crops and Livestock Products, 2005 Data. URL: http://faostat.fao.org/site/535/default.aspx#ancor. Accessed 2008/11/21.

Food and Nutrition Board, Institute of Medicine, National Academy of Science, Dietary Reference Intakes (DRIs): Recommended Intakes for Individuals, Vitamins. Washington, DC. 2004.

Friends of the Earth International. Malaysian palm oil greenwash report. Available from: URL: http://www.foei.org/en/media. Accessed 2008/12/06.

Gomez-Lim, MA. Mango fruit ripening: Physiology and molecular biology. *Acta Horticulture,* 1993, 341, 489-499.

Gouado, I; Schweigert, FJ; Ejoh, RA; Tchouanguep, MF; Camp, JV. Systemic levels of carotenoids from mangoes and papaya consumed in three forms (juice, fresh and dry slice). *European Journal of Clinical Nutrition,* 2007, 61, 1180-1188

Greenpeace. Failures of Golden Rice: all glitter, no gold. Available from URL: http://www.greenpeace.org/international/news/failures-of-golden-rice. Accessed 2008/11/30.

Greenpeace. Palm oil: Cooking the Climate. Available from: URL: http://www.greenpeace. org/international/news/palm-oil_cooking. Accessed 2008/11/12.

Haskell, MJ; Jamil, KM; Hassan, F; Peerson, JM; Hossain, MI; Fuchs, GJ; Brown, KH. Daily consumption of Indian spinach (Basella alba) or sweet potatoes has a positive effect on total-body vitamin A stores in Bangladeshi men. *American Journal of Clinical Nutrition,* 2004, 80, 705-714. Comment in: *American Journal of Clinical Nutrition,* 2005, 81, 943-935, author reply 945-946.

Haskell, MJ; Pandey, P; Graham, JM; Peerson, JM; Shrestha, RK; Brown KH. Recovery from impaired dark adaptation in nightblind pregnant Nepali women who receive small daily doses of vitamin A as amaranth leaves, carrots, goat liver, vitamin A-fortified rice, or retinyl palmitate. *American Journal of Clinical Nutrition,* 2005, 81, 461-471.

Hussein, MZB; Kuang, D; Zaina, Z; Teck, TK. Kaolin–carbon adsorbents for carotene removal of red palm oil. *Journal of Colloid and Interface Science,* 2001, 235, 93-100.

Khor, GL. Micronutrient status and intervention programs in Malaysia. *Food and Nutrition Bulletin,* 2005, 26, Suppl 2, S281-285.

Lietz, G; Henry, CJ; Mulokozi, G; Mugyabuso, JK; Ballart, A; Ndossi, GD; Lorri, W; Tomkins, A. Comparison of the effects of supplemental red palm oil and sunflower oil on maternal vitamin A status. *American Journal of Clinical Nutrition,* 2001, 74, 501-509.

Low, JW; Arimond, M; Osman, N; Cunguara, B; Zano, F; Tschirley, D. A food-based approach introducing orange-fleshed sweet potatoes increased vitamin A intake and serum retinol concentrations in young children in rural Mozambique. *Journal of Nutrition,* 2007, 137, 1320-1327.

Mahapatra, S; Manorama, R. The protective effect of red palm oil in comparison with massive vitamin A dose in combating vitamin A deficiency in Orissa, India. *Asia Pacific Journal of Clinical Nutrition,* 1997, 6, 246-250.

Matsuda-Inoguchi, N; Date, C; Sakurai, K; Kuwazoe, M; Watanabe, T; Toji, C; Furukawa, Y; Shimbo, S; Nakatsuka, H; Ikeda, M. Reduction in estimated vitamin A intake induced by new food composition tables in Japan, where vitamin A is taken mostly from plant foods. *International Journal of Food Science and Nutrition,* 2006, 57, 279-291.

Mudur, G. Deaths trigger fresh controversy over vitamin A programme in India. *British Medical Journal,* 2001, 323, 1206.

Mwaniki, A. Biofortification as a vitamin A deficiency intervention in Kenya. Ithica NY: Cornell Univeristy, 2007.

Nana, CP; Brouwer, ID; Zagré, NM; Kok, FJ; Traoré AS. Impact of promotion of mango and liver as sources of vitamin A for young children: a pilot study in Burkina Faso. *Public Health Nutrition*, 2006, 9, 808-813.

Nestel, P; Nalubola, R. Red Palm Oil is a Feasible and Effective Alternative Source of Dietary vitamin A , ILSI Human Nutrition Institute, Washington DC, 2003.

Paine, JA; Chaggar, S; Howells, RM; Kennedy, MJ; Vernon, G; Wright, SY; Hinchliffe, E; Adams, JL; Silverstone, AL; Drake, R. Improving the nutritional value of Golden Rice through increased pro-vitamin A content. *Nature Biotechnology,* 2005, 23: 482-487.

Pangaribuan, R; Erhardt, JG; Scherbaum, V; Biesalski, HK. Vitamin A capsule distribution to control vitamin A deficiency in Indonesia: effect of supplementation in pre-school children and compliance with the programme. *Public Health Nutrition* 2003, 6, 209-216.

Potrykus, I. Golden Rice and beyond. *Plant Physiology,* 2001, 125, 1157-1161

Radhika, MS; Bhaskaram, P; Balakrishna, N; Ramalakshmi, BA. Red palm oil supplementation: a feasible diet-based approach to improve the vitamin A status of pregnant women and their infants. *Food and Nutrition Bulletin,* 2003, 24, 208-217.

Ray, RC; Ravi, V. Post harvest spoilage of sweet potato in tropics and control measures. *Critical Reviews of Food Science and Nutrition*, 2005, 45, 623-644

Rodriquez-Amaya, DB. Assessment of the provitamin A contents of foods - the Brazilian experience. *Journal of Food Composition and Analysis,* 1996, 9, 196-230.

Rosen, S; Shapouri, S. Rising food prices intensify food insecurity in developing countries, *Amber Waves*, United States Department of Agriculture, 2008, 16-21.

Ruel, MT. Can food-based strategies help reduce vitamin A and iron deficiencies? A review of recent evidence. Washington, DC: International Food Policy Research Institute; 2001.

Sauco, VG. Mango production and world market: current situation and future prospects. *Proceedings of the 7th International Mango symposium*, 2004, ISHS, *Acta Horticulturae*, Belguim, 107-111.

Sitorus, RS; Abidin, MS; Prihartono, J. Causes and temporal trends of childhood blindness in Indonesia: study at schools for the blind in Java. *British Journal of Ophthalmology*, 2007, 91, 1109-1113.

Sommer, A; West, KP. Vitamin A deficiency: health, survival and vision. New York: Oxford University Press; 1996.

Stapleton P. Combating vitamin A deficiency with orange-fleshed sweet potato. 26 June, 2008. Biodiversity International, the International Plant Genetic Resources Institute (IPGRI) and the International Network for Improvement of Banana and Plantain (INIBAP). Available from: URL: http://www.bioversityinternational.org/index.php?id=21&tx_ttnews%5Btt_news%5D=560&tx_ttnews%5BbackPID%5D=%7Bpage:uid%7D&no_cache=1. Accessed 2008/10/27.

Stein, AJ; Qaim JV; Meenakshi P; Nestel P; Sachde HPS; Bhutta ZA. Analyzing the health benefits of biofortified staple crops by means of other disability adjusted life years approach. HarvestPlus Technical Monograph 4. Washington DC: International Food Policy Research Institute; 2005.

Stein, AJ; Sachdev, HPS; Qaim. M. Potential impact and cost-effectiveness of Golden Rice. *Nature Biotechnology*, 2006, 28, 1200-1201.

Strobel, M; Tinz, J; Biesalski, HK. The importance of beta-carotene as a source of vitamin A with special regard to pregnant and breastfeeding women. *European Journal of Nutrition*, 2007, 46 Suppl 1, 1-20.

United States Department of Agriculture, Agricultural Research Service, National Nutrient Database for Standard Reference, Release 21. 2008. URL: http://www.nal.usda.gov/fnic/foodcomp.html Accessed 2008/11/15. Accessed 2008/09/20.

United States Department of Agriculture, Economic Research Service. Mangoes: U.S. import-eligible countries; world production and exports, 2005. URL: www.ers.usda.gov/Data/FruitVegPhyto/Data/fr-mangoes.xls. Accessed 2008/11/01.

United States Department of Agriculture, Economic Research Service, IPC, Agricultural Projections to 2017, 2007. URL: www. ers.usda.gov/Publications/OCE081/OCE20081a.pdf. Accessed 2008/11/01.

van Jaarsveld, PJ; Faber, M; Tanumihardjo, SA; Nestel, P; Lombard, CJ; Benadé, AJ. Beta-carotene-rich orange-fleshed sweet potato improves the vitamin A status of primary school children assessed with the modified-relative-dose-response test. *American Journal of Clinical Nutrition*, 2005, 81, 1080-1087.

van Stuijvenberg, ME; Dhansay, MA; Lombard, CJ; Faber, M; Benadé, AJ. The effect of a biscuit with red palm oil as a source of beta-carotene on the vitamin A status of primary school children: a comparison with beta-carotene from a synthetic source in a randomized controlled trial. *European Journal of Clinical Nutrition*, 2001, 55, 657-662.

Veda, S; Platel, K; Srinivasan, K. Varietal differences in the bioaccessibility of beta-carotene from mango (Mangifera indica) and papaya (Carica papaya) fruits. *Journal of Agricultural and Food Chemistry*, 2007, 55, 7931-7935.

West, KP Jr; Katz, J; Khatry, SK; LeClerq, SC; Pradhan, EK; Shrestha, SR; Connor, PB; Dali, SM; Christian, P; Pokhrel, RP; Sommer, A. Double blind, cluster randomized trial of low dose supplementation with vitamin A or beta carotene on mortality related to pregnancy in Nepal. *British Medical Journal*, 1999, 318, 570-575. Comments in: *British Medical Journal*, 1999, 318, 551-552; *British Medical Journal*, 1999, 319, 1201-1203; author reply *British Medical Journal*, 1999, 319, 1203.

West, KP Jr; Sommer A. Vitamin A programme in Assam probably caused hysteria. *British Medical Journal*, 2002, 324, 791.

World Health Organization. Vitamin and mineral requirements in human nutrition. 2004. 2nd ed. Vitamin A. Available from URL: http://wholibdoc.who.int/publication/2004/9241546123-chap2.pdf. Accessed 2008/11/19.

World Health Organization. WHO global database on vitamin A deficiency. Vitamin and Mineral Nutrition Information System. Updated 2007-08-09. Bangladesh. China. India. Indonesia. Malaysia. Nigeria. Tanzania. URL: http://www.who.int/VMNIS/vitamina/data/en/indexhtml. Accessed 2008/11/19.

Young, T. First batch of "sustainable" palm oil on way to UK – but environmental standards are still not rigorous enough, claims Greenpeace Available from URL: http://www.businessgreen.com/business-green/news/2230512/first-batch-sustainable-palm. Accessed 2008/12/12.

In: Encyclopedia of Vitamin Research
Editor: Joshua T. Mayer

ISBN 978-1-61761-928-1
© 2011 Nova Science Publishers, Inc.

Chapter 31

β-Carotene Production under Greenhouse Conditions[*]

Ramón Gerardo Guevara-González[†], Irineo Torres-Pacheco,
Enrique Rico-García, Rosalía Virginia Ocampo-Velázquez,
Adán Mercado-Luna, Rodrigo Castañeda-Miranda,
Luis Octavio Solís-Sánchez, Daniel Alaniz-Lumbreras,
Roberto Gómez-Loenzo, Gilberto Herrera-Ruíz
and Genaro Martin Soto-Zarazúa

Facultad de Ingeniería, Universidad Autónoma de Querétaro,
Centro Universitario Cerro de las Campanas, S/N, Colonia Las Campanas,
C.P. 76010, Santiago de Querétaro, Querétaro, México

Abstract

β-carotene is a secondary metabolite that is a hydrocarbon carotene predominantly located in lower concentrations in PS II functioning as a helper to harvest light pigment during photosynthesis and to dissipate excess energy before damage occurs. As other carotenes, β-carotene is uniquely synthesized in plants, algae, fungi and bacteria. β-carotene is the main diet precursor of pro-vitamin A. Additionally, β-carotene serves as an essential nutrient and is in high demand in the market as a natural food colouring agent, as an additive to cosmetics and also as a health food. Several approaches have been carried out in order to increase β-carotene production in algae, bacteria, fungi and plants using biotechnological and engineering focuses. In the case of plants, such species

---

[*] A version of this chapter was also published in *Beta Carotene: Dietary Sources, Cancer and Cognition, edited by Leiv Haugen and Terje Bjornson* published by Nova Science Publishers, Inc. It was submitted for appropriate modifications in an effort to encourage wider dissemination of research.

[†] Corresponding author: ramon.guevara@uaq.mx

as tomato have important β-carotene contents, which are theoretically amenable to management using approaches such as fertilization, growth conditions and mild stress. On the other hand, greenhouse structures can protect crops from wind and rain, and can also protect from insects when fitted with insect exclusion screens. β-carotene production could potentially be improved and enhanced in greenhouse conditions in plants as well as in algae, based on the exclusion of the structure, and the possibility of controlling aspects such as climate, fertilization and stress management, among others. Production of β-carotene (and other secondary metabolites) from several organisms in greenhouse conditions should be an interesting future approach, visualizing the greenhouse as a "factory" using frontier technologies such as biotechnology and mechatronics in order to optimize this production.

Introduction

The bright colours found in nature and the molecules that cause them have always fascinated organic chemists. The earliest studies on carotenoids date back to the beginning of the nineteenth century. β-carotene was first isolated by Wackenroder in 1831, and many other carotenoids were discovered and named during the 1800s, although their structures were still unknown. Not until 1907 was the empirical formula of β-carotene, $C_{40}H_{56}$, established by Willstatter and Mieg (Coultate, 1996). The structure was elucidated by Karrer in 1930–31, which was the first time that the structure of any vitamin or provitamin had been established, and he received a Nobel Prize for his work (Middleton et al., 2000). Steenbock suggested in 1919 that there could be a relationship between β-carotene and vitamin A. The concept of provitamins (molecules that are converted into vitamins by the body) was entirely new, and proved to have great significance scientifically and commercially (Coultate, 1996). The first total syntheses of β-carotene were achieved in 1950; various studies were carried out throughout the 1970s–80s to determine its suitability for use in food and its activity in the body. In the early 1980s it was suggested that β-carotene might be useful in preventing cancer, and it was found to be an antioxidant (Burton and Ingold, 1984; Aggarwal et al., 2008). More recently, β-carotene has been claimed to prevent a number of diseases, including several types of cancer, cystic fibrosis and arthritis, and there is a flourishing trade in vitamin supplements containing β-carotene (Coultate, 1996; Middleton et al., 2000; Czeczuga et al., 2007; Veloz-García et al., 2004; Guevara-González et al., 2006; Guzmán-Maldonado & Mora-Avilés, 2006; Aggarwal et al., 2008; Marín-Martínez et al., 2009).

Carotenoids are lipid-soluble yellow, orange and red pigments that are uniquely synthesized in plants, algae, fungi and bacteria (Sandmann, 2001). They are secondary plant compounds that are divided into two groups: the oxygenated xanthophylls such as lutein (3R, 3'R, 6'R β,β-carotene-3,3'diol) and zeaxanthin (3, 3'R-β,β-carotene-3,3'diol) and the hydrocarbon carotenes such as β-carotene (β-β-carotene), α-carotene (6'R,β,β-carotene), and lycopene (Ψ,Ψ-carotene) (Zaripheh and Erdman, Jr., 2002). Carotenoid C_{40} biosynthesis is a branch of the isoprenoid pathway. To begin the process of biosynthesis, isoprene (2-methyl-1,3-butadiene; C_5) is converted into isopentenyl diphosphate (IPP; C_5) which then in turn is converted into dimethylallyl diphosphate (DMAPP; C_5) (see Figure 1). Combining four DMAPP molecules together results in the formation of geranylgeranyl pyrophosphate (GGPP). The first step considered as part of carotenoid biosynthesis is the condensation of two molecules of the C_{20} GGPP to form the first C_{40} carotenoid, phytoene. Desaturation of phytoene then produces in sequence four acyclic compounds: phytofluene, ζ-carotene, neurosporene and lycopene. Cyclization of lycopene can occur on one end, producing monocyclic γ-carotene or δ-carotene, or to both ends, producing dicyclic α-carotene or β-carotene. Further modification of the pathway can occur with the addition of oxygen functions in the form of hydroxyl, epoxide or keto groups, resulting in the xanthophylls. The carotenoid pathway can be further modified with other structural end groups, such as esterification. Approximately 700 different types of carotenoids have been discovered and characterized (Baransky et al., 2005; Beyer et al., 2002; Hornero-Mendez and Britton, 2002; Niyogi et al., 2001). β-carotene functions in several organisms as an osmotic regulator, protector against irradiance stress, antioxidant agent, and accessory pigment in photosynthesis, among others. In order to increase the carotenoids, especially β-carotene, several approaches have been carried out, including transgenic organisms, gene silencing strategies and fermentation technologies (Diretto et al., 2007; Nanou et al., 2007). Another interesting and promising possibility in this sense is the use of mechatronic methodologies in order to phytomonitor and optimize crop production, especially under greenhouse conditions (van Henten and Bonsema, 1995; Schmitd, 2005; Castañeda et al., 2006). Thus, several strategies, such as process automation (plant nutrition, climate control, light quality, pest and pathogen detection, etc.), sensor development, image analysis of crop and fruit development, among others, together with biotechnological approaches, will promote reaching higher β-carotene (and other secondary metabolites) production in living systems under protected environments such as greenhouses. Finally, understanding and controlling environmental and genetic factors that may contribute to the nutritional value of food (such as production of β-carotene in living systems) will therefore be important when making cultural management decisions in order to increase production.

Role of β-Carotene in Living Systems

Carotenoids are naturally-occurring pigments that are responsible for the different colours of fruits, vegetables and other plants (Ben-Amotz and Fishler, 1998; Raja et al., 2007). So far, more than 700 types of carotenoids have been reported in nature, and about 50 are provitamin-A, which includes α-carotene, β-carotene and β-cryptoxanthin (Faure et al., 1999; Raja et al., 2007). In plants, carotenoids play critical roles in both light harvesting and energy dissipation for the photosynthetic mechanism. Within the thylakoid membranes of chloroplast organelles, carotenoids are found bound to specific protein complexes of photosystem I (PSI) and photosystem II (PS II). β-carotene is the predominant carotenoid in PS I, while it is presented in lower concentrations in PS II (Demmig-Adams et al., 1996; Thayer and Bjorkman, 1992).

Within each photosystem, β-carotene is associated with antenna pigments and photosynthetic reaction centers (Peng and Gilmore, 2003; Taiz and Zaiger, 2003). In PS II complex, β-carotene is highly concentrated close to the reaction center (Niyogi et al., 1997). In humans, carotenoids have been associated with reduced risk of lung cancer and chronic eye diseases such as cataracts and age-related macular degeneration (Raja et al., 2007). Kale (*Brassicae oleraceae* L.) ranks highest and spinach (*Spinacia oleraceae* L.) ranks second among vegetable crops for the accumulation of the carotenoids lutein and β-carotene (Lefsrud, 2006). The results clearly indicate that increasing carotenoid level using different approaches in plants (i.e., spinach and tomato, among others) commonly consumed in the diet would impart health benefits without changing the dietary habits of individuals (Diretto et al., 2007). In the halotolerant microalgae *Dunaliella*, β-carotene production is enhanced as an environmental adaptation in which β-carotene and glycerol are produced in excess to maintain its osmotic balance in saline stress as well as in irradiance stress (Raja et al., 2007). In this latter case, *Dunaliella* produces β-carotene in excess to overcome irradiance stress and inhibits high photoinhibitory activity when blue light is used, intermediate with white and non-existent with red light (Ben-Amotz et al., 1989; Raja et al., 2007). In addition, β-carotene is a purported anticancer agent that is believed by some to have antioxidant action of a radical-trapping type. However, definitive experimental support for such action has been lacking. New experiments in vitro show that β-carotene belongs to a previously unknown class of biological antioxidants. Specifically, it exhibits good radical-trapping antioxidant behavior only at partial pressures of oxygen significantly less than 150 torr, the pressure of oxygen in normal air. Such low oxygen partial pressures are found in most tissues under physiological conditions. At higher oxygen pressures, β-carotene loses its antioxidant activity and shows an autocatalytic prooxidant effect, particularly at relatively high concentrations. Similar oxygen-pressure-dependent behavior may be shown by other compounds containing many conjugated double bonds (Burton and Ingold, 1984; Meyer et al., 2007; Guruvayoorappan and Kuttan, 2007). The potential ability of β-carotene as an antioxidant, immunomodulatory and anticancer agent led to more active research studies of its application for the prevention of human cancers. During recent years there have been reported elsewhere a myriad of papers in which β-carotene has generally been associated with reducing the risk of lung, gastric, brain and breast cancer, as well as Alzheimer's and heart diseases (Dai et al., 2006; Polus et al., 2006; Voutilanen et al., 2006; Larsson et al., 2007; Czeczuga et al., 2007; Aggarwal et al., 2008).

β-Carotene Production in Several Organisms

As mentioned elsewhere, β-carotene serves as an essential nutrient and is in high demand in the market as a natural food colouring agent, as an additive to cosmetics and also as a health food. It occurs naturally as its isomers, namely all-*trans* (Figure 2a), 9-*cis* (Figure 2b), 13-*cis* and 15-*cis* forms (Wang et al., 1994) and functions as an accessory light harvesting pigment, thereby protecting the photosynthetic apparatus against photo damage in all green plants, including algae (Ben-Amotz et al., 1987).

β-carotene, as a component of photosynthetic reaction centre is accumulated as lipid globules in the interthylakoid spaces of the chloroplasts in *Dunaliella* (Vorst et al., 1994). They protect the algae from damage obtained during excessive irradiances by preventing the formation of reactive oxygen species, by quenching the triplet-state chlorophyll or by reacting with singlet oxygen ($^1O_2$), and also, it acts as a light filter (Telfer, 2002). Only few reports are available on the enzymes and proteins involved in β-carotene regulation. In *Dunaliella*, β-carotene is accumulated into extraplastid lipid globules (García-González et al., 2005), which are stabilized and maintained by a peripherally associated 38 KD protein called carotene globule protein (CgP). Probably, CgP is involved in stabilizing the globules within chloroplast (Katz et al., 1995; Raja et al., 2007). Induction of CgP and deposition of triacylglycerol are in parallel with β-carotene accumulation (Raja et al., 2007). The biosynthetic pathway for β-carotene has been determined for fungi such as *Phycomyces blakesleeanus* and *Neurospora crassa* (Cerdá-Olmedo, 1987; Rodríguez-Sáiz et al., 2004). It contains three enzymatic activities: 1) phytoene synthase, which links two molecules of geranylgeranyl pyrophosphate to form phytoene; 2) phytoene dehydrogenase, which introduces four double bonds in the phytoene molecule to yield lycopene; and 3) lycopene cyclase, which sequentially converts the acyclic ends of lycopene to β-rings to form α-carotene and β-carotene. A similar biosynthetic pathway is known in all carotenogenic organisms (Lee and Schmidt-Dannert, 2002).

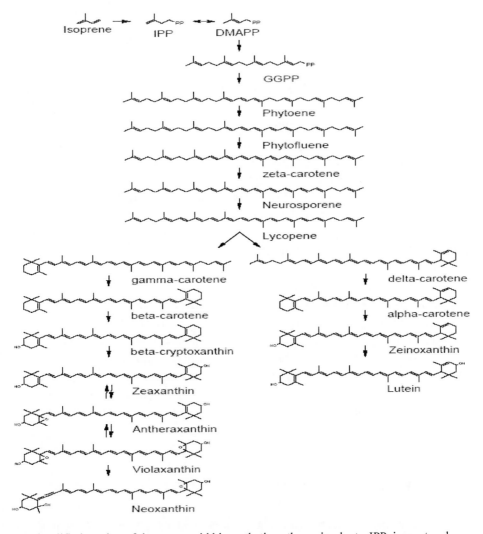

Figure 1. Simplified version of the carotenoid biosynthetic pathway in plants. IPP, isopentenyl diphosphate; DMAPP, dimethylallyl diphosphate; GGPP, geranylgeranyl pyrophosphate.

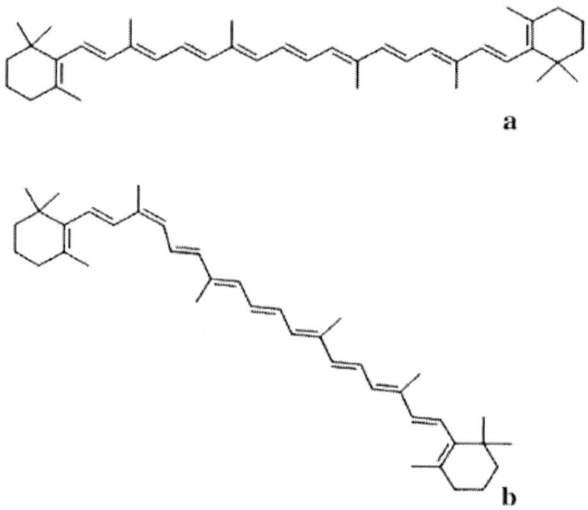

Figure 2. Chemical structures of β-carotene isomers. Panel a, 9-*cis*-b-carotene; Panel b, all-*trans*-β-carotene.

All-*trans* β-carotene is responsible for the light-yellow color of *Phycomyces blakesleeanus*, a heterothallic fungus of the class Zygomycetes and the order Mucorales (Cerdá-Olmedo, 1987; Mehta et al., 1997). In this fungus, many external factors influence the color of the mycelium because they activate or inhibit carotene biosynthesis. Among these factors, sexual stimulation, blue illumination, and the addition of retinol and dimethyl phthalate to the medium represent four separate mechanisms of activation (Mehta et al., 1997). In the red yeast *Xanthophyllomyces dendrorhous* (formerly named as *Phaffia rhodozyma*), β-carotene accumulates as an intermediary of the astaxanthin biosynthesis pathway (Girard et al., 1994; Verwaal et al., 2007). The genes involved in β-carotene production in *X. dendrorhous* have been cloned previously (Verdoes et al., 1999$_{a,b}$). Carotenogenesis in prokaryotes is constitutive or photoinducible. Several prokaryotes, including *Erwinia herbicola* and *Rhodobacter capsulatus* produce Carotenoids constitutively, whereas organisms such as *Myxococcus xanthus*, *Flavobacterium dehydrogenans* and *Sulfolobus* spp., produce carotenoids in a photoinducible manner (Armstrong et al., 1990$_{a,b}$; Burchard and Dworkin, 1966; Grogan, 1989; Weeks and Garner, 1967; Takano et al., 2005). The control mechanisms of carotenogenesis have been studied in phototrophic bacteria such as *Rhodobacter* spp., which revealed the involvement of global signal transduction initiated by light capture in the bacteriochlorophyll (Takano et al., 2005). On the other hand, the molecular mechanism in nonphototrophic bacteria has not yet been fully studied except in *M. xanthus*, a gram-negative gliding bacterium characterized by a unique life cycle (Takano et al., 2005).

Commercial Importance of β-Carotene

The market for ingredients basically found in the food and pharmaceutical area continues to grow much faster than related markets, such as those for feed or industrial chemicals. Examples of highly demanded ingredients are the carotenoids. For many years, the most prominent representative of carotenoids, β-carotene, was used as a food colorant.

Additionally, due to the antioxidative properties of carotenoids, this sector has become one of the fastest growing outlets for such products. In addition, the feed area still is a large sector, demanding all entire range of carotenoids to color fish, broilers and eggs. The worldwide market value of all commercially-used carotenoids was estimated at $887 million for 2004 and expected to rise at an average annual growth rate (AAGR) of 2.9% to just over $1 billion. Specifically, more recent data mentioned that the global market for carotenoids was $766 million in 2007. This is expected to increase to $919 million by 2015, a compound annual growth rate (CAGR) of 2.3% (bcc Research, March 2008; Figure 3). β-carotene has the largest share of the market. Valued at $247 million in 2007, this segment is expected to be worth $285 million by 2015, a CAGR of 1.8% (*Bussiness Wire, 2008; Focus on the Global Market for Carotenoids*).

As mentioned, carotenoids (including β-carotene) are an important group of natural pigments with specific applications as colorants, feed supplements and nutraceuticals; they are also used for medical, cosmetic and biotechnological purposes. A few of the variety of natural and synthetic carotenoids available have been exploited commercially, these includes β-carotene, lycopene, astaxanthin, canthaxanthin, lutein, annatto and capxanthin (Bhosale, 2004; Martín et al., 2008). Although more than 600 different Carotenoids have been described from carotenogenic microorganisms, only a few of them are produced industrially, and β-carotene is the most prominent (Rodríguez-Saíz et al., 2004). β-carotene is still the most prominent carotenoid used in foods and supplements, but due to a changing consumer perception, primarily in Europe, the product is suffering from natural replacements, specifically carrot juice, and market growth in the past few years was much lower than expected. In parallel, the number of producers of synthetic and algae derived β-carotene rose sharply, which added to the imbalance of supply and demand, driving prices down (*Bussiness Wire, 2008; Focus on the Global Market for Carotenoids*). Despite the mentioned before, based on data presented before, it is expected that β-carotene will continue to be the most prominent carotenoid in the market, with an increased value in the next years as the future market projections to the year 2015 (Figure 3).

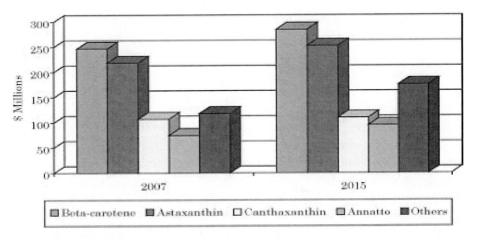

Figure 3. Global carotenoid market value by product 2007 and 2015 (USD $ millions). Source: bcc Research, 2008.

Increasing β-Carotene Production using Biotechnological Approaches

As it has been pointed out previously, the advent of biotechnology has brought the opportunity to accelerate the development of methodologies to investigate and clarify the biosynthesis pathways of carotenoids in general and in particular β-carotene (Umeno et al., 2005). The work and analysis of mutants was a key tool for rough outline of the biochemical reactions that constitute the biosynthetic pathway of carotenoids in the first half of the 1960s (Spurgeon and Porter, 1981). Characterization of biochemical reactions in the cell-free systems and in vivo using radiolabeled precursors generated important information and more details were known. However, it was only possible to capitalize on the knowledge acquired until relevant enzymes involved were identified (Dogbo and Camara, 1987). A concomitant use of this knowledge and the tools of biotechnology have generated methods to increase the amount of β-carotene that occurred in some systems or to produce it in significant levels in biological systems in which this compound is normally not produced (Ye et al., 2000; Kim., et al., 2006; Diretto et al., 2007). Some biotechnological approaches that have been used in order to increase β-carotene contents are the following:

a. Induction of Mutations

One way for increasing the quantity of β-carotene in fungi has been through mutations. As early as 1976, even with emerging knowledge about the route of biosynthesis of carotenoids and the involved genes were reported encouraging results by inducing mutations in *Phycomyces blakesleeanus*. It was handled evidence that there were two genes involved; carS and carA, and β-carotene overproduction was associated with the induced mutation in carS (Murillo and Cerda-Olmedo, 1976). Recessive carS gene mutations abolished the end product regulation of the pathway, and these strains could contain 2 to 5 mg of β-carotene per g of dry mycelium, that is, up to 100 times the wild-type level (Murillo et al., 1978).

b. Methods to Induce Mutations

The most common means to induce mutations have been: N-methyl-N'-nitro-N-nitrosogua-nidine, ethyl methanesulfonate and UV light (An et al., 1989). Nitrosoguanidine (N-methyl-N'-nitro-N-nitrosoguanidine) has been most frequently used for the induction of mutations in a lot of organisms (Gichner and Veleminsky, 1982). The mutations are preferentially produced in DNA regions being replicated at the time of the mutagen exposition in cases such as yeasts and bacteria (Cerda-Olmedo et al., 1968; Dawes, and Carter , 1974; Casadesus and Cerda Olmedo, 1985). In bacteria this results in relatively high rates of closely linked double mutants (Gichner and Veleminsky, 1982). The induction of mutations in bacteria and fungi also has been conducted with the use of UV radiation. However nitrosoguanidine is a more effective mutagen than UV radiation (Casadesus and Cerda Olmedo, 1985). Spores of *Phycomyces blakesleeanus* (strain NRRL 1555) at a concentration of 1 X 10^7 spores/mL were treated with 0.5 mg/mL of N-methyl-N-nitroso-N'-nitroguanidine in 0.2 M acetate buffer at pH 5 for 80 minutes at 220°C. The suspension was shaken occasionally to prevent the sedimentation of spores. The spores were washed and seeded at a concentration of 50 viable spores per petri dish on agar plates containing glucose-asparagine medium (1/7) supplemented with 0.1 % yeast extract (Meissner and Delbruck, 1968). Mutants were isolated after treatment with 100 ug of N-methyl-N'-nitro-N-nitrosoguanidine (NTG) per ml in pH 7.0 citrate-phosphate buffer, as previously described (Cerdá-Olmedo and Reau, 1970).

c. Microorganisms with Greater Success in the Production of β-carotene

Among the carotenoid-producing microorganisms, bacteria, filamentous fungi and unicellular algae have been extensively examined in order to evaluate their possible industrial interest. The most successful cases have been with the halophilic alga *Dunaliella*, phycomycetes fungi *Blakeslea trispora*, *Phycomyces blakesleeanus* (Ninet and Renaut 1979; Weete 1980) and the yeast *Phaffia rhodozyma* (Girard et al., 1994).

d. Metabolic Engineering

Summary of the biosynthesis pathway

With genes and cDNAs encoding nearly all the enzymes required for carotenoid biosynthesis in a lot of organisms, sequenced, and their products characterized, it was possible to use genetic engineering to introduce the ability to synthesize the β-carotene in plants or organisms that did not produce it and enhance this capacity in other. In order to place in context the actions undertaken we will briefly describe the general elements of the biosynthetic pathway of carotenoids. Carotenoids as before mentioned, share with the rest of the isoprenoids the basic molecule: isopentenyl pyrophosphate. This is a 5-carbon compound which is the unit of synthesis for the formation of compounds 5, 10, 15, 20 or more carbon (always multiples of 5). By this way arises the skeleton of many isoprenoids through a reduced number of steps of basic reactions (McGarvey and Croteau, 1995). Carotenoids have a skeleton of 40 carbons (C40), which is produced by joining two 20 carbon-molecules of geranylgeranyl pyrophosphate (GGPP). Strictly, the carotenoid biosynthetic pathway begins with the isomerization of IPP to its allylic isomer, dimethylallyl pyrophosphate (DMAPP). DMAPP is the initial, activated substrate in synthesis of long chain polyisoprenoid compounds such as GGPP. The formation of DMAPP from IPP is a reversible reaction that is catalyzed by the enzyme IPP isomerase (EC 5.3.3.2) (Cunningham Jr. and Gantt, 1998.). Introduction of any of a number of different plant, algal, or yeast IPP isomerase cDNAs, or additional copies of the *E. coli* gene for this enzyme, enhances several folds the accumulation of carotenoid pigments within these cells (Sun et al., 1996; Kajiwara et al., 1997). The GGPP molecule is the next precursor in the synthesis of carotenoids; the enzyme that catalyzes its formation is the GGPP synthase (GGPS; EC 2.5.1.29) (Dogbo and Camara, 1987; Ogura et al., 1997). The formation of the symmetrical 40-carbon phytoene (7,8,11,12,7',8',11',12'-octahydro-ψ,ψ carotene) from two molecules of GGPP is the first specific reaction in the pathway of carotenoid biosynthesis. The biosynthesis of phytoene from GGPP is a two-step reaction catalyzed by the enzyme phytoene synthase (PSY; EC 2.5.1.32).

The next compound in the route of synthesis of β-carotene is lycopene, which originates through four successive desaturation reactions of phytoene (Karvouni, 1995). These desaturation reactions serve to lengthen the conjugated series of carbon-carbon double bonds that constitutes the chromophore in carotenoid pigments, and thereby transform the colorless phytoene into the pink-colored lycopene. The desaturations undergone by phytoene are catalyzed by two related enzymes in plants: phytoene desaturase (PDS) and ζ-carotene desaturase (ZDS). In bacteria and fungi achieve the same result with a single gene product (Armstrong G. A. 1994; Sandmann, 1994). Later lycopene β-cyclase (LCYB), catalyzes the formation of the bicyclic β-carotene from the linear, symmetrical lycopene in plants and cyanobacteria (Cunningham et al., 1994; Cunningham et al., 1996; Hugueney et al., 1996). Xanthophylls comprise most of the carotenoid pigment in the thylakoid membranes of plants. Hydroxylation at the number three carbon of each ring of the hydrocarbons β-carotene and α-carotene will produce xanthophyll pigments zeaxanthin (β,β-carotene- 3,3′-diol) and lutein (β,ε-carotene-3,3′-diol), respectively. Finally, the evidence has shown that a similar biosynthetic pathway is present in all carotenogenic organisms (Sun et al., 1996; Lee and Schmidt-Dannert 2002). The biosynthetic pathway, in all the carotenoid producing organisms follows similar routes with minor variations in the final steps leading to different carotenoids (Umeno et al., 2005). Logically, most of the enzymes involved can be expressed in heterologous host. For more details, several reviews on aspects of biosynthesis and function of carotenoids are available (Hirschberg, 2001; Sandmann, 2002; DellaPenna, 2005). This situation offers multiple opportunities for the use of different approaches using biotechnology tools to increase the production of β-carotene.

e. New Processes and Products Using Genetic Engineering

Although there was not previously carotenoid synthesis capacity, availability of FPP among microorganisms has been utilized at various events which has been successful in producing β-carotene as major carotenoid product in various microorganisms including *Escherichia coli, Zymomonas mobilis, Agrobacterium tumefaciens and Saccharomyces cerevisiae* carrying the *Erwinia uredovora* carotenogenic genes (Figure 4). Expression of β-carotene was achieved through introduction of genes crtE, crtB, crtI and crtY, encoding the four enzymes required, in the genome of the microorganisms mentioned. In these cases, the transferred genes were flanked by promoters and terminators derived from the corresponding organisms (Mizawa et al., 1990; Mizawa et al., 1991; Yamano et al., 1994).

Although the production of vitamin A by chemical means could be cheap, its use as a therapeutic element by oral delivery is erratic and therefore the results are often not as expected (Pirie, 1983). Success might be reached if the provitamin A is integral component of food. As already mentioned, the shortage in the intake of vitamin A is associated with many diseases in developing countries. In some of these countries, rice is the staple food.

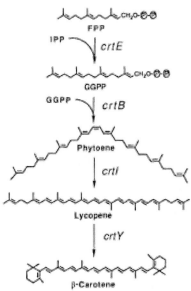

Figure 4. β-carotene biosynthetic pathway of non-photosyntetic bacterium *Erwinia* (Yamano et al., 1994).

Rice cultivars did not produce this provitamin in the endosperm, but immature rice endosperm is capable of synthesizing the early intermediate geranylgeranyl diphosphate; thus, Burkhardt et al., (1997) achieved produce the uncolored carotene phytoene by expressing the enzyme phytoene synthase in rice endosperm. Shortly afterwards, the same group completed the biosynthetic pathway to produce β-carotene in transgenic rice plants (Ye et al., 2000; Beyer et al., 2002). With regard to rice, efforts have been made subsequently to increase the level of β-carotene in the grain (Al-Babili, et al., 2006), and possibly in the near future this effort could be reached. In turn, the potato is a major staple food, and changing its content of provitamin is a possible means of alleviating nutritional deficiencies in the West hemisphere. Potato tubers contain low levels of carotenoids, mainly xanthophylls lutein, antheraxanthin, violaxanthin, and of xanthophyll esters. None of these carotenoids have provitamin A activity. Potato tubers contain low levels of carotenoids, mainly xanthophylls lutein, antheraxanthin, violaxanthin, and xanthophyll esters. Diretto et al., (2006) silenced the lycopene epsilon cyclase, by introducing, via Agrobacterium-mediated transformation, an antisense fragment of this gene under the control of the patatin promoter. The results showed significant increases in β-β-carotenoid levels, with β-carotene showing the maximum increase (up to 14-fold). The same group, achieved through silencing β-carotene hydroxylase increases total carotenoid and β-carotene levels in potato tubers (Diretto et al., 2007).

The availability of a large number of carotenoid biosynthetic genes has facilitated the recent progress in the metabolic engineering of carotenogenesis in other plants (Fraser and Bramley, 2004; Taylor and Ramsay, 2005), such as in the cases of Golden Canola seeds (Shewmaker et al., 1999), yellow potato (Ducreux et al., 2005), and plants with high-economic-value carotenoids (Stalberget al., 2003; Ralley et al., 2004; Lu et al., 2006). Looking ahead, researchers have been highlighted new complementary strategies to enhance expression of carotenoids in general and β-carotene in particular in plants of interest: gene assembly, directed enzyme evolution, and these combined approaches (Umeno et al., 2005).

f. Biotechnology, Greenhouses and β-carotene

Curiously, in countries where there is greater biodiversity, there are also problems of diseases related to deficiency of β-carotene in food (Ye et al., 2000). Under the argument does not affect biodiversity (Quist and Chapela, 2001), the use of genetically modified organisms (GMOs) in these countries is restricted or forbidden, unless it is conducted in conditions of confinement. Greenhouses are an option, in terms of the exclusion, for the production of GMOs, including maize and other crops. Another interesting approach using biotechnological knowledge in greenhouses is the elicitation of β -carotene production with specific compounds in no-transgenic systems. The effect of exogenous methyl jasmonate (MeJA) on antioxidative compounds of romaine lettuce (*Lactuca sativa* L.) has been investigated. Lettuces were treated with various MeJA solutions (0, 0.05, 0.1, 0.25, and 0.5 mM) before harvest. Total phenolic compounds content and antioxidant capacity of romaine lettuce significantly increased after MeJA treatments (0.1, 0.25, and 0.5 mM). The total content of phenolic compounds of the romaine lettuce treated with 0.5 mM MeJA (31.6 μg of gallic acid equivalents/mg of dry weight) was 35% higher than that of the control. The increase in phenolic compound content was attributed to a caffeic acid derivative and an unknown phenolic compound, which also contributed to increased antioxidant capacity. The induction of phenylalanine ammonia-lyase (PAL) activity by the MeJA treatment indicated that phenolic compounds were altered due to the activation of the phenylpropandoid pathway. Total content of carotenoids, including lutein and β -carotene, of the MeJA-treated lettuce did not change after 8 days of treatment, whereas the content of the control without MeJA decreased after 8 days (Kim et al., 2007).

Mechatronic Approaches
to Improve β-Carotene Production

Mechatronics involves the synergy of mechanics, electronics and computer science applied to the development of electromechanical products and systems by means of an integrated design. Mechatronics is not the union but the intersection of these three fields within the context of system design (see Figure 5).

Originally conceived by engineers from the Yaskawa Electic Company as the conjunction of the words 'mechanics' and 'electronics' [Mori, 1996; Harashima et al., 2005], the mechatronics concept has been redefined to include an interdisciplinary field of engineering now also covering other engineering areas such as electricity, control, computer science, robotics, chemical and nuclear instrumentation and even other areas like medicine and biotechnology. This new approach promotes the design and development of advanced electromechanical systems controlled by embedded systems. The end product is, thus, an advanced electromechanical system whose design is not a sequential process iterating over different fields of engineering but a concurrent process where the product is designed optimally in all these fields of engineering simultaneously. In this sense, the mechatronics is not a new field of engineering but it is the result of its natural evolution towards integral design and implementation of advanced electromechanical systems [Grimheden y Hansen, 2005].

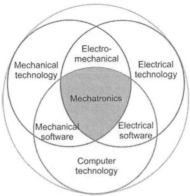

Figure 5. Mechatronics: synergy of mechanics, electronics and computer science.

Mechatronic design has been widely used to provide solutions to diverse problems. For example Lee (1999) developed a device capable of determining certain properties of an object such as shape, texture, temperature, stiffness among others; Tandon et al. (2002) used a predictive model based on an artificial neural network to optimize cutting forces in numerically controlled machine-tools; Xiaoli and Shiu (2000) used *fuzzy logic* techniques along with the wavelet transform to monitor real time wear and breakage conditions by means of current sensors in drilling; Jae and Yun (2005) a highly effective velocity profile generator using polynomial techniques that can produce profiles with different acceleration characteristics; Alaniz et al. (2006) developed a sensorless system to detect tool breakage by means of the wavelet transform applied to monitoring signals of the machine motors; Castañeda et al. (2006) developed an intelligent climate control system for greenhouses based on *fuzzy logic* and FPGAs (*Field Programmable Gate Arrays*) for low cost monitoring.

A typical mechatronic system is structured with a mechanical frame, actuators, sensors, signal conditioning and processing devices, computers, device interfaces and power sources. The sophistication of these systems and the incorporation of new technologies, such as intelligent sensors, control techniques, microelectromechanical systems (MEMS), have provided more maturity to mechatronic solutions. Among the fields where engineering has evolved to integrate areas that did not seem to converge previously is climate control systems or biotronic systems. In this context, biotronic systems is the application of mechatronic technologies to biological systems, especially when referred to intensive production under greenhouses. The application of new technologies and automation systems for biotronic systems has provided engineers with better construction technologies and enhanced designs, intelligent sensors, fitomonitoring and control strategies. This biotronic approach has had a positive effect in critical areas of climate control system for intensive production under greenhouses by increasing its cost-effectiveness:

a. Greater energy efficiency. Having enhanced greenhouse designs and a more precise climate control system can reduce heating and electricity costs.
b. Increased productivity. Automation increases productivity of workers by providing time for more important tasks.
c. Improved administration. Automation offers the value added of real time information to improve administrative decisions and invest time on strategic administration rather than on quantitative administration.

d.   Water requirements reduction. Automatic watering systems provide a more precise water dosification control reducing water consumption by providing the right amounts of water on time and in precise amounts.

e.   Fertilizer requirements reduction. By having an automated dosification, monitoring and high precision system the amount of required fertilizer can be reduced and used more effectively.

f.   Reduced use of chemicals. Having a climate (temperature, humidity and watering) control system for intensive production helps reduce stress in the crops and reduces the risk of diseases caused by pests and, thus, the need for fungicides, pesticides y herbicides.

g.   Improved crop quality and uniformity. A climate control system enables the producer to handle the crop properly with uniform grow conditions, simplifying the shipping, handling and commercialization. Moreover, biotronic system provide effective watering and fertilizing systems offering better product quality given the controlled climate and nutrition of the plant that causes it to generate a better content of vitamins, antioxidants and other nutrients. For example, under a controlled climate and nutrition the tomato fruit can be induced to produce a greater content of lycopene and β-carotene.

h.   Less equipement wear and damage. A control system with low performance increases the amount of work the artificial climate system requires; on the other hand, a well designed control system simplifies the equipment administration and its lifetime.

i.   Continuous monitoring and alarms. A system that automatically informs the producer of inusual situations at an early stage can reduce risks for the crop and the production system.

j.   Better decision making. A good control system stores greenhouse climatic data during the crop growth providing feedback for better decisions.

In general, mechatronics applied to greenhouse production (greenhouse automation and mechanization of production processes, climate control system and irrigation system design, greenhouse structural design, etc.) have improved production quality and quantity, and increasing the contents of lycopene and β-carotene in the case of the tomato fruit (Schmidt, 2008). A few examples of relevant work in the field are discussed next.

Greenhouse Mechanisation

International competition demand low cost, high quality and safe horticultural produce, issues that are not new in industrial production (aeronautics and automobile industry, electro domestic etc.). Also, quality management and the improvement of the over-all efficiency of the production process have received considerable attention in industrial production it is not the exception in the greenhouse crop production process which is composed of various steps (Figure 6). Depending on the crop grown, a whole production cycle may take a few weeks (e.g., lettuce), several months (e.g., tomatoes, etc.) up to several years (roses). In this sense, greenhouse mechanization has impact on the plant production such as seeding and cutting (where the greenhouse crop production process and most of the times seedlings or cuttings are produced by highly specialised companies), grafting (grafting is a necessary step to assure production quality and quantity or prevent diseases) and transplanting (plants are seeded in substrate or soil and then transplanted into or onto the final growing substrate: soil, tezontle, perlite, coco fibre etc.) as well as on the crop production including sorting and packing the harvested produce (the harvested produce is collected, sorted, and packed before shipment to the auction or retailer). In this way crop maintenance and harvest (for single harvest crops the production is finished at harvest time) does not show much automation yet because they are much more difficult to automate (van Henten, 2003).

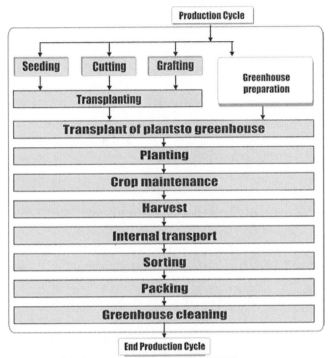

Figure 6. Greenhouse crop production process (Van Henten, 2003).

Nowadays, seeding is a highly mechanised process. A fully automated seeding line consists of a tray washer, a tray de-stacker, a tray filling machine, a seeding machine, a machine covering the trays, a watering machine and a tray stacking machine and to improve product quality and uniformity as well as efficient use of the production area, camera assisted tray inspection and filling machines are used to achieve 100% filling with good quality plant material. Rose cutting production robotic that use machine vision and industrial manipulators is in the market (Rombouts and Rombouts, 2002). The development of Geranium and Chrysanthemum cutting sticking robots were reported by Simonton (1990) and Kondo and Monta (1999), respectively. Grafting is a delicate process which requires a high degree of skill and the operation is physically and mentally demanding. A grafting robot was developed by Nishiura et al. (1996). The grafting robot achieved a success rate of 97% at a speed 10 times faster than human workers (Kondo and Ting, 1998). This machine is commercially available and can be used for grafting cucumber, water melon, melon, tomato and egg-plant at a capacity of 800 plants per hour. A robot for sorting and transplanting of Orchid seedlings in tissue culture was reported by Kaidu et al. (1998) and Okamoto (1996). For seedling production, transplanting machines are common practice nowadays. The development of transplanting robots has been reported in the USA, Korea and Japan (Yang et al., 1991; Sakaue, 1996; Ryu et al., 2001). Mobile growing systems and internal transport systems have been developed especially for potted plants and seedling production throughout the last two decades. More, recently also roses and gerbera's are produced at relatively small scale in a mobile growing system (van Henten, 2003). Automatic in row pesticide sprayers are commonly used in greenhouse vegetable production. Automatic over head pesticide sprayers are used during the production of seedlings, flowers and potted plants. Hand-tool has been developed to attach the plants to the wire with a copper ring significantly reducing the amount of labour needed for this task. Machines for lettuce and radish harvesting are commercially available. A robot prototype for leaf picking of cucumbers in greenhouse was reported by Van Henten et al. (2004). There are some researches of harvesting robots for harvesting cucumbers (Arima and Kondo, 1999; Van Henten 2003), tomatoes (Kondo, 1996; Monta et al., 1998) without having these machines commercially available. Automatic grading lines for tomatoes (colour, weight and diameter), cucumber (weight) and sweet pepper (weight) are commonly used in combination with automated box fillers and stacking machines. Sorting lines consisting of buffered feeders, maturity measurement, length and thickness measurement and automatic bunching (Van Henten 2003).

Mechanical and Structural Design of Greenhouses

Greenhouse design, structure, topology and cover provides a barrier between the external environment and the crop, which creates a microclimate that protects crops from wind, rain, pests, diseases, weeds and animals. Likewise, such protection enables control of the climate variables (temperature, humidity, CO_2, etc.) and allows to effectively implement chemical and biological monitoring to protect the crop. All these characteristics make the production under greenhouse have higher yields than conventional open field production.

Research related to the design of the structures of greenhouses and fluid mechanics involved in them have been conducted from a mechanical and structural point of view as a means of improving the climate inside the greenhouse (Critten, 2002). Baptista et al., (1999) mention that ventilation is one of the most important tools for controlling the climate in the greenhouse. In order to understand more clearly the physical processes associated with natural ventilation several research works have been carried out. Earlier works were merely experimental, employing mainly the tracing gas technique (Boulard & Draoui, 1995; Baptista et al., 1999). On the other hand, purely theoric approaches have also been used, as in the case of energy balance models (Seginer, 1997; Roy et al, 2002). However, these techniques provide information only about the rate of overall ventilation without giving details of the spatial distribution of lines of air flow, temperature or humidity inside the greenhouse. In recent years, computer simulations have reinforced the theoretical and experimental research. The numerical simulations made using the CFD technique have always been accompanied by an experimental stage that has served to give certainty (validating) the results obtained by CFD. Recent advances in CFD programs facilitate the study of vector and scalar fields in the present climate in the greenhouse through the solution of the equations governing the flow of fluids (Navier-Stokes equations). This technique also allows consideration of all the climate variables (temperature, relative humidity, CO_2 concentration), as well as the geometry of the greenhouse together with the crop in question (Molina-Aiz et al., 2004). Norton et al. (2007) reviewed the use of CFD for modelling and designing of ventilation systems for farm buildings. Bartzanas et al. (2002) carried out an analysis of the process of ventilation in a tunnel greenhouse equipped with anti-insect mesh on the side windows. Fatnassi et al. (2003) studied the patterns of air flow, temperature and humidity in a tomato greenhouse using a three-dimensional model. Campen y Bot (2003) employed a three-dimensional model to study the ventilation of a "parral" type greenhouse taking into consideration the presence of the surrounding greenhouses. Molina-Aiz et al. (2004) carried out measurements of velocity and temperature inside an Almeria type greenhouse to determine the effect of wind speed on natural ventilation. Ortiz (2004) carried out the numerical simulation of natural ventilation in a greenhouse of 10 Colombian ships, without considering the presence of the crop. The results showed the impact of exterior climate upon the pasive climate control of greenhouses using natural ventilation. Rico-Garcia et al. (2006) studied the effect of wind on the ventilation of two configurations of greenhouse using two-dimensional simulations and experiments to validate the simulations. Ould Khaoua et al. (2006) a two-dimensional model used in CFD to study the effect of wind speed and the configuration of the vents on the patterns of ventilation and temperature inside a greenhouse of glass.

Currently, there are greenhouses on the market with different topologies and cover materials (glass, plastic, etc.) developed in different countries (Mexico, Netherlands, France, Israel, etc.), which have been successfully applied to production in greenhouse in different climates, however, innovation and technological development in this area is vital for efficient energy use and improve the quantity and quality of production.

Modeling and Climate Control of Greenhouses

In particular, climate control in a greenhouse is one of the tools used for the improving of the production. According to Challa (1990), strict control of different climate variables (temperature, radiation, the amount of CO_2 in the atmosphere, humidity, etc.). which have an effect on plant growth, results in increased production and quality. The climate control in a greenhouse should be considered as part of general management rather than an isolated activity. The administration can be defined as a collection of activities aimed at achieving certain goals. One of the goals of the farmer as a businessman, is generally maximize the profits. The optimal control of the climate of a greenhouse has been the subject of many philosophical thoughts throughout the past two decades. One of the first qualitative analysis on this subject dates from 1978, when Udink ten Cate, Van Dixhoorn and Bot considered the climate control of a greenhouse and the administration of the crop from an integral point of view (Udink ten Cate, 1978). Their ideas changed in different ways during the following years (Challa et al., 1988; Challa and Van Straten, 1991; van Henten, 1994, 2000, 2003), but the fundamental concept is still the same. Within this concept of integral control, a greenhouse is seen as a process in which multilevel hierarchical levels are distinguished by different time scales. The main reason for this hierarchical decomposition of the administration of a greenhouse is the inherent complexity of the process being considered, there are a lot of variables in the process related to the cultivation and the climate of the greenhouse, and their complex interactions, which would inevitably demand decomposition into sub-problems, which is more desirable in the design of control systems; this hierarchical decomposition in a greenhouse can be compared to that found in industrial production systems where automatic control concepts can be applied.

The main objective of this kind of hierarchical control is the treatment of the raw information produced by the sensors, this treatment can be addressed with simple empirical relationships or through simulation models of the relations established between climate and the physiological response of the crop. The commercial greenhouse control systems and research in this area revolve around this outline of the production system in a greenhouse. Research has been conducted at all levels of the hierarchical pattern, either in every particular level, or as a whole, i.e., covering two or all levels. At the lowest level is the shorter-term monitoring of climatic conditions of the greenhouse, which operates with a time scale of seconds or minutes. This level has to do with the efficient operation of the valves of both heating and CO2, and the mechanisms of the ventilation system, etc., which has to do with controlling climate variables in the greenhouse, such as air temperature, concentration of carbon dioxide and moisture. In this lower level, research in climate control of greenhouses have been mainly focused on the control of air temperature by applying different control strategies. Classic control schemes were used by Kamp (1996) and Bontsema (1994) studied predictive control schemes, which are based on measuring the disturbance and act immediately on the process before it affects the variable that is controlling. For this kind of control it is necessary to have a model of behavior of the process to calculate the control action necessary to compensate the effect of the disturbance. Tanatu (1989) showed that with the use of models to predict the impact of changes in outside weather conditions on the interior environment, it is possible take corrective actions in advance rather than waiting until the change in internal climatic conditions is detected. Young (1994) showed that substantial improvements could be made on the controllers if the PID control algorithm directly took into account the real response of the greenhouse. At this level, studies have been conducted on more advanced control schemes based on changing controller behavior under new circumstances such as the open loop adaptive control (Kamp, 1996) and model-based closed loop adaptive schemes (Udink ten Cate, 1983; Rodriguez, 1996). Davis (1984) designed an algorithm to control the temperature with ventilation which performs better than with a PI controller with fixed parameters. Ehrlich (1996) studied the use of an intelligent controller to control the temperature of a greenhouse, and based on this concept used two approaches for modifying and determining the set points.

The middle level is responsible for the control of vegetative development, where the time scales are set by physiological processes and can range from one hour to several days. The main task at this level is to generate the optimal trajectory of climate variables that are controlled at the lower level to achieve the required outcome at the top level. It is at this stage where contributions have been reported regarding the increase in lycopene and β-carotene content in the production of greenhouse tomato (Schmidt, 2008). Of course, there is the need to have information on the plant, either through growth models and development of the plant or fitomonitoring techniques, and we must optimize an objective function so as to maximize production and minimize the economic costs. Most research at this level have been developed around the interaction of the crop with the climate in the greenhouse to get the ideal conditions for the development of the crop in an optimal way. This second level, essentially open-loop, may become a closed loop process when the growth of plants is quantified using sensors or machine vision (van Henten, 1995; Schmitd, etc.). This way, it is possible to modify the lower level set points to improbé the overall behavior. Kozai (1985) and Jacobson (1988) studied greenhouse control on the basis of expert systems, where the response of crops to their environment is indirectly represented by means of the preset set points as knowledge rules. In learning based control (based on the model of decision of a farmer) both logic and decision rules made by the farmer have a paramount importance. This integration of a subsystem of decision or model of "decision-action" is aimed at evaluating the interventions of human beings in the biophysical sub-system. Clouaire (1996) studied this kind of heuristic modeling (expert systems) based on artificial intelligence techniques. At this stage Hashimoto (1985) proposed a scheme of control depending on the response of the plant (speaking-plant), where the plant is considered as a black box and identification techniques are used in the system to determine the responses of plants to changes in the microclimate. This type of approach has been being conducted due to advances in the field of sensors and hardware technology, which allowed for continuous monitoring of the dynamic response of the plant (Schmitd, 2003). Some experimental studies have been released independently on the variables that affect the development of the plant. To cite some examples, the ratio of wind in controlling the temperature has been studied theoretically (Bailey, 1985), this being one of the few approaches that has been formally proven in practice in commercial greenhouses in production (Chalabi, 1996). This concept is based on the performance of the crop, which uses a simple model which only defines a band of temperature that does not lead to production losses and a physical model that deals with the energy balance of the greenhouse and includes solar radiation, wind speed and the exchanges of radiation in the greenhouse. The physical model is used to determine the trajectory of the operation point of warming that minimizes the total consumed heat loss. There is also work done on the use of models applied to the control of humidity based on transpiration control strategies (Stanghellini, 1992), where the idea is that the requirements of the quality of the crop are based on the rate of transpiration. Schmidt (2008) developed an study on levels 1 and 2 by means of fitomonitoring and Mollier diagrams, where the comparision between different controllers is shown and this is one of the first works where the importance of humidity on the quality of the fruit is quantitatively determined. Results show a significant increase in the average fruit yield per plant, as well as a considerable increase in the content of Lycopene and β-carotene in the tomato fruit.

At the highest level, decisions are made regarding the planning of the overall production of the crop, where the scale of time is likely to range from weeks to months. Models are used for the development of the crop, and even market models are used to optimize profitability. Based on the experience of the manager or purely economic criteria, the implications of changes in dates of harvest are explored, of reducing production costs, and so on. This level communicates the middle level the production goals so that it generates paths to be followed by the climatic variables to meet the main objective. At the highest level is where decisions are made regarding the planning of the overall production of the crop. Only in some researchs has been considered a global approach, which tends toward the optimal integration of climate control. This approach is fairly complex, first because it considers different time scales: 1 to 2 months at the level of cultivation, 1 to 2 days at ground level and some processes in the cultivation, and 10 to 20 minutes at the level of greenhouse climate. And, secondly, the rapid dynamics of the system is influenced by the strong interactions of the greenhouse climate and the rapid fluctuations in the external environment, especially natural radiation. Moreover, accurate predictions of climate over the long term are not usually available. A final problem is the need for measurements of the crop online. To make optimal control suitable for the production of crops in a greenhouse all these difficulties must be considered and resolved. Most research studies have dealt by parts with the optimal control of production under greenhouse conditions. Sengier (1998) considered the problem of the slow sub-system, whereas Hwang (1993) focused efforts on the rapid sub-problem. Chalabi et al. (1996) and Tchamitchian et al. (1992) optimized part of the greenhouse production system. Seginer (1997) studied the optimal control based on neural models and neural controllers. Among the first ones to address the problem of optimal control in general is Van Renten (1994, 2003), who presented a methodology to decompose the system in two different time sacles despite the presence of strong influences and rapid fluctuations of the external inputs. According to this methodology, long-term problem must first be resolved, and then using the results of it, the problem of short-term can be addressed. To practically apply the methodology of Van Henten, two problems must be solved, the first is related to exogenous inputs, that is, the climate must be known over the full range of optimization for calculating the optimal control; secondly, because that the best control is essentially open-loop, feedback is required to deal with initial states, modeling errors and flaws in climate prediction. There is still a problem inherent in this type of control proposals, namely, the practical solution. Tap (2000) used the decomposition in two time scales proposed by Van Henten and combined it with two kinds of climate prediction and online adaptive optimal control, based on the use of an integrated model of the greenhouse-crop (tomatoes) to solve the problems of the methodology proposed by Van Henten. The combination of these approaches (two times-scale receding horizon optimal control algorithm) represents the state of the art when it comes to implementing optimal control in the production of vegetables in greenhouses.

On the other hand, the biggest drawback for the development of techniques for monitoring, lies in the need for an appropriate model of the greenhouse climate, as the algorithm design is based on prior knowledge of the model and is independent of it. The kindness of the controller will depend on the differences between the actual process and the model used. This is the reason that justifies the great efforts being undertaken to design, calibrate and validate a good model of the greenhouse climate. During the last two decades, a large amount of scientific knowledge has been accumulated and expressed in mathematical models with regard to greenhouses. In the literature, several climate models have been submitted, some are based on the physical laws involved in the process (thermodynamic properties), models in which the processes responsible for the transfer of energy and mass are to be examined. Such models provide a detailed description of the climate in a greenhouse in connection with the weather outside, the physical properties of the greenhouse and its equipment, and therefore are of a high order, such as the models by Bot (1983), Zwart (1996), Tap (2000), Tavares (2001), and Castañeda et al. (2007). On the other hand in this kind of models, there are simplified models based on the linearization of the exchange of sensible and latent head, such as the models by Boulard (1993 and 2000). There are other models based on transference functions, in which the nonlinear greenhouse system is linearized by selecting an operation point and assuming first order outcomes, such as in models by Udkin Ten Cate (1985b). Some others are black box models, which are based on analysis of data into and out of the process such as the model by Boaventura et al.(1992), López et al. (2007) or special cases of black box models based on neural networks such as the model by Seginer (1994) or based on fuzzy logic (Boaventura et al., 2006). There are research studies of simplified physical models, where the greenhouse is considered a solar collector and its thermal performance can be described by an equation of energy balance. These kinds of models are based on the linearization of the Exchange of sensible and latent heat and use only a limited number of parameters (Boulard and Baille, 1993; Boulard and Wang, 2000; Castañeda et al., 2002).

A large number of solutions have been proposed to improve climate control in the direction of the requirements set above. However, these solutions have been only partial ones, and have not been fully implemented commercially and all have been developed around a hierarchy of a decision-making process. Climate commercial controllers are mainly based on looping only at level 1 of the hiearchical schema. A few commercial controllers have incorporated heuristic rules and some other more advanced commercial systems that— although also rely on a lot of heuristic knowledge and are focused only to control the climate in the greenhouse without taking into account the physiological processes or the second level of the hierarchical schema—unlike the first ones, allow us to make more efficient use of energy and integrate advanced models in which the climate control system takes into account the climatic conditions of both the exterior and interior control system, and the ventilation is based on a model that calculates the energy balance. It is worth to mention that the option of integrating models, is not widespread because it works only for certain structural designs of glass greenhouses, so it can not be applied to other types of greenhouses with different types of covers.

Irrigation and Dosage of Nutrients in Greenhouses

The contribution of adequate water and fertilizer is one of the key elements in improving production and quality of the crop in the greenhouse. Providing the plants with the right amount and enough water and nutrients requires an irrigation system with the following four components: System for feeding nutrients and water, keeping a record of events, sensors and a method for making decisions. If any of the four components is missing, then the efficiency of the system is reduced and the yield and quality of production decreases (Waller, 2004). With a proper irrigation system the quality and quantity of crops can be considerably increased (Domínguez A., 1996). An optimal irrigation is a complex process: the amounts of water and nutrients must be enough to avoid stoping the photosyntesis process and, thus, the growth, but at the same time an excessive amount of water and nutrients can cause an exaggerated vegetal growth damaging the product among other consequences (Howard M, 1992). Work has been carried out on the determination of the optimum amount of water to be used in greenhouses (Guang-Cheng et al 2008; Chun-Zhi et al, 2008) and, in the development of automatic control systems for fertigation (Michels & Feyen, 1994; Kell et al., 1999; Yunseop et al., 2008). Likewise, work on intelligent controllers for fertigation has been developed (Bahat et al., 2000; Caprarico et al., 2008). However, most of the current commercial fertirrigation equipment provide a medium degree of automation based on classic controllers, and allow control over the mixture of fertilizer and water, controlling the pH and the electrical conductivity through feedback from sensors that return an online measurement of these two variables and not for each nutrient (e.g., calcium, potassium, phosphorus, etc.). Moreover, these systems usually have some type of feedback (pressure, radiation sensors, etc.) to determine the amount of water to supply.

Other Technologies Applied to Agriculture

The integrated pest management has a direct relationship with production in the greenhouse. The pest detection and monitoring activity is a tedious and time consuming task (Thomas, 1995; Stansly et al., 2004). IPM is a management strategy to optimize dealing with the pests in an economic and environment-friendly way (Koumpouros et al., 2004). In practice, the most common detection procedure is the visual exploration of plants or the use of sticky colored screens able to trap flying insects (Tang, 2008; Smith et al., 1983) and it is done once a day, it requires a number of well trained and well equipped personal. Some works related with the development of automatic systems based on machine vision for pest detection have been reported (Neethirajan et al., 2007; Zayas et al., 1989; Zayas and Flinn, 1998; Ridgway et al., 2002). However, the vast majority of these works have not been brought to commercial products.

Other important aspects of electronic technologies applied to agriculture are ruggedness and low cost which are a necessity for its implementation (Zhang, 2002). In this regard, new technologies such as FPGAs are presented as a good alternative for many real-life applications, a technology that has been under a lot of contributions in different fields of application in image processing and signals (Reyneri, 2004; Sklyarov's, 2004), multimedia (Ramachandran, 2004), robotics (Sridhara, 2004), telecommunications, cryptography (Daly, 2004), network systems (Martins et al., 2005; Moon et al., 2005) and computing in general (Salcic, Z., 1997; Gschwind et al., 2001; Chains and Megson, 2004; Ali et al., 2004). There are successful applications in detecting fracture and wear inserts in machine-tools (Troncoso, 2004), real-time monitoring of climatic variables (Mendoza-Jasso, et al., 2005) and intelligent climate control in greenhouses (Castañeda et al., 2006).

Greenhouse Possibilities in β-Carotene Production

Greenhouse production systems are an important tool for improving the quantity and quality of production (considering the increase in β-carotene as part of the quality). As mentioned, there has been a lot of work on the system of production in greenhouses and today there is a vast area of opportunity in different areas of engineering of greenhouses to increase the quality and quantity of production.

Having reviewed the various areas that are closely related to improvement in quality and quantity of crop production in greenhouses—such as the design and development of structures, the production process of growing in a greenhouse, and climate control systems and other related technologies—it is interesting to note that only the synergy of different fields will enable us to improve the quantity and quality of production, in particular climate control and irrigation (Castañeda et al., 2006). In this sense, from the analyzed fields follow some discussions and future prospects.

In the same vein, a new control system must meet certain requirements in relation to the goal of climate control according to the following criteria: production, quality of the crop, product quality, time of the production process, costs and risks of production. In addition, at the same time it must eliminate the drawbacks and deficiencies of the current controllers. However, monitoring systems have evolved into complex systems in which a large quantity of knowledge is implemented: control algorithms, instrumentation and various climate processes. Despite the great success of these automated systems for control of greenhouses that are now available, the control systems today are focused on environmental monitoring; information about the plant growth as a function of climate variables is used only in an indirect way through a generic pattern of the desired trajectory of operation, which are sometimes changed every day depending on the performance of the crop. If knowledge about the physiology of the plant and the physical processes can be incorporated, new improvements in control systems can be achieved (Castañeda et al., 2005). In this sense, progress in the coming years in the fitomonitoring technology, artificial intelligence, sensors and mechanical systems, modeling and control techniques will enable the development of control systems that involve the hierarchical control scheme of production in greenhouses.

In terms of fertigation systems, most of the current specific ion sensors are only available for off-line measurements; in this sense, the coming years—with the development of specific ion sensors (e.g., phosphorus, potassium and calcium) for online measurements, as well as the improvement of mechanical, hydraulic and electronic systems for fertigation—will allow a more precise dosage of each nutrient. Likewise, advances in fitomonitoring systems allow the control system to make decisions on the amount of water and nutrients based on the best response of the plant.

Concluding Remarks

Taken together, the data presented in this review display an interesting future in the production of β-carotene (and other secondary metabolites) exploiting methodologies based on biotechnology and mechatronics. Biotechnology approaches must be used in order to increase β-carotene content in living systems and even produce it in those in which it is not naturally possible. Plant or algae systems are obvious candidates to be used as "β-carotene factories" in greenhouses. Thus, mechatronics tools will be fundamental in order to control and optimize β-carotene production. Nowadays, the available machines are largely based on principles of industrial automation. It is expected that the next generation of technologies for greenhouse production will be the result of combined innovations in the field of biotechnology, mechatronics and robot technology, mechatronic sensing and control hardware and software, electronics technologies, ion selective sensors, machine vision pest scouting sensors, cultivation systems, plant physiology and plant breeding, among others.

Acknowledgments

The authors thank Fondo de Investigación de la Facultad de Ingeniería (FIFI-2008), PROMEP/103.5/08/3320 and Fondos Mixtos CONACyT-Gobierno del Estado de Querétaro-2008, for supporting the elaboration of this review.

References

Aggarwal, S; Subberwal, M; kumar, S; Sharma, M. Brain tumor and role of β-carotene, α–tocopherol, superoxide dismutase and glutathione peroxidase. *J Cancer Res Ther.*, 2006, 2(1), 24-27.

Alaniz Lumbreras, D; Gómez Loenzo, R; Romero Troncoso, R; Herrera Ruiz, G. Sensorless Detection of Tool Breakage in Milling Process. *Machining Science and Technology*, 2006.

Al-Babili, S; Tran, H; Thi, C; Schaub, P. Exploring the potential of the bacterial carotene desaturase CrtI to increase the β-carotene content in Golden Rice. *J Exp Bot*, 57(4), 1007-1014

Allen, W; Rajotte, E. The changing role of extension entomology in the IPM era. *Annu Rev Entoml.*, 1990, 35, 379-397.

Arima, S; Kondo, N. Cucumber harvesting robot and plant training system. *Journal of Robotic and Mechatronics*, 1999, 11(3), 208-212.

Armstrong, GA; Alberti, M; Hearst, JE. Conserved enzymes mediate the early reactions of carotenoid biosynthesis in nonphotosynthetic and photosynthetic prokaryotes. *Proc Natl Acad Sci.*, U.S.A., 1990_a, 87, 9975-9979.

Armstrong, GA; Schmidt, A; Sandmann, G; Hearst, JE. Genetic and biochemical characterization of carotenoid biosynthesis mutants of Rhodobacter capsulatus. *J Biol Chem.*, 1990_b, 265 (14), 8329-8338.

Armstrong, GA. Eubacteria shows their true colors: genetics of carotenoid pigment biosynthesis from microbes to plants. *J. Bacteriol.*, 1994, 176, 4795-802.

Baptista, F; Bailey, B; Randall, J; Meneses, J. Greenhouse ventilation rate: theory and measurement with tracer gas techniques. *Journal of Agricultural Engineering Research*, 1999, 72, 363-374.

Baranski, RM; Baranska, Schulz, H. Changes in carotenoid content and distribution in living plant tissue can be observed and mapped in situ using NIR-FT-Raman spectroscopy. *Planta*, 2005, 222(3), 448-457.

Bartzanas, T; Boulard, T; Kittas, C. Effect of Vent Arrangement on Windward Ventilation of a Tunnel Greenhouse. *Biosystems Engineering*, 2004.

Ben-Amotz, A; Fishler, R. Analysis of carotenoids with emphasis on 9-cis-β-carotene in vegetables and fruits commonly consumed in Israel. *Food Chem.*, 1998, 62, 515-520.

Ben-Amotz, A; Gressel, J; Avron, M. Massive accumulation of phytoene induced by norflurazon in *Dunaliella bardawil* (Chlorophyceae) prevents recovery from photoinhibition. *J Phycol.*, 1987, 23, 176-181.

Ben-Amotz, A; Shaish, A; Avron, M. Mode of action of the massively accumulated b-carotene of Dunaliella bardawil in protecting the alga against damage by excess irradiation. *Plant Physiol.*, 1989, 91, 1040-1043.

Beyer, P; Al-babili, S; Ye, X; Lucca, P; Schaub, P; Welsch, R; Potrykus, I. Golden rice: Introducing the β-carotene biosynthesis pathway into rice endosperm—by genetic engineering to defeat vitamin A deficiency. *J. Nutr.*, 2002, 132(3), 506-510.

Bhosale, P; Larson, AJ; Frederick, JM; Southwick, K; Thulin, CD; Bernstein, PS. Identification and Characterization of a Pi Isoform of Glutathione S-Transferase (GSTP1) as a Zeaxanthin-binding Protein in the Macula of the Human Eye. *J. Biol. Chem.*, 2004, 279, 49447-49454.

Boaventura, J; Ruano, A; Couta, C. Identification of greenhouse climate dymanic models. *Computer in Agriculture*, 1992, 43, 1-10.

Boaventura, J; Salgado, P. Greenhouse. *Control Engineering Practice*, 2005, 13(5), 613-628.

Bot, G. Greenhouse climate: form physical processes to a dynamic model. PhD thesis, Wageningen Agricultural University, The Netherlands. 1983.

Boulard, T; Baille, A. A simple greenhouse climate control model incorporating effects of ventilation an evaporative cooling. *Agricultural and Forest Meteorology*, 1993, 65, 145-157.

Boulard, T; Draoui, B. Natural ventilation of a greenhouse with continuous roof vents: measurements and data analysis. *J. Agric. Eng.*, 1995, 61, 27-36.

Boulard, T; Wang, S. Greenhouse crop traspiration simulation from external climate conditions. *Agricultural and Forest Meteorology*, 2000, 100, 25-34.

Burchard, RP; Dworkin, M. Light-Induced lysis and carotenogenesis in *Myxococcus xanthus*. *J Bacteriol*, 1966, 91(2), 535-545.

Burkhardt, PK; Beyer, P; WQnn, J; Klbti, A; Armstrong, GA.; Schledz, M; von Lintig, J; Potrykus, I. Transgenic rice (*Oryza sativa*) endosperm expressing daffodil (*Narcissus pseudonarcissus*) phytoene synthase accumulates phytoene, a key intermediate of provitamin A biosynthesis. *Plant J*, 1997, 11(5), 1071-1078.

Burton, GW; Ingold, KU. Beta-Carotene: an unusual type of lipid antioxidant. *Science*, 1984, 224(4649), 569-573.

Campen, J; Bot, G. Determination of greenhouse-specific aspects of ventilation using three-dimensional computational fluid dynamics. *Biosystems Engineering*, 2003.

Castañeda-Miranda, R. Elementos de instrumentación y control para la simulación del balance de energía en un invernadero. Master's thesis, Universidad Autónoma de Querétaro. 2002.

Castañeda-Miranda, R; Ventura-Ramos, E; Peniche-Vera, RR; Herrera-Ruíz, G. Fuzzy greenhouse climate control system based on a field programmable gate array. *Biosys Eng.*, 94 (2), 165-177.

Castañeda-Miranda, R; Ventura-Ramos, E; Peniche-Vera, R; Herrera-Ruiz, G. Análisis y simulación del modelo físico de un invernadero bajo condiciones climáticas de la región central de México, *Agrociencia*, 2007, 41(3), 317-335.

Cerdá-Olmedo, E. Standard growth conditions and variations. P.337-339. In E. Cerdá-Olmedo, & E. D. Lipson (Eds.), *Phycomyces*. Cold Spring Harbor Laboratory, Cold Spring Harbor, N.Y.

Chalabí, Z; Bailey, B; Wilkinson, D. A real-time optimal control algorithm for greenhouse heating. *Computers and Electronics in Agriculture*, 1996, 15, 1-13.

Challa, H; Bot, G; Van der Braak, N. Crop growth models for greenhouse climate control. *Theoretical Production Ecology*, 1988, 125-145.

Challa, H; Van Straten, G. Reflections about optimal climate control in greenhouse cultivation. In: Hashimoto Y., Mathematical and control applications in agriculture and horticulture. *IFAC Workshop series*, 1991, 1, 13-18.

Challa, H. Crop growth models for greenhouse climate control. *Theoretical Production Ecology*, 1990, 125-145.

Clouaire, M; Schotman, R; Tchamitchian, M. Survey of computer-based approachess for greenhouse climate management. *Acta Horticulturae*, 1996, 406, 409-423.

Coultate, T. *Food: The Chemistry of Its Components*, 3rd Edition. *Royal Society of Chemistry*, 1996.

Critten, D; Bailey, B. A review of greenhouse engineering developments during the 1990s. *Agricultural and Forest Meteorology*. 2002.

Cunningham, FX Jr; Pogson, B; Sun, ZR; McDonald, KA; DellaPenna, D; Gantt, E. Functional analysis of the β and ε–lycopene cyclase enzymes of Arabidopsis reveals a mechanism for control of cyclic carotenoid formation. *Plant Cell*, 1996, 8, 1613-26.

Cunningham, FX Jr; Sun, ZR; Chamovitz, D; Hirschberg, J; Gantt, E. Molecular.structure and enzymatic function.of lycopene cyclase from the.cyanobacterium *Synechococcus* sp. Strain.PCC7942. *Plant Cell*, 1994, 6, 1107-21.

Czeczuga-Semeniuk, E; Lemancewicz, D; Wolczynski, S. Can vitamin A modify the activity of docetaxel in MCF-7 breast cancer cells? *Folia Histochem Cytobiol.*, 2007, 45(1), 169-174.

Dai, Q; Borenstein, AR; Wu, Y; Jackson, JC; Larson, EB. Fruit and vegetables Juices and Alzheimer´s Disease: The Kame Project. *Am J Med.*, 2006, 119(9), 751-759.

Davis, P. A technique of adaptive control of the temperature in a greenhouse using ventilator adjustement. *Journal of Agricultural Engineering Research*, 1984, 29, 241-248.

De Zwart. Analyzing Energy-Saving Options in Greenhouse Cultivation Using a Simulation Model. Ph.D, Dissertation, Wageningen Agricultural University, Wageningen, Netherlands, 1996.

DellaPenna, D; Pogson, BJ. Vitamin Synthesis in Plants: Tocopherols and Carotenoids. *Annu. Rev. Plant Biol.* 2006, 57, 711-738.

DellaPenna, D. A decade of progress in understanding vitamin E synthesis in plants. *J Plant Physiol.*, 2005, 162, 729-37.

Demmig-Adams, B; Gilmore, AM; Adams III. WW. In vivo functions of carotenoids in higher plants. *FASEB J.*, 1996, 10, 403-412.

Diretto, G; Tavazza, R; Welsch, R; Pizzichini, D; Mourges, F; Papacchioli, V; Beyer, P; Giuliano, G. Silencing of beta-carotene hydroxylase increases total carotenoid and beta-carotene levels in potato tubers. *BMC Plant Biology*, 2007, 7, 11.

Diretto, G; Tavazza, R; Welsch, R; Pizzichini, D; Mourgues, F; Papacchioli, V; Beyer, P; Giuliano, G. Metabolic engineering of potato tuber carotenoids through tuber-specific silencing of lycopene epsilon cyclase. *BMC Plant Biol.*, 2006, 6, 13.

Domínguez, A. *Fertirrigación*. Ediciones Mundi-Prensa, segunda edición. 1996.

Ducreux, LJM; Morris, WL; Hedley, PE; Shepherd, T; Davies, HV; Millam, S; Taylor, MA. Metabolic engineering of high carotenoid potato tubers containing enhanced levels of b-carotene and lutein. *J. Exp. Bot.*, 2005, 56, 81-89.

Ehrlich, H; Khne, M; Jakel, J. Development of a fuzzy control system for greenhouses. *Acta Horticulturae*, 1996, 406, 125-145.

Fatnassi, H; Boulard, T; Bouirden, L. Simulation of climatic conditions in full-scale greenhouse fitted with insect-proof screens. *Agricultural & Forest Meteorology*, 2003.

Faure, H; Fayol, V; Galabert, C; Grolier, P; Moel, GL; Steghens, J; Kappel, AV; Nabet, F. Carotenoids: 1. Metabolism and physiology. *Ann Biol Clin* (Paris), 1999, 57, 169-183.

Fraser, PD; Bramley, PM. The biosynthesis and nutritional uses of carotenoids. *Prog. Lipid Res.*, 2004, 43, 228-265.

García-Gonzalez, M; Moreno, J; Manzano, JC; Florencio, FJ; Guerrero, MG. Production of Dunaliella salina biomass rich in 9-cis-b-carotene and lutein in a closed tubular photo bioreactor. *J Biotech*, 115, 81-90.

Girard, P; Falconnier, B; Brocout, J; Vladescu, B. Beta-carotene producing mutants of Phaffia rhodozyma. *Appl Microbiol Biotechnol*, 1994, 41, 183-191.

Grimheden, M; Hansen, M. Mechatronics—the evolution of an academic discipline in engineering education. *Int. J Mechatronics*, 2005, 15.

Grogan, DW. Phenotypic characterization of the archaebacterial genus Sulfolobus: comparison of five wild-type strains. *J Bacteriol*, 1989, 171, 6710-6719.

Guevara-González, RG; Guzmán-Maldonado, SH; Veloz-Rodríguez, R; Cardador-Martínez, A; Loarca-Piña, G; Veloz-García, RA; Marín-Martínez, R; Guevara-Olvera, L; Torres-Pacheco, I; Miranda-López, R; Villaseñor-Ortega, F; González-Chavira, MM. Antimicrobial, Antimutagenic and Antioxidant Properties of Tannins from Mexican 'Cascalote' Tree (*Caesalpinia cacalaco*). In: *Recent Progress in Medicinal Plants*. Vol. 14. Biopharmaceuticals. J. N. Govil, V. K. Singh, & Khalil Ahmad. (Eds.), Pp. 13-30. (ISBN: 0-9761849-6-6, series ISBN: 0-9656038-5-7). Studium Press, LLC, U.S.A. 2006.

Guruvayoorappan, C; Kuttan, G. "Beta-carotene inhibits tumor-specific angiogenesis by altering the cytokine profile and inhibits the nuclear translocation of transcription factors in B16F-10 melanoma cells." *Integr Cancer Ther.*, 2007 Sep, 6(3), 258-70.

Guruvayoorappan, C; Kuttan, G. Beta-carotene inhibits tumor-specific angiogenesis by altering the cytokine profile and inhibits the nuclear translocation of transcription factors in B16F-10 melanoma cells. *Integr Cancer Ther.*, 2007, 6(3), 258-70.

Guzmán-Maldonado, SH; Mora-Avilés, A. Molecular breeding for nutritionally and healthy food components. In: *Advances in Agricultural and Food Biotechnology*. Eds. Ramón G. Guevara-González and Irineo Torres-Pacheco. Research Signpost, ISBN: 81-7736-269-0. Kerala, India. 2006.

Harashima, F; Tomizuka, M; Fukuda, T. Mechatronics: What Is It? Why and How? IEEE/ASME Trans. on Mechatronics, (1). 1996.

Hashimoto, Y; Marimoto, T; Fukuyama, T. Some speaking plant approach to the synthesis of control systems in greenhouses. *Acta Horticulturae*, 1985, 174, 219-226.

Hirschberg, J. Carotenoid biosynthesis in flowering plants. *Curr. Opin. Plant Biol.*, 2001, 4, 210-18.

Hornero-Mendez, D; Britton, G. Involvement of NADPH in the cyclization reaction of carotenoid biosynthesis. *FEBS Lett.*, 2002, 515, 133-136.

Howard, M. *Cultivos Hidropónicos*. Ediciones Mundi-Prensa, cuarta edición. 1992.

Hugueney, P; Badillo, A; Chen, HC; Klein, A; Hirschberg, J. Metabolism of cyclic carotenoids: a model for the alteration of this biosynthetic pathway in *Capsicum annuum* chromoplasts. *Plant J.*, 1995, 8, 417-24.

Hwang, Y. Optimization of greenhouse temperature and carbon dioxide in subtropical climate. PhD thesis, University of Florida, Florida, 1993.

Jae, W; Yun-Ki, K. FPGA based acceleration and deceleration circuit for industrial robots and CNC machine tools. *Mechatronics*, 2002.

Kaidu, Y; Okamoto, T; Torii, T. Robotic system for sorting and transplanting orchid seedlings in tissue culture. *Journal of Japanese Society of Agricultural Machines*, 1998, 60, 55-62.

Kamp, P. Computerized Environmental Control in Greenhouses. IPC-Plant, Ede, the Netherlands, 1996.

Karvouni, Z; John, I; Taylor, JE; Watson, CF; Turner, AJ; Grierson, D. Isolation and characterization of a melon cDNA clone encoding phytoene synthase. *Plant. Mol. Biol.*, 1995, 27, 1153-62.

Katz, A; Jimenez, C; Pick, U. Isolation and characterization of a protein associated with carotene globules in the alga, Dunaliella bardawil. *Plant Physiol.*, 108, 1657-1664.

Kim, HJ; Fonseca, JM; Choi, JH; Kubota, C. Effect of methyl jasmonate on phenolic compounds and carotenoids of romaine lettuce (Lactuca sativa L.). *J Agri Food Chem.*, 55(25), 10366-10372.

Kondo, N; Monta, M. Chrysanthemum cutting sticking robot system. *J Rob Mech.*, 1999, 11(3), 220-224.

Kondo, N; Ting, K. *Robotics for bioproduction systems.* ASAE, St. Joseph, USA. 1998.

Kondo, N. Visual feedback guided robotic cherry tomato harvesting. *Transactions*, 1996, 2331-2338.

Koumpouros, Y; Mahaman, B; Maliappis, M; Passam, H; Sideridis, A; Zorkadis, V. Imagen processing for distance diagnosis in pest management. *Comput Electron Agr.*, 2004, 44, 121-131.

Larson, S; Bergkvist, L; Naslund, I; Rutegard, J; Wolk, A. Vitamin A, retinol, and carotenoids and the risk of gastric cancer: a prospective cohort study. *Am J Clin Nutr.*, 2007, 85, 497-503.

Lee, M; Nicholls, H. Review Article. Tactile sensing for mechatronics-a state of the art survey. *Mechatronics*, 1999, 9.

Lee, P; Schmidt-Dannert, C. Metabolic engineering towards biotechnological production of carotenoids in microorganisms. *Appl Microbiol and Biotechnol*, 2002, 60, 1-11.

Lefsrud, MG. Environmental manipulation to increase the nutritional content in leafy vegetables. Ph.D Dissertation, the University of Tennessee, Knoxville, 2006, Pp. 1-12.

López-Cruz, I; Rojano Aguilar, A; Ojeda Bustamante, W; Salazar Moreno, R. Modelos ARX para predecir la temperatura del aire de un invernadero: una metodología. *Agrociencia*, 2007, 41(2), 181-192.

Lu, S; Van Eck, J; Zhou, X; Lopez, AB; O'Halloran, DM; Cosman, KM; Conlin, BJ; Paolillo, DJ; Garvin, DF; Vrebalov, J; Kochian, LV; Kupper, H; Earle, ED; Cao, J; Li, L. The Cauliflower Or Gene Encodes a DnaJ Cysteine-Rich Domain-Containing Protein That Mediates High Levels of β-Carotene Accumulation. *The Plant Cell*, 2006, 18, 3594-3605.

Marín-Martinez, R; Veloz-García, R; Veloz-Rodríguez, R; Guzmán-Maldonado, SH; Loarca-Piña, G; Cardador-Martínez, A; Villagómez-Torres, AF; Guevara-Olvera, L; Muñoz-Sánchez, CI; Torres-Pacheco, I; González-Chavira, MM; Herrera-Hernández, G; Guevara-Gonzalez, RG. Antimutagenic and antioxidant activities of quebracho phenolics (*Schinopsis balansae*) recovered from tannery wastewaters. *Bioresource Technology*, 2009, 100(1), 434-439.

Mehta, BJ; Salgado, LM; Bejarano, ER; Cerdá-Olmedo, E. New mutants of Phycomyces blakesleeanus for β -carotene production. *Appl Environ Microbiol.*, 1997, 63 (9), 3657-3661.

Meyer, F; Bairati, I; Jobin, E; Gélinas, M; Fortin, A; Nabid, A; Têtu, B. Acute adverse effects of radiation therapy and local recurrence in relation to dietary and plasma β-carotene and α-tocopherol in head and neck cancer patients. *Nutr Cancer*, 2007, 59(1), 29-35.

Middleton, E Jr; Kandaswami, C; Theoharides, T. The effects of plant flavonoids on mammalian cells: Implications for inflammation, heart disease, and cancer. *Pharmacol Rev.*, 2000, 52(4), 673-751.

Misawa, N; Nakagawa, M; Kobayashi, K; Yamano, S; Izawa, Y; Nakamura, K; Harashima, K. Elucidation of pathway the *Erwinia uredovora* carotenoid biosynthetic by functional analysis of gene products expressed in Escherichia coli. *J Bacteriol.*, 1990, 172, 6704-6712.

Misawa, N; Yamano, S; Ikenaga, H. Production of 1-Carotene in *Zymomonas mobilis* and Agrobacterium tumefaciens by Introduction of the Biosynthesis Genes from Erwinia uredovora. *Applied and Environmental Microbiology*, 1991, 1847-1849.

Molina-Aiz, F; Valera, D; Alvarez, A. Measurement and simulation of climate inside Almeria-type greenhouse using computational fluid dynamics. *Agric. Forest Meteorol.*, 2004, 125.

Monta, M; Kondo, N. Ting, K. End-effectors for tomato harvesting robot. *Artificial Intelligence Review*, 1998, 12, 11-25.

Mori, T. Mechatronics, Yaskawa International Trademark Application Memo. 1969.

Nanou, K; Roukas, T; Kotzekidou, P. Role of hydrolytic enzymes and oxidative stress in autolysis and morphology of Blakeslea trispora during β-carotene production in submerged fermentation. *Appl Microbiol Biotechnol*, 2007, 74, 447-453.

Neethirajan, S; Karunakaran, C; Jayas, D; White, N. Detection techniques for stored-product insects in grain. *Foodcont*, 2007, 18, 157-162.

Nishiura, Y; Murase, H; Honami, N; Taira, T; Wadano, A. Development of a gripper for a plug-in grafting robot system. *Acta Horticulturae*, 1996, 440, 475-480.

Niyog,i, KK; Björkman, O; Grossman, AR. The roles of specific xanthophylls in photoprotection. *Proc. Natl. Acad. Sci.*, 1997, 94, 14162-14167.

Norton, T; Sun, D; Grant, J; Fallon, R; Dodd, V. Applications of computational fluid dynamics (CFD) in the modelling and design of ventilation systems in agricultural industry: A review. *Bioresource Technology*, 2007, 98, 2386-2414.

Okamoto, T. Robotization of orchid protocorm transplanting in tissue culture. *Japan Agricultural Research Quarterly*, 1996, 30(4), 213-220.

Ortiz, D. Simulación numérica de la ventilación natural en un invernadero colombiano de 10 naves. Congreso Iberoamericano para el Desarrollo y Aplicación de los Plásticos en Agricultura, Bogotá, Colombia, 2004, 99-104.

Ould Khaoua, S; Bournet, P; Migeon, C; Boulard, T; Chassériaux, G. Analysis of greenhouse ventilation efficiency based on computational fluid dynamics. *Biosystems Engineering*, 2006, 95.

Peng, CL; Gilmore, AM. Contrasting changes of photosystem 2 efficiency in Arabidopsis xanthophylls mutants at room or low temperature under high irradiance stress. *Photosynthetica*, 2003, 41(2), 233-239.

Pirie, A. Vitamin A deficiency and child blindness in the developing world. *Proc. Nutr. Soc.*, 1983, 42, 53.

Polus, A; Kiec-Wilk, B; Hartwich, J; Balwierz, A; Stachura, J; Dyduch, G; Laidler, P; Zagajewski, Langman, T; Schnitz, G; Goralczyk, R; Wertz, K; Riss, G; Keijer, J; Dembinska-Kiec. The chemotactic activity of beta-carotene in endothelial cell progenitors and human umbilical vein endothelial cells: A microarray analysis. *Exp Clin Cardiol*, 2006, 11(2), 117-122.

Quist, D; Chapela, I. Transgenic DNA introgressed into traditional maize landraces in Oaxaca, Mexico. *Nature*, 2001, 414, 541-543.

Raja, R; Hemaiswarya, S; Rengasamy, R. Exploitation of *Dunaliella* for β-carotene production. *Appl Microbiol Biotechnol*, 2007, 74, 517-523.

Ralley, L; Enfissi, EMA; Misawa, N; Schuch, W; Bramley, PM; Fraser, PD. Metabolic engineering of ketocarotenoid formation in higher plants. *Plant J.*, 2004, 39, 477-486.

Rico-García, E; Reyes-Araiza, J; Herrera-Ruiz, G. Simulation of the climate in tow different greenhouses. *Acta Hortc.*, 2006.

Ridgway, C; Davies, E; Chambers, J; Mason, D; Bateman, M. Rapid machine vision method for the detection of insects and other particulate biocontaminants of bulk grain in transit. *Biosyst Eng.*, 2002, 83(1), 21-30.

Rodríguez, E. Efecto de la poda y densidad de población en el rendimiento y calidad de fruto de jitomate. PhD thesis, Universidad de Chapingo, 1996.

Rodríguez-Saíz, M; Paz, B; de la Fuente, JL; López-Nieto, MJ; Cabri, W; Barredo, JL. Blakeslea trispora Genes for Carotene Biosynthesis. *Appl Environ Microbiol*, 2004, 70(9), 5589-5594.

Rombouts, N; Rombouts, P. Inrichting voor het machinaal afscheiden Van stekken Van een plantentak. Patent NL1017794C, 29 p. 2002.

Roy, C; Boulard, T; Kittas, C; Wang, S. Convective and ventilation transfers in greenhouses. Part 1. The greenhouse considered as a perfectly stirred tank. *Biosyst. Eng.*, 2002, 83 (1), 1-20.

Ryu, K; Kim, G. Han, J. Development of a robotic transplanter for bedding plants. *J Agric Eng Res.*, 2001, 78(2), 141-146.

Sakaue, O. Development of seedling production robot and automated transplanter system. *Japanese Agric Res Quart*, 1996, 30(4), 221-226.

Sandmann, G. Carotenoid biosynthesis in microorganisms and plants. *Eur. J. Biochem.*, 1994, 223, 7-24.

Sandmann, G. Molecular evolution of carotenoid biosynthesis from bacteria to plants. *Physiol. Plantarum*, 2002, 116, 431-40.

Sandmann, G. Carotenoid biosynthesis and biotechnological application. *Arch. Biochem. Biophys.*, 2001, 385(1), 4-12.

Schmidt, U. Microclimate Control in Greenhouses Based on Phytomonitoring Data and Mollier Phase Diagram. *Acta Hort*, 691, ISHS 2005.

Seginer, I; Ioslovich, I. Seasonal optimization of the greenhouse environment for a simple two-stages cropgrowth model. *Journal of Agricultural Engineering Research*, 1998, 70, 145-155.

Seginer, I. Some artificial neural network applications to greenhouse environmental control. *Computers and Electronics in Agriculture*, 1997, 18, 167-186.

Shewmaker, CK; Sheeh,y, JA; Daley, M; Colburn, S; Ke, DY. Seed-specific overexpression of phytoene synthase: Increase in carotenoids and other metabolic effects. *Plant J.*, 1999, 20, 401-412.

Simonton, W. Automatic Geranium stock processing in a robotic workcell. *Transactions of the ASAE*, 1990, 33(6), 2074-2080.

Smith, R; Boutwell, J; Allen, J. Evaluating practice adoption: one approach, *Journal of Extension*, 1983.

Stalberg, K; Lindgren, O; Ek, B; Hoglund AS. Synthesis of ketocarotenoids in the seed of *Arabidopsis thaliana*. *Plant J.*, 2003, 36, 771-779.

Stanghellini, C. Van Meurs T. Environmental control of greenhouse crop trnspiration. *J Agric Eng Res.*, 1992, 51, 297-311.

Stansly, P; Sánchez, P; Rodríguez, J; Cañizares, F; Nieto, A; López, M; Fajardo, M; Suárez, V; Urbaneja. Prospects for biological control of Bemisia tabaci (Homoptera, Aleyrodidae) in greenhouse tomatoes of southern Spain. *Crop Prot.*, 2004, 23(8), 701-712.

Taiz, L; Zeiger, E. *Plant Physiology*. 3d edition. Sinauer Associates, Inc; Publishers. Sunderland, Massacusetts, 2002, 690-715.

Takano, H; Obitsu, S; Beppu, T; Ueda, K. Light-induced carotenogenesis en streptomyces coelicolor A3 (2): Identification of an Extracytoplasmic function sigma factor that directs photodependent transcription of the carotenoid biosynthesis gene cluster. *J Bacteriol*, 2005, 187(5), 1825-1832.

Tanatu, H. Models for greenhouse climate control. *Acta Horticulturae*, 1989, 245, 397-404.

Tandon, V; El-Mounayri, H; Kishawy, H. NC end milling optimization using evolutionary computation, *International Journal of Machine Tools & Manufacture*, 2002.

Tang, S; Chepe, R. Models for integrated pest control and their biological implications. *Math Biosci.*, 2008.

Tap, F. Economics-based optimal control of greenhouse tomato crop production. PhD thesis, Wageningen Agricultural University, the Netherlands. 2000.

Tavares, C; Goncalves, A; Castro, P; Loureiro, D; Joyce, A. Modelling an agriculture production greenhouse. *Renewable Energy*, 2001, 22, 15-20.

Taylor, M; Ramsay, G. Carotenoid biosynthesis in plant storage organs: Recent advances and prospects for improving plant food quality. *Physiol. Plant*, 2005, 124, 143-151.

Tchamitchian, M; Van Willigenburg, L; Van Straten, G. Short term dynamic optimal control of the greenhouse climate. *MRS Report*, 1992, 92(3).

Telfer, A. What is β-carotene doing in the photosystem II reaction centre? *Philos Trans R Soc Lond B Biol Sci.*, 357, 1431-1439.

Thayer, SS; Bjorkman. O. Carotenoid distribution and deepoxidation in thylakoid pigment-protein complexes from cotton leaves and bundle-sheath cells of maize. *Photosynthesis Res.*, 1992, 33(3), 213-235.

Thomas, M. Developing computer-based expert diagnostic systems for diseases, disorders and pest damage of citrus and tropical fruit crops. Master Thesis, University of Florida, Gainesville. 1995.

Udink Ten Cat, A; Bot, G; Van Dixhoorn, J. Computer control of greenhouse climates, *Acta Hort*, 1978, 87, 265-272.

Udink Ten Cate, A. Greenhouse climate control in the nineties. *Acta Hort*, 1985, 230, 459-470.

Udink Ten Cate, A. *Simulation models for greenhouse climate control*. In Proceedings, 7th IFAC Symposium. Identification and System Parameter Estimation, York, England. Pergamon, Oxford. 1983.

Umeno, D; Tobias, AV; Arnold, FH. Diversifying Carotenoid Biosynthetic Pathways by Directed Evolution. *Microbiol Mol Biol Rev.*, 2005, 69(1), 51-78.

Van Henten, E; Van Tuijl, B; Hemming, J; Bontsema, J. An Autonomous Robot for De-leafing Cucumber Plants Grown in a High-wire Cultivation System. *Proceedings of Greensys*, 2004, 12-16.

Van Henten, E. *Greenhouse climate management: an optimal control approach*. PhD thesis, Wageningen Agricultural University, the Netherlands. 1994.

Van Henten, E. Greenhouse Mechanization, Greenhouse Technology Group, Agrotechnology & Food Innovations B.V., Netherlands, 2003.

Van Henten, E. Non-destructive crop measurements by image processing for crop grow control. *J Agric Eng Res.*, 1995, 61, 97-105.

Van Henten, E. Sensitivity analisys of an optimal control problem in greenhouse climate management. *Biosys Eng.*, 2000, 85, 335-364.

Van Henten, EJ; y Bontsema, J. Non-destuctrive Crop Measurements by Image Processing for Crop Growth Control. *J. Agric. Eng Res.*, 1995, 61, 97-105.

Veloz-García, RA; Marín-Martínez, R; Veloz-Rodríguez, R; Muñoz-Sánchez, CI; Guevara-Olvera, L; Miranda-López, R; González-Chavira, MM; Irineo Torres-Pacheco, I; Guzmán-Maldonado, SH; Cardador-Martínez, A; Loarca-Piña, G; Guevara-González, RG. Antimutagenic and antioxidant activities of Cascalote (*Caesalpinia cacalaco*) phenolics. *J Sci Food Agric.*, 2004, 84, 1632-1638.

Verdoe,s, J C; Krubasik, KP; Sandmann, G; Van Ooyen, AJJ; Echavarri-Erasun, C; Johnson, EA. Isolation and functional characterisation of a novel type of carotenoid biosynthetic gene from Xanthophyllomyces dendrorhous. *Mol. Gen. Genet.*, 1999$_a$, 262, 453-461.

Verdoes, JC; Misawa, N; Van Ooyen, AJJ. Cloning and characterization of the astaxanthin biosynthetic gene encoding phytoene desaturase of *Xanthophyllomyces dendrorhous*. *Biotechnol. Bioeng.*, 1999$_b$, 63, 750-755.

Verwaal, R; Wang, J; Meijnen, JP; Visser, H; Sandmann, G; Van den Berg, JA; Van Ooyen, JJ. High-level production of beta-carotene in Saccharomyces cerevisiae by succesive transformation with carotenogenic genes from Xanthophyllomyces dendrorhous. *Appl Env Microbiol.*, 2007, 73(13), 4342-4350.

Vorst, P; Baard, RL; Mur, LR; Korthals, HJ; Van, D. Effect of growth arrest on carotene accumulation photosynthesis in Dunaliella. *Microbiol.*, 1994, 140, 1411-1417.

Voutilainen, S; Nurmi, T; Mursu, J; Rissanen. Carotenoids and cardiovascular health. *Am J Clin Nutr.*, 2006, 83, 1265-1271.

Weeks, OB; Garner, RJ. Biosynthesis of carotenoids in Flavobacterium dehydrogenans Arnaudi. *Arch Biochem Biophys.*, 1967, 121(1), 35-49.

Xiaoli, L; Shiu Kit, T. Real-Time Tool Condition Monitoring Using Wavelet Transforms and Fuzzy Techniques, *IEEE Transactions on Systems, Man, and Cybernetics*, 2000, 30(3).

Yamano, S; Ishii, T; Nakagawa, M; Ikenaga, H; Misawa, N. Metabolic engineering for production of b-carotene and lycopene in *Saccharomyces cerevisiae. Biosci. Biotechnol. Biochem.*, 1994, 58, 1112-1114.

Yang, Y; Ting, K; Giacomelli, G. Factors affecting performance of sliding-needles gripper during robotic transplanting of seedlings. *Appl Eng Agric.*, 1991, 7(4), 493-498.

Ye, X; Al-Babili, S; Klbti, A; Zhang, J; Lucca, P; Beyer, P; Potrykus, I. Engineering the Provitamin A (β-Carotene) Biosynthetic Pathway into (Carotenoid-Free) Rice Endosperm. *Science*, 2000, 287, 303-305.

Young, P. Modelling an PIP control of glasshouse micro-climate. *Control Engineering Practice*, 1994, 65, 591-604.

Zaripheh, S; Erdman, JW Jr. Factors that influence the bioavailability of xanthophylls. *J. Nutr.*, 2002, 132, 531-534.

Zayas, I; Flinn, P. Detection of insects in bulk wheat samples with machine vision. *Transactions of the ASAE.*, 1998, 41(3), 88.

Zayas, I; Pomeranz, Y; Lai, F. Discrimination of wheat and nonwheat components in grain samples by image analysis. *Cereal Chem.*, 1989, 66(3), 233.

In: Encyclopedia of Vitamin Research
Editor: Joshua T. Mayer

ISBN 978-1-61761-928-1
© 2011 Nova Science Publishers, Inc.

Chapter 32

Water Soluble Supramolecular Complexes of β-Carotene and Other Carotenoids[*]

Nikolay E. Polyakov[1,2] and Lowell D. Kispert[1]
[1]Chemistry Department, University of Alabama, Tuscaloosa, AL 35487-0336, USA
[2]Institute of Chemical Kinetics & Combustion, Novosibirsk, 630090, Russia

Abstract

It is well known, that the wide practical application of β-carotene and other carotenoids as antioxidants or food colorants is substantially hampered by their hydrophobic properties, instability in the presence of oxygen and metal ions, and high photosensitivity. The majority of carotenoids are lipophilic molecules with near zero inherent aqueous solubility. Moving carotenoids into a pharmaceutical application requires a chemical delivery system that overcomes the problems with parenteral administration of a highly lipophilic, low molecular weight compound. Many different methods have been developed to make the carotenoids "water dispersible", as true water solubility has not been described. Most of the attempts to increase in solubility of carotenoids are related to the preparation of cyclodextrin inclusion complexes. Application of inclusion complexes was first related to an attempt to minimize the aforementioned disadvantages of carotenoids when these compounds are used in food processing (colors and antioxidant capacity) as well as for production of therapeutic formulations considering the better solubility and consequently higher bioavailability. In this chapter we present three examples of supramolecular complexes of carotenoids with natural oligosaccharides and polysaccharides: cyclodextrin, glycyrrhizin and arabinogalactan. It was demonstrated that incorporation of carotenoids into the "host" macromolecule results in significant change in their properties. In particular, we present

---

[*] A version of this chapter was also published in *Beta Carotene: Dietary Sources, Cancer and Cognition, edited by Leiv Haugen and Terje Bjornson* published by Nova Science Publishers, Inc. It was submitted for appropriate modifications in an effort to encourage wider dissemination of research.

the first example of water soluble complexes of carotenoids with natural polysaccharide arabinogalactan, a branched polymer with molecular mass 15000-20000. Compared to pure carotenoids, polysaccharide complexes show enhanced photostability in water solutions. A significant decrease in the reactivity towards metal ions (Fe^{3+}) and reactive oxygen species in solution was also detected.

Introduction

Carotenoids are a class of pigments widely found in nature. These essential nutrients are synthesized by plants and microorganisms and exist in many foods including vegetables, fruits, and fish. About 600 various carotenoids are known. However, only a few (about 20) have been found in human tissues. These include β-carotene, canthaxanthin, zeaxanthin, etc. The presence of a polyene chain and various terminal substituents in carotenoid molecules determines their color, redox properties and location inside the lipid layers in biological media.

Recently much attention has been focused on the reactions between carotenoids and free radicals [1-7] because of the ability of carotenoids to prevent the development of diseases caused by toxic free radicals [8]. One factor contributing to the development of various diseases, including infarction, cerebral thrombosis, and tumors has been attributed to the action of free radicals and the toxic forms of oxygen [9]. Carotenoids are assumed to protect cells by scavenging either free radicals or excited oxygen that have a severe impact on cells. Of no less significance are the membrane-stabilizing and immunostimulating functions of carotenoids as well as their provitamin A activity. Vitamin A and carotenoids favor normal metabolism, enhance the resistance of an organism against infections, provide normal operation of the organ of vision, exert beneficial effect on the performance of skin and mucous membranes and are involved in redox processes. At the same time, wide practical application of carotenoids as antioxidants or food colorants is substantially hampered by their hydrophobic properties, instability in the presence of oxygen and high photosensitivity.

One of the promising way to overcome there problems is the preparation of supramolecular inclusion complexes. Complex formation is widely used in medicine to improve the solubility of preparations, to deliver drugs, and to decrease their toxicity (see Figure 1) [10-12].

Fundamental and applied research has recently been devoted to the inclusion complexes of carotenoids with natural compounds, specifically the cyclodextrins (CD) [13-21], which are assumed to possess protective properties and to decrease the hydrophobic behavior of the included molecules. Application of inclusion complexes was first related to an attempt to minimize the aforementioned disadvantages of carotenoids when used in the food industry, cosmetology, and medicine.

At present, it can be stated with confidence that it is the chemical and physicochemical studies of the reactivity of carotenoids in redox processes in organized media that are most promising. In particular, this refers to a study of supramolecular inclusion complexes of active compounds that can be of interest in medicine, pharmacology, artifical light-harvesting, and other areas. As it was mentioned above, most studies concern the inclusion complexes of cyclodextrins that are widely used in practice as agents for transporting and conserving drugs. The main difficulty in practical applications of "host-guest" complexes of cyclodextrins is that the rigidly fixed volume of the cyclodextrin cavity prevents binding of either very small or very large molecules including many compounds that are of interest in medicine and pharmacology. Therefore, the search is being continued for complexing agents devoid of these disadvantages. One of the compounds that appear to be promising is glycyrrhizic acid (or glycyrrhizin). β-glycyrrhizic acid (GA) belongs to the triterpene glycosides and contains both hydrophilic (glucuronic acid) and hydrophobic (glycyrrhetic acid) regions. GA is extracted from the Ural licorice root (*Glyzyrrhiza glabra L*).

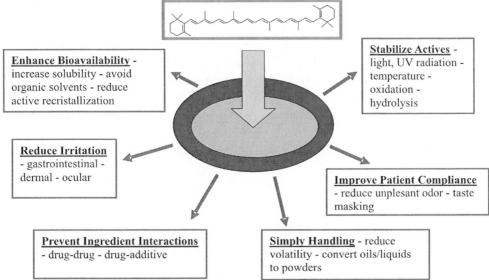

Enhance Bioavailability - increase solubility - avoid organic solvents - reduce active recristallization

Stabilize Actives - light, UV radiation - temperature - oxidation - hydrolysis

Reduce Irritation - gastrointestinal - dermal - ocular

Improve Patient Compliance - reduce unplesant odor - taste masking

Prevent Ingredient Interactions - drug-drug - drug-additive

Simply Handling - reduce volatility - convert oils/liquids to powders

Figure 1. Application spectrum of the inclusion complexes in medicine.

β-glycyrrhizic acid (GA)

It was suggested in many studies that glycyrrhizic acid in solution can create cyclic structures that can form inclusion complexes with various organic compounds [22, 23]. GA is of considerable interest to pharmacologists because of its unique physiological activity. In particular, its preparations are very popular in connection with AIDS treatment [24]. This compound is particularly attractive for three main reasons. First, GA in contrast to the cyclodextrins has an open chain structure and thus, for complex formation, there are no rigorous restrictions on the size of a "guest" molecule. Second, all authors indicate unusual stability of GA complexes [22, 23, 25, 26]. The stability constants of GA complexes are in the range of 10^5 M^{-1}, which are two orders of magnitude higher than a mean stability constant of cyclodextrin complexes [27]. And third, it was demonstrated that application of glycyrrhizic acid together with other medicines strengthens their therapeutic efficiency by orders of magnitude and reduces side effects, e.g., the toxic action on the alimentary canal [28-30].

Another imperfection of carotenoid-cyclodextrin complexes is their poor solubility. In reality, these complexes form water dispersions, rather than solutions. According to the studies of Mele with coauthors [16-17], carotenoid-cyclodextrin complexes in water form large aggregates with size 100-200 nm. This results in weakly colored opalescent solution [20]. The reduced color intensity significantly decreases the application area of carotenoids, in particular as food colorants.

Now we can present the first example of water soluble complex of β-carotene and some other carotenoids. The present chapter describes the complex formation between carotenoids and natural polysaccharide arabinogalactan (AG), a branched polymer with molecular mass 15000-20000.

Arabinogalactans are found in a variety of plants but are more abundant in the Larix genus, primarily Western and Siberian Larch [31,32]. Larch arabinogalactan is approved by the U.S. Food and Drug Administration (FDA) as a source of dietary fiber, but also has potential therapeutic benefits as an immune stimulating agent and cancer protocol adjunct. The immune-enhancing herb echinacea also contains AG, as do leeks, carrots, radishes, pears, wheat, red wine, and tomatoes. AG is an important source of dietary fiber. It is known that AG increases the production of short-chain fatty acids, principally butyrate and proprionate, which are essential for the health of the colon. AG also acts as a food supply for "friendly" bacteria, such as bifidobacteria and lactobacillus, while eliminating "bad" bacteria. AG has a beneficial effect upon the immune system as it increases the activity of natural killer cells and other immune system components, thus helping the body to fight infection [32]. The increased aqueous solubility of a number of carotenoids will likely find utility in their introduction into mammalian cell culture systems that have previously been dependent upon liposomes, or toxic organic solvents, for the introduction of carotenoids into aqueous solution [21]. Also water soluble carotenoids displays several technological applications that could be used in food processing to enhance color and antioxidant capacity as well as for the production of therapeutic formulations considering the better solubility and consequently higher bioavailability [13-15, 33]. It is worth noting that at present, progress in developing novel forms of medicines has been related not only to a search for new active substances but also to regulating the effect of already available preparations. Complexation is one method for regulating this effect.

The present chapter describes our studies of the inclusion complexes of a number of natural and synthetic carotenoids with natural oligosaccharides and polysaccharides, namely with cyclodextrins, glycyrrhizin and arabinogalactan. We have studied the solubility of these complexes of carotenoids in water and their reactivity in redox processes. The reactivity was studied using important electron transfer reactions with metal ions and quinones as well as in the reactions with free radicals. These processes have been previously studied in detail in homogeneous solutions [34-35].

Fragment of Arabinogalactan

Results and Discussion

1. Inclusion Complexes of Carotenoids with Cyclodextrins (CD) [20].

Since carotenoids are highly hydrophobic, air- and light-sensitive compounds, developing methods for increasing their bioavailability and stability towards irradiation and reactive oxygen species is essential. One can find several examples of practical application of carotenoid-cyclodextrin complexes in the food, cosmetics and pharmaceutical industry [13-15]. In the food industry, carotenoids are mainly used as food colorants and antioxidants. The application of their CD complexes instead of pure carotenoids results in increasing stability of colorants under storage and simplicity in using without preliminary solubilization in organic solvents. In cosmetics, carotenoids are used as antioxidants, but limited in application by the intense color of carotenoids. Incorporation of carotenoids into cyclodextrin cavity reduces significantly their color intensity. In particular, the cosmetic cream with β-carotene-cyclodextrin complex has a nice pink color instead of the saturated red color for pure carotene [15]. However, in spite of this practical application, there is still no strong evidence of real inclusion complex formation, and only a few attempts of structural studies of such complexes have been reported [16-17]. Previous studies of short-chain analogues of carotenoids, β-ionone [36], and retinoids [37], demonstrated the formation of stable inclusion complexes of these substrates with different cyclodextrins (β-CD), 2-hydroxypropyl-β-cyclodextrin (HP-β-CD), 2-hydroxypropyl-γ-cyclodextrin (HP-γ-CD). It was shown that the terminal cyclohexene fragment of β-ionone, which is present in most carotenoids (Figure 2), has the requisite size for incorporation into the CD cavity. It seemed likely that carotenoids, which are even more hydrophobic, should also form inclusion complexes with CDs.

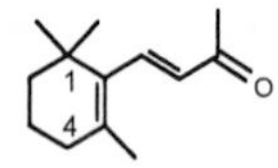

β–Ionone

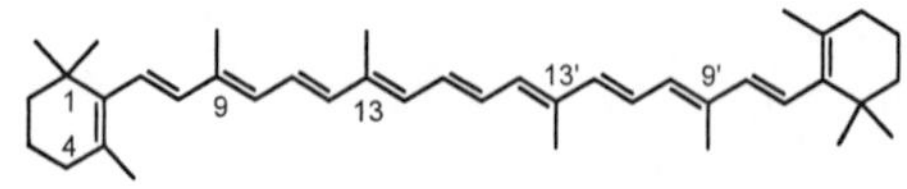

β–Carotene (I)

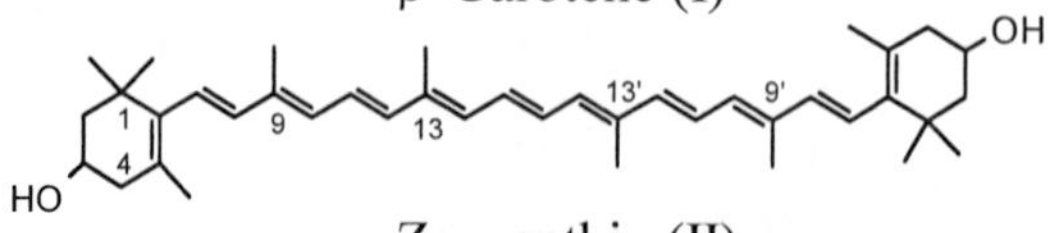

Zeaxanthin (II)

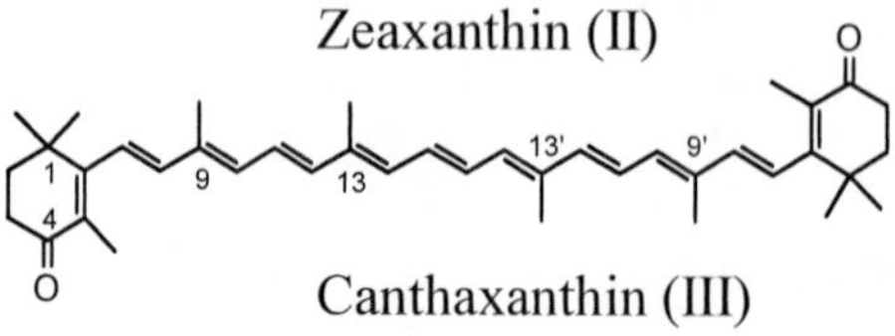

Canthaxanthin (III)

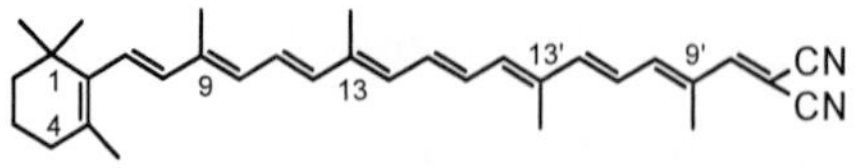

7'-Apo-7',7'-dicyano-β–carotene (IV)

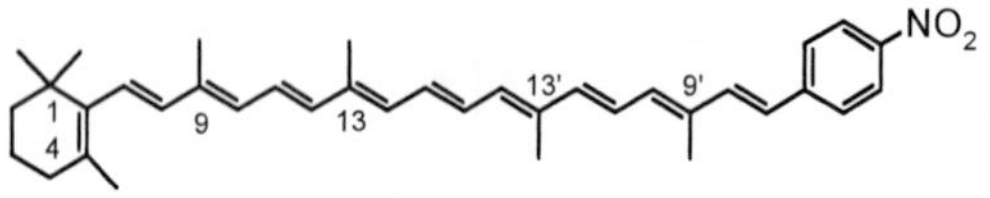

7'-Apo-7'-(p-NO$_2$-C$_6$H$_4$)-β–carotene (V)

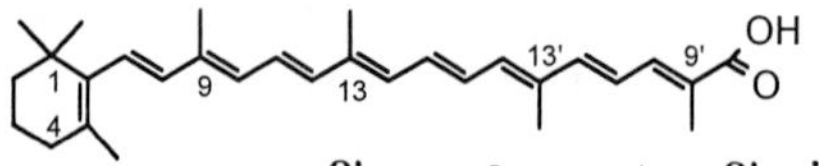

8'-apo-β–caroten-8'-oic acid (VI)

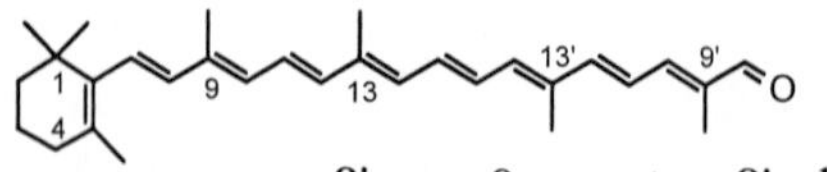

8'-apo-β–caroten-8'-al (VII)

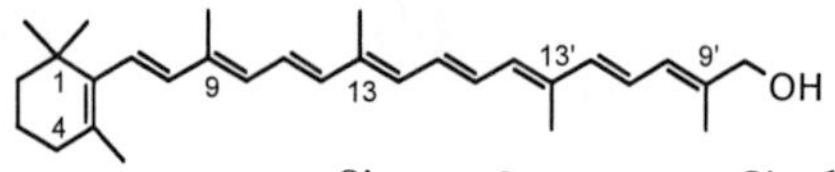

8'-apo-β–caroten-8'-ol (VIII)

Figure 2. The structures of β-ionone and some natural and synthetic carotenoids.

In our study we have focused on two aspects. The first aim was to obtain direct evidence of inclusion complex formation. For this purpose we applied standard approaches using ^{1}H-NMR and UV-Vis absorption spectroscopy. The second aim was the investigation of the reactivity of carotenoid-CD inclusion complexes towards peroxyl radicals (antioxidant activity). It was earlier suggested that β-carotene and other carotenoids react with peroxyl radicals primarily at the 4-C position of the cyclohexene ring (see Figure 2) [2, 6, 7]. One can expect that the reactivity of carotenoids towards free radicals may decrease if the cyclohexene ring is embedded in the CD cavity. This investigation was beneficial for the purpose of application of the carotenoid-CD complexes to protect carotenoids against damage caused by O_2 and free radicals.

In our study we used two methods of complex preparation, described in details in the literature [13-16]. In the first method, "solid mixture" (SM), solid carotenoid and requisite amounts of CD (1 or 2 equiv) were ground together until a homogeneous powder was obtained. Grinding was continued after adding a small amount of deionized water to give a paste, which was then stored overnight under nitrogen, treated with water to obtain a final carotenoid concentration of 1 mM, and the suspension was stirred for several hours. In the second method, "liquid mixture" (LM), the solution of carotenoid in methanol (or other organic solvent) was added to the aqueous CD solution.

UV-Vis absorption study. All carotenoid-CD complexes prepared in water by the SM method show a considerable change in color compared to carotenoid solutions in organic solvents. Note that with the exception of **VI**, all carotenoids are completely insoluble in water. For example, **I**-CD complex has opalescent intensely pink-orange in aqueous solution. The **IV**-CD complex is black, while the MeOH or CH_2Cl_2 solutions of **IV** are violet. All complexes have a very broad absorption band up to 1100 nm with reduced intensity (about one order of magnitude). We suggest that the broadening of the absorption band is due to aggregation of complexes in aqueous solution. Such aggregate formation was previously detected by light scattering spectroscopy [16, 17]. Assuming that only a cyclohexene ring of the carotenoid can be embedded in the CD cavity, we suggest that aggregates of the complexes have a micelle-like structure in the aqueous media.

Aggregate formation could be observed by changes occurring in the UV-Vis spectra when mixing separately prepared solutions of CD in H_2O and carotenoid in ethanol. For the highly water soluble HP-β-CD and HP-γ-CD used in UV-Vis experiments, similar effects were observed. The maximum absorption of Car-CD complexes in water is at a much shorter wavelength than that of the pure carotenoids in ethanol. The most significant blue shifts were observed for carotenoids with polar terminal groups: -CN, -Ph-NO_2, -COOH. For example, carotenoid **V** shows the blue shift of the absorption maximum from 485 nm in ethanol to 315 nm in water with simultaneous considerable decrease of extinction coefficient. The spectrum of the Car-CD mixture gradually changed with time due to aggregate formation. With large excess (50 eq.) of HP-β-CD, the changes with time were greatly attenuated (see Figure 3). We suggest that this is due to the existence of an equilibrium between individual complexes and aggregates of the complexes. Compounds with other polar groups (**IV** and **VI**) showed similar behavior, an increase of complex solubility with increase of CD concentration.

However, β-carotene (**I**), which does not contain polar groups, displayed divergent spectral changes (Figure 4). No large blue shift was observed in this case, and the presumed equilibrium favors the formation of complex aggregates. According to published phase-solubility diagrams [38], two types of complex can exist. The first type demonstrates the increase of solubility with increased CD concentration, and the second type shows the opposite effect. Figures 3 and 4 show that both types of complexes take place for the carotenoids under study. Different behavior of various carotenoids could be explained by the difference in their structure, namely the structure of terminal groups. Assuming that the Car-CD complex has a hydrophilic CD head and hydrophobic carotenoid tail, one can suggest the formation of more stable aggregates for complexes with non-polar carotenoids.

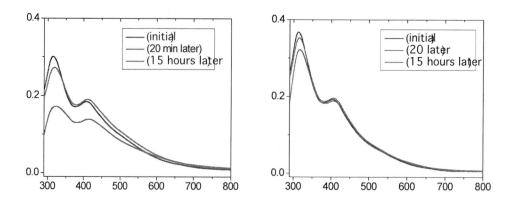

Figure 3. Transformation of UV-Vis. absorption spectrum of V-HP-β-CD (a) 1:1 mixture and (b) 1:50 mixture in water-ethanol solution as a function of time (adopted from [20], Figure 1).

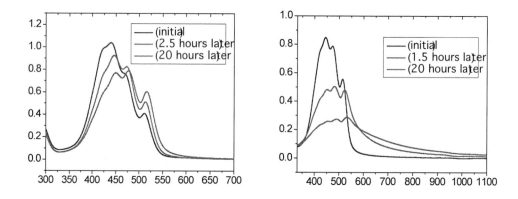

Figure 4. Transformation of UV-Vis. absorption spectrum of β-carotene-HP-β-CD (a) 1:1mixture and (b) 1:50 mixture in water-ethanol solution as a function of time (adopted from [20], Figure 2).

The presence of aggregation makes elucidation of the structure of CD complexes difficult for most of carotenoids. For this purpose we used the partly water soluble carotenoid **VI** with acid terminal group. It is known that the solubility of CD complexes with organic acids can be increased dramatically by changing the pH of the solution [39]. Indeed, the presence of 4 mM NaOH in 2 mM aqueous complex solution resulted in increased complex solubility so that the monomers of the **VI**-CD complex could be observed by UV-Vis as well as NMR techniques. The absorption maximum of **VI** in water shows a strong blue shift (λ_{max} = 285 nm) compared to that in ethanol (λ_{max} = 400 nm). The spectrum of the **VI**-CD complex in the presence of NaOH is nearly identical to that of **VI** in ethanol (see Figure 5). This observation might be considered as proof of incorporation of carotenoid within the CD cavity, since it is known that the polarity of the CD interior is similar to that of an ethanolic solution [40]. No changes were detected in the absorption spectrum after addition of NaOH in the absence of CD.

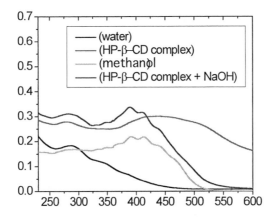

Figure 5. UV-Vis. absorption spectra of VI in different media. The concentrations of carotenoid were different in each case (adopted from [20], Figure 3).

H-NMR study of CD complex. Usually ^{1}H-NMR experiments can provide information about the stoichiometry, stability, and the structure of CD complexes [27, 40, 41]. In particular, Job's plot, which correlates the chemical shift and the host/guest ratio, has been widely used to determine complex stoichiometry [42, 43]. The possibility of detecting inclusion complexes by NMR spectroscopy is based on the expectation that if a guest molecule is incorporated into the CD cavity, the screening constants of the CD protons inside the cavity (H_3 and H_5) should be sensitive to the changed environment, but the outside protons (H_1, H_2, and H_4) should not (Figure 6).

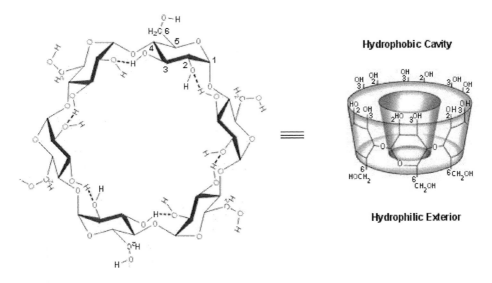

Figure 6. Schematic presentation of the structure of cyclodextrin.

As stated above, sufficiently high concentrations of carotenoid-CD complex (1 mM) needed for NMR measurements could be obtained only for carotenoid **VI** in the presence of NaOH. As it was earlier detected for β-ionone-CD complex [36], the shift of the internal protons of the CD cavity was detected in the presence of carotenoid **VI** (see Figure 7).

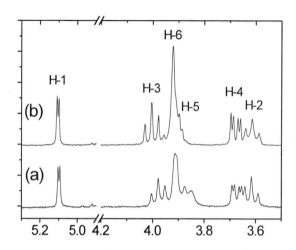

Figure 7. ^{1}H-NMR (360 MHz) spectra of aqueous solution of β-CD with addition of 4 mM NaOH in the presence (a) and absence (b) of VI. See Figure 6 for identification of CD protons. Concentrations of CD and carotenoid are 2 mM (adopted from [20], Figure 4).

For calculation of stoichiometry of this inclusion complex and its association constant, the variation of NMR chemical shifts of CD protons was measured with changes of carotenoid concentration. This approach is widely used by many authors for analysis of an inclusion complex [44, 45]. Let's consider the equilibrium process of complex (C_{nm}) formation between **n** cyclodextrin (CD) molecules and **m** guest (G) molecules (1):

$$mG + nCD \rightleftharpoons C_{nm} \tag{1}$$

The association constant of this complex is described as:

$$K_{nm} = \frac{[C_{nm}]}{[G]^m [CD]^n} \tag{2}$$

Since the association-dissociation process is rapid relative to the NMR time scale (in the microsecond to millisecond range), the chemical shift of CD protons can be determined as follows:

$$\delta_{obs} = f_{CD}\, \delta_{CD} + f_{Cnm}\delta_{Cnm} \tag{3}$$

where δ_{CD} and δ_{Cnm} are the chemical shifts of the free and complexed CD, and f_{CD} and f_{Cnm} are their molar fractions. Substituting $\Delta\delta_{obs} = \delta_{obs} - \delta_{CD}$ and $\Delta\delta_{Cnm} = \delta_{Cnm} - \delta_{CD}$ we obtain:

$$\Delta\delta_{obs} = n\Delta\delta_{Cnm} \frac{[C_{nm}]}{[CD]_o} \tag{4}$$

From the mass balance, the initial concentrations of carotinoid $[G]_0 = [G] + m[C_{nm}]$ and cyclodextrin $[CD]_0 = [CD] + n[C_{nm}]$. If $m = n = 1$, from eq. (2) the following equation for concentration of a 1:1 complex can be obtained:

$$[C_{11}]^2 - ([G]_0 + [CD]_0 + 1/K_{11})[C_{11}] + ([G]_0 [CD]_0 = 0 \tag{5}$$

Combination of eqs (4) and (5) results in the expression (6) from which the value K_{11} can be obtained from the G_0 concentration dependence of $\Delta\delta_{obs}$ (CD).

$$\Delta\delta_{obs} = \frac{n\Delta\delta_{Cnm}}{2[CD]_0} \left\{ [G]_0 + [CD]_0 + 1/K_{11} - \left(\left([G]_0 + [CD]_0 + 1/K_{11}\right)^2 - 4[G]_0[CD]_0 \right)^{1/2} \right\}$$

$$\tag{6}$$

The observed values of $\Delta\delta_{obs}$(CD) were measured at varying carotenoid concentration and constant concentration of CD. To increase the accuracy of the measurements, a small amount of CH_3OH (~ 1 mM) was added to all samples as reference. It is known that methanol is a good internal reference due to its low association constant with cyclodextrins [46]. The stoichiometry of this complex was obtained by the continuous variation technique (Job's plot) [41]. The position of the maximum at R = 0.5 on the Job's plot (Figure 8) indicates that carotenoid **VI** forms a 1:1 complex with β-CD. The value of the association constant (K_{11} = 1536 ± 75 M^{-1}) was extracted using equation (3) from the dependence of the chemical shifts of CD protons on carotenoid concentration (Figure 9). Taking into account that the sodium salt of **IV** itself is water soluble, one can expect even higher complex stability for carotenoid **IV** in the absence of NaOH. This example is the first direct evidence of inclusion complex formation of a carotenoid.

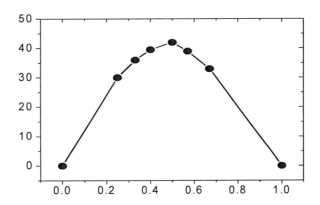

Figure 8. Job's plot corresponding to the chemical shift displacement of 3-H protons of β-CD in the presence of VI. The total concentration of CD plus carotenoid was 2 mM in this experiment (adopted from [20], Figure 5).

EPR study of scavenging ability of carotenoids towards peroxyl radicals. For investigation of the scavenging ability of carotenoid IV and its complex with CD we used the well known Fenton reaction for generation of free peroxyl radicals [47-49].

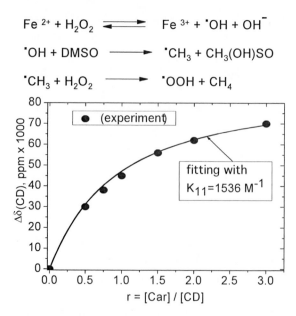

$$Fe^{2+} + H_2O_2 \;\rightleftharpoons\; Fe^{3+} + {}^\bullet OH + OH^-$$

$${}^\bullet OH + DMSO \;\longrightarrow\; {}^\bullet CH_3 + CH_3(OH)SO$$

$${}^\bullet CH_3 + H_2O_2 \;\longrightarrow\; {}^\bullet OOH + CH_4$$

Figure 9. Dependence of chemical shift of 3-H β-CD protons on VI:CD ratio in D_2O: experimental points and calculated curves for association constant $K_{11} = 1536$ M^{-1}. [β-CD] = 2 mM, and [NaOH] = 4 mM (adopted from [20], Figure 6).

At low H_2O_2 concentration (H_2O_2] ~ [FeCl$_2$] = 1 mM) only one spin adduct PBN-CH$_3$ was detected with ESR parameters a(H) = 3.4 G and a(N) = 14.9 G. However, at higher H_2O_2 concentration (0.5 M) the reaction of CH$_3$ radicals with H_2O_2 results in disappearance of the PBN-CH$_3$ adduct, and appearance of another adduct with higher yield which was assigned to the PBN-OOH spin adduct (a(H) = 2.3 G and a(N) = 13.9 G) [7]. On the other hand, it is known that the ${}^\bullet$OOR spin adducts are relatively unstable especially in the presence of transition metal ions which can reduce ${}^\bullet$OOR radicals yielding the ${}^\bullet$OR spin adduct [50, 51]. However, these facts are mainly related to alkyl peroxyl radicals. We have found several examples in the literature of the observation of the PBN-OOH adducts at normal conditions [52-54]. The additional confirmation of the PBN-OOH adduct formation was obtained using the superoxide dismutase (SOD) test [55]. Both the PBN-OOH and the PBN-CH$_3$ adducts were observe in the absence of SOD at concentration of hydrogen peroxide 200 mM (Figure 10, bottom). The addition of SOD (200 U/ml) completely suppressed the PBN-OOH signal, but had no influence on the PBN-CH$_3$ adduct (Figure 10, top).

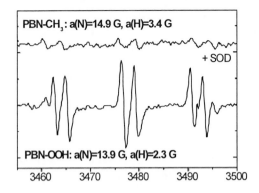

Figure 10. ESR spectra of PBN–OOH and PBN–CH₃ adducts detected in the presence (at the top), and in the absence of 200 U/ml SOD in DMSO (contained 10% H_2O). Experimental conditions: [PBN] = 5 mM, [FeSO₄] = 1 mM, [H₂O₂] = 0.2 M. Experiments with SOD (Sigma, EC 1.15.1.1) were carried out using ER-200D SRC (X-band, 9.5 GHz) ESR spectrometer (from [55], Figure 3).

Note that the Fenton reaction has been suggested as one of the possible sources of reactive species in living cells [56, 57].

The ability of carotenoid **VI** to scavenge peroxyl radicals was compared in the absence and presence of CD. In previous studies, the EPR spin trapping technique was applied to measure the scavenging rates of carotenoids towards free radicals [7, 58]. The scavenging ability was measured as a relative scavenging rate of carotenoid (Car) and spin trap (ST). These values were determined from concentration dependence of spin adduct yield (A) by using the equation (7):

$$\frac{A_0}{A} = \frac{k_{ST}[ST] + k_{Car}[Car]}{k_{ST}[ST]} \tag{7}$$

Here k_{Car} and k_{ST} are the reaction rate constants of carotenoid and spin trap with a free radical, and A_0 is spin adduct yield at zero carotenoid concentration. It was observed that k_{Car} values depend on the redox properties of carotenoid and increase with increasing of their oxidation potentials [7]. According to our results, β-carotene shows the worst antioxidant ability among the carotenoids under study. The values of k_{Car}/k_{ST} change from 0.6 for **I** to 24 for **IV**. Figure 11 demonstrates the decrease of PBN-OOH spin adduct yield with increase carotenoid **VI** concentration as a result of scavenging process.

Plot $(A_0/A - 1)$ vs. [Car]x[CD] shows linear dependence. The value $k_{Car}/k_{ST} = 40$ was calculated from this plot. This is the highest value from all carotenoids previously studied.

The same technique was applied to study the scavenging ability of the inclusion complex of **VI** in water. The highly water soluble hydroxypropyl substituted CDs were used for these EPR experiments. In contrast with Figure 11, no decrease in spin adduct yield was observed for CD complex of this carotenoid (see Figure 12). Moreover, one can see the appearance of the pro-oxidant effect (increase of spin adduct yield) in the presence of carotenoid.

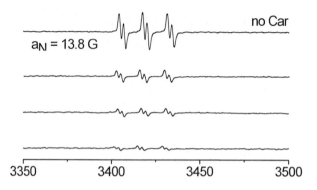

Figure 11. Variation of PBN-OOH spin adduct EPR spectrum in the presence of VI. Concentration of PBN = 10 mM; Fe^{2+} = 1 mM; H_2O_2 = 500 mM in DMSO (from [20], Figure 7).

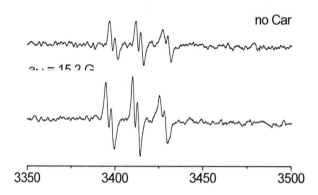

Figure 12. Variation of PBN/OOH spin adduct EPR spectrum in the presence of VI-HP-β-CD complex. Concentration of PBN = 10 mM; Fe^{2+} = 1 mM; H_2O_2 = 500 mM; HP-β-CD = 4 mM in H_2O (from [20], Figure 9).

To confirm that this observation is not due to encapsulation of the spin trap by CD the same measurement was made in the absence of carotenoid. The presence of CD does not result in a change of spin adduct yield in this case. We suggested that the absence of the antioxidant effect is due to protection of the radical sensitive site of the carotenoid (cyclohexene ring) by the CD. This result confirms our suggestion that peroxyl radicals attack mainly the cyclohexene ring of carotenoid. The occurrence of the pro-oxidant effect for the Car-CD complex was attributed to chain elongation by reaction of carotenoid with Fe^{3+} ions. Fe^{3+} ions, present in solution as the product of the Fenton reaction, oxidize the carotenoid and regenerate Fe^{2+}:

$$Car + Fe^{3+} \rightarrow Car^{+\bullet} + Fe^{2+}$$

The radical cation of carotenoid, $Car^{+\bullet}$, was detected as a product of this reaction. In the presence of excess of H_2O_2 this reaction will results in repetition of the redox cycle of the Fenton process and production of additional portion of free radicals.

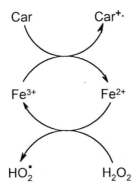

Due to their biological importance for living systems, the reaction of electron transfer between carotenoids and other metal ions such as Cu, Ti, and Ni have been intensively studied [59-62]. In particular, transition-metal complexes of carotenoids were detected in these studies. The role of Fenton-like processes in *in vivo* generation of toxic free radicals is now being widely discussed [56, 57, 63-68].

The results of our study [20] show that complexation with CD protects the carotenoid during transportation to the target, but to be an effective antioxidant, the carotenoid should be extracted from the CD cavity after delivery to the membrane. It is an important consideration in using carotenoid-CD complexes in medical practice. Recent *in vivo* and *in vitro* experimental data demonstrated that cyclodextrins can be used as carriers for the incorporation of dietary carotenoids into plasma and mitochondrial and microsomal cell membranes. Cyclodextrins, in contrast to dimethylsulfoxide, stabilize carotenoids and allow efficient cellular uptake [18, 19, 69]. At the same time, carotenoids encapsulated in the CD cavity show no photoprotection of human skin fibroblasts against UV irradiation [70].

2. Host-Guest Complexes of Carotenoids with β-Glycyrrhizic Acid [55, 71]

This section deals with the complexation of carotenoids with β-glycyrrhizic acid (GA). Glycyrrhizic acid is an unique natural compound of considerable interest to pharmacologists not only due to its physiological activity, but also due to its ability to enhance the activity of some drugs by non-covalent complex formation. The purpose of our study was the investigation of the structure of these complexes as well as the influence of GA on radical processes involving carotenoids. Special attention was paid to the antioxidant activity of carotenoids in the complexes.

Measurement of the stability and stoichiometry of GA complexes in aqueous solutions [71]. First of all we have have shown that complex formation occurs between the carotenoid and glycyrrhizic acid, and the structure of this complex has been estimated. The high extinction coefficients of carotenoids ($\sim 10^5$ $M^{-1}cm^{-1}$) make it convenient to use optical methods and thus allow us to work with very low concentrations. Note that the using of optical methods for inclusion complex analysis is more convenient compared to NMR techniques in the case of carotenoids. This is due to two reasons. First is the very low solubility of carotenoids even in water-alcohol solutions. Since carotenoids are insoluble in water, in these experiments we used water-ethanol mixtures. From our experience, the addition of small amounts of alcohol can slightly decrease complex stability but has no effect on its stoichiometry. Second, the sensitivity of NMR spectra to complex formation decreases considerably in the presence of alcohol or other organic solvents. NMR techniques are widely used for studying the stability and stoichiometry of cyclodextrin inclusion complexes, but in the case of GA complexes the changes in chemical shifts are much lower even in aqueous solutions.

To calculate the stability constant and stoichiometry of GA complexes, we used an approach similar to the analysis of CD complexes. In this case it was used to analyze the concentration dependence of the absorption and fluorescence spectra of the carotenoids [40, 72]. In our experiments all carotenoids showed nearly the same change in extinction coefficient at a fixed wave length in the presence of GA (~10%). The stoichiometry of the complexes was calculated using Job's plot of the dependence of the optical density of the solution with mole fraction of carotenoid. The measurements were performed with only two carotenoids **VII** and **VIII** that displayed the best solubility in alcohols. Both carotenoids have the same Job's plot. The position of a maximum of the curve at R = [Car] / ([Car] + [GA]) = 0.33 corresponds to the 1:2 ratio between carotenoid and GA molecules in the complex. It was earlier suggested that in aqueous solutions GA molecules form cyclic dimers of either torus [22] or podant [23] type.

To estimate the complex stability constant, the changes in optical density of the solution were measured at a fixed concentration of carotenoids with varying GA concentration (Figure 13).

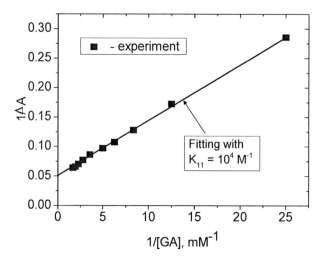

Figure 13. Benesi-Hildebrand plot of optical density changes (ΔA) of carotenoid I (2.5 μM) at 440 nm vs. GA concentration in 20% aqueous ethanol solution (adopted from [71], Figure 2).

The Benesi-Hildebrand plot (8) allows one to estimate both the complex stability constant and the order of complexation from a single experiment:

$$A/\Delta A - 1 = 1/[GA]^n \times 1/K \quad (8)$$

Here $\Delta A = \Delta\varepsilon \times [Car]$, and K is the stability constant of the complex for the reaction:

$$Car + nGA \overset{K}{\rightleftharpoons} CarGa_n$$

$$K = \frac{[CarGA_n]}{[Car] \times [GA]^n}$$

In our experiments, in all cases, the plot of $A/\Delta A$ versus $1/[GA]^n$ provides the linear dependence only for $n = 1$. Taking into account the result of the analysis of Job's plot, it was concluded that the reaction of complexation is second order between one carotenoid molecule and one dimer of glycyrrhizic acid.

$$Car + GA_2 \underset{}{\overset{K}{\rightleftharpoons}} CarGa_2$$

The complex structure is suggested to consist of a carotenoid molecule located within a torus formed by the glycyrrhizic acid dimer (Figure14).

Computer simulation of the experimental concentration dependence in Figure 13 provide the value $K = 10^4$ ($\pm 10^3$) M^{-1} for the β-carotene-GA complex. Carotenoids **VII** and **VIII**, whose solubility in water-alcohol solutions is greater than that of β-carotene, form less stable complexes ($K \sim 10^3$ M^{-1}), as expected from the hypothesis that hydrophobic interactions are essential for complex formation with GA. To elucidate the role of hydrophobic interactions in the formation of the carotenoid-GA complex, a thermodynamics study was carried out for carotenoid **VII** in the temperature interval $293 - 306$ K°. Thermodynamic parameters were estimated using the relevant equations (9-11):

$$- \Delta G = RTlnK \tag{9}$$

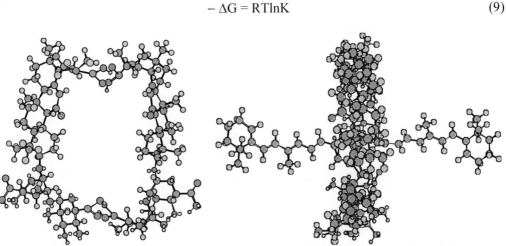

Figure 14. Schematic Chem3D Pro (Cambridge Software, Cambridge, MA) presentation of the suggested structures of the GA dimer and their inclusion complex with carotenoid (from [71], Figure 9).

$$\Delta G = \Delta H - T\Delta S \tag{10}$$

$$ln(K_2/K_1) = -(\Delta H/R)(1/T_2 - 1/T_1) \tag{11}$$

Here $K_i = K(T_i)$ are the values of the stability constants at different temperatures. Enthalpy of this complex formation was determined equals +42.9 kJ/mol, $\Delta G = 19.9$ kJ/mol and $\Delta S = +211$ J/(mol·K) at T = 293 K°. Experimental error in this study was about 25%. Positive values of both enthalpy and entropy contributions point out that hydrophobic interactions are an important factor in the binding, and that complex formation follows considerable desolvation of the carotenoid molecules. This feature is characteristic of inclusion complexes. We have found several examples of thermodynamic measurements of molecular complexes of β-glycyrrhizic acid with various organic molecules [23, 25]. It should be noted the heat of formation of molecular complexes is generally dependent on the electronegativity of the donor group in the 'host' molecule. A linear correlation was found between the formation enthalpies of GA complexes and the Hammett constants of the substituents in the nitro derivatives [23]. A thermodynamic study of the GA complex with two drugs, 8-hydroxy-5-nitroquinoline and nitroglycerin shows the presence of both enthalpy and entropy contribution to the complex stability [25]. Indeed, the presence of a number of carboxy and hydroxy groups in the GA and guests molecules is favorable for intermolecular H-bond formation in these cases.

Stability and stoichiometry of carotenoid-GA complexes in non-aqueous solutions [71]. A very important question for understanding the behavior of these complexes in living systems is their stability in non-aqueous media. For this purpose we investigated the possibility of complex formation between carotenoids and GA in several organic solvents, namely in alcohols, acetonitrile and DMSO. Since the optical absorption spectra of carotenoids are insensitive to the presence of GA in non-aqueous media, an attempt was made to study the influence of GA on the fluorescence spectrum of carotenoids. Due to high sensitivity of fluorescence intensity to the media properties, this approach is widely used to study inclusion complexes of the "guest-host" type [73-75]. The luminescence of molecules imbedded in the cavity of cyclodextrin is strengthened by the protection against quenching and other processes occurring in solution. Carotenoid canthaxanthin (**III**) was used in this investigation. The increase of fluorescence intensity of canthaxanthin in the presence of 1 mM GA in pure DMSO was about 15% from the value in the absence of GA. The addition of a small amount of water (5%) to DMSO had no influence on the fluorescence intensity in the absence of GA, but leads to an increase of the effect up to 50% in the presence of 1 mM of GA. The complex stability constant in DMSO was estimated by the methods of analysis applied to aqueous solutions. Over this concentration range (0-1 mM of GA), the calculation provides the value $K = 0.3\text{-}1 \times 10^4$ M^{-1}. The large error in the calculation of the stability constant is due to superposition of two processes. One can see that in the plot of the concentration dependence, the fluorescence intensity does not reach the plateau but starts to increase linearly when the GA concentration exceeds 1 mM (Figure 15).

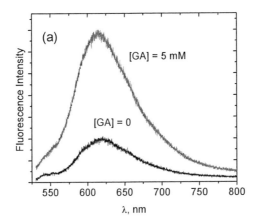

Figure 15. (a) Fluorescence spectrum of canthaxanthin (III) solution, 0.02 mM with and without GA in DMSO containing 5% of water. The excitation wave length is 470 nm, the detection wave length is 620 nm. (b) Dependence of fluorescence intensity of carotenoid III on GA concentration in solution (adopted from [71], Figure3).

The changes in the properties of GA solutions at the same concentration point (1 mM) have been observed in several studies, and this effect was explained by GA micelles formation [76, 77]. This hypothesis for micelle formation in water solution was confirmed by studying the processes of micelle formation of water-soluble GA derivatives, in particular, their sodium sulfates[24]. There is no evidence of micelle formation in other solvents at this time.

Interaction of carotenoids and their GA complexes with Fe ions and quinones [71]. An important question we tried to answer in our work was the influence of complex formation on carotenoid reactivity. The reactivity of carotenoids towards metal ions, quinones and free radicals is closely related to their antioxidant activity as well as stability in living systems, food and medical preparations. One of the most important natural processes involving carotenoids is electron transfer from carotenoids to acceptors. The mechanism of the reaction between carotenoids and Fe^{3+} ions has been studied in detail in our previous work [35]. As it was mentioned above, the reaction with Fe ions is considered by a number of authors to be one of the possible mechanisms of the pro-oxidant activity of β-carotene. The first step of this reaction is the electron transfer from carotenoid to acceptor resulting in formation of the carotenoid radical cation. The latter also can react with Fe^{3+}:

$$Car^{+\cdot} + Fe^{3+} \rightleftharpoons Car^{2+} + Fe^{2+}$$

Carotenoid radical cation and dication can undergo *cis-trans* isomerization. In the presence of oxygen, the oxidation of carotenoids leads to a stable product, a 5,8-epoxide. In acetonitrile, all carotenoids form relatively stable radical cations according to their absorption spectra, but are not detectable in aqueous solutions. The strongest radical cation signal was observed for β-carotene that has the lowest redox potential, $E^{ox}_{1/2} = 0.54$ V vs. SCE [78], (Figure 16). For other carotenoids, the signal intensity at room temperature was about 10% of that recorded for β-carotene.

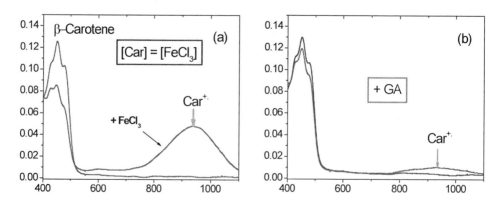

Figure 16. Absorption spectra of β-carotene, 1.3 μM, recorded before and after mixing with FeCl₃, 1.3 μM, in acetonitrile at room temperature. (a) in the absence of GA; (b) in the presence of 0.1 mM GA (adopted from [71], Figure4).

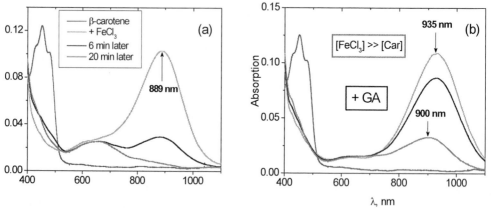

Figure 17. Absorption spectra of β-carotene, 1.3 μM, recorded before and after the mixing with FeCl₃, 7 μM, in acetonitrile at room temperature. (a) in the absence of GA; (b) in the presence of 0.1 mM GA. Signal at 935 nm is due to β-carotene radical cation, that at 889 nm – dication of β-carotene (adopted from [71], Figure6).

Figure 16b shows the absorption spectra of the β-carotene-GA complex recorded before and after mixing with FeCl₃. The absorption of radical cation resulting from the reaction is observed at 935 nm. A considerable decrease in the yield of β-carotene radical cation was observed in the presence of GA. It can be attributed to a decrease in the electron transfer rate in the case of complexation. With excess FeCl₃, all carotenoid is relatively rapidly transformed into the radical cation both with and without GA (Figure 17).

One can see that the behavior of β-carotene radical cation is quite different in the absence or presence of GA (Figure 17). Since the first and second redox potentials of β-carotene nearly coincide [78], both radical cation and dication are present when oxidation occurs and are in comproportionation equilibrium.

$$2Car^{+\cdot} \rightleftharpoons Car^{2+} + Car$$

Whereas a free radical cation transforms rapidly into dication (absorption at 889 nm), in the complex the radical cation is stabilized, i.e., it can be observed for a much longer period (tens of minutes). Since the rates of electron transfer (both the first and the second) decrease significantly, it means that the charged forms of carotenoids (cations and dications) do not leave the complex after the reaction and are also stabilized inside the cavity.

Control measurements (the addition of acetic acid with $pK_a \sim 4.6$ to a carotenoid solution which is close to that of GA) indicate that none of the observations can be attributed to changes in medium acidity.

Another example of the influence of GA on the reactivity of carotenoids is the electron transfer from carotenoid to quinone. Quinones are known to be important natural electron acceptors in photosynthetic centers [79, 80]. As a model system for studying the reactivity of inclusion compounds, we used dichloro-dicyano-benzoquinone (DDQ), which, owing to its low reduction potential, reacts with carotenoids without additional initiation by either light or temperature. Formation of a radical ion pair (RIP) in this reaction occurs via an intermediate charge transfer complex (CTC) [34]:

$$\text{Car} + \text{Q} \rightleftharpoons \text{CTC} \rightleftharpoons \text{Car}^{+\cdot} + \text{Q}^{-\cdot} \longrightarrow cis\text{-isomers} + \text{Car-Q}$$

The product of RIP recombination is the quinone–carotenoid adduct, whereas the radical cations escaping recombination result in the formation of cis-isomers [81]. Since the radical cations of β-carotene are stable in acetonitrile solution, we used optical absorption spectroscopy for monitoring their behavior in the reaction with quinone. Figure 18a demonstrates the difference in the form of the kinetic curves describing the carotenoid radical cation decay with and without GA. Whereas for a free carotenoid the radical cation signal decays exponentially with a half-life τ of ~20 s, in the presence of GA biexponential decay was observed. The fast process exhibits exponential decay with τ ~20 s, and the slow process is described by eq.: $I = a/(1 + t/\tau)$, with τ ~1000 s.

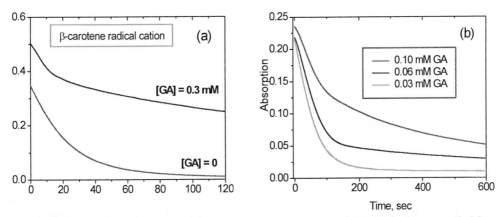

Figure 18. Kinetics of the decay of β-carotene radical cation at 935 nm. (a) 4 μM β-carotene + 4 μM DDQ with and without GA; (b) 2 μM β-carotene + 5 μM DDQ for various GA concentrations (adopted from [71], Figure7).

The contribution of a slow component of the kinetic increases nonlinear with increase of GA concentration (Figure 18b). It was suggested that the slow decay component is due to the radical cation in the complex. The observed ratio of fast and slow components is proportional to the square GA concentration, so we can estimate the stability constant of GA complex with radical cation in acetonitrile from the ratio of slow and fast kinetics components using equation (12).

$$K_{12} \times [GA]^2 = \frac{[CarGA_2^{+\bullet}]}{[Car^{+\bullet}]} \qquad (12)$$

The estimated stability constant in acetonitrile is near 10^8 M^{-2}. The two-component kinetics of the radical cation signal decay indicates the absence of a fast exchange between complexed and free radical cations.

How will the increase in the lifetime of the radical cation influence the yield of main reaction products? We propose that the changes in the ratio of the reaction products depend on whether only radical cation or CTC is imbedded in GA complex. To elucidate this question, we compared the yields of the reaction products for two carotenoids (**III, IV**) using HPLC method. As a result, a substantial increase in the yield of carotenoid-quinone adduct was observed for these carotenoids in the presence of GA (Figure 19).

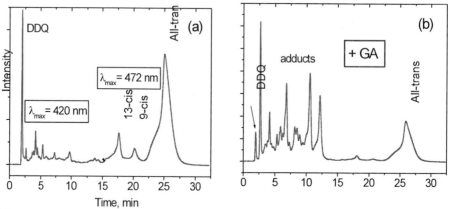

Figure 19. HPLC spectrum detected at 420 nm in acetonitrile of the products of the reaction between carotenoid III and dichloro-dicyano-benzoquinone (concentrations of 0.06 mM) (a) without and (b) with 0.2 mM GA (adopted from [71], Figure 8).

As an example, Figure 19 demonstrates HPLC spectra of the products of the reaction between carotenoid **III** and DDQ with and without 0.2 mM GA. One can see the decrease of the amount of initial compounds (quinone and carotenoid) in the presence of GA as well as carotenoid isomers (17 – 27 min). Simultaneously an increase of the yield of adducts (3 -10 min) was detected. Several peaks of adducts appear due to addition of quinone at the various double bonds of the conjugated canthaxanthin chain. This observation allowed us to conclude that GA can form stable complexes not only with individual compounds and their ions but also with charge transfer complexes. In the case of carotenoids, this leads to a change in both the reaction direction and the ratio of products. The important point is also the possibility to control the life time of carotenoid radical cations by the formation of "host-guest" complexes.

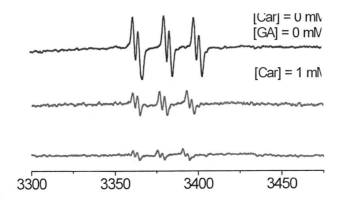

Figure 20. ESR spectra of PBN–OOH adduct detected without carotenoid (top), and in the presence of canthaxanthin or its complex with GA in DMSO. Experimental conditions: [PBN] = 5 mM, [FeCl$_2$] = 1 mM, [H$_2$O$_2$] = 0.5 M (adopted from [55], Figure2).

*Antioxidant and redox properties of supramolecular complexes of carotenoids with glycyrrhizic acid_*[55]. Antioxidant activity is known to be one of the most important biological properties of carotenoids, because they react with toxic free radicals and thus prevent damage to living organism [2-4]. From a practical point of view, it is interesting to know how the complexation of carotenoids with glycyrrhizic acid will affect their ability to scavenge free radicals. As it was stated above, the complexes of carotenoids with cyclodextrin is used to improve their solubility, and to increase bioavailability, however, it has failed to improve their antioxidant properties. As it was shown in the first part of this chapter, measuring the scavenging rate of peroxide radicals by carotenoids in solutions indicates that the reaction can be almost totally inhibited by cyclodextrin due to embedding the cyclohexene fragment in the cyclodextrin cavity [20].

The antioxidant activity of carotenoids and their complexes with GA was studied by the same EPR spin-trapping technique. EPR spectra of the spin adduct of OOH radical with the spin trap *N-tert*-butyl-α-phenylnitrone (PBN) were recorded using an ESR Varian E-12 (X-band, 9.5 GHz) spectrometer. Note: the method involves measuring the yield of the stable spin adduct of peroxyl radicals as a function of carotenoid concentration. Because of the two competing processes, i.e., reactions of the radical with carotenoid and spin trap, the yield of the spin adduct is proportional to the carotenoid concentration (see Figure 20 and Eq. 7).

The relative rates of radical scavenging (k_{Car}/k_{ST}) by carotenoids were calculated from the dependence of the spin adduct yield with carotenoid concentration. The absolute value of the rate constant can be estimated using the available kinetic database (Spin Trap Data Base: http://epr.niehs.nih.gov) which provides the value of the rate constant k_{ST} measured in water ($k_{ST} \leq 10^6$ M^{-1}s^{-1} for the PBN spin trap). Using the same approach we have measured the reaction rates of the OOH radical with GA complexes of carotenoids. Our experiments show that GA itself displays a substantial antioxidant activity with k/k$_{ST}$ = 12 (Table 1). Note that the rate constant of the reaction between GA and peroxyl radicals is independent of GA concentration. On the other hand, comparison of the scavenging rates of peroxyl radicals by free carotenoids and their complexes in DMSO shows a strong dependence of the rate constants on the concentration of GA.

Table 1. Relative rate constants of OOH radicals scavenging by glycyrrhizic acid, carotenoids, and their complexes (k/k_{ST}) in DMSO. Experimental error ~10%. $E_{1/2}$ are the redox potentials of carotenoids (in V vs. SCE) [78].

[GA] mM	GA	II ($E_{1/2}$ = 0.56 V)	III ($E_{1/2}$ = 0.68 V)	IV ($E_{1/2}$ = 0.72 V)
0		4	2	7
0.5	12	4	59	133
1	12	4	46	116
2	12	4	6	38

The k_{Car}/k_{ST} values given in Table 1 were obtained by subtracting the GA contribution from the total rate constant measured in the presence of glycyrrhizic acid. From these values, it is possible to determine whether a synergetic effect of GA on the scavenging ability of carotenoids III and IV occurs. Of importance is the absence of this effect for zeaxanthin (II). Analyzing the oxidation potentials of these three carotenoids (see Table 1) and the dependence of the carotenoids scavenging rate [7] on their $E_{1/2}$, points out that GA can affect the oxidation potential of the carotenoids. This hypothesis was verified by CV measurement of the oxidation potential of two carotenoids II and III in the presence of GA. In both cases, we have observed an increase in $E_{1/2}$: by 0.05 V for canthaxanthin (Figure 21) and by 0.03 V for zeaxanthin.

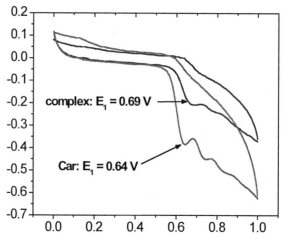

Figure 21. Cyclic voltammetry (CV) plot of canthaxathin (0.1 mM) and its complex with GA (0.2 mM of GA) in acetonitrile. Scan rate is 10 mV/s (adopted from [55], Figure4).

Using this result and the diagram in Figure 22 we can explain the different behavior of carotenoids II - IV in the presence of GA. As one can see in Figure 22, the dependence of the rate constant of the reaction of peroxyl radicals with oxidation potential of carotenoids is nonlinear. A negligible change in the oxidation potential for beta-carotene and zeaxanthin (<0.05 V) should cause no changes in their antioxidant activity. At the same time, this diagram allows us to predict a substantial increase in the reaction rate for carotenoids with $E_{1/2}$ ~ 0.7 V when their oxidation potential increases due to complexation.

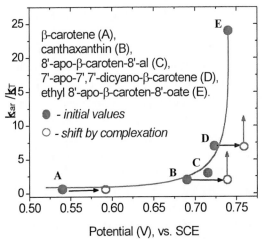

Figure 22. Diagram of the dependence of the carotenoid scavenging rate toward peroxyl radicals on the oxidation potential of carotenoids [7]. Arrows denote the shifts in oxidation potentials due to complexation (adopted from [55], Figure5).

These experimental results verify the hypothesis for the role of electron transfer in the scavenging of free radicals by carotenoids. A very important observation is determining the effect of GA on the oxidation potential of carotenoids [55]. An increase in the oxidation potential of carotenoids can serve the main reason for a decrease in their oxidation rate in reactions with electron acceptors. Note also, that the rate constants of peroxyl radical scavenging by carotenoids (Table 1) are different at various GA concentrations. The scavenging rates measured at low GA concentrations (0.5 мM) considerably exceed those measured at high concentrations (2 мM). This fact confirms the hypothesis for the dependence of the structure and properties of GA complexes on its concentration. It was shown that in aqueous solutions, at a concentration of above 1 мM, GA forms micelle type aggregates [76, 77]. However, the data on the micelle formation in non-aqueous solvents are unavailable in the literature. As it was described in the previous paragraph, the stability constant of GA complex with canthaxanthin in DMSO estimated from fluorescence measurements is about 10^4 M^{-1} for low GA concentrations and $<10^2$ M^{-1} for high concentrations. Below GA concentration of 1 mM, the GA-carotenoid complex stoichiometry was determined to be 2:1. The differences in the scavenging rates of peroxyl radicals for various GA concentrations indicate that the properties of 2:1 complexes really differ from those for carotenoids in the assumed micellar solution. The reason for these differences is still unknown.

3. Water Soluble Complexes of Carotenoids with Arabinogalactan [82]

The majority of carotenoids are lipophilic molecules with near zero inherent aqueous solubility. Moving carotenoids into a pharmaceutical application requires a chemical delivery system that overcomes the problems with parenteral administration of a highly lipophilic, low molecular weight compound. Increase water solubility of carotenoids opens several technological applications that could be provided in food processing (colors and antioxidant capacity) as well as for production of therapeutic formulations considering the better solubility and consequently higher bioavailability.

In this chapter we present the first example of water soluble complexes of carotenoids. The stability and reactivity of carotenoids in the complexes with natural polysaccharide arabinogalactan (AG) were investigated by different physicochemical techniques: optical absorption, HPLC, and pulsed EPR spectroscopy. Polysaccharide complexes of carotenoids showed enhanced photostability compared to pure carotenoids as well as reduced reactivity towards metal ions (Fe^{3+}) and reactive oxygen species. On the other hand, the yield and stability of carotenoid radical cations produced on titanium dioxide nanoparticles were greatly increased in the solid state complex of arabinogalactan. Canthaxanthin radical cations was stable for 10 days at room temperature in this system. We suggest that these results are important for a variety of carotenoid applications.

Arabinogalactan was extracted from *Larix sibirica* [83]. Arabinogalactans are long, highly branched polysaccharides composed of galactose and arabinose molecules in a 6:1 ratio. Pharmaceutical-grade larch arabinogalactan is a fine, dry, off-white powder with a slightly sweet taste and mild pine-like odor. It is low in viscosity, dissolves completely in water or juice, and therefore easy to administer, even to children.

Solubility of carotenoids in water as a criterion of complex formation. It is well known that carotenoids are highly hydrophobic, air- and light-sensitive compounds. Earlier there were several attempts to prepare water soluble complexes of carotenoids using water-oil emulsion or cyclodextrin solutions. However, this products when placed in water forms an obvious dispersion, with particles visible to the naked eye and the β-carotene separates from the water within a few days. While water dispersible β-carotenes are suitable for some applications (e.g., beverages) they are not suitable for others (e.g., fat substitutes) because the beta-carotene itself is still oil soluble. Also, the solutions of all carotenoid-cyclodextrin complexes show a considerable decrease in color intensity as compared to carotenoid solutions in organic solvents [20]. This fact significantly constricts the application of these complexes as food colorants.

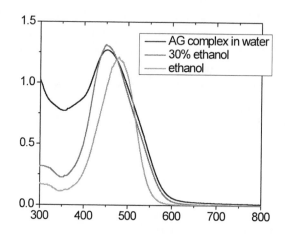

Figure 23. Absorption spectra of carotenoid III in different solvents. The increase of optical density at λ < 400 nm is due to arabinogalactan absorbance (adopted from [82], Figure1).

The estimated solubility of the complexes of carotenoids **I**, **III** and **IV** with arabinogalactan prepared mechanochemically in solid state with molar stoichiometry 1:1, is 2-5 mM in water solution. The carotenoid-arabinogalactan complexes maintain their original color and show insignificant changes in absorption spectra. UV-Vis spectrum of aqueous solutions of canthaxanthin-AG complex has the same absorption maximum as the spectrum of canthaxanthin solution in 30% ethanol (Figure 23).

The formation of carotenoid complexes of arabinogalactan were monitored by X-ray diffraction phase analysis and differential scanning calorimetry (DSC) techniques (Figure 24).

In the mixture of initial compounds before treatment one can see the characteristic peaks of the crystal structure of carotenoid (plot 1), which disappears during complex formation (plot 3). We suggested that the absence of crystal structure in this case is due to molecular penetration of carotenoid into arabinogalactan polymer matrix. It means that complex formation occurs in the solid state without using any toxic organic solvents. Further solubilization in water results in preservation of the complex structure. This is confirmed by significant increase in solubility of the complex as compared with traditional solvent-mediated methods.

Photostability of carotenoids and their AG complexes in water solution. One of the main problems in the practical application of carotenoids is their photosensitivity and instability, especially in the presence of oxygen and water. The photostability of drugs and vitamins attracts increasing attention since serious toxic reactions produced by many pharmacologically important chemicals occur under sunlight irradiation [84]. Photoallergic and photomutagenic effects are also of current concern. Photogenerated intermediates can interact with cell components and lead to cell degeneration or death. Control of the drug photostability and preparation of protective strategies against the light-induced damage requires understanding of the structural and environmental factors determining their photoreactivity.

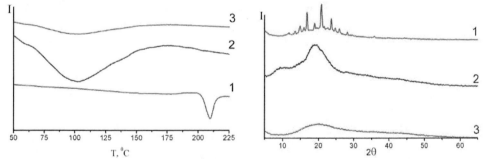

Figure 24. X-ray diffraction phase analysis (right) and differential scanning calorimetry analysis (left) of solid canthaxanthin-arabinogalactan complex prepared mechanochemically. 1 - canthaxanthin; 2 - arabinogalactan; 3 - complex (from [82], Figure2).

We have studied the relative photodegradation rate of carotenoids and their complex with AG using canthaxanthin as an example. The photolysis of pure canthaxanthin and its complex in aerated water-ethanol mixture shows a significant increase in the photostability of canthaxanthin when incorporated into an AG complex (Figure 25). The estimated decrease in the photodegradation rate is ten times for this system.

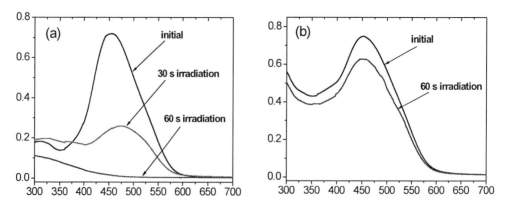

Figure 25. Photodegradation of canthaxanthin. Absorption spectra were recorded after different irradiation times in aerated 30% ethanol solution by the full light of a xenon lamp. (a) Pure canthaxanthin; (b) Canthaxanthin-AG complex (adopted from [82], Figure3).

It is thought but not proven that the decrease in stability of the carotenoids when redox processes occur in the presence of water is due to deprotonation of their radical cations and dications with formation of neutral radicals. Earlier we have demonstrated that the carotenoid neutral radicals are formed from the corresponding radical cations generated electrochemically or photochemically by proton loss [85-87]. Electrochemical measurements showed that the radical cations of a majority of carotenoids have pK's ranging between 4-7 and, therefore, can deprotonate spontaneously even without photoexcitation [81, 88]. We propose that incorporation of carotenoids into the hydrophobic polymer environment reduces their interaction with water molecules. It was confirmed by the absence of a considerable blue shift in the absorption spectra of the AG complex of carotenoid containing a polar group (canthaxanthin, for example) observed earlier in the presence of water in homogeneous solutions [20].

Reactivity of the carotenoid complexes of AG in solution. One of the most important natural processes involving carotenoids is the electron transfer from carotenoids to a variety of acceptors. In the previous section, we have shown that complexation with natural oligosaccharide glycyrrhizin (GA) has a noticeable effect on the reactivity of carotenoids, such as a decrease in the electron transfer rates in the reaction with ferric chloride, and an increase in the lifetime of the complexing radical cations [71]. To study a single electron transfer reaction of carotenoids in aqueous solution, we have chosen a ferric citrate complex (Fe:cit) as an electron acceptor [89]. The first step of this reaction is the electron transfer with formation of the carotenoid radical cation. In the presence of water carotenoid radical cations can undergo deprotonation reaction resulting in neutral carotenoid radicals with further dimerization:

$$Car^{+\cdot} \rightleftharpoons \dot{Car} + H^+$$

$$2\dot{Car} \longrightarrow Car_2$$

The formation of carotenoid dimers was detected from the broadening of the carotenoid absorption spectra with the shift of absorption maxima to higher wavelength (see Figure 26, for example). In the absence of water, in pure ethanol, reaction of β-carotene with Fe:cit results in its degradation without dimer formation (Figure 27).

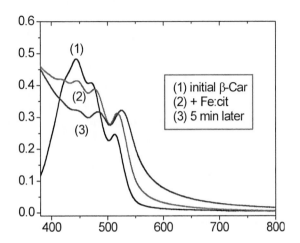

Figure 26. Transformation of the absorption spectra of β-carotene during the reaction with ferric citrate (0.5 mM) in 30% ethanol (adopted from [82], Figure4).

In contrast to a homogeneous solution, AG complexes of carotenoids under study (**I, III** and **IV**) show no change in the absorption spectra in the presence of ferric citrate during a 20 minute observation period in 30% aqueous ethanol solution, as well as in water solution. We suggest that two factors play an important role in the stabilization of carotenoids in AG complexes, namely, isolation from water molecules and isolation from metal ions. The important conclusion that be can made from this result, is that the Fe:cit complex does not penetrate into the polysaccharide matrix.

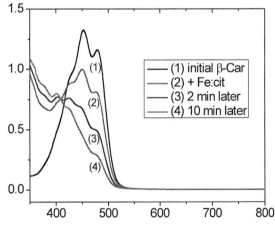

Figure 27. Absorption spectra of β-carotene in the presence of ferric citrate (0.5 mM) in ethanol solution (adopted from [82], Figure4).

Another important reaction of carotenoids which was investigated in the presence of AG is the interaction with active oxygen species. This reaction attracts great attention in relation to antioxidant and pro-oxidant activities of carotenoids. In the present study we used the photo-Fenton reaction [89, 90] listed below and Fe(III):cit for generation of free radicals.

$$Fe^{3+} + H_2O \xrightarrow{\;h\nu\;} Fe^{2+} + H^+ + \dot{O}H$$

$$H_2O_2 + Fe^{2+} \longrightarrow Fe^{3+} + OH^- + \dot{O}H$$

UV irradiation of a water solution of Fe(III):cit shows only a decrease of the Fe^{3+} absorption spectrum band due to a low extinction coefficient of Fe^{2+}. Irradiation of the same solution in the presence of hydrogen peroxide results in the appearance of a new absorption peak near 500 nm (Figure 28). A modern interpretation of the Fenton (and photo-Fenton) mechanism [90] assumes that other oxidizing intermediates such as highly valent iron complexes (Fe^{4+}) are formed during oxidation of Fe^{2+} to Fe^{3+}.

$$H_2O_2 + Fe^{2+}(aq) \longrightarrow [H_2O_2 + Fe^{2+}] \longrightarrow Fe^{4+}(aq) \longrightarrow Fe^{3+} + OH^- + OH^\cdot$$

It is suggested that the long lived species observed at 500 nm (life time more than one hour) might be a citrate complex with highly valent iron ion.

The Fenton reaction is widely used for generation of free radicals in solution for model experiments. According EPR spin-trapping study, only peroxyl radicals were detected in this system at high H_2O_2 concentration (more then 0.1 M) [7]. The interaction of OOH radicals with the carotenoid polyene chain results in fast bleaching of the solution. As an example, Figure 29 shows a rapid decrease of the β-carotene absorption immediately after addition of H_2O_2 to the mixture of β-carotene with Fe(II):cit.

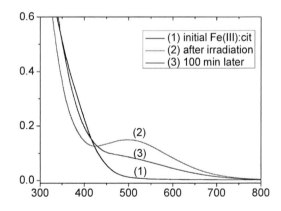

Figure 28. Absorption spectra of Fe:cit complex (0.5 mM) irradiated 1 min in the presence of H_2O_2 (0.25 M) in 30% ethanol(adopted from [82], Figure5).

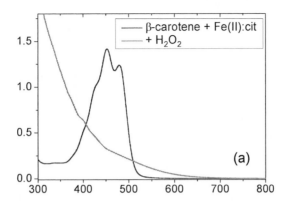

Figure 29. Absorption spectra of β-carotene in the presence of Fe(II):cit (0.5 mM) and H_2O_2 (0.25 M) in ethanol (adopted from [82], Figure6).

A big difference was observed in the behavior of β-carotene when it is incorporated into the AG complex. Figure 30 shows the significant effect of complexation, namely the stability of β-carotene in the AG complex in the presence of Fe^{3+} ions (plot (2)) as well as in the presence of peroxyl radicals generated by irradiation of the reaction mixture (plots (3) and (4)).

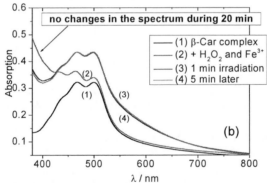

Figure 30. Absorption spectra of β-carotene in the presence of Fe(III):cit (0.5 mM) and H_2O_2 (0.25 M) in AG complex in 30% ethanol solution. The observed increase in optical density after irradiation of the sample is due to formation of Fe^{4+} (adopted from [82], Figure6).

A decrease in absorption at 300-450 nm and an increase of absorption at 450-700 nm after irradiation is due to formation of Fe^{4+} from Fe^{3+} during the reaction (see Figure 28). Similar effect of increasing stability was also observed for the other two carotenoids, **III** and **IV**. Figures 31a and 31b show the difference in decay rates for carotenoid **III** and its AG complex respectively in thr presence of the photo-Fenton reaction. The estimated ratio of decay rates equals 20 for this system. Ethanol was chosen as a solvent for the homogeneous reaction to decrease the contribution of the carotenoid – Fe^{3+} interaction to the decay rate.

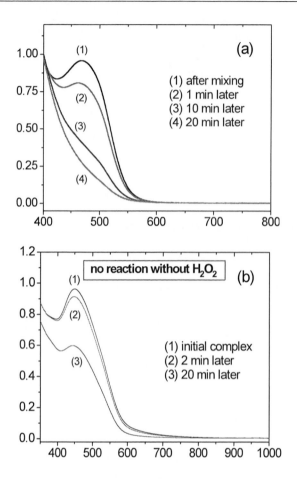

Figure 31. Absorption spectra of Canthaxanthin in the presence of Fe(II):cit (0.5 mM) and H_2O_2 (0.25 M) (a) in ethanol; (b) in AG complex in water solution (adopted from [82], Figure7).

It is proposed that the stability of the carotenoids incorporated into the AG macromolecule might have wide practical application. A decrease in reaction rate towards free radicals does not mean a decrease in antioxidant activity of a complex in living systems since polysaccharides are easily assimilated by living media.

Photo-induced electron transfer from carotenoid in the solid state [82]. The next study was devoted to the electron transfer processes from carotenoids to acceptors in the solid state. The main question of interest concerns the properties of the carotenoid radical cations in the AG complex in the solid state. The properties of carotenoid radical cations in organized media have been intensively investigated [91-93] because of the importance of carotenoids in photosynthesis and their possible use in artificial solar cells. In this study we have succeeded in detecting the canthaxanthin radical cation incorporated in a AG macromolecule during photoirradiation on the surface of TiO_2 nanoparticles. Among the semiconductors, titanium dioxide is the most suitable for many environmental applications. Due to its ability to absorb light, TiO_2 is widely used in photocatalysis and in artificial solar cells [94-98]. Figure 32 provides the schematic illustrations of the photocatalytic reactions of Carotenoid (Car) adsorbed on the surfaces of TiO_2 nanoparticles.

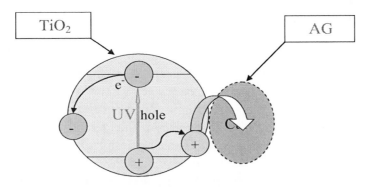

Figure 32. Schematic illustrations of the photocatalytic processes on the surfaces of the TiO_2 nanoparticles in the presence of carotenoid (Car) (adopted from [82], Figure8).

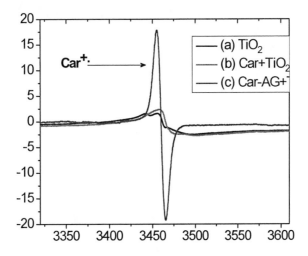

Figure 33. EPR spectra detected after irradiation of TiO_2 powder (a); TiO_2 in the presence of canthaxanthin (b); and TiO_2 in the presence of canthaxanthin-AG complex in solid state at 20 K (c); (adopted from [82], Figure9).

Irradiation of TiO_2 nanoparticles (T = 77° K, λ > 350 nm) in the absence of carotenoid results in the appearance of an EPR signal which we attributed to Ti^{3+} (Figure 33a). Irradiation of pure canthaxanthin at the same conditions (without AG) adsorbed on the TiO_2 surface shows only a weak signal with $g = 2.0028 \pm 0.0002$ and $\Delta H_{pp} = 13.0 \pm 0.5$ G, which is characteristic of carotenoid radical cations [99-101] (Figure 33b). In contrast, carotenoid-AG complex irradiated on TiO_2 shows a significant increase in the intensity of EPR signal (Figure 33c) compared to that of the pure carotenoid.

It is suggested that the low yield of the charge separated state in the absence of AG might be due to efficient back electron transfer on semiconductor materials. The "redox cycling", where a product of the hole transfer acts, in turn, as scavenger for the photogenerated electrons, appears as a frequent cause of weak photocurrents [102,103]. The isolation of the carotenoid radical cation from the TiO_2 surface by incorporation into the polysaccharide matrix allows more efficient charge separation, reducing the rate of back electron transfer. A number of authors used the same approach for design of the "donor-bridge-acceptor" molecular triads as a model of the light harvesting complex [104-106]. In these studies porphyrin was chosen as the initial electron donor, and quinone (or fullerene) as an electron acceptor. Initial charge separation in such triads was accomplished by photoinduced electron transfer from the excited porphyrin to the attached quinone to generate the charge-separated species $CP^{.+}\ Q^{.-}$. In a second step, an electron is donated by the attached carotenoid moiety to the porphyrin to form the species $C^{.+}P\ Q^{.-}$. This species lives long enough to transfer an electron to a freely diffusing secondary quinone which act as a proton shuttle [104, 105]. Apparently, such a way of light energy transformation is similar to the mechanism used by plants for utilisation of solar energy in photosynthesis. The life time of the model molecular triads has an order of tens nanoseconds, and is mainly restricted by back electron transfer reaction [106]. Previous studies on the use of a carotenoid-sensitized TiO_2 nanocrystalline mesoporous electrode in the preparation of a photovoltaic cell, indicated that the cell efficiency also was partially limited by the recombination of the injected electron with the oxidized form of the carotenoid radical cation. The current results suggest the use of the polysaccharide complex in the preparation of a more efficient cell. Stabilization of the carotenoid radical cation would reduce the recombination rate. Simultaneously AG matrix provides the defense of the carotenoid from degradation decay.

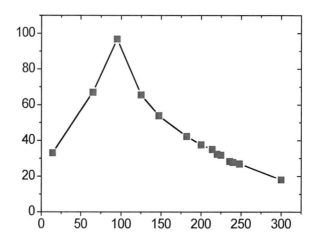

Figure 34. Temperature dependence of EPR intensity of Canthaxanthin radical cation in solid state complex of arabinogalactan on TiO_2 surface.

According to earlier published results [107], carotenoid radical cations generated on the surface of TiO_2 are stable at 77° K, but disappear when the temperature is increased above 250° K. The most important design feature of the carotenoid-AG complex is the significant increase in stability of the carotenoid radical cation. Increasing the temperature up to room temperature does not lead to disappearance of the spectrum (Figure 34).

The estimated life time of the canthaxanthin radical cation in the solid state complex of arabinogalactan on TiO_2 surface is approximately 10 days at room temperature. The increase in lifetime of such molecular devices opens up wide possibilities for their use in molecular electronics as the nanosized means of communication and data processing as well as in sensors.

Conclusion

In conclusion we can summarize that incorporation of carotenoids into the oligosaccharide or polysaccharide macromolecules result in significant change in their physical and chemical properties. This result opens new possibilities to control the reactivity of carotenoids in living systems as well as for wide practical application in various fields. In addition to cyclodextrins inclusion complexes which are already used in pharmacology, cosmetics and food industry, we propose two new compounds, glycyrrhizin and arabinogalactan which form more stable complexes with carotenoids and demonstrate some unique properties useful for many applications. In particular, complexes of glycyrrhizin with some carotenoids show enhanced ability to scavenge free radicals. In practice it means a significant reduction in the required dosage of antioxidants in medical preparations and enriched drinks. Complexes with arabinogalactan are unique water soluble compositions which provide enhanced stability of carotenoids at room temperature in the presence of sunlight and water, and significantly reduce their interaction with different additives including metal ions.

Another important field of carotenoid application is photosynthesis and artificial solar cells. The increased stability of carotenoid radical cations in solution (in GA complex) and in the solid state (in AG complex) at room temperature may results in new discoveries in design of artificial light-harvesting, photoredox and catalytic systems.

It was demonstrated that the mechanochemical method of solid state complex preparation has significant advantages as compared with traditional techniques. Primarily, the interest in solvent-free conditions stems from the possibility of obtaining the same product as that from solution *without solvent* because the process is cheaper, less time consuming and often more environmentally friendly. In the case of carotenoid chemistry the solvent-free conditions open the possibility of obtaining products not otherwise accessible from solvents.

Finally, it is worth noting that the creation of novel, more effective compositions based on the complexes of tested medicines and vitamins with natural compounds is now an intensively developed field of medicinal chemistry, cosmetology, and food industry. Fundamental studies substantially lag behind the nature of the complexation and physicochemical properties of complexes. At the same time, these studies are highly important from the point of view of their predictive potential. In medicine, screening of new drugs is, as a rule, performed using animals. Therefore, the possibility to control the reactivity of chemical compounds by complexation and equally important, to predict the range of either an increase or decrease in therapeutic activity, would allow one to substantially reduce the number of *in vivo* experiments.

References

[1]   Jørgensen, K; Skibsted, LHZ. Lebensm. Unters. *Forsch.* 1993, 196, 423-429.

[2]   Edge, R; McGarvey, DJ; Truscott, TGJ. Photochem. Photobiol., *B: Biol.*, 1997, 41, 189-200.

[3]   Woodall, AA; Lee, S. WM; Weesie, RJ; Jackson, MJ; Britton, G. *Biochim. Biophys. Acta*, 1997, 1336, 33-42.

[4]   Al-Agamey, A; Lowe, GM; McGarvey, DJ; Mortensen, A; Phillip, DM; Truscott, TG; Young, AJ. *Arch. Biochim. Biophys.*, 2004, 430, 37-48.

[5]   Palozza, P; Calviello, G; Serini, S; Maggiano, N; Lanza, P; Ranelletti, FO; Bartoli, GM. *Free Rad. Biol. Med.*, 2001, 30, 1000-1007.

[6]   Hill, TJ; Land, EJ; McGarvey, DJ; Schalch, W; Tinkler, JH; Truscott, TGJ. *Am. Chem. Soc.*, 1995, 117, 8322-8326.

[7]   Polyakov, NE; Kruppa, AI; Leshina, TV; Konovalova, TA; Kispert, LD. *Free Rad. Biol. Med.*, 2001, 31, 43-52.

[8]   Cross, CE; Halliwell, B; Borish, ET. *Annals Int. Med.*, 1987, 107, 526-545.

[9]   Halliwell, B. *Nutr. Rev.*, 1997, 55, 44-52.

[10] Loftsson, T; Brewster, MEJ. *Pharm. Sci.*, 1996, 85, 1017-1025.

[11] Buschmann, HJ; Schollmayer, EJ. *Cosmet. Sci.*, 2002, 53, 185-191.

[12] Szejtli, J. Cyclodextrin technology; Kluwer Academic: Dordrecht, 1988.

[13] Hasebe, K; Ando, Y; Chikamatsu, Y; Hayashi, K. Patent JP 62267261, 1987.

[14] Murao, T; Maruyama, T; Yamamoto, Y. Patent JP 04244059, 1992.

[15] Schwartz, JL; Shklar, G; Sikorski, C. Patent WO 9513047, 1995.

[16] Mele, A; Mendichi, R; Selva, A. *Carbohydr. Res.*, 1998, 310, 261-267.

[17] Mele, A; Mendichi, R; Selva, A; Molnar, P; Toth, G. *Carbohydr. Res.*, 2002, 337, 1129-1136.

[18] Szente, L; Mikuni, K; Hashimoto, H; Szejtli, JJ. *Inclusion Phenom. Mol. Recognit. Chem.*, 1998, 32, 81-89.

[19] Lancrajan, I; Diehl, HA; Socaciu, C; Engelke, M; Zorn-Kruppa, M. *Chem. Phys. Lipids*, 2001, 112, 1-10.

[20] Polyakov, NE; Leshina, TV; Konovalova, TA; Hand, EO; Kispert, LD. *Free Rad. Biol. Med.*, 2004, 36, 872-880.

[21] Lockwood, SF; O'Malley, S; Mosher GL. *J. Pharm. Sci.*, 2003, 92, 922-926.

[22] Sangalov, E. *Yu. Russ. J. Gen. Chem.* (Engl. Transl.) 1999, 64, 641-644.

[23] Gusakov, VN; Maistrenko, VN; Safiullin, PP. *Russ. J. Gen. Chem.* (Engl. Transl.) 2001, 71, 1307-1316.

[24] Saito, S; Furumoto, T; Ochiai, M; Hosono, A; Hoshino, H; Haraguchi, U; Ikeda, R; Shimada, N. *Eur. J. Med. Chem.*, 1996, 31, 365-381.

[25] Maistrenko, VN; Gusakov, VN; Rusakov, IA; Murinov, Yu. I; Tolstikov, GA. *Dokl. Akad. Nauk.*, 1994, 335, 329-331.

[26] Polyakov, NE; Khan, VK; Taraban, MB; Leshina, TV; Salakhutdinov, NF; Tolstikov, GA. *J. Phys. Chem. B.*, 2005, 109, 24526-24530.

[27] Connors, KA. *Chem. Rev.*, 1996, 97, 1325-1357.

[28] Kondratenko, RM; Baltina, LA; Mustafina, SR; Ismagilova, AF; Zarudii, FS; Davydova, VA; Basekin, GV; Suleimanova, GF; Tolstikov, GA. *Pharm. Chem. J.*, 2003, 37, 485-488.

[29] Tolstikova, TG; Bryzgalov, AO; Sorokina, IV; Hvostov, MV; Ratushnyak, AS; Zapara, TA; Simonova, OG. *Lett. Drug Design Discovery*, 2007, 4, 168-170.

[30] Sorokina, IV; Tolstikova, TG; Dolgikh, MP; Shul'ts, EE; Dushkin, AV; Karnatovskaya, LM; Chabueva, EN; Boldyrev, VV. *Pharm. Chem. J.*, 2002, 36, 11-13.

[31] Odonmazig, P; Ebringerova, A; Machova, E; Alfoldi, J. *Carbohydr. Res.*, 1994, 252, 317-324.

[32] D'Adamo, PJ. *Naturopath. Med.*, 1996, 6, 33-37.

[33] Fortier, NE. *US Patent*, 5552009, 1996.

[34] Polyakov, NE; Konovalov, VV; Leshina, TV; Luzina, OA; Salakhutdinov, NF; Konovalova, TA; Kispert, LD. *J. Photochem. Photobiol.*, A 2001, 141, 117-126.

[35] Gao, Y; Kispert, LD. *J. Phys. Chem.*, B 2003, 107, 5333-5338.

[36] Polyakov, NE; Leshina, TV; Petrenko, A; Hand, E; Kispert, LD. *J. Photochem. Photobiol. A: Chem.*, 2004, 161, 261–267.

[37] Munoz-Botella, S; Martin, MA; del Castillo, B; Lerner, DA; Menendez, JC. *Anal. Chim. Acta*, 2002, 468, 161-170.

[38] Higuchi, T; Connors, KA. *Adv. Anal. Chem. Instrum.*, 1965, 4, 117-212.

[39] Redenti, E; Szente, L; Szejtli, J. *J. Pharm. Sci.*, 2001, 90, 979-986.

[40] Szejtli, J; Osa, T. In *Comprehensive Supramolecular Chemistry*; Atwood, J.L; Davies, J.E.D; MacNicol, D.D; Vögtle, F; Ed; Elsevier Sci. Ltd.: Oxford, UK, 1996. vol. 3, pp 5-41.

[41] Yamamoto, Y; Inoue, Y. *J. Carbohydr. Chem.*, 1989, 8, 29-46.

[42] Greatbanks, D; Pickford, R. *Magn. Res. Chem.*, 1987, 25, 208-215.

[43] Casy, AR; Cooper, AD; Jefferies, TM; Gaskell, RM; Greatbanks, D; Pickford, RJ. *Pharm. Biomed. Anal.*, 1991, 9, 787-792.

[44] Schneider, HJ; Hacket, F; Rudiger, V. *Chem. Rev.*, 1998, 98, 1755-1785.

[45] Cabrer, PR; Alvares-Parrilla, E; Meijide, F; Seijas, JA; Nunez, ER; Tato, JV. *Langmuir*, 1999, 15, 5489-5495.

[46] Matsui, Y; Tokunada, S. *Bull. Chem. Soc.*, Jpn. 1996, 69, 2477-2480.

[47] Lai, C; Piette, LH. *Tetrahedron Lett.*, 1979, 9, 775-778.

[48] Saprin, AN; Piette, LH. *Arch. Biochem. Biophys.*, 1977, 180, 480-492.

[49] Walling, C. *Acc. Chem. Res.*, 1998, 31, 55-157.

[50] Buetter, GR. In *Handbook of methods of oxygen radical research*; R. A. Greenwald, (Ed.), CRC Press: Boca Raton, FL, 1986, pp 151-155.

[51] Dicalov, SI; Mason, RP. *Free Radic. Biol. Med.*, 1999, 27, 864-872.

[52] Buettner, GR. *Free Radic. Biol. Med.*, 1987, 3, 259-303.

[53] Harbour, JR; Chow, V; Bolton, JR. *Can. J. Chem.*, 1974, 52, 3549-3554.

[54] Yoshimura, Y; Inomata, T; Nakazawa, H. *J. Liq. Chromatogr. Rel. Technol.*, 1999, 22, 419-428.

[55] Polyakov, NE; Leshina, TV; Salakhutdinov, NF; Konovalova, TA; Kispert, LD. *Free Rad. Biol. Med.*, 2006, 40, 1804-1809.

[56] Welch, KD; Davis, TZ; Van Eden, ME; Aust, SD. *Free Rad. Biol. Med.*, 2001, 32, 577-583.

[57] Barbouti, A; Doulias, PT; Zhu, BZ; Frei, B; Galaris, D. *Free Rad. Biol. Med.*, 2002, 32, 93-101.

[58] Polyakov, NE; Leshina, TV; Konovalova, TA; Kispert, LD. *Free Rad. Biol. Med.*, 2001, 31, 398-404.

[59] Konovalova, TA; Gao, Y; Kispert, LD; van Tol, J; Brunel, LC. *J. Phys. Chem.*, B 2003, 107, 1006-1011.

[60] Konovalova, TA; Gao, Y; Schad, R; Kispert, LD. *J. Phys. Chem.*, B 2001, 105, 7459-7464.

[61] Gao, Y; Konovalova, TA; Xu, T; Kispert, LD. *J. Phys. Chem.*, B 2002, 106, 10808-10815.

[62] Gao, Y; Konovalova, TA; Lawrence, JN; Smitha, MA; Nunley, J; Schad, R; Kispert, LD. *J. Phys. Chem.*, B 2003, 107, 2459-2465.

[63] Persson, HL; Yu, Z; Tirosh, O; Eaton, JW; Brunk, UT. *Free Rad. Biol. Med.*, 2003, 34, 1295-1305.

[64] Suh, J; Zhu, BZ; Frei, B. *Free Rad. Biol. Med.*, 2003, 34, 1306-1314.

[65] Celander, DW; Cech, TR. *Biochem.*, 1990, 29, 1355-1361.

[66] Li, S; Nguyen, TH; Schoneich, C; Borchardt, RT. *Biochem.*, 1995, 34, 5762-5772.

[67] Platis, IE; Ermacora, MR; Fox, RO. *Biochem.*, 1993, 32, 12761-12767.

[68] Rana, TM; Meares, CF. *J. Am. Chem. Soc.*, 1990, 112, 2457-2458.

[69] Francz, PI; Biesalski, HK; Pfitzner, I. *Biochim. Biophys. Acta*, 2000, 1474, 163-168.

[70] Offord, EA; Gautier, JC; Avanti, O; Scaletta, C; Runge, F; Kramer, K; Applegate, LA. *Free Rad. Biol. Med.*, 2002, 32, 1293-1303.

[71] Polyakov, NE; Leshina, TV; Salakhutdinov, NF; Kispert, LD. *J. Phys. Chem.*, B. 2006, 110, 6991-6998.

[72] Martı́n, L; Leo´n, A; Olives, AI; del Castillo, B; Martı́n, MA. *Talanta*, 2003, 60, 493-503.

[73] Lopez, EA; Bosque-Sendra, JM; Rodriguez, LC; Campana, AMG; Aaron, J. *J. Anal. Bioanal. Chem.*, 2003, 375, 414-423.

[74] Rekharsky, MV; Inoue, Y. *Chem. Rev.*, 1998, 98, 1875-1917.

[75] Maafi, M; Laassis, B; Aaron, JJ; Mahedero, MC; Munoz de la Pena, A; Salinas, F. *J. Inclusion Phenom. Mol. Recogn.*, 1995, 22, 235-247.

[76] Kornievskaya, VS; Kruppa, AI; Polyakov, NE; Leshina TV. *J. Phys. Chem.*, B 2007, 111, 11447-11452.

[77] Polyakov, NE; Khan, VK; Taraban, MB; Leshina, TV. *J. Phys. Chem.*, B 2008, 112, 4435-4440.

[78] Liu, D; Kispert, LD. In Recent research developments in electrochemistry; S. G. Pandalai, (Ed), Transworld Research Network: Trivandrum, India, 1999, pp 139-157.

[79] Lawlor, DW. *Photosynthesis: Metabolism, Control and Physiology*, Wiley: New York, 1987.

[80] Kohl, DH. In Biological Applications of Electron Spin Resonance; H. M. Swartz, J. R. Bolton, & D. C. Berg (Eds.), Wiley: New York, 1972.

[81] Kispert, LD; Konovalova, TA; Gao, Y. *Arch. Biochim. Biophys.*, 2004, 430, 49-60.

[82] Polyakov, NE; Leshina, TV; Meteleva, ES., Dushkin, AV; Konovalova, TA; Kispert, LD. *J. Phys. Chem.*, B, 2008, in press.

[83] Babkin, VA; Kolzunova, LG; Medvedeva, EN; Malkov, YuA; Ostroukhova, LA. Russian Patent, 2256668, 2005.

[84] Tonnesen, HH; Ed; *Photostability Of Drugs And Drug Formulations*; CRC Press: Orlando, FL, 2004.

[85] Wu, Y; Piekara-Sady, L; Kispert, LD. *Chem. Phys. Lett.*, 1991, 180, 573-577.

[86] Piekara-Sady, L; Khaled, MM; Bradford, E; Kispert, LD; Plato, M. *Chem. Phys. Lett.*, 1991, 186, 143-148.

[87] Gao, Y; Webb, S; Kispert, LD. *J. Phys. Chem.*, B. 2003, 107, 13237-13240.

[88] Liu, D; Gao, Y; Kispert, LD. *J. Electroanal. Chem.*, 2000, 488, 140-150.

[89] Silva, MRA; Trovó, AG; Nogueira, RFP. *J. Photochem. Photobiol.*, A: Chem. 2007, 191, 187-192.

[90] Bacardit, J; Stötzner, J; Chamarro, E; Esplugas, S. *Ind. Eng. Chem. Res.*, 2007, 46, 7615-7619.

[91] Konovalova, TA; Krzystek, J; Bratt, PJ; van Tol, J; Brunel, LC; Kispert, LD. *J. Phys. Chem.*, B 1999, 103, 5782-5786.

[92] Konovalova, TA; Dikanov, SA; Bowman, MK; Kispert, LD. *J. Phys. Chem.*, B 2001, 105, 8361-8368.

[93] Focsan, AL; Bowman, MK; Konovalova, TA; Molnár, P; Deli, J; Dixon, DA; Kispert, LD. *J. Phys. Chem.*, B 2008, 112, 1806-1819.

[94] Hoffmann, MR; Martin, ST; Choi, W; Bahnemann, DW. *Chem. Rev.*, 1995, 95, 69-96.

[95] Chen, LX; Rajh, T; Wang, Z; Thurnauer, MC. *J. Phys. Chem.*, B 1997, 101, 10688-10697.

[96] Mills, A; Hunte, SL. *J. Photochem. Photobiol.*, A 1997, 108, 1-35.

[97] Hagfeld, A; Grätzel, M. *Chem. Rev.*, 1995, 95, 49-68.

[98] Bard, AJ. *J. Phys. Chem.*, 1982, 86, 172-177.

[99] Jeevarajan, AS; Kispert, LD; Piekara-Sady, L. *Chem. Phys. Lett.*, 1993, 209, 269-274.

[100] Konovalova, TA; Kispert, LD; Konovalov, VV. *J. Phys. Chem.*, B 1997, 101, 7858-7862.

[101] Konovalova, TA; Kispert, LD. *J. Chem. Soc., Faraday Trans.*, 1998, 94, 1465-1468.

[102] Solarska, R; Rutkowska, I; Morand, R. Augustynski, *J. Electrochim. Acta*, 2006, 51, 2230-2236.

[103] Nakade, S; Saito, Y; Kubo, W; Kanzaki, T; Kitamura, T; Wada, Y; Yanagida, S. *Electrochem. Commun.*, 2003, 5, 804-808.

[104] Kuciauskas, D; Liddell, PA; Hung, SC; Lin, S; Stone, S; Seely, GR; Moore, AL; Moore, TA; Gust, D. *J. Phys. Chem.*, B, 1997, 101, 429-440.

[105] Liddell, PA; Kuciauskas, D; Simuda, JP; Nash, B; Nguyen, D; Moore, AL; Moore, TA; Gust, D. *J. Am. Chem. Soc.*, 1997, 119, 1400-1405.

[106] Kodis, G; Liddell, PA; Moore, AL; Moore, TA; Gust, D. *J. Phys. Org. Chem.*, 2004, 17, 724-734.

[107] Konovalova, TA; Kispert, LD. *J. Phys. Chem.*, B, 1999, 103, 4672-4677.

In: Encyclopedia of Vitamin Research
Editor: Joshua T. Mayer

ISBN 978-1-61761-928-1
© 2011 Nova Science Publishers, Inc.

Chapter 33

Carotene Dispersion in Liquid Media[*]

Cao-Hoang Lan[1,2†] and Waché Yves[1†]

[1]Laboratoire GPMA, AgroSup Dijon & Université de Bourgogne,
1, esplanade Erasme, 21000 Dijon
[2]Institute of Biotechnology and Food Technology, Hanoi University of Technology,
1 Dai Co Viet road, Hanoi, Vietnam

Abstract

β-Carotene is a highly hydrophobic compound that is almost insoluble in aqueous media. Due to its biological interest, it is the constant subject of researches on absorption, cleavage etc. However, in most experiments, the technical problem of β-carotene dispersion in liquid media arises. This non-polar compound possesses a very high LogP_octanol/water (around 15). From this value, it can be deduced that in an emulsion, there is practically no partition between the two phases and all the carotene is extracted by the organic phase. In the food ingestion system, the carotene present in food is extracted by the lipidic phases and especially the bile acids. In the present chapter, after a presentation of some ways β-carotene is dispersed or transported in cells and organisms (especially in biological membranes) we propose to review various methods that have been used to disperse carotene for different purposes (e.g. food, medical, etc.) This includes dispersion in surfactant micelles, use of alkane/water biphasic systems, reverse micelles and formulation of β-carotene nanoparticles.

---

[*] A version of this chapter was also published in *Beta Carotene: Dietary Sources, Cancer and Cognition, edited by Leiv Haugen and Terje Bjornson* published by Nova Science Publishers, Inc. It was submitted for appropriate modifications in an effort to encourage wider dissemination of research.
[†] Correspondance: [*] Email: hoanglan_cao@yahoo.fr
[†] Email: ywache@u-bourgogne.fr., Tel: + 33 (0) 3 80 39 66 80, Fax: + 33 (0) 3 80 39 66 41

1. Introduction

Carotenoids, particularly β-carotene, are gaining interest in the food industry due to their nutritional and antioxidant properties. β-Carotene is an important compound in many fields of food, nutrition and pharmacy. It is the most commonly used source of vitamin A for nutritional supplementation and has been known as a powerful singlet oxygen scavenging antioxidant [1, 2]. Some of its interests are presented in other parts of this book and include many health and nutritional aspects. We can also cite its role as a food ingredient as it is one of the main natural color used in the food industry, or precursor of aroma compounds (among its cleavage products are β-cyclocitral, β-ionone, 5,6-epoxy-β-ionone and dihydro-actinidiolide, which are compounds possessing fruity, flower and woody-sensorial notes) [3, 4]. In a physiological point of view, the main interests of β-carotene are related to its role of precursor of vitamin and to its behavior toward oxygen and its reactive species [5-9]. This chemical reactivity is also a source of problems due to the instability of this pigment and to the possibility to slide from an antioxidant to a prooxidant effect depending on the environmental conditions. As a consequence, β-carotene is usually considered as a positive nutritional compound as long as it is targeted to the right tissue and not degraded before [10]. A main concern for all applications is the high hydrophobicity of this carotenoid. It possesses a Log P (octanol-water partition coefficient, which represents carotenoid hydrophobicity) around 15. However, in most applications it has to be dispersed in aqueous phases to be stable and to be absorbable. A good deal of research is being carried out in this field and this chapter proposes to review the main principles and techniques used to overcome the low water solubility problem of β-carotene. After a brief presentation of the solutions proposed by nature itself (i.e. the way β-carotene is encountered in nature aqueous systems), dispersion in surfactant micelles, biphasic systems and formulation of nanoparticles of β-carotene will be presented.

2. Carotenoids in Cells and Organisms

2.1. Presence of Carotene in Cells and Higher Organism Tissues

β-Carotene is almost insoluble in water but it is present in many organisms from microorganisms to higher organisms. Due to its highly lipophilic character, it is mainly encountered in the lipid portions of tissues and cells including membranes, but it is also present in blood serum where it is transported by lipoproteins [6, 11]. The various dispersion forms of carotenoids that can be encountered during digestion are summerized in Figure 1. In blood, carotenoids are transported by LDL (low density lipoprotein) particles with a difference between nonpolar or monopolar carotenoids, which are localized in the larger, less dense LDL particles, and dipolar ones, which are localized preferentially in the smaller more dense LDL particles [12].

2.2. Interactions of Carotenoids with Membranes

The incorporation of carotenoids into membranes is an important point to understand. From about the 20 carotenoids circulating in blood, only lutein and zeaxanthine selectively accumulate in membranes [13, 14]. This phenomenon might involve specific carotenoid binding proteins but it may also be explained by structural characteristics of carotenoids and membranes. Carotenoids (xanthophylls) bearing hydroxyl groups at the extremity (on the cycles) can be incorporated into membranes. Due to the polar group at the extremities, their orientation is almost normal to the bilayer surface [15], although lutein could also be present in another orientation [16]. Actually, with xanthophylls with two hydroxyl groups (lutein or zeaxanthine), the size of the molecule permits a localization inside the bilayer with the two polar groups anchoring the compound in the two head-group regions from one side to the other of the lipid bilayer (Figure 2). This good fitting between lipid bilayers and xanthophylls results in high incorporation of these carotenoids inside membranes, as it can be estimated that carotenoids solubilize as monomers at concentration up to 10 mol% [14]. However, this fitting is strongly dependent on the thickness of the phosphatidylcholine (PC) bilayer: with DilauroylPC (DLPC) or DimyristoylPC (DMPC), the thickness of the membrane is less important than the length of the dihydroxycarotenoids which remain therefore inclined with respect to the bilayer surface [15], whereas for DipalmitoylPC (DPPC) and DistearoylPC (DSPC) membranes, the match is better and the incorporation can reach up to 28 mol% [17]. With only one hydroxyl group (e.g. cryptoxanthin), the solubility decreases drastically but in a way dependent on the thickness of the membrane: only 3 mol% in DLPC, between 5 and 10 mol% for DMPC and comparable to lutein for thicker membranes [14]. In contrast, the apolar carotene is poorly incorporated and could already crystallize in the aqueous phase outside the membrane from 0.5 to 1 mol% [18-20]. Its orientation can be both parallel and perpendicular to the surface of the lipid bilayer, especially in DMPC membranes, but it can be mainly perpendicular in DioleylPC membranes [21]. In conclusion, the incorporation and solubility of carotenoids are strongly dependent on the size of the hydrophobic layer as compounds tend to orientate parallel to the acyl chains of the phosphatidylcholine, as illustrated in Figure 2.

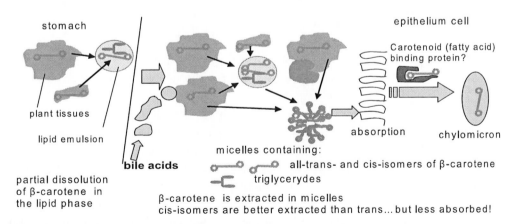

Figure 1. Different forms of dispersion of β-carotene during intestinal absorption. Carotenoids are lipophilic and their metabolism is therefore related to lipids. In the stomach, they are partially dissolved and transferred to micelles, then, they form emulsions with bile acids, are absorbed into epithelial cells and are transferred to the serum.

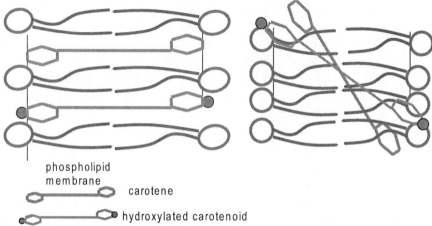

phospholipid
membrane

carotene

hydroxylated carotenoid

Figure 2. Schematic representation of the localization of carotenoids in membranes made of C18-acyl (left) and shorter acyl (right) phospholipids. There is a low solubility of carotene in C18 membranes where the hydrophobic molecule may be incorporated and almost no solubility in thinner membranes. For the hydroxylated carotenoid, the size between the two polar groups matches well with the intramembranar distance of C18 membranes, the two polar groups anchoring the compound in the two head-group regions from one side to the other of the lipid bilayer. This results in a very good solubility whereas with thinner membranes the solubility is lower. In blue: hydrophobic parts; in red: hydrophilic parts.

3. Dispersion of β-carotene

As seen above, carotenoids in general and β-carotene in particular can find hydrophobic cores to be transported and dispersed in cells and organisms. However, when attempting to disperse β-carotene in solutions, it forms readily aggregates (for a review on aggregation of carotenoids, see [22]). The next part will deal with several techniques for preparation of β-carotene dispersion to improve its solubility and to avoid its aggregation in aqueous solution.

3.1. Dispersion in Surfactant Micelles

Carotenoids are insoluble in water but can be dissolved in fat solvent such as alcohol, ether, chloroform etc. For instance, carotenes are readily soluble in petroleum ether and hexane; xanthophylls dissolve best in methanol and ethanol. The choice of solvent is highly dependent on the nature of the carotenoid and more important, on the field of application. In food applications, the organic solvent chosen must boil below boiling point of water, (e.g. butane, ethanol, ethyl acetate etc). Other solvents can also be used, but the conditions of utilization must be restrictly respected (e.g. maximum residual concentration in final products). Such solvents include hexane, dichloromethane, methanol etc.

To improve the solubility and bioavailability of carotenoids such as β-carotene, formation of water dispersible β-carotene is needed. The common method is first forming solution of β-carotene in a volatile organic solvent then emulsifying with an aqueous solution containing a surfactant (surface-active agent). The solvent is evaporated after emulsification. Surfactants play an important role in the dispersion of carotenoids as they will increase the specific surface area by surrounding carotenoid droplets, thus avoiding their aggregation. They are indeed amphiphilic molecules composed of a hydrophilic and a hydrophobic moieties. They can be generally classified according to the nature of their hydrophilic head group, as anionic (e.g. fatty alcohol sulfate, sulfonic acid salts), cationic (e.g. polyamines and their salts) and nonionic (e.g. polyoxyethylenated alkyphenols, polysorbates). Some typical surfactants widely used in biochemistry and food applications can be found in Figure 3.

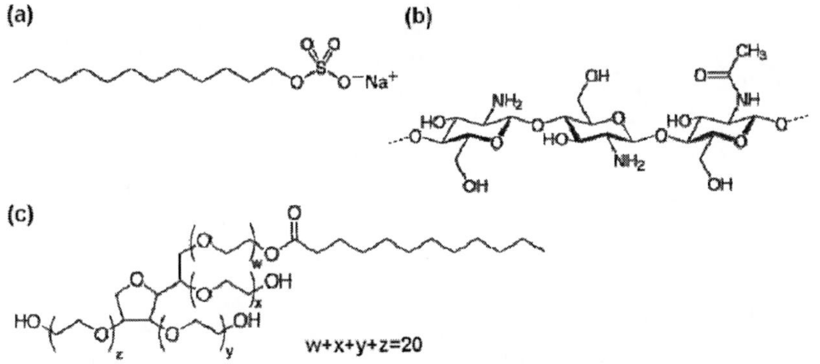

Figure 3. Chemical structures of some surfactants/emulsifiers commonly used for β-carotene dispersion. (a) Sodium dodecyl sulfate (SDS), an anionic surfactant; (b) Chitosan, a weak cationic emulsifier; (c) Tween 20, a nonionic surfactant.

The dispersion technique of β-carotene was first proposed by Ben-Aziz *et al.* [23] using Tween 80 as a surfactant. Since then, numerous other surfactants were studied to improve β-carotene dispersion such as different Spans (sorbitan esters), Tweens (polyoxyethylene derivatives of the Spans), saccharides or other surface-active compounds [24-27]. When these substances are present in an aqueous medium at concentrations above a certain value, called the critical micelle concentration (CMC), they form aggregates known as micelles. An important function of surfactants is to stabilize in micelles and thereby allow β-carotene to disperse in aqueous media. This occurs because β-carotene can be incorporated into the micelle core, which is itself solubilized in the aqueous medium by virtue of the head groups' favorable interactions with the medium. Without micellization, β-carotene would be insoluble and could only be suspended as particles in the aqueous phase, as illustrated in Figure 4a. Different steps in common preparation of β-carotene solution can be schematically illustrated in Figure 4b. Interaction between β-carotene and the micellar solution is strongly dependent on the characteristics of the surfactant chosen. As described above, a surfactant molecule is composed of a hydrophilic and a hydrophobic portions, and the relationship between these two portions which determines the overall characteristics of the compound is characterized by the hydrophile-lipophile balance (HLB) value. This provides an indication of the relative strength of the hydrophilic and hydrophobic portions of the surfactant and a relative affinity of the surfactant for aqueous and organic phases. The higher the HLB of a surfactant, the more hydrophilic it is. In general, when the HLB is less than 10, the lipophilic property is stronger and inversely. For instance, the Spans are lipophilic (low HLB values ranging from 1.8 - 8.6), while the Tweens are hydrophilic and have high HLB values ranging from 9.6 - 16.7.

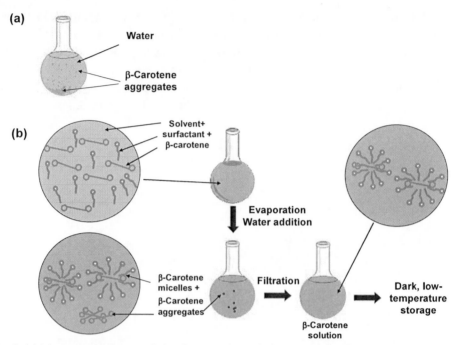

Figure 4. (a) Macroscopic characteristic of an aqueous solution containing β-carotene: without entrapment in micelle cores, β-carotene molecules remain suspended in water and tend to form molecular aggregates by themselves. (b) Schematic representation of preparation of β-carotene solution by dispersion in surfactant micelle.

In the previous section 2.2., the important role of the size of the membrane acyl chain in the solubilization of carotenoids such as β-carotene is discussed. Besides this parameter, the ratio between the hydrophilic and hydrophobic nature of the molecule, i.e. the HLB value, is also an important criterion when choosing a surfactant for β-carotene dispersion. For instance, difference in entrapment efficiency for β-carotene was found when various Tweens were used [28]. The maximum entrapment efficiency was reached with Tween 60, while the lowest was observed in presence of Tween 20. Such a different dispersion level can be presumably due to a different HLB, being the HLB of Tween 60 = 14.9 and that of Tween 20 = 16.7, thus making Tween 60 more efficient in solubilizing lipophilic compounds such as β-carotene. The β-carotene particle sizes were shown to depend also on the surfactant used, and this is an important point in production of β-carotene micro or nanoemulsion. For instance, Yuan *et al.* [29] pointed out that of four surfactants used Tween 20, Tween 40, Tween 60 and Tween 80, Tween 20 produced the smallest particle sizes in an oil in water (O/W) emulsion. The HLB values of these four surfactants are 16.7, 16.5, 14.9 and 15.0 for Tweens 20, 40, 60 and 80, respectively. It is shown that emulsifiers with greater hydrophilicity could wrap and stabilize the particles in an O/W emulsion more efficiently, resulting in smaller particles [30]. The higher HLB value of Tween 20 could be responsible for the smaller particle sizes in the emulsions produced with this surfactant, while the relatively small differences in the HLB values among the other three Tween emulsifiers might explain the lack of a consistent pattern in the particle size of the emulsions prepared with them [29].

In conclusion, β-carotene is water insoluble but can be dissolved in organic solvents and dispersed in aqueous media in presence of surfactants. Besides the hydrophobic part length, it is important to take into account the HLB value, one of the most important properties of the surfactant, which has a great impact on the characteristic of the β-carotene solution obtained.

3.2. Degradation of Dispersed β-carotene

The high reactivity of β-carotene confers to this molecule its anti/pro-oxidant properties, but it results also in a high instability. Therefore, for the various utilizations of β-carotene, the stability or degradation must be checked. This field is a constant subject of investigation aiming at understanding the antioxidant and radical scavenging properties, the mechanism and the products of cleavage and conservation of carotene or carotene-rich food products [31, 32]. Although the question of degradation is not always addressed in studies concerning the dispersion or encapsulation of β-carotene, some interesting data have been provided by projects dealing with the free radicals degradation of β-carotene in order to produce aroma compounds such as β-ionone, its 5,6-epoxy and dihydroactinidiolide. The degradation of the pigment dispersed in surfactant micelles by xanthine oxidase (XO) generated radicals has been investigated depending on the nature of the surfactant and thus, on the structure of the micelle [33-35]. Results obtained with Tween compounds pointed out that for Tween 20, which possesses a short acyl tail, the degradation of carotene is very rapid compared to the results obtained with longer acyl-chain Tweens. Moreover, for Tweens 20 and 40, no ionone-cycle-containing-cleavage-compounds were detected whereas these compounds constitute a good proportion of the cleavage compounds obtained with longer acyl-chain Tweens [24, 35]. This suggests that β-carotene may be incorporated in short acyl-chain Tween micelles but, in this case, the ionone cycles jut out from the micelle and the pigment molecule is less protected.

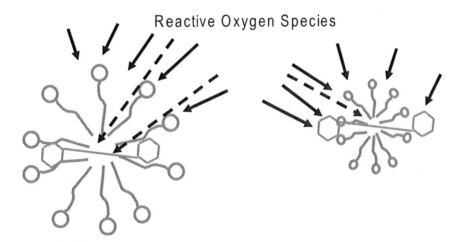

Figure 5. Hypothetical scheme of structure of Tween micelles of β-carotene deduced from β-carotene degradation. The reactive oxygen species (ROS) are represented by black arrows. Left: Tween 80 micelle; Right: Tween 20 micelle. Most ROS have reacted before entering micelles resulting in a slow degradation of β-carotene for left micelles with cleavage of the C9-10 double bond and in a rapid degradation in right micelles with cleavage of the β-ionone cycle.

3.3. Dispersion of β-carotene in Multiphasic Media

To overcome the lack of water solubility of β-carotene, some work has tried to solubilize it in organic solvents in multiphasic systems. However, in these studies the question of dispersion was not addressed directly but as for the previous paragraph, indirectly, through the enzyme-generated reactive oxygen species (ROS) degradation of the pigment. These studies have been realized from the 1990ies in order to investigate the production of volatile compounds deriving from β-carotene [33, 36]. Several aroma compounds can accumulate following oxidative cleavage of β-carotene and the chemical pathway was elucidated from experiments using Tween 80 micelles to disperse the precursor [34, 37]. However, in a biotechnological goal, solvents were used to improve the dispersion of the carotenoid. A first attempt was made with a water soluble solvent, acetone, to increase the solubility of β-carotene in water [38]. However, such a polar solvent inhibited the free radical generating enzyme used: xanthine oxidase. More apolar solvents forming two phases in water were used. For low LogP solvents (acetone or dichloromethane), the enzymatic activity was inhibited and no β-carotene degradation occurred [38]. However, even for higher LogP, β-carotene was not degraded if dispersed in the solvent, suggesting that the free radicals generated in the aqueous phase were inactive in the solvent phase. Moreover, these results can give rise to a second hypothesis. As this free radical system can degrade β-carotene dispersed in Tween 80 micelles, it can be assumed that β-carotene can be degraded at the interface. However, no degradation was detected when the pigment was solubilized in solvents, suggesting that this molecule was located in the solvent phase and not at the interface. Similar results were obtained with more apolar ROS generated by lipoxygenase. The following experiments were carried out in the presence of a solvent phase but with carotene dispersed in micelles in the aqueous phase. With this system, there was a good degradation of carotene and the cleavage products were well extracted in the solvent part (up to 35 mol%, see [39]). Interactions between carotene micelles and the aqueous/solvent interface were likely to occur and this could explain the good extraction of ionone products before any degradation (this hypothesis is schematized in Figure 5). A second experiment using reversed micelles confirmed this hypothesis: carotene micelles were present in the aqueous phase but, as the reversed micelles were homogeneous, they were too small to contain Tween micelles and it is thus likely that Tween micelles interacted with the surfactant-rich water/solvent interface (Figure 6). It can be noted that in this case, the hydrophobic carotene stays localized at the interface, embedded in surfactant molecules and does not go deep inside the solvent phase in which it would not be degraded by ROS.

4. β-Carotene Nanoparticles

Different techniques have been developed to overcome the insolubility in water of β-carotene and to increase its bioavailability which considerably limits its applications, among which those that we presented in the previous paragraphs. In this part, formulation of β-carotene nanoparticles will be presented as an important step in the development of nanotechnology. Nanotechnology refers to the development of functional materials at a length scale of less than 100 nm. This latter has been explored significantly over the last five years [40] and is rapidly emerging as one of the most active research fields with potential applications in many food industries. Size greatly relates to functionality of food materials. It has been shown that formulating nanostructured particles may increase the apparent solubility of the active ingredient, the rate of mass transfer, the retention time or the absorption via direct uptake by the intestinal epithelium [41-45]. Due to their sub-cellular size, nanoparticles offer promising means of improving the bioavailability and the uptake of nutraceutical compounds, especially poorly soluble substances such as β-carotene and numerous other compounds that are widely used as active ingredients in various food products. Figure 7 illustrates uptake mechanisms of β-carotene molecules depending on their particle size.

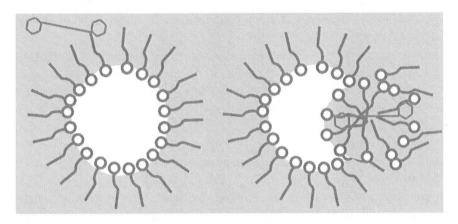

Figure 6. Interaction of β-carotene and reversed micelles. Left: A reversed aqueous micelle is present in a solvent containing β-carotene. Right: The same reversed micelle contains micelles of β-carotene. Hypothetical localization of β-carotene micelle at the interface between the two phases.

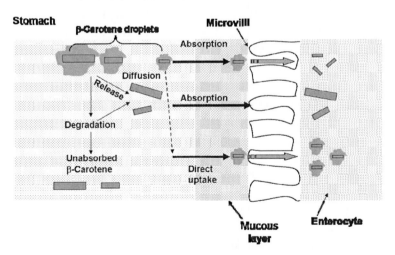

Figure 7. Schematic representation of different absorption mechanisms of β-carotene depending on its particle size. Bigger β-carotene droplets need to be released from the matrix to allow absorption by the intestinal wall. Intestinal absorption is increased with β-carotene nanodroplets due to (i) the increase in their retention time thanks to entrapment in the mucous layer and (ii) the direct uptake of the particle by the intestinal epithelium.

Contrary to macroemulsions that are thermodynamically unstable systems, which means that they must end at a coalesced system [46], micro and nanoemulsions (also called miniemulsions, ultrafine emulsions, submicron emulsions or translucent emulsions) possess a high preservation of stability against sedimentation over certain storage time. Indeed, nanoemulsions are emulsions with an extremely small droplet size which can overlap those of microemulsions. The fundamental difference between microemulsions and nanoemulsions is that microemulsions are equilibrium systems (i.e. thermodynamically stable) while nanoemulsions are non-equilibrium systems with a spontaneous tendency to separate into the constituent phases. Nevertheless, nanoemulsions may possess a relatively high kinetic stability, even for several years due to their small droplet size [47]. Moreover, nanoemulsions can be prepared using a small surfactant concentration comprised between 3-10%, while microemulsions need a higher surfactant concentration of about 20% to decrease their interfacial tension and to achieve their narrow size distribution [48].

β-Carotene nanoparticles can be produced either by mechanical (*top-down*) or by chemical (*bottom-up*) processes [40]. The principle of mechanical processes is using shear or particle collisions as the energy source to break down larger entities into smaller nano-scale aggregates, then small particles are produced through different size reduction [26, 27, 29, 30, 41]. Chemical processes consist in the self-assembly of smaller molecules such as lipids and proteins to produce nanoparticles [49-53]. Combination of these two approaches to generate nanoparticle systems has also been investigated to improve the quality, e.g. stability, bioavailability, sensory aspects, of the final product [54].

High-pressure homogenization is one of the techniques (*top-down* approach or *mechanical process*) used for preparing the nanosized dispersion of β-carotene. By varying different parameters, e.g. the power density applied (pressure) and the number of homogenization cycles, a desired particle size distribution can be obtained. In general, the particle diameter decreases with increasing the homogenization pressures and cycles [29]. For instance, Tan and Nakajima (2005) showed that the particle diameter of β-carotene nanodispersions is about 80 nm and 60 nm with samples prepared from 60 MPa/1 cycle and 140 MPa/1 cycle, respectively. The role of the surfactants, such as Tweens, Spans, is also indispensable due to its ability to stabilize the produced nanoparticles, thus avoiding coalescence of the formed β-carotene particles. Differences observed between different surfactants or surfactant concentrations have been correlated with their ability to prevent aggregation [26, 48]. High pressure homogenization is thus a relatively simple and effective technique for producing β-carotene nanoemulsions. However, one technological problem still remains: the β-carotene nanoemulsions have usually good physical stabilities but, chemically, significant degradation of β-carotene is observed during storage even at low temperatures [29]. Two major factors that could be responsible for the degradation of β-carotene in nanodispersions during storage were identified: (i) large surface area of the emulsion particles as a result of their size reduction to the nanometer range, which may significantly reduce the stability of β-carotene nanodispersions by providing more contact surface between β-carotene particles and the aqueous environment; and (ii) possible formation of free radicals during the high pressure homogenization process, that may induce a loss of β-carotene in the prepared nanodispersions [29, 30].

Besides the mechanical high pressure homogenization for the preparation of β-carotene nanodispersions, emulsification-solvent displacement method is one of *chemical processes* (or *bottom-up* approach) widely used for formulation of β-carotene nanoparticles [48, 51]. This method consists of dissolving the hydrophobic substance (β-carotene) in a polar organic solvent such as acetone (in some cases a polymer such as polylactic acid is also dissolved in the solvent with β-carotene particles), then mixing this system with an aqueous solution (e.g. water) containing a surfactant. Spontaneous emulsification will occur due to the affinity between the polar organic solvent and the continuous phase (aqueous phase), and upon addition of more water, the organic solvent diffuses out of the emulsion drop and into the aqueous phase, inducing the formation of β-carotene nanoparticles in the continuous phase. This methods is capable of producing 20-80 nm β-carotene nanoparticles using acetone as organic solvent and poly(lactic) and poly (lactic-co-glycolic) acids as polymer carriers [51]. This method shows several advantages such as low energy input, high entrapment efficiency and high stability of β-carotene nanodispersions over five month storage, compared with *mechanical process* such as high pressure homogenization.

Recently, there has been a growing interest to encapsulate bioactive compounds into protein microbead structures, based on self-assembly of proteins, for drug delivery applications. This method consists in the transformation of proteins such as globular proteins (e.g. egg white, whey protein) and casein micelles in nanocapsules to entrap molecules of interest such as β-carotene. Various kinds of animal and vegetal proteins have been investigated, including gelatin [55], collagen [56, 57], casein [50, 58], or plant proteins such as zein [59]. Multiple component matrix such as protein–polysaccharide [50, 60, 61] or protein-synthetic polymer [62, 63] particles have also been studied. With acquired knowledge of protein physical chemistry, one could currently build protein nanoparticles using the *bottom-up* approach. Casein-*graft*-dextran coated β-carotene nanoparticles (around 200 nm) have been recently developed by first forming casein-*g*-dextran copolymer through Maillard reaction.

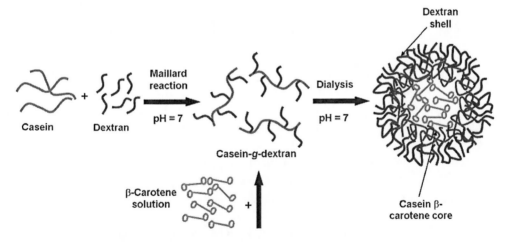

Figure 8. Schematic representation of formation of nanoparticle β-carotene encapsulated in casein-*graft*-dextran.

The copolymers form micelles at the pI of casein and the micelles dissociate when pH is away from the pI [64]. The second step is dialysis of organic solvent containing β-carotene and the copolymer against distilled water [50]. β-Carotene is encapsulated in the copolymer micelles while the solvent is changed to water, resulted in the formation of nanoparticles with casein and β-carotene core and dextran shell (Figure 8). The encapsulation of β-carotene in protein nanogels appears to be due to the hydrophobic interaction between β-carotene and hydrophobic segments of casein, forming the hydrophobic particle core [50]. This strong interaction gives the nanoparticle encapsulation a high stability against dilution, storage, β-carotene becomes thus much more stable after being encapsulated and can even be stored in dried form after preparation. The encapsulated β-carotene can then be released by hydrolysis of digestive enzymes (e.g. pepsin or trypsin) without decrease in β-carotene activity [50]. This technology reveals a potential for a broad range of applications requiring biocompatible formulation of active ingredients, e.g. human and animal nutrition, cosmetics, pharma, crop protection etc [49].

Conclusion

Interest in carotenoids, particularly β-carotene, has increased over the past decade from scientific researchers involved in a variety of disciplines. However, owing to the strong hydrophobic character of β-carotene, it is nearly impossible to directly dissolve it in aqueous media, and therefore, its bioavailability and its absorption are reduced considerably. Various strategies have been proposed as alternative solutions to its indispersibility in water, such as the "pseudosolubilization" of β-carotene in micelles of surfactant in water, use of multiphasic systems to disperse β-carotene or preparation of nanoemulsion of β-carotene. Further investigations are still required to achieve better stabilization of the β-carotene structures formed and better understanding of the mechanisms involved in the processes at the molecular level, e.g. protein-β-carotene interactions, to ensure industrial applications.

References

[1]   Choe, E. & Min, D. B. (2006). Chemistry and Reactions of Reactive Oxygen Species in Foods. *Critical Reviews in Food Science and Nutrition, 46(1)*, 1-22.

[2]   Lee, J. H., Ozcelik, B. & Min, D. B. (2003). Electron Donation Mechanisms of Beta-Carotene as a Free Radical Scavenger. *Journal of Food Science, 68(3)*, 861-865.

[3]   Aguedo, M., Ly, M. H., Belo, I., Texeira, J., Belin, J. M. & Waché, Y. (2004). The use of enzymes and microorganisms for the production of aroma compounds from lipids. *Food Technology and Biotechnology, 42(4)*, 327-336.

[4]   Enzell, C. (1985). Biodegradation of carotenoids-an important route to aroma compounds. *Pure and Applied Chemistry, 57(5)*, 693-700.

[5]   Astorg, P. (1997). Food carotenoids and cancer prevention: an overview of current research. *Trends in Food Science & Technology, 8*, 406-413.

[6]   Bendich, A. & Olson, J. A. (1989). Biological actions of carotenoids. *Federation of American Societies for Experimental Biology Journal, 3(8)*, 1927-1932.

[7]   Krinsky, N. I. & Yeum, K. J. (2003). Carotenoid-radical interactions. *Biochemical and Biophysical Research Communications, 305(3)*, 754-760.

[8]   Mortensen, A., Skibsted, L. H. & Truscott, T. G. (2001). The interaction of dietary carotenoids with radical species. *Archives of Biochemistry and Biophysics, 385(1)*, 13-19.

[9]   Parker, R. S. (1996). Absorption, metabolism, and transport of carotenoids. *Federation of American Societies for Experimental Biology Journal, 10(5)*, 542-551.

[10] Biesalski, H. K., Tinz, J. & Steve, L. T. (2008) Nutritargeting. In: editor. *Advances in Food and Nutrition Research*: Academic Press, 179-217.

[11] Borel, P., Drai, J., Faure, H., Fayol, V., Galabert, C., Laromiguière, M. & Le Moël, G. (2005). Données récentes sur l'absorption et le catabolisme des caroténoïdes. *Annales de Biologie Clinique*, *63(2)*, 165-177.

[12] Lowe, G. M., Bilton, R. F., Davies, I. G., Ford, T. C., Billington, D. & Young, A. J. (1999). Carotenoid composition and antioxidant potential in subfractions of human low-density lipoprotein. *Annals of Clinical Biochemistry*, *36(Pt 3)*, 323-332.

[13] Krinsky, N. I. (2002). Possible Biologic Mechanisms for a Protective Role of Xanthophylls. *Journal of Nutrition*, *132(3)*, 540S-542.

[14] Wisniewska, A., Widomska, J. & Subczynski, W. K. (2006). Carotenoid-membrane interactions in liposomes: effect of dipolar, monopolar, and nonpolar carotenoids. *Acta Biochimica Polonica*, *53(3)*, 475-484.

[15] Gruszecki, W. I. & Sielewiesiuk, J. (1990). Orientation of xanthophylls in phosphatidylcholine multibilayers. *Biochimica et Biophysica Acta (BBA) - Biomembranes*, *1023(3)*, 405-412.

[16] Gruszecki, W. I. & Strzalka, K. (2005). Carotenoids as modulators of lipid membrane physical properties. *Biochimica et Biophysica Acta (BBA) - Molecular Basis of Disease*, *1740(2)*, 108-115.

[17] Kolev, V. D. & Kafalieva, D. N. (1986). Miscibility of beta-carotene and zeaxanthin with dipalmitoylphosphatidylcholine in multilamellar vesicles: a calorimetric and spectroscopic study. *Photobiochemical Photobiophysical*, *11*, 257-267.

[18] Kennedy, T. A. & Liebler, D. C. (1992). Peroxyl radical scavenging by beta-carotene in lipid bilayers. Effect of oxygen partial pressure. *Journal of Biological Chemistry*, *267(7)*, 4658-4663.

[19] Woodall, A. A., Britton, G. & Jackson, M. J. (1995). Antioxidant activity of carotenoids in phosphatidylcholine vesicles: chemical and structural considerations. *Biochemical Society Transactions*, *23(1)*, 133S.

[20] Socaciu, C., Jessel, R. & Diehl, H. A. (2000). Competitive carotenoid and cholesterol incorporation into liposomes: effects on membrane phase transition, fluidity, polarity and anisotropy. *Chemistry and Physics of Lipids*, *106(1)*, 79-88.

[21] van de Ven, M., Kattenberg, M., van Ginkel, G. & Levine, Y. K. (1984). Study of the orientational ordering of carotenoids in lipid bilayers by resonance-Raman spectroscopy. *Biophysical Journal*, *45(6)*, 1203-1209.

[22] Köhn, S., Kolbe, H., Korger, M., Köpsel, C., Mayer, B., Auweter, H., Lüddecke, E., Bettermann, H. & Martin, H. D. (2008). Aggregation and Interface Behaviour of Carotenoids. In: Basel B, editor. *Carotenoids: Natural Functions*, 3-98.

[23] Ben-Aziz, A., Grossman, S., Ascarelli, I. & Budowski, P. (1971). Carotene-bleaching activities of lipoxygenase and heme proteins as studied by a direct spectrophotometric method. *Phytochemistry*, *10(7)*, 1445-1452.

[24] Waché, Y., Bosser-De Ratuld, A. & Belin, J. M. (2006). Dispersion of beta-carotene in processes of production of beta-ionone by cooxidation using enzyme-generated reactive oxygen species. *Process Biochemistry*, *41(11)*, 2337-2341.

[25] Bertau, M. & Jörg, G. (2004). Saccharides as efficacious solubilisers for highly lipophilic compounds in aqueous media. *Bioorganic and Medicinal Chemistry*, *12(11)*, 2973-2983.

[26] Anantachoke, N., Makha, M., Raston, C. L., Reutrakul, V., Smith, N. C. & Saunders, M. (2006). Fine tuning the production of nanosized beta-carotene particles using spinning disk processing. *Journal of the American Chemical Society, 128(42)*, 13847-13853.

[27] Tan, C. P. & Nakajima, M. (2005). Effect of polyglycerol esters of fatty acids on physicochemical properties and stability of beta-carotene nanodispersions prepared by emulsification/evaporation method. *Journal of the Science of Food and Agriculture, 85(1)*, 121-126.

[28] Palozza, P., Muzzalupo, R., Trombino, S., Valdannini, A. & Picci, N. (2006). Solubilization and stabilization of [beta]-carotene in niosomes: delivery to cultured cells. *Chemistry and Physics of Lipids, 139(1)*, 32-42.

[29] Yuan, Y., Gao, Y., Zhao, J. & Mao, L. (2008). Characterization and stability evaluation of [beta]-carotene nanoemulsions prepared by high pressure homogenization under various emulsifying conditions. *Food Research International, 41(1)*, 61-68.

[30] Tan, C. P. & Nakajima, M. (2005). [beta]-Carotene nanodispersions: preparation, characterization and stability evaluation. *Food Chemistry, 92(4)*, 661-671.

[31] Mordi, R. C. & Walton, J. C. (1993). Oxidative degradation of beta-carotene and beta-apo-8'-carotenal. *Tetrahedron, 49(4)*, 911-928.

[32] Mordi, R. C., Walton, J. C., Burton, G. W., Hughes, L., Ingold, K. U. & Lindsay, D. A. (1991). Exploratory study of Beta-carotene autoxidation. *Tetrahedron Letters, 32(33)*, 4203-4206.

[33] Bosser, A. & Belin, J. M. (1994). Synthesis of beta-ionone in an aldehyde/xanthine oxidase/beta-carotene system involving free radical formation. *Biotechnology Progress, 10*, 129-133.

[34] Waché, Y., Bosser-DeRatuld, A., Lhuguenot, J. C. & Belin, J. M. (2003). Effect of cis/trans Isomerism of β-Carotene on the Ratios of Volatile Compounds Produced during Oxidative Degradation. *Journal of Agricultural and Food Chemistry, 51(7)*, 1984-1987.

[35] Bosser, A. (1995). Production de béta-ionone par voie enzymatique [Thèse de doctorat]. Dijon: Université de Bourgogne.

[36] Belin, J. M., Dumont, B., Ropert, F., inventors; Procédé de fabrication, par voie enzymatique, d'arômes, notamment des ionones et des aldéhydes en C6 à C10. France patent WO 94/08028. 1994 14/04/1994.

[37] Bosser, A., Paplorey, E. & Belin, J. M. (1995). A simple way to (+/-)-dihydroactinidiolide from beta-ionone related to the enzymic co-oxidation of beta-carotene in aqueous solution. *Biotechnology Progress, 11*, 689-692.

[38] Waché, Y., Bosser-DeRatuld, A., Ly, H. M. & Belin, J. M. (2002). Co-oxidation of beta-carotene in biphasic media. *Journal of Molecular Catalysis B: Enzymatic, 19-20*, 197-201.

[39] Ly, M. H., Cao-Hoang, L., Belin, J. M. & Waché, Y. (2008). Improved co-oxidation of beta-carotene to beta-ionone using xanthine oxidase-generated reactive oxygen species in a multiphasic system. *Biotechnology Journal, 3(2)*, 220-225.

[40] Acosta, E. (2009). Bioavailability of nanoparticles in nutrient and nutraceutical delivery. *Current Opinion in Colloid & Interface Science, 14(1)*, 3-15.

[41] Krause, K. P. & Müller, R. H. (2001). Production and characterisation of highly concentrated nanosuspensions by high pressure homogenisation. *International Journal of Pharmaceutics, 214(1-2)*, 21-24.

[42] Jacobs, C., Kayser, O. & Müller, R. H. (2001). Production and characterisation of mucoadhesive nanosuspensions for the formulation of bupravaquone. *International Journal of Pharmaceutics, 214(1-2)*, 3-7.

[43] Desai, M. P., Labhasetwar, V., Amidon, G. L. & Levy, R. J. (1996). Gastrointestinal Uptake of Biodegradable Microparticles: Effect of Particle Size. *Pharmaceutical Research, 13(12)*, 1838-1845.

[44] Desai, M. P., Labhasetwar, V., Walter, E., Levy, R. J. & Amidon, G. L. (1997). The Mechanism of Uptake of Biodegradable Microparticles in Caco-2 Cells Is Size Dependent. *Pharmaceutical Research, 14(11)*, 1568-1573.

[45] Hussain, N., Jaitley, V. & Florence, A. T. (2001). Recent advances in the understanding of uptake of microparticulates across the gastrointestinal lymphatics. *Advanced Drug Delivery Reviews, 50(1-2)*, 107-142.

[46] Overbeek, J. T. G. (1978). The First Rideal Lecture. Microemulsions, a field at the border between lyophobic and lyophilic colloids. *Faraday Discussions of the Chemical Society, 65*, 7-19.

[47] Solans, C., Izquierdo, P., Nolla, J., Azemar, N. & Garcia-Celma, M. J. (2005). Nano-emulsions. *Current Opinion in Colloid & Interface Science, 10(3-4)*, 102-110.

[48] Bouchemal, K., Briançon, S., Perrier, E. & Fessi, H. (2004). Nano-emulsion formulation using spontaneous emulsification: solvent, oil and surfactant optimisation. *International Journal of Pharmaceutics, 280(1-2)*, 241-251.

[49] Liebmann, B., Hümmerich, D., Scheibel, T. & Fehr, M. (2008). Formulation of poorly water-soluble substances using self-assembling spider silk protein. *Colloids and Surfaces A: Physicochemical and Engineering Aspects, In Press, Corrected Proof.*

[50] Pan, X., Yao, P. & Jiang, M. (2007). Simultaneous nanoparticle formation and encapsulation driven by hydrophobic interaction of casein-graft-dextran and [beta]-carotene. *Journal of Colloid and Interface Science, 315(2)*, 456-463.

[51] Ribeiro, H. S., Chu, B. S., Ichikawa, S. & Nakajima, M. (2008). Preparation of nanodispersions containing [beta]-carotene by solvent displacement method. *Food Hydrocolloids, 22(1)*, 12-17.

[52] Amar, I., Aserin, A. & Garti, N. (2003). Solubilization patterns of lutein and lutein esters in food grade nonionic microemulsions. *Journal of Agricultural and Food Chemistry, 51(16)*, 4775-4781.

[53] Chu, B. S., Ichikawa, S., Kanafusa, S. & Nakajima, M. (2007). Preparation of Protein-Stabilized β-Carotene Nanodispersions by Emulsification–Evaporation Method. *Journal of the American Oil Chemists' Society, 84(11)*, 1053-1062.

[54] Horn, D. & Rieger, J. (2001). Organic Nanoparticles in the Aqueous Phase - Theory, Experiment, and Use. *Angewandte Chemie International Edition, 40(23)*, 4330-4361.

[55] Franz, J., Pokorová, D., Hampl, J. & Dittrich, M. (1998). Adjuvant efficacy of gelatin particles and microparticles. *International Journal of Pharmaceutics, 168(2)*, 153-161.

[56] Alex, R. & Bodmeier, R. (1990). Encapsulation of water-soluble drugs by a modified solvent evaporation method. I. Effect of process and formulation variables on drug entrapment. *Journal of Microencapsulation, 7(3)*, 347-355.

[57] Swatschek, D., Schatton, W., Müller, W. E. G. & Kreuter, J. (2002). Microparticles derived from marine sponge collagen (SCMPs): preparation, characterization and suitability for dermal delivery of all-trans retinol. *European Journal of Pharmaceutics and Biopharmaceutics, 54(2)*, 125-133.

[58] Latha, M. S., Lal, A. V., Kumary, T. V., Sreekumar, R. & Jayakrishnan, A. (2000). Progesterone release from glutaraldehyde cross-linked casein microspheres: In vitro studies and in vivo response in rabbits. *Contraception, 61(5)*, 329-334.

[59] Liu, X., Sun, Q., Wang, H., Zhang, L. & Wang, J. Y. (2005). Microspheres of corn protein, zein, for an ivermectin drug delivery system. *Biomaterials, 26(1)*, 109-115.

[60] Chen, L. & Subirade, M. (2005). Chitosan/beta-lactoglobulin core-shell nanoparticles as nutraceutical carriers. *Biomaterials, 26(30)*, 6041-6053.

[61] Guerin, D., Vuillemard, J. C. & Subirade, M. (2003). Protection of bifidobacteria encapsulated in polysaccharide-protein gel beads against gastric juice and bile. *Journal of Food Protection, 66(11)*, 2076-2084.

[62] Kasper, F. K., Kushibiki, T., Kimura, Y., Mikos, A. G. & Tabata, Y. (2005). In vivo release of plasmid DNA from composites of oligo(poly(ethylene glycol)fumarate) and cationized gelatin microspheres. *Journal of Controlled Release, 107(3)*, 547-561.

[63] Arbós, P., Arangoa, M. A., Campanero, M. A. & Irache, J. M. (2002). Quantification of the bioadhesive properties of protein-coated PVM/MA nanoparticles. *International Journal of Pharmaceutics, 242(1-2)*, 129-136.

[64] Yu, S., Hu, J., Pan, X., Yao, P. & Jiang, M. (2006). Stable and pH-sensitive nanogels prepared by self-assembly of chitosan and ovalbumin. *Langmuir, 22(6)*, 2754-2759.

In: Encyclopedia of Vitamin Research
Editor: Joshua T. Mayer

ISBN 978-1-61761-928-1
© 2011 Nova Science Publishers, Inc.

Chapter 34

Comparing Local Fruits and Vegetables and β-carotene Supplements as a Vitamin A Source for Honduran Mothers and Infants[*,†,‡]

Douglas L Taren[1#], Rina G. Kaminsky[2], Jackeline Alger[3], Monica Mourra[3], Rahul Mhaskar[1] and Louise M. Canfield[1,4]

[1]The Mel and Enid Zuckerman College of Public Health,
University of Arizona, Tucson, Arizona, USA
[2]The Universidad Nacional Autónoma de Honduras, Tegucigalpa, Honduras
[3] Servicio de Parasitología, Departamento de Laboratorios Clínicos,
Hospital Escuela, Tegucigalpa, Honduras
[4] The Arizona Cancer Center, College of Medicine, University of Arizona,
Tucson, Arizona, USA

Abstract

Background

To evaluate the feasibility of fruits and vegetables as a longterm strategy to combat vitamin A deficiency we compared the effects of dietary levels of local fruits and

---

[*] A version of this chapter was also published in *Beta Carotene: Dietary Sources, Cancer and Cognition, edited by Leiv Haugen and Terje Bjornson* published by Nova Science Publishers, Inc. It was submitted for appropriate modifications in an effort to encourage wider dissemination of research.
[†] Supported by a grant from The International Life Sciences Institute (ILSI), Washington, DC
[‡] Presented in part at the XIX Meeting of the International Vitamin A Consultive Group Durban, S. Africa
[#] Corresponding author: Mel and Enid Zuckerman College of Public Health, 1295 N. Martin Ave., PO Box 245163, Tucson, Arizona USA, 85724. Phone: 520-626-8375, Fax: 520-626-6093, email: taren@email.arizona.edu.

vegetables, an equivalent amount of β-carotene supplements and placebo on serum vitamin A concentrations of lactating mothers and infants in a periurban community in Honduras.

Methods

Mothers and their nursing infants were randomly assigned to receive β-carotene supplements, foods high in β-carotene or placebo three times/wk for four wk. Each treatment day, mothers in the supplement group received 7.5 mg β-carotene beadlets with a breakfast of local foods providing ~8 g fat. The placebo group received the same breakfast without the supplement. Mothers in the food group received lunch furnishing 7.5 mg β-carotene from local foods. Mothers and infants donated blood samples on days 1, 14 and 30. Milk samples were obtained at days 1 and 30 and maternal dietary intake was estimated by 24-hour dietary recalls on days 1, 14 and 30.

Results

Local foods high in β-carotene resulted in significant increases in maternal and infant serum retinol compared to the other two treatment groups. Increases in serum retinol of mothers and infants following β-carotene supplements were not significantly different from placebo. ß-Carotene supplements increased maternal serum and milk concentrations but did not increase infant serum ß-carotene levels.

Conclusions

Foods in the local diet increased circulating retinol levels of both mothers and infants. The importance of including food-based approaches in strategies to combat vitamin A deficiency is discussed.

Keywords: β-carotene, infant nutrition, lactation, deficiency, vitamin A

Introduction

Vitamin A deficiency (VAD) persists worldwide. Currently over 140 million preschool-aged children and at least 7.2 million pregnant women are vitamin A deficient (serum or breast-milk vitamin A concentrations < 0.70 µMol/L). Vitamin A supplementation alone has not been sufficient to eliminate VAD and a sustainable solution will require a comprehensive effort including nutrition education, fortification, supplementation and consumption of local foods high in provitamin A carotenoids [1-2].

Early studies focused on increased consumption of dietary sources of vitamin A and β-carotene as the most sustainable solution to vitamin A deficiency in children in developing countries. However, we now know that it is difficult for young children in low income countries where vitamin A deficiency exists to consume sufficient vitamin A and β-carotene-containing foods to prevent vitamin A deficiency [1]. Nevertheless, as part of an overall program, consumption of foods high in pro-vitamin A carotenoids is important for lactating mothers who provide a significant vitamin A source for nursing infants. However, since bioavilability and bioconversion of available foods, their acceptability, and methods of food preparation differ greatly among populations [3-5], a food-based strategy is irrelevant unless foods providing a sufficient source of vitamin A can be readily obtained and are culturally acceptable. The goal of this research was therefore to test the efficacy of local fruits and vegetables provided to lactating mothers in a community setting to improve the vitamin A status of the mother-infant dyad.

Methods

Study Design –This randomized placebo-controlled dietary intervention of lactating mothers and their infants compared the effects of ß-carotene supplements (Hoffman LaRoche) and β-carotene in local foods on concentrations of ß-carotene and retinol in serum of mothers and infants and in milk of mothers. The study design is presented in Figure 1. We administered 90 mg β-carotene as twelve 7.5 mg supplements or in lunches containing food high in β-carotene to study groups, evenly spaced over a four-week period in the month of April. This time period was chosen to avoid the rainy season in Honduras and the supplementation phase of the study was completed within one month to control for seasonal variation in consumption of fruits and vegetables. Meals and supplements containing the equivalent of 7.5 mg of purified β-carotene or placebo were provided three times per week (Mondays, Wednesdays, Fridays) for four weeks to all study participants. This dosage was chosen based on our previous results [6-7] demonstrating an increase in vitamin A status in Honduran mothers and infants in response to a 90 mg β-carotene supplement, the work of others using a comparable dosage in another vitamin A-low population [8] and an evaluation by our dietician (MM) of a realistic β-carotene intake from the local food supply. Ages, heights, and weights of mothers and infants and parity of mothers were recorded on the first day of the study. Twenty-four hour dietary recalls were administered on days 1, 14 and 30. Blood samples were collected from mothers and infants on the first day of the study, after 14 days and after 30 days. Mothers donated milk samples on day 1 and day 30. At the conclusion of the study, all mothers were provided multi-vitamins and instruction on preparation of local β-carotene containing foods served in the study. All instructions (verbal or written) and consent forms were in the Spanish language.

Study population - Lactating women and their infants were recruited from a Ministry of Health clinic in Colonia Alemania, a community near Tegucigalpa, with a population of slightly over 20,000 at the time of our study. One month prior to the study, local field staff visited physicians at local clinics to obtain permission to recruit study participants from their clinics. Mothers were recruited by flyers, radio broadcasts and by personal visits at clinics. Mothers were Spanish-speaking, of low socio-economic status and had the equivalent of middle school education or less.

Sample Size - Power calculations were based on expected changes in outcome variables in data gathered in our previous studies of Honduran women and infants [6, 7]. To quantitate a statistical difference of 20% among groups, assuming a dropout rate of 15%, we estimated that we would require a minimum of 44 subjects per group, or 132 lactating mothers and infants to achieve a 95% confidence interval, power = 80, significance level, $\alpha = 0.05$ (two-sided). One hundred ninety-five mother-infant pairs were recruited.

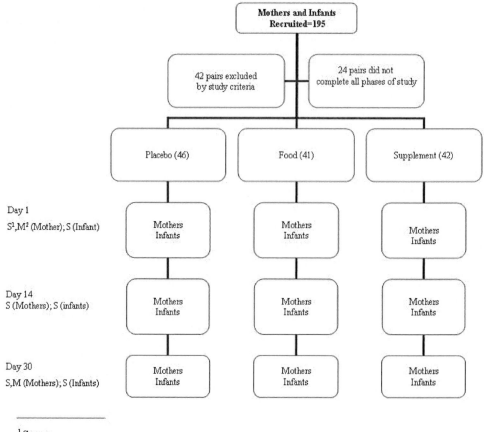

¹ Serum

² Milk

Figure 1. Mother-Child Pairs Recruited and Participating in Study.

Inclusion/exclusion criteria - At the time of the study, the Honduran Ministry of Health provided vitamin A supplements to children at 9 months of age when they received immunization against measles. Therefore, we excluded mothers of nursing infants who were either older than 9 months or had received vitamin A supplements as documented on the mother's health care certificate, provided by the Honduran Ministry of Health. Women who were ill, had infants with illness, who declined to participate for the full duration of the study, or who declined to sign an Informed Consent Form as well as mothers of infants less than 1 month, were also excluded. Infants were full-term without any known congenital or chronic disease. The included mothers were aged 15 - 45 years, parity $\leq$ 6, and by self-report, non-pregnant, non-smoking, not suffering from any chronic disease or infection, and not consuming other vitamin or mineral supplements.

Compliance - Of the 195 mother-infant pairs, 129 presented at all study visits to obtain supplements and contribute samples. However, analyte concentrations in some samples were below the level of detection by our analytical method and some infant serum samples sizes were insufficient for accurate analysis. Each mother who completed the study received gifts, the total value of which was approximately $50 (U.S. currency). In addition, lectures on health and nutrition were provided by one of our Tucson-based staff. A day-long ceremony was held at the end of the study in which lectures and literature in Spanish were provided emphasizing the importance of vitamin A in the diet. Certificates were awarded to the mothers in a ceremony at the end of the study.

Human Subjects Assurance - All procedures were conducted in accordance with regulations of the Human Subjects Protection Program at the University of Arizona and were approved by the Biomedical Committee of the University of Arizona Institutional Review Board. At least one member of the Arizona-based research team was present in the field for the duration of the study. All mothers were provided detailed information in Spanish about the study including risks, benefits and expectations of participation before they signed Informed Consent Forms in Spanish language in accordance with regulations of the University of Arizona and of the Honduran Ministry of Health. Physical examination findings, tests and sample analyses results were recorded in laboratory notebooks and computer disks with a coded identification number. Personal information about subjects was available only to the Principal Investigator and Field Coordinator. Code numbers were assigned at the time the samples were labeled for shipping in the field. Samples were analyzed by code number and technical staff were unaware of the treatment group to which the samples belonged.

Randomization of subjects - On arrival at the clinic, field researchers or study nurses greeted mothers and randomly assigned them to one of three groups using a simple random sampling method. The mothers' names were recorded on a blank, colored 3" X 5" card representing a specific study group; e.g., blue for Placebo Group, orange for mothers receiving β-carotene-containing foods (Food Group) and green for those receiving β-carotene supplements (Supplement Group). Mothers were asked to bring their cards for each clinic visit and the dates of each visit were recorded by the study nurse.

Physical Characteristics - Heights and weights of mothers were measured by field staff using tape measures and gravimetric balances. Infant weight was measured using an infant balance and length recorded by field staff. Brief medical histories for mothers and infants were recorded by field nurses or physicians.

Diet - Twenty-four hour dietary recall questionnaires were administered orally by experienced local dietitians or nurses who had been instructed in procedures for collecting dietary data. Mothers were shown pictures of foods or food models when asked to estimate the amount of food they consumed. Amounts were then converted to servings using standard conversion factors. The usual diet of this population is fairly monotonous and does not typically include foods high in carotenoids in large quantities. However, to minimize contamination of the study with sources of dietary β-carotene and vitamin A from food outside the research study meals, mothers were furnished a list of local foods high in carotenoids by our Honduras-based nutritionist and asked not to consume more than one portion per day of these for the duration of the study.

Supplementation - Mothers were served meals at our field site within walking distance from their homes. The study was conducted on Monday, Wednesday and Friday of each week. Mothers in the β-carotene supplementation group received a capsule containing 7.5 mg purified β-carotene as beadlets (Hoffman LaRoche) with a breakfast containing foods typical for this population; e.g., tortillas with sour cream, black beans, and eggs. Because dietary fat is required for absorption of carotenoids, we provided ~8g of fat as butter or ("crema") a local product similar to sour cream, in the meal. Mothers in the placebo group received the same meal as the β-carotene supplementation group, with a dextrose-filled placebo capsule. (Dextrose was substituted for lactose because of lactose intolerance in Honduras.) Placebo capsules were assembled in the University of Arizona Pharmacy and were encased in a capsule having the same shape and color as the β-carotene-containing capsules supplied by Hoffman LaRoche.

To avoid food trading between the groups and to minimize the placebo effect, meals in the food supplement group were given at lunch instead of breakfast. Mothers in the food supplement group were served lunch containing an amount of foods high in pro-vitamin A carotenoids calculated to deliver 7.5 mg of β-carotene in the meal [9, 10]. Foods were chosen for which food composition data were available and these data were used to estimate the amount of β-carotene in the meal. Foods were prepared in a kitchen near the field site using local recipes and menus varied on each study day. A sample lunch menu consisted of eggs with raidsh leaves (120 g), 3 tablespoons of black beans, 1 fried plantain, 2 ounces of white cheese, sweet potato and honey (150 g), 3 six inch diameter tortillas, and 8 ounces of orange juice. Mothers consumed their meals under supervision of field staff to assure that they consumed the entire meal. No adverse effects to any of the treatments were reported.

Sample Collection - As a control on the method, prior to traveling to Honduras, Arizona staff provided blood samples for serum analysis. Blood samples were again collected from the staff at the collection sites each day when blood was drawn from subjects, and samples were treated identically. Blood (5-10 mL) was obtained from the antecubital vein of mothers and approximately 1 mL of infant blood was taken by an experienced Spanish-speaking phlebotomist using "butterfly needles." If the phlebotomist was unable to obtain sufficient blood for analysis after two attempts, the procedure was aborted and the sample discarded in biological waste. Samples were light-protected and transported at ambient temperature (~25°C) within two hours to Laboratorios Medicos, a private clinical laboratory in Tegucigalpa, for preparation of serum. Blood samples were allowed to clot and serum was removed by centrifugation, and samples (~1 mL) stored at -70° C until they could be transported to Arizona.

Milk - These women nursed on demand, several times per hour. Therefore, hind milk did not accumulate and the supply to the infant was essentially midstream milk. Since a single mid-morning sample provides a reliable estimate of a 24-hour collection for an individual mother [11], milk samples (5–20 mL) were collected by manual expression into polypropylene or glass bottles at mid-morning. Electric breast pumps were culturally unacceptable in this community. Samples were light protected on ice in insulated coolers and transported to Laboratorios Medicos, and were stored at -70° C.

Transport of milk and serum samples - Authorization to transport biological samples was obtained prior to the study from the Center for Disease Control (CDC) and signed authorizations presented to Honduran and U.S. customs agents. Because dry ice was unavailable, samples were maintained frozen at -20°C in light-protected styrofoam shipping crates and hand-delivered to the Department of Biochemistry at the University of Arizona where they were immediately stored at -70° C until they could be analyzed. All protocols were documented in our laboratory instruction manual and were available to all project staff. Procedures for analysis of human samples followed University of Arizona biomedical safety guidelines (Bio-Safety level II; BL-2).

Extraction of retinol - Retinol was extracted from serum as previously described [11, 12]. Retinyl esters in milk were solubilized with bile salts and released from milk fat globules by enzymatic and/or alkaline hydrolysis using modifications of methods previously described [13]. Total milk lipid was determined by the "creamatocrit" method [14]. Analysts were blinded to allocation of study group and identity of participants.

Data Analysis - Twenty-four hour dietary records were evaluated for content of foods high in retinol and provitamin A carotenoids (β-cryptoxanthin, β-carotene and α-carotene). Intake was recorded as the number of servings of foods containing provitamin A, fruits and vegetables high in provitamin A, meat, eggs, fish, and sugar using food tables for use in developing countries [9, 10]. Intake records were ranked by number of servings of foods high in retinol or pro-vitamin A carotenoids. We used deductive imputation for editing questionnaires and filling in those questions for which data was missing; e.g., sex of respondent by using other information in the questionnaire (his or her name).

Accuracy of data entry was verified using independent entry by two analysts. Data was stored on hard disk and protected by backup discs. Because this population was transitory, data were not analyzed on an intention to treat basis, however, preliminary results were presented to the Honduran government upon completion of the data analysis [15].

Descriptive statistical analyses were performed using Stata Statistical Software, Version 6.0 (STATA Corp, College Stn, TX) or Microsoft Excel, Version 5.0, (Microsoft Corp). Paired t-tests, ANOVA or ANCOVA analyses were used to determine the significance of increases in retinol concentrations following supplementation and to compare the changes among the treatment groups. In calculating changes in serum and milk retinol concentrations, all data were controlled for baseline values. Dietary intake for foods high in β-carotene was also considered as a covariate for these analyses. However, dietary intakes for foods consumed outside the study meals were not included in the final analyses because they were not associated with the initial retinal or β-carotene concentrations in milk or blood or with the changes in the values after the intervention.

Analyses were repeated with all subjects using linear mixed effects models but these analyses did not result in any differences in significant results among groups. Thus, for interpretation of the results we present only those subjects who completed the protocols and we considered $p < 0.05$ to represent a statistically significant change.

Results

Baseline characteristics - The mean age of all mothers was 24.9 years. Parity ranged from one to six, and was strongly correlated with age (Pearson Correlation Coefficient = 0.76, p<0.0001.) Mean body mass index (BMI) was 24.5 kg/m^2, ranged from 15.9 to 47.0 kg/m^2 and was at the low normal range of weight for height [16]. Age and body mass index were not correlated and neither was significantly different among the treatment groups.

The average age of the infants in the Supplement Group (3.96 ± 2.1) was about one month less than Food and Placebo Groups (5.19 ± 2.3 and 4.59 ± 2.2 respectively, **Table 1**). To avoid any effect of age, we controlled for baseline values when calculating changes in changes in serum β-carotene and retinol concentrations.

Table 1. Baseline data for all subjects who participated in the study.

Measurement	Study Group							
	Beta-Carotene	n	Food	n	Placebo	n	All groups	n
Mothers								
Age, yr ± SD[1]	24 ± 6.4	52	25.0 ± 5.8	56	25.1 ± 5.87	54	24.86 ± 6.0	162
Height, cm	152.5 ± 4	52	147.5 ± 6	56	148.82 ±4.24	54	149.17± 4.86	162
Weight, kg	56.74 ± 10.34	52	54.36 ± 8.22	56	52.25 ± 7.59	54	54.42 ± 8.90	162
Parity	2.29 ± 1.38	52	2.68 ± 1.42	56	2.59 ± 1.55	54	2.52 ± 1.45	162
Serum retinol, µMol/l ± SEM[2]	1.17 ± 0.04	52	1.12 ± 0.05	47	1.17 ± 0.04	54	1.15 ± 0.03	153
Serum β-carotene, µMol/l ± SEM	0.30 ± 0.02	52	0.37 ± 0.02	47	0.31 ± .02	54	0.33 ± 0.01	153
Milk retinol µMol/L	0.99 ± 0.09	46	1.13 ± 0.11	43	1.1 ± 0.08	46	1.06 ± 0.05	135
Milk retinol, µMol/g fat	0.029 ± 0.003	46	0.03 ± 0.003	43	0.03 ± 0.002	46	0.03 ± 0.01	135
Milk β-carotene µMol/L	29.6 ± 3.4	46	32.5 ± 3.4	43	38.8 ± 3.3	46	33.7 ± 1.9	135
Milk β-carotene, µMol/g fat	0.90 ± 0.12	46	0.89 ± 0.11	43	1.0 ± 0.11	46	0.93 ± 0.06	135
Infants								
Age, mo.	3.96 ±2.14	51	5.19 ± 2.28	53	4.59 ± 2.20	54	4.59 ± 2.25	158
Length, cm.	60.47 ± 4.74	50	62.52 ± 2.10	53	60.87 ± 1.53	52	61.3 ± 3.12	155
Weight, kg	6.30 ± 1.55	47	6.66 ± 1.53	47	6.47 ± 0.34	41	6.48 ± 1.53	135
Serum retinol µMol/l	0.48 ± 0.02	45	0.53 ± 0.02	42	0.56 ± 0.02	45	0.52 ±0.01	132
Serum β-carotene µMol/l	0.10 ± 0.01	45	0.10 ± 0.01	40	0.13 ± 0.004	34	0.11 ± 0.006	119

1. SD = all values are standard deviation unless otherwise noted; 2 = standard error of the mean

Diet - **Table 2** provides a qualitative estimate of maternal intake of foods furnishing significant sources of vitamin A. Only data from mothers that supplied three 24-hour recalls was used to estimate dietary intake. The records were averaged and data grouped by numbers of servings. More than a third of the mothers reported no intake of fruits and vegetables on the three days we collected data and only five reported five or more servings. None of the mothers reported more than three servings per day of fruits and vegetables considered to be good sources of vitamin A.

At the time the study was conducted, the Honduran sugar supply was fortified with retinol (6.6 mg/kg) [17] and we confirmed this concentration of retinol in sugar samples randomly collected in Honduras [6]. Thus sugar and soft drinks were included as vitamin A-containing foods. Only seven mothers reported consuming more than two servings per day of refined sugar. Since the mandated supplement was 6.6 mg retinol/kg sugar, assuming a teaspoon to be five g, the maximum daily amount consumed by the mothers based on their self-report would have been around 70 µg of retinol or less than 10% of the current US Recommended Daily Intake (RDI) for lactating women [18].

We first analyzed the mothers' diets quantitatively using the USDA database modified for use in the Nutritionist IV nutrient analysis program [19, 20]. However, even after modifying the program with the aid of a Honduran nutritionist to reflect local recipes for preparation of salads, vegetables, etc., and using international food composition tables, exhaustive comparisons of carotenoid and retinol intakes with serum and milk concentrations resulted in no associations. However, we and others have previously demonstrated that serum carotenoids and qualitiative rankings of intake and serum concentrations were significantly correlated [21-23]. Thus since diet was not the primary focus of this report, and there was no association between the nutrients from the diet and the biochemical values, we estimated dietary intake of vitamin A by quantitating numbers of servings of foods containing vitamin A and provitamin A carotenoids.

Table 2. Maternal intake of foods furnishing significant sources of vitamin A[1].

Food group	Study Group					
	Supplement	n	Food	n	Placebo	n
	No of servings, Average ± SD					
Fruits and vegetables containing provitamin A[2]	1.53 ± 1.55	50	1.77±1.67	43	1.16 ± 0.80	46
Fruits and vegetables high in provitamin A[2a]	0.09± 0.27	50	0.24±0.59	43	0.10 ± 0.27	46
Dairy products containing vitamin A or provitamin A carotenoids[3]	0.41±0.49	50	0.62±0.62	43	0.51 ± 0.47	46
Meat, eggs and fish[4]	1.55±0.80	50	1.71±0.92	43	1.75 ±1.00	46
Foods containing sugar fortified with vitamin A[5]	0.70±0.81	50	0.84±0.70	43	0.63 ± 0.72	46

[1]Average daily intake of mothers on three days as estimated by dietary recall records.
[2]Foods included carrots, watermelon, oranges, tomatoes, potatoes, mangos, plantains, bananas, onions, cabbage, lettuce, plums, avocadoes, cauliflower, spaghetti, salsa, and vegetable soup. One serving of fruits or vegetables was approximately 100g. One serving of vegetable soup or spaghetti was approximately 200g. One serving of salsa was approximately 60 grams.
[a]Carrot, mixed vegetables (containing carrots) pumpkin, sweet potato, spinach, squash, broccoli, apricot, papaya and mango were considered high in provitamin A carotenoids. (Subset of fruits and vegetables containing provitamin A)
[3]Milk, cheese, margarine, ice cream, "crema" and butter were considered to contain vitamin A or provitamin A carotenoids. Serving sizes were 1 pat of butter or margarine, 1tbsp (15mL) "crema", 1 cup milk (~225mL), 1 cup ice cream (~150g), 1 oz (~28g) cheese.
[4]Meats included chicken, eggs, beef bologna, sardines, squid, and pork. One serving was approximately 100 g meat or one egg.
[5]At the time of the study, sugar in Honduras was fortified with 6.6 mg retinol/kg sugar (12). One soft drink or fruit drink (8oz) was estimated to contain1 tsp (~5g) refined sugar. Servings for sweet bread (pan dulce) were counted as 1 tsp refined sugar/100 g product.

Maternal Serum β-Carotene - One hundred twenty-nine mothers contributed usable blood samples for all three days of the study (**Table 3**). Initial serum carotenoid concentrations were not correlated with age or parity, were slightly less than those of Tucson mothers we studied earlier, but higher than those measured in Honduran communities in our previous studies [6, 7]. One-way ANOVA analyses showed that changes in maternal serum β-carotene concentrations were greatest in mothers receiving β-carotene supplements relative to the other groups ($p < 0.001$). After two weeks, serum β-carotene was increased more than two-fold relative to baseline ($p < 0.0001$) in this group. Over the four-week treatment period, serum β-carotene concentrations of mothers who received β-carotene supplements were approximately four fold greater than those who received food supplements. Serum β-carotene concentrations continued to increase throughout the study in the Supplement Group, but in mothers receiving foods high in β-carotene (Food Group), concentrations were not increased after 14 days.

   Milk β-Carotene - Because carotenoid and lipid concentrations co-vary [24], milk β-carotene concentrations are expressed relative to total milk lipid. β-Carotene concentrations were not different among the treatment groups at baseline by one-way ANOVA. Increases in milk β-carotene concentrations were greater in mothers with the lower baseline concentrations and for all mothers baseline milk β-carotene concentrations were negatively correlated with changes in β-carotene concentrations (r = -0.60, p <0.001). Thus, ANCOVA analyses controlling for baseline milk β-carotene concentrations was used to determine how supplementation affected 30-day changes. These analyses showed that milk β-carotene concentrations were significantly greater in the Supplement Group compared to the other two groups at day 30 (p < 0.001). Milk carotenoid/lipid ratios were higher in the present study than in those of Tucson mothers due to the lower milk lipid concentrations of the Honduran mothers, (3- 4 g/dl; cf. 5-6 in Tucson mothers).

Table 3. Changes in β-carotene concentrations in serum and milk following β-carotene supplementation or intake of β-carotene–containing foods.

Study day	Supplement	n	Food	n	Placebo	n
	Mothers serum					
	μMol/L ± SD					
0	0.28 ± 0.11	40	0.37 ±0.14	41	0.33 ± 0.15	46
14	0.66 ± 0.25	40	0.47 ± 0.16	41	0.38 ± 0.20	46
30	0.76 ± 0.35	40	0.47 ± 0.19	41	0.40 ± 0.23	46
Change	0.48 ± 0.33[a,b]		0.10 ± 0.21[b]		0.07 ± 0.21	
	Milk					
	nMol/g lipid ± SD					
0	0.89 ± 0.83	42	0.91 ± 0.71	38	1.04 ± 0.73	42
30	1.83 ± 0.84	42	1.23 ± 0.73	38	1.03 ± 0.72	42
Change	0.94 ± 1.09[a,b]		0.32 ± 0.83[a,b]		0.07 ± 0.90	
	Infant serum					
	μMol/L ± SD					
0	0.09 ± 0.05	20	0.10 ± 0.06	18	0.12 ± 0.09	22
14	0.13 ± 0.88	20	0.12 ± 0.08	18	0.14 ± 0.10	22
30	0.15 ± 0.07	20	0.16 ± 0.10	18	0.18 ± 0.11	22
Change	0.06 ± 0.06		0.06 ± 0.12		0.06 ± 0.11	

a. Changes in concentration after 30 days were significantly different from placebo when controlled for baseline β-carotene concentrations (p < 0.001).
b. Changes in concentration after 30 days were significantly different from each other when controlled for baseline β-carotene concentrations (p < 0.001).

Infant Serum β-Carotene - Twenty-two (17%) of the 131 infants from whom we obtained sufficient blood for analysis on day one of the study had serum β-carotene concentrations below the level of detection of our HPLC system (2.5 nMol/L). At 14 and 30 days of the study respectively, only 88 and 78 usable samples were obtained from infants. Due to these constraints, we obtained complete data sets for serum carotenoids for only 60 infants on all three-study days.

Neither baseline concentrations of infant serum β-carotene nor changes in their serum β-carotene levels over the period of the study were different among the groups.

Maternal Serum Retinol - Initial maternal serum retinol concentrations (1.1 – 1.2 μMol/L) were low (**Table 4**) but within the range of vitamin A adequacy [1, 28]. One-way ANOVA analysis showed no significant differences in maternal serum retinol concentrations among the groups at the beginning of the study. Initial serum retinol concentrations were not correlated with age or parity. ANCOVA analyses of maternal serum retinol concentrations showed that changes in serum retinol concentrations were not different between the Supplement and the Placebo Groups. In contrast, the retinol concentrations were significantly higher in the food group compared to the supplement and placebo groups at day 30 (p <0.05).

Table 4. Changes in retinol concentrations in serum and milk following β-carotene supplementation or intake of foods containing β-carotene.

Study day	Supplement	n	Food	n	Placebo	n
Mothers serum	μMol/L ± SD					
0	1.12 ± 0.24	40^1	1.12 ± 0.33	41	1.16 ± 0.30	46
14	1.05 ± 0.28	40	1.04 ± 0.32	41	0.99 ± 0.28	46
30	1.24 ± 0.34	40	1.42 ± 0.44	41	1.29 ± 0.43	46
Change	0.13 ± 0.29^a		$0.30 \pm 0.40^{a,b}$		0.14 ± 0.37^b	
Milk	μMol/g lipid ± SD					
0	0.028 ± 0.15	42	0.031 ± 0.18	38	0.027 ± 0.014	42
30	0.032 ± 0.02	42	0.033 ± 0.15	38	0.030 ± 0.013	42
Change	0.004 ± 0.03		0.001 ± 0.02		0.004 ± 0.02	
Infant serum	μMol/L ± SD					
0	0.48 ± 0.15	26	0.52 ± 0.12	20	0.55 ± 0.14	32
14	0.44 ± 0.13	26	0.54 ± 0.15	20	0.54 ± 0.15	32
30	0.54 ± 0.13	26	0.65 ± 0.14	20	0.56 ± 0.19	32
Change	0.07 ± 0.15		0.14 ± 0.12^c		0.01 ± 0.15^c	

Values with the same alpha superscripts are significantly different from each other, (p < 0.05).
[1] Two mothers declined to provide serum samples on d1 but participated in all other phases of the study.

Milk retinol - (**Table 4**) Initial milk retinol concentrations were within the range of adequacy (~1μMol/L, **Table 1**). Baseline concentrations were negatively correlated with the changes in milk retinol concentrations for all groups (r = -0.64, p < 0.001). One-way ANOVA analysis revealed no significant difference in milk retinol concentrations among the groups at baseline or at day 30. Similarly, using ANCOVA, changes in milk retinol levels over the study period were not different among the groups.

Infant serum retinol - At baseline, 94% of the infants had inadequate serum vitamin A (≤ 0.7 μMol/L) and 10% of the infants were severely vitamin A deficient (serum levels ≤ 0.35 μMol/l). Infants with low serum retinol also had low β-carotene concentrations (r = 0.26). Possibly due to the small age range (85% of the infants between two and seven months), there was no significant association between serum retinol concentrations and age ($R^2 = 0.08$).

Only data from mother-infant pairs who completed all phases of the study are reported here. Thus to insure that the data we reported is representative of the entire sample pool, we compared the average baseline retinol concentrations for theose who completed the study with the average of the samples from infants who had missed either one or two followup data points. The differences were not significant among the groups.

Infants with the lower initial serum retinol concentrations had the greater increases after supplemention in both treatment groups after 30 days (r = -0.38, p<0.001). The greatest increase occurred in the Food Group compared with the Placebo (p < 0.05). Increases in infant serum retinol were not different between the Supplement and Placebo groups (**Table 4**).

Discussion

To our knowledge, this is the first study directly comparing the efficacy of local foods and ß-carotene supplements of mothers in a community setting to improve vitamin A status of their breastfed infants. In addition, supplementation of mothers with foods high in ß-carotene produced the greatest increases in their serum retinol and that of their nursing infants. This was done by using foods that were culturally acceptable in amounts available to this community. The success of this intervention was partially due to the inclusion requirement that mothers were breastfeeding five times/d, so that breastmilk would account for the major share of the infant's vitamin A intake.

Interestingly, serum retinol concentrations of mothers in the Supplement Group were not significantly increased relative to placebo. The most logical explanation of this result is that when administered over time, ß-carotene was more bioavailable in foods than from supplements. A definitive explanation will require pharmacokinetic studies over a longer period of time with larger sample sizes.

Our results are consistent with an earlier report from the Honduran Ministry of Health that approximately 30% of children aged 12 - 71 months in Tegucigalpa [17] had serum vitamin A concentrations in the vitamin A low range (≤0.70 μMol/L.) As presented in the results, over 90% of the infants had low vitamin A levels and 10% were severely vitamin A deficient. The β-carotene concentrations for infant serum are lower than U.S. values and similar to those we reported previously from a neighboring village in Honduras [6-7]. Furthermore, the serum retinol concentrations of the infants in this study were less than or comparable to areas of the world in which vitamin A deficiency is considered prevalent; e.g.,

Bangladesh (0.80 μMol/L) (24) and Nigeria (0.50 μMol/L) [2]. Thus vitamin A deficiency remains a concern for Honduran children.

Milk β-carotene concentrations were increased in both treatment groups, but more significantly in the supplement group compared with the food group. This is consistent with other reports that water miscible ß-carotene supplements result in greater acute changes in ß-carotene serum and milk compared with food [8].

We might have expected to see a greater increase in infant serum carotenoid concentrations given the increase in their mother's milk β-carotene concentrations. A possible explanation is that the infants converted the increased ß-carotene available to them in milk to retinol because of their low vitamin A status. On the other hand, maternal serum retinol concentrations were in the range of vitamin A sufficiency and thus substantial bioconversion of the ß-carotene from supplements would not be required to replenish vitamin A stores. Alternatively, a longer period of supplementation may be required to produce substantial increases in serum carotenoids from maternal milk.

In summary, mothers consuming local fruits and vegetables furnishing 90 mg β-carotene over a one month period significantly increased their concentrations of serum retinol as well as that of their infants relative to placebo. The data imply that β-carotene provided as food could be an effective source of retinol for mothers as well as for their nursing infants. Given the practical limitation of obtaining sufficient β-carotene from the local diet, foods alone cannot provide a reliable source of vitamin A for this population. However, data from this study supports the inclusion of dietary intake of local fruits and vegetables in the overall strategy for improving the vitamin A status of mothers and infants in Honduras.

References

[1] Sommer, A. & Davidson, F. R. (2002). Assessment and control of vitamin A deficiency: The Annecy Accords. *J. Nutr.*, *132*, 2845S-2850S.

[2] Oso, O. O., Abiodum, P. O., Omotade, O. O. & Oyewole, D. (2003). Vitamin A status and nutritional intake of carotenoids of preschool children in Ijaye Orile Community in Nigeria. *Journal of Tropical Pediatrics*, *49*, 42-47.

[3] Vuong, L. T., Ducker, S. R. & Murphy, S. P. (2002). Plasma ß-carotene and retinol concentrations of children increase after a 30-d supplementation with the fruit *Momordica cochinchinensis* (*gac*). *Am J Clin Nutr.*, *75*, 872-879.

[4] Yeum, K. J. & Russell, R. M. (2002). Carotenoid bioavailability and bioconversion. *Ann Rev Nutr.*, *22*, 483-504.

[5] West, C. E., Eilander, A. & van Lieshout, M. (2002). Consequences of revised estimates of carotenoid bioefficacy for dietary control of vitamin A deficiency in developing countries. *J. Nutr.*, *132*, 2920S-2926S.

[6] Canfield, L. M., DeKaminsky, R., Taren, D. & Mahal, Z. (1999). Maternal ß-carotene supplementation: A strategy for improving the vitamin A status of the mother-infant dyad. *J Nutr Biochem.*, *10*, 523-538.

[7] Canfield, L. M., Kaminsky, R. G., Taren, D. I., Shaw, E. & Sander, J. K. (2001). Red palm oil in the maternal diet increases provitamin A carotenoids in breastmilk and serum of the mother-infant dyad. *Eur J Nutr.*, *40*, 30-38.

[8]   de Pee, S., West, C. E., Muhilal, Karyadi, D. & Hautvast, J. G. (1995). Lack of improvement in vitamin A status with increased consumption of dark-green leafy vegetables. *Lancet, 346*, 75-81.

[9]   West, C. E. & Poortvliet, E. J. (1993). The carotenoid content of foods with special reference to developing countries. Arlington, VA: Isti, Inc.

[10] United States Department of Agriculture USDA National Nutrient Database for Standard Reference. 2003.

[11] Giuliano, A. R., Neilson, E. M., Yap, H., Baier, M. & Canfield, L. M. (1994). Quantitation of and inter/intraindividual variability in major carotenoids of mature human milk. *J Nutr Biochem.*, 5, 551-556.

[12] Giuliano, A. R., Matzner, M. B. & Canfield, L. M. (1993). Assessing variability in the quantitation of carotenoids in human plasma: variance component model. In: *Methods in Enzymology* (Packer, L. ed.), Academic Press, San Diego, CA., 94-101.

[13] Giuliano, A. R., Neilson, E. M., Kelly, B. E. & Canfield, L. M. (1992). Simultaneous quantitation and separation of carotenoids and retinol in human milk by high-performance liquid chromatography. In: *Methods in Enzymology* (Packer, L. ed.). Academic Press, San Diego, CA., 391-399.

[14] Lucas, A., Gibbs, J. A. H., Lyster, R. L. J. & Baum, J. D. (1978). Creamatocrit: Simple clinical technique for estimating fat concentration and energy value of human milk. *Br Med J.*, 1, 1018-1020.

[15] Canfield, L. M., Kaminsky, R. G., Alger, J., Zavala, G. & Mourra, M. (2004). Suplementación con betacaroteno a madres y lactantes hondureños: Intervencionces dietéticas en barrios marginales. Journal Cientifica de las Ciencias Biologicas y de la salud, Tegucigalpa, Honduras(IV).

[16] Heymsfield, S. B., Tighe, A. & Wang, Z. M. (1994). Nutritional Assessment by Anthropometric and Biochemical Methods. In: *Modern Nutrition in Health and Disease* (Shils, M. E., Olson, J. A. & Shike, M. eds.). Philadelphia, Lea & Febiger., 812-841.

[17] Secretaria de Salud, T. H. (1998). *Encuesta nacional sobre micronutrientes* (National Honduran micronutrient survey). Tegucigalpa, Honduras, C.A.

[18] Olson, J. A. (1987). Recommended dietary intakes (RDI) of vitamin A in humans. *Am J Clin Nutr.*, 45, 704-716.

[19] US Department of Agriculture (USDA) CSF II-85 reference. Nutrition Monitoring Division, Human Nutrition Information Service, Hyattsville, Md Report no. 1987, 85-4, 182.

[20] Granado, F., Olmedilla, B., Blanco, I., Gil-Martinez, E. & Rojas-Hadalgo, E. (1997). Variability in the intercomparison of food carotenoid content data: a user's point of view. *Crit Rev Food Sci Nutr.*, 37, 621-633.

[21] Canfield, L. M., Clandinin, M. T., Davies, D. P., Fernandez, M. C., Jackson, J., Gibson, R., Goldman, W. J., Pramuk, K., Reyes, H., Sablan, B., Sonobe, T. & Xu, B. (2003). Multinational study of major breast milk carotenoids of healthy mothers, *Eur J. Nutr*, 42, 133-141.

[22] Sloan, N. L. D., Rosen, D. M., de la Paz, T. M., Arita, M., Temalilwa, C. & Solomons, N. W. M. (1997). Identifying areas with vitamin A deficiency: The validity of a semiquantitative food frequency method. *American Journal of Public Health, 87*, 186-191.

[23] Neuhouser, M. L., Patterson, R. E., Kristal, A. R., Eldridge, A. L. & Vizenor, N. C. (2001). A brief dietary assessment instrument for assessing target foods, nutrients and eating patterns. *Public Health Nutr.*, 4, 73-78.

[24] Rice, A. L., Stoltzfus, R. J., deFrancisco, A., Chakraborty, J., Kjolhede, C. L. & Wahed, M. A. (1999). Maternal vitamin A or β-carotene supplementation in lactating Bangladeshi women benefits mother and infants but does not prevent subclinical deficiency. *J Nutr.*, *192*, 356-365.

[25] Drammeh, B. S., Marquis, G. S., Funkhouser, E., Bates, C., Eto, I. & Stephensen, C. B. A. (2002). Randomized, 4-month mango and fat supplementation trial improved vitamin A status among young Gambian children. *J. Nutr.*, *132*, 3693-3699.

[26] dePee, S., West, C. E., Permaesih, D., Martuti, S., Muhilal, J. & Hautvast, G. (1998). Orange fruit is more effective than are dark-green, leafy vegetables in increasing serum concentrations of retinol and beta-carotene in schoolchildren in Indonesia. *Am J Clin Nutr.*, *68(5)*, 1058-1067.

[27] Ncube, T. K., Greiner, T., Malaba, L. C. & Gebre-Medhin, M. (2001). Supplementing lactating women with puréed papaya and grated carrots improved vitamin A status in a placebo-controlled trial[1]. *J Nutr.*, *131*, 1497-1502.

[28] dePee, S. & Dary, O. (2002). Biochemical indicators of vitamin A deficiency: Serum retinol and serum retinol binding protein. *J. Nutr.*, *132*, 2857S-2866S.

In: Encyclopedia of Vitamin Research
Editor: Joshua T. Mayer

ISBN 978-1-61761-928-1
© 2011 Nova Science Publishers, Inc.

Chapter 35

The Role of Small-Sized Tomatoes in Carotenoid Uptake[*]

Fabio Licciardello[†] and Giuseppe Muratore
Section of Food Technologies, DOFATA, University of Catania, Italy
Via Santa Sofia 98, 95123 Catania, Italy

Abstract

The nutritional value of the tomato owes to the beneficial effects that some of its components have on human health, particularly the prevention of some types of cancer and cardiovascular disease and, in general, contributing to the inhibition of oxidative processes. Among these, β-carotene and lycopene are the most important, the former represented at levels four to eight times lower than the latter. The tomato is an irreplaceable component of the Mediterranean diet, to which it contributes antioxidants, vitamins, minerals, fibre and carotenoids. The preference of consumers has recently increased towards small-sized tomato varieties, which nowadays represent an emergent product in Italy, where different cultivars are produced and delivered almost entirely for fresh consumption. Many authors have studied the nutritional characteristics of cherry tomatoes, but no study, other than the one presented in this chapter, deals with plum tomatoes, which turn out to be a tomato type even more valuable than the cherry tomato in terms of its carotenoid content. All of the studies, including the one presented hereafter, confirm that small-sized tomatoes, with differences among varieties, are richer in dry matter and in antioxidant compounds, which accumulate especially in the external parts of the fruits and are, therefore, more concentrated in small berries having a higher surface/volume ratio. A literature survey of the tomato's nutritional content points out that if, on one hand, it is difficult to correlate the lycopene content with the tomato size,

---

[*] A version of this chapter was also published in *Beta Carotene: Dietary Sources, Cancer and Cognition, edited by Leiv Haugen and Terje Bjornson* published by Nova Science Publishers, Inc. It was submitted for appropriate modifications in an effort to encourage wider dissemination of research.

[†] Corresponding author: Tel. +39 957580210; fax: +39 957141960; email: fabio.licciardello@unict.it

as some large-sized varieties are rich in this carotenoid, it is more evident that small-sized varieties are characterized by higher β-carotene levels.

Tomato antioxidants are relatively stable in the presence of heat treatment. The partial drying of cherry tomatoes represents a novel preservation technology with the ability to increase the opportunity for consumption of tomatoes. Semi-dry cherry tomatoes obtained at higher temperatures with short drying times show a nutritional content, with special regard for β-carotene, very close to the fresh product. The slight heat damage produced is easily counterbalanced by the concentration of dry matter which, in turn, allows increased consumption of the tomato's nutritive compounds.

Introduction

The tomato (*Lycopersicum esculentum*) is worldwide the most cultivated and consumed vegetable. Its diffusion is prevalent in the Mediterranean basin, thanks to the mild temperatures that allow the optimization of yields and the availability of the produce year-round.

World production amounts to about 12 million tons, mostly represented by China, the United States, Turkey and Egypt (FAO, crop statistics, 2007). Italy, among European countries, has the highest tomato production, which is concentrated especially in the southern regions. In particular, Sicily, according to statistics for 2000–2007, offers only about 7% of the overall Italian tomato production but more than 40% of the national produce cultivated in greenhouses, which is addressed to fresh consumption (ISTAT, crop statistics, 2007). Slightly less than 10% of the national tomato production comes from protected cultivation, while a major part is represented by field production for the purpose of industrial processing.

Increased interest in tomatoes and tomato products owes to the verification of the beneficial effects that some of its ingredients have on human health. Previous research (Russo et al., 2000; Nakagawa et al., 2002; Hadley et al., 2003) has proven the effect of tomatoes and tomato product consumption on the inhibition of oxidative processes in the human organism. Oxidative stress induced by reactive oxygen species (ROS), with special concern for the oxidation of circulating low-density lipoprotein (LDL), is considered to play an important role in the aetiology of atherosclerosis and coronary artery disease.

The antioxidative power of its compounds, which have been found in blood plasma following consumption, has assigned to the tomato a role in the prevention of atherosclerosis and cardiovascular disease (Parfitt et al., 1994; Agarwal & Rao, 2000).

Moreover, tomato consumption has been inversely correlated with the risk of contracting degenerative diseases such as digestive tract cancer, lung and prostate cancer (Franceschi et al., 1994; Clinton et al., 1996; Giovannucci, 1999; Stacewicz-Sapuntzakis & Bowen, 2005).

Factors contributing to disease protection are believed to correspond to tomato antioxidants. This class is represented by phenolic compounds, ascorbic acid and carotenoids. Among the former group, the most represented are chlorogenic acid, a hydroxycinnamic acid; and the flavonoids rutin, naringenin, chalconaringenin, kaempferol and myricetin (Stewart et al., 2000; Martinez-Valverde et al., 2002, Shen et al., 2007, Slimestad et al., 2008), most of which are in the glycolylated form and can be found in the free form after processing, therefore in tomato-based products. All of these, except chlorogenic acid, are available at a higher concentration in the peel than in the pulp (Peng et al., 2008).

Tomato is a rich source of carotenoids; among these, β-carotene and lycopene are the most important, the former being represented at levels four to eight times lower than the latter. Tomatoes and tomato products represent the primary source of lycopene in the human diet. This compound, the major carotenoid of the tomato, represents about 80% of the total carotenoids, is responsible for the intense red colour of the berries, and is characterized by high antioxidant and anticarcinogenic activity which has been extensively studied and assessed in vivo (Di Mascio et al., 1989; Agarwal & Rao, 2000; Gerster, 1993). Both lycopene and β-carotene accumulate in plasma and tissues in relation to dietary uptake and exert antioxidant activity (Oshima et al., 1996), while only β-carotene has provitaminic importance, being the precursor of vitamin A. Tomato poliphenols and carotenoids are much more concentrated in the external part of the berries than in the flesh (about five fold) (Dumas et al., 2003).

The tomato is an irreplaceable component of the so-called "Mediterranean diet", consisting of fruits and vegetables, especially cooked tomatoes and considerable amounts of olive oil. This diet, to which tomatoes make a contribution in terms of antioxidants, vitamins, fibre and carotenoids, has been associated with a lower risk of several important chronic diseases and is regarded as a model of a good life-style. A recent study carried out on a wide sample of the Spanish population (García-Closas et al., 2004) classified tomatoes as the main source of lycopene (71.6%), the second most important source of vitamin C (12.0%), pro-vitamin A carotenoids (14.6%) and β-carotene (17.2%).

Tomatoes find various uses in both fresh and processed forms. Processed products include ketchup, sauces, pastes and juice. Drying is not a popular way to process tomatoes due to its negative effect on the quality of the final product (Lewicki et al., 2002), such as fruit tissue browning and remarkable change of the flavour profile. Processed fruits and vegetables have been considered to have a lower nutritional value than their respective fresh commodities due to the loss of vitamin C and other phytochemicals. The tomato represents a particular case, as thermal processing often enhances the nutritional quality by increasing the bioavailability of carotenoids (Gartner et al., 1997; Tonucci et al., 1995; Dewanto et al., 2002). The wide range of available tomato products implies a great number of occasions for tomato consumption and for uptake of its precious phytochemicals. As a result of this variety of tomato-containing foods, it is not easy to estimate the consumption of tomatoes. However, a study on the Italian food consumption patterns in the years 1994–1996 estimated consumption of tomatoes (both salad and ripe) at 75.5 g/day/capita (Turrini et al., 2001).

Due to its relatively high average consumption, the tomato is an important source of these dietary antioxidants. Tomatoes are the most highly consumed vegetable in Italy, with the highest average consumption among European countries (NETTOX, 1998). In Italy, cherry tomatoes are largely used for fresh consumption (more than 25% of the market) and their commercial importance is continuously increasing (Leonardi et al., 2000).

This chapter presents some results concerning the nutritional value of small-sized tomato varieties, such as plum and cherry tomatoes, with a focus on carotenoids and their role in the β-carotene and lycopene uptake. Six different plum tomato cultivars were compared with one cherry tomato, chosen as a reference for its reknowned high quality and wide distribution worldwide: both types of small-sized tomato were grown in the same greenhouse under the same conditions of cultivation and harvested at the same commercial ripening.

Moreover, the chapter points out the effect of partial drying on the nutritional aspects of small-sized tomatoes: this process offers an alternative to fresh consumption and represents a mild technology able to preserve the chemical and sensory characteristics, offering advantages in terms of product stability. The effects of different drying temperatures and of a pre-treating solution on cherry tomato quality was assessed, with special attention to the changes in the main physical, chemical and organoleptic characteristics of the products — namely colour, water activity, dry matter, L-ascorbic acid, lycopene, β-carotene, 5-hydroxy-methylfurfural and total antioxidant capacity.

Furthermore, this chapter offers an updated state-of-the-art report on research dealing with the nutritional assessment of tomato varieties, outlining some general considerations regarding the carotenoids and nutritional content of small-sized tomatoes in comparison with normal-sized varieties.

Results

Nutritional Assessment of small-sized Tomatoes

It is well established that small-sized tomatoes are characterized by higher levels of dry matter and soluble solids than normal-sized tomatoes; these differences are due to the higher content of sugars and organic acids, which are the main factor responsible for the greater sweetness, sourness and overall flavour intensity (Picha, 1986; Leonardi et al., 2000). The preference of consumers has recently increased towards small-sized tomato varieties (Pagliarini et al., 2001), which nowadays represent the prevalent greenhouse production in southern Italy, where different cultivars are grown and intended almost entirely for fresh consumption, and fill about 25% of the national fresh tomato demand (Siviero et al., 1999). This preference is based both on the simplicity of use, on the "charming" appeal which makes them suitable for starter dishes, ready-to-eat salads and as a decoration, and on the sensory characteristics; moreover, from a commercial point of view, these products are characterized by reduced price floating and constant availability on markets. *Lycopersicon esculentum* includes *L. esculenturn* var. *cerasiforme* (cherry tomato), a species characterized by its small size and round shape, with fruit size ranging from 1.5 to 3.0 cm in diameter (Warhock, 1988). Many authors have studied the nutritional characteristics of cherry tomatoes (Picha, 1986; Hart & Scott, 1995; Leonardi et al., 2000; Raffo et al., 2002), which is the most popular among small-sized tomatoes and is available in a wide number of cultivars.

The "plum tomato", also referred to as the "grape tomato", is a relatively new hybrid of tomato, originating from the inter-specific crossbreed among *Lycopersicon lycopersicum*, *Lycopersicon pimpinellifolium* (red currant type) and *Lycopersicon chesmanii*. The peculiar shape of the berry, similar to a small plum or date, hence the Italian name "Datterino"; the "bite-sized shape" (Sugarman, 2001) (10–15 g); and its very pleasant taste make it a valuable and refined product. Thanks to these characteristics, plum tomato demand has increased rapidly in the more recent years, despite the unsuitability to be commercialized as clusters (like cherry tomato) (Muratore et al., 2005b). Plum-type tomatoes are smaller on average than cherry tomatoes, and this attribute makes them more appealing from a mere aesthetic point of view.

No study has been performed on the nutritional quality of plum tomatoes, apart from a recent study on the effect of packaging on the shelf-life (Muratore et al., 2005a). The chemical composition of six plum tomato cultivars was assessed—namely Dasher, Iride, Navidad, Sabor, 292, and 738, in comparison with a cherry tomato cultivar, Cherubino; all of these were grown in the same greenhouse under the same organic farming conditions and harvested at commercial ripening stage, throughout the productive season which runs from December to April.

Acidity values were similar for all plum tomatoes, ranging from 0.64 to 0.78 g citric acid/100 g. Cherry Cherubino was the most acidic, showing mean values of 0.85, statistically different from those of plum tomatoes. Sabor showed the lowest values of soluble solids and dry matter, and 738 the highest ones (9.1 and 11.1%, respectively). Cherry type showed mean values that are very close to those of plum tomato, but lower than cultivar 738.

Glucose and fructose were always present in high amounts, with a slight prevalence of fructose (~7%). The cultivar 738 showed the highest content of total sugars, according to the highest value of dry matter, of which sugars represented about 55%, respectively.

The phenolic fraction of tomato includes different flavonoid glycosides and esters of hydroxycinnamic acids, prevalently represented by the derivatives of naringenin and caffeic acid, both characterized by high antioxidant capacity (Raffo et al., 2002; Hollman et al., 1996; Stewart et al., 2000). The plum and cherry tomatoes contained a remarkable amount of total phenolics, but Sabor was the poorest and 738 the richest.

The distribution of the major carotenoids showed a different trend between the plum cultivars and the cherry variety. The former showed a mean content of lycopene higher than the latter (4.65 and 3.43 mg/100g, respectively). **Table 1** shows the average lycopene and β-carotene content for each cultivar examined. The highest concentration was measured in Sabor, followed by Navidad and 738. On the other hand, the cherry variety was marked by a content of β-carotene (0.99 mg/100g) higher than that observed in plum type (averagely, 0.77 mg/100g). Lycopene represented the 81% of total carotenoids in the plum cultivars, while in cherry Cherubino it was 73%. Conversely, β-carotene amounted to 13.5% and 21.1% in plum and cherry type, respectively (**Figure 1**). Minor carotenoids, such as lutein and the colourless phytoene and phytophluene, were also present in about 0.1 mg/100g each.

A comparison with a study carried out on cherry tomatoes grown in a Norwegian greenhouse points out higher values for every nutritional compound in cherry and plum tomatoes grown in a Sicilian greenhouse. In particular, the average lycopene content in the former study is 2.73 mg/100 g, which is lower than the lowest lycopene content observed in our study in cherry samples (2.90 mg/100g). The mean lycopene and β-carotene values in our cherry tomato samples were 3.43 and 0.99 mg/100 g, respectively. It is worth noting that the average β-carotene content in cherry tomatoes grown in the Norwegian greenhouse is 0.44 mg/100 g, which is less than half the mean values that we found.

Table 1. Lycopene and β-carotene contents in six plum tomato cultivars (Dasher, Iride, Navidad, Sabor, 292 and 738), and one cherry variety (Cherubino).

	Dasher	Iride	Navidad	Sabor	292	738	Cherubino
Lycopene	3.98ab	4.45bc	4.89bc	5.22c	4.57bc	4.77bc	3.43a
β-carotene	0.68ab	0.80cd	0.89de	0.67a	0.78bc	0.80cd	0.99e

Different letters indicate significant differences for P<0.05.

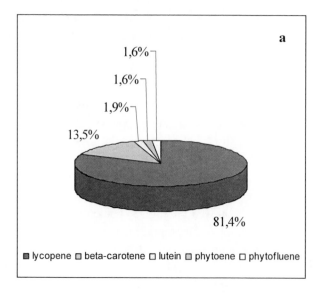

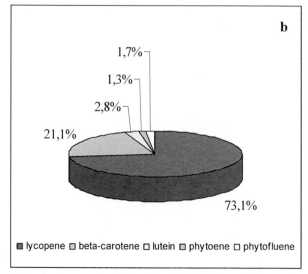

Figure 1. Distribution of the major carotenoids in plum (a) and cherry (b) type tomatoes.

A comparison with literature data appears appropriate in some cases, in other cases it might be influenced by different extraction yields. However, the fact that small-sized tomatoes are richer in dry matter than normal-sized tomatoes, is well established. In particular, small-sized berries are richer in antioxidant compounds, such as phenols, ascorbic acid, and carotenoids. The reason for this has to be found in a higher skin/volume ratio of the small-sized berries (Stewart et al., 2000), which guarantees a higher concentration of compounds that are mostly present in the external parts of tomatoes. It has been demonstrated that the highest amount of lycopene accumulates in the tomato skin and that the skin and the seeds are important contributors to the major antioxidants of tomatoes (Al-Wandawi et al., 1985; Sharma & Le Maguer, 1996; Dumas et al., 2003; Toor & Savage, 2005; Peng et al., 2008).

Table 2. Lycopene, β-carotene, ascorbic acid and total phenols content of different tomato types, from a literature survey. Values in parentheses following a range (minimum-maximum) represent the average in cases where several cultivars were considered.

Tomato type	Lycopene mg/100g	β-carotene mg/100g	Ascorbic acid mg/100g	Total phenols mg/100g	Reference
Not specified	9.27	0.23	—	—	Tonucci et al., 1995
Normal-sized	1.7–5.77 [b]	0.11–0.37	22.0–48.0	—	Abushita et al., 1997
Salad	5.3–8.5 (6.0)	0.28–0.62 (0.42)	15.0–21.0 (17.0)	—	Abushita et al., 2000
Industrial	5.1–11.6 (7.9)	0.21–0.44 (0.31)	17.0–22.0 (19.0)	—	Abushita et al., 2000
Normal-sized	5.00–6.63	0.13–0.18	20.1		Arias et el., 2000
Normal-sized	4.59 [a]	0.35 [a]	18.9 [a]	20.7 [a]	Lavelli et al., 2000
Normal-sized	6.82 [a]	0.95 [a]	9.1 [a]	27.3 [a]	Lavelli et al., 2000
Cherry	7.20	0.92	—	—	Leonardi et al., 2000
Cherry	10.80	1.05	—	—	Leonardi et al., 2000
Salad	0.11	0.08	—	—	Leonardi et al., 2000
Elongated	1.00	0.29	—	—	Leonardi et al., 2000
Cluster	7.9	0.49	—	—	Leonardi et al., 2000
Cherry	10.4	1.07	11.0	—	Raffo et al., 2002
Cherry cvs	4.3–12.0	0.5–1.1	14.0–30.5	97.0–137.0	Lenucci et al., 2003
Cherry	6.94	—	32.4	—	George et al., 2004
Normal-sized	5.26	0.35	—	—	Seybold et al., 2004
Cherry	1.60–5.54	0.38–0.55	5.6–20.0	17.5–32.6	Slimestad and Verheul, 2005
Plum	3.98–5.22	0.67–0.89	13.4–28.5	42.5–74.9	Muratore et al., 2005b
Cherry	3.43	0.99	31.3	63.9	Muratore et al., 2005b
Cherry	7.06–12.0	0.5–1.06	31.0–71.0	—	Raffo et al., 2006

[a] Values originally expressed on dry weight basis, are converted into fresh weight basis by means of the relative dry matter value provided.

[b] Lycopene values are approximated by subtraction of β-carotene from total carotenoids.

— : data not available.

As can be observed from **Table 2** and from the comparison of the different studies listed, the lycopene content varies significantly, and a clear correlation between this parameter and the berry size cannot be observed. Even big-sized varieties show high levels of lycopene (Leonardi et al., 2000; Abushita et al., 2000). What seems to stand out more clearly, on the other hand, is the highest β-carotene content in the small-sized varieties (cherry and plum). Indeed, β-carotene in the normal-sized tomatoes ranges between 0.2 and 0.5 mg/100 g, with some rare exceptions, while most studies dealing with small-sized varieties report higher levels, ranging to about 1 mg/100 g. The most evident exception to this generalization is represented by a study on cherry tomatoes cultivated in greenhouse in Norway (Slimestad & Verheul, 2005): in this case tomatoes show lower levels for every nutritional constituent, and the reason might be found in the environmental conditions, not suitable for the full expression of the plant potential, rather than in varietal factors. As a conclusion, it seems that no correlation can be found between the lycopene and β-carotene contents. As a matter of fact, a recent study on cherry and high pigmented cultivars (Lenucci et al., 2006) pointed out lycopene levels which are about 3-folds higher in the latter cultivars than in the cherry type, while the β-carotene content, with just one exception, is comparable or lower than that of the small-sized tomatoes.

Our data confirmed that cherry tomatoes are important source of carotenoids, not only lycopene but also β-carotene, one serving providing from 13% to 27% of the recommended daily intake of vitamin A (Società Italiana di Nutrizione Umana, 1996).

Effect of Partial Drying on the Nutritional Quality of Cherry Tomatoes

A relevant part of the cherry tomatoes production is concentrated in a short period of the year during which the price of the product becomes so low that it doesn't cover agronomical costs. For this reason, producers aim at alternative ways to commercialise the excess production, possibly obtaining an economical benefit. This aim can be achieved by creating a new transformed product, stable and marketable all year round. Partial dehydration represents a suitable solution, being a mild preservation technology able to yield a product with good organoleptic characteristics, softer than the conventionally dried tomatoes, with better colour and aroma.

Lycopene, according to the findings of Stahl & Sies (1992) and Gartner et al. (1997), is stable during heating and industrial treatments which, indeed, are able to improve lycopene bioavailability. Nevertheless, a research carried out by Shi et al. (1999), showed significant losses in the lycopene content during the dehydration of tomato products. Processes like cooking, cooling and canning usually do not cause large changes in the total lycopene content but, during tomatoes conventional management, the biggest part of lycopene can be converted from the *all-trans* form into the *cis* isomer, the last having a lower bioactivity.

Many studies are concerned with the drying process of tomatoes, but none of these has considered the small sized cherry tomatoes as a raw material for obtaining a partially dehydrated product. Results discussed hereafter concern cherry tomatoes dried in a forced air oven at 40, 60 and 80°C, with and without a dipping treatment into a solution containing citric acid, sodium chloride and calcium chloride (Muratore et al., 2008). The research aimed at evaluating the optimal process conditions, which would allow obtaining a product with the highest nutrional characteristics, with special regards for lycopene, β-carotene and ascorbic acid contents, and for the thermal damage indexes, such as hydroxymethylfuraldehyde (HMF) and browning.

Minimum browning effects of drying, evaluated either by the a*/b* or the b*L*/a* ratios, were observed for treated samples dehydrated at 60 and 80°C, while the highest colour degradation was caused when drying untreated samples. The colour parameters highlighted, therefore, a clear positive effect of pre-treatment by dipping into a solution containing citric acid, sodium chloride and calcium chloride.

The effect of drying on the carotenoid content of cherry tomatoes is highlighted in **Figure 2**. The highest lycopene value in semi-dry samples was for the untreated sample dehydrated at 80°C (76.4 mg/100g d.m.), while the lowest was relative to those treated at 60°C (54.9 mg/100g d.m.). In the untreated sample, lycopene was damaged by the length of the drying process at the lower temperature.

β-carotene shows large resistance at low temperature with long process time (40°C for 24 hours) in treated samples, on the contrary, the untreated ones gave the best results in the opposite conditions (80°C for 5 hours). β-carotene was found to be more stable in comparison with lycopene, its content decreases from 38.0 mg/100 g d.m. in fresh cherry tomatoes to 25.9 mg/100 g d.m. reached in untreated products dried at 60°C. The β-carotene content is minimum after drying at 60°C, with losses ranging to 32% and 28% in treated and untreated tomatoes, respectively.

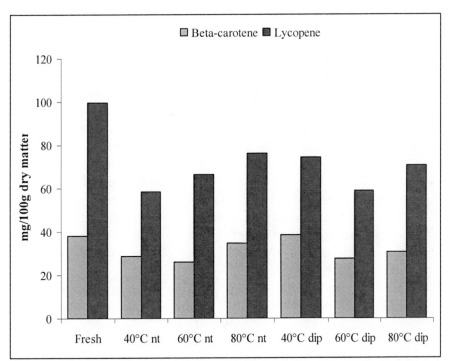

Figure 2. β-carotene and lycopene contents in fresh and semi-dry cherry tomatoes obtained at different temperatures (40, 60 or 80°C), not-treated (nt) and pre-treated (dip) by immersion in a dipping solution.

No clear relation was found between the loss of these compounds and temperature and/or whether pre-treatment was performed. In any case, the worst results were observed at 60°C. The use of a dipping solution has only slight advantages in preserving the carotenoid content of semi-dry cherry tomatoes. Drying tomatoes at 80°C without pre-treatment allows considerable energy and time savings and yields a product with a β-carotene content very close to the fresh material.

Ascorbic acid was always higher in the treated tomatoes than in untreated ones. The use of mild temperatures allowed to maintain ascorbic acid levels closer to that of fresh tomatoes, while at 80°C the vitamin C loss reached 59% and 74% in treated and untreated samples, respectively.

The HMF contents, even if statistically different in the different treatments, thus confirming the effect of temperature on its formation, were so low that they can be considered insignificant.

Tomatoes and their derivatives are important in human diet for their contribution in terms of carotenoids, and represent the almost exclusive source of lycopene and a good source of β-carotene, especially in the small-sized varieties. After partial dehydration of tomatoes, the loss of carotenoids was not related to time of treatment or to temperature. The only slight carotenoid loss after dehydration at 80°C suggests that this temperature is the best condition for obtaining a product with nutritional characteristics close to the fresh product, on a dry weight basis, but with a much higher concentration of nutritional compounds, due to water loss, which would increase the phytochemical uptake level.

Conclusion

Various studies have investigated the nutritional characteristics of cherry tomatoes, while only a few seem to deal with plum tomatoes, which turn out to be a tomato type even more valuable than the cherry tomato in terms of its carotenoid content. All studies, including the one presented in this contribution, confirm that small-sized tomatoes, with differences among varieties, contribute to carotenoid uptake at a higher extent than normal-sized ones.

Being established that tomato and tomato derivatives consumption positively contributes to human health, the choice should be addressed towards smaller-sized tomato varieties, which are richer in the antioxidants lycopene and β-carotene. Tomatoes do not contain high amounts of vitamin C and β-carotene; however, considering the relevant consumption of this vegetable in its fresh and processed forms, it represents the second greatest source of these two compounds in the Mediterranean diet. A thorough comparison of literature data points out that small-sized varieties (cherry and plum) have a β-carotene content from 2 to 5 folds higher compared to normal-sized types, while the lycopene content cannot be clearly correlated with the berry size.

Today, the market demonstrates an increasing interest in products with intermediate humidity, which combine increased stability (due to decreased water activity) with good nutritional and organoleptic characteristics. Partially dehydrated cherry tomatoes could be utilized as a seasoning or main ingredient in the preparation of starters and typical dishes, similarly to the fresh product, or as snacks with high phytochemical content. The use of tomato varieties with high levels of nutritional and antioxidant compounds is suggested for processing in order to obtain products that still offer high levels of phytochemicals. The heat damage to the lycopene and β-carotene content caused by drying the tomato is low, and is easily counterbalanced by the concentration of dry matter in the dried product which, in turn, allows increased uptake of tomato nutritive compounds.

References

Abushita, A. A., Daood, H. G. & Biacs, P. A. (2000). Change in carotenoids and antioxidant vitamins in tomato as a function of varietal and technological factors. *Journal of Agriculture and Food Chemistry*, *48*, 2075-2081.

Abushita, A. A., Hebshi, E. A., Daood, H. G. & Biacs, P. G. (1997). Determination of antioxidant vitamins in tomatoes. *Food Chemistry*, *60*, 207-212.

Agarwal, S. & Rao, A. V. (2000). Tomato lycopene and its role in human health and chronic diseases. *Canadian Medical Association Journal*, *163*, 739-744.

Al-Wandawi, H., Abul Rahman, M. H. & Al Shaikhly, K. A. (1985). Tomato processing wastes as essential raw materials source. *Journal of Agricultural and Food Chemistry*, *33*, 804-807.

Arias, R., Lee, T. C., Specca, D. & Janes, H. (2000). Quality comparison of hydroponic tomatoes (*Lycopersicon esculentum*) ripened on and off vine. *Journal of Food Science*, *65*, 545-548.

Clinton, S. K., Emenhiser, C., Schwartz, S. J., Bostwick, D. G., Williams, A. W., Moore, B. J. & Erdman, J. W. (1996). Cistrans lycopene isomers, carotenoids, and retinol in the human prostate. *Cancer Epidemiology Biomarkers and Prevention*, *5*, 823-833.

Dewanto, V., Wu X., Adom K. K. & Liu, R. H. (2002). Thermal processing enhances the nutritional value of tomatoes by increasing total antioxidant activity. *Journal of Agricultural and Food Chemistry*, *50*, 3010-3014.

Di Mascio, P., Kaiser, S. & Sies, H. (1989). Lycopene as the most efficient biological carotenoid singlet oxygen quencher. *Archives of Biochemistry and Biophysics*, *274*, 532-538.

Dumas, Y., Dadomo, M., DiLucca, G. & Grolier, P. (2003). Effects of environmental factors and agricultural techniques on antioxidant content of tomatoes. *Journal of the Science of Food and Agriculture*, *83*, 369-382.

FAO –Food and Agriculture Organization of the United Nations - Statistics on crops. Available from: URL: http://faostat.fao.org/site/567/default.aspx#ancor

Franceschi, S., Bidoli, E., La Vecchia, C., Talamini, R., D'Avanzo, B. & Negri, E. (1994). Tomatoes and risk of digestive-tract cancers. *International Journal of Cancer*, *59*, 181-184.

García-Closas, R., Berenguer, A., Tormo, M. J., Sanchez, M. J., Quirós, J. R., Navarro, C., Arnaud, R., Dorronsoro, M., Chirlaque, M.D., Barricarte, A., Ardanaz, E., Amiano, P., Martinez, C., Agudo, A. & González, C. A. (2004). Dietary sources of vitamin C, vitamin E and specific carotenoids in Spain. *British Journal of Nutrition*, *91*, 1005-1011.

Gartner, C., Stahl, W. & Sies, H. (1997). Lycopene is more bioavailable from tomato paste than from fresh tomatoes. *American Journal of Clinical Nutrition*, *66*, 116-122.

George, B., Kaur, C., Khurdiya, D. S. & Kapoor, H. C. (2004). Antioxidants in tomato (*Lycopersium esculentum*) as a function of genotype. *Food Chemistry 84*, 45-51.

Gerster, H. (1993). Anticarcinogenic effect of common carotenoids. *International Journal of Vitamin and Nutrition Research*, *63*, 93-121.

Giovannucci, E. (1999). Tomatoes, tomato-based products, lycopene and cancer. Review of the epidemiologic literature. *Journal of the National Cancer Institute*, *91*, 317-331.

Hadley, C. W., Clinton, S. K. & Schwartz, S. J. (2003). The consumption of processed tomato products enhances plasma lycopene concentrations in association with a reduced lipoprotein sensitivity to oxidative damage. *Journal of Nutrition, 133*, 727-732.

Hollman, P. C. H., Hertog, M. G. L. & Katan, M. B. (1996). Analysis of health effects of flavonoids. *Food Chemistry, 57*, 43-46.

ISTAT (Italian Institute of Statistics). Available from: URL: http://www.istat.it/agricoltura/datiagri/coltivazioni/anno2007.

Lenucci, M. S., Cadinu, D., Taurino, M., Piro, G. & Dalessandro, G. (2006). Antioxidant composition in cherry and high-pigment tomato cultivars. *Journal of Agricultural and Food Chemistry, 54*, 2606-2613.

Leonardi, C., Ambrosino, P., Esposito, F. & Fogliano, V. (2000). Antioxidative activity and carotenoid and tomatine contents in different typologies of fresh consumption tomatoes. *Journal of Agricultural and Food Chemistry, 48*, 4723-4727.

Lewicki, P. P., Vu Le, H. & Pomarańska-Lazuka, W. (2002). Effect of pre-treatment on convective drying of tomatoes. *Journal of Food Engineering, 54*, 141-146.

Martinez-Valverde, I., Periago, M. J., Provan, G. & Chesson, A. (2002). Phenolic compounds, lycopene and antioxidant activity in commercial varieties of tomato (*Lycopersicon esculentum*). *Journal of the Science of Food and Agriculture, 82*, 323-330.

Muratore, G., Del Nobile, M. A., Buonocore, G. G., Lanza, C. M. & Nicolosi Asmundo, C. (2005a). The influence of using biodegradable packaging films on the quality decay kinetic of plum tomato (PomodorinoDatterino®). *Journal of Food Engineering, 67*, 393-399.

Muratore, G., Licciardello, F. & Maccarone, E. (2005b). Evaluation of the chemical quality of a new type of small-sized tomato cultivar, the plum tomato (*Lycopersicon lycopersicum*). *Italian Journal of Food Science, 17(1)*, 75-81.

Muratore, G., Rizzo, V., Licciardello, F. & Maccarone, E. (2008). Partial dehydration of cherry tomato at different temperature, and nutritional quality of the products. *Food Chemistry, 111*, 887-891.

NETTOX, 1998. Compilation of Consumption Data, EU Report No. 4. Danish Veterinary and Food Administration.

Oshima, S., Ojima, F., Sakamoto, H., Ishiguro, Y. & Terao, J. (1996). Supplementation with carotenoids inhibits singlet-oxigen-mediated oxidation of human plasma low density lipoprotein. *Journal of Agricultural and Food Chemistry, 44*, 2306-2309.

Pagliarini, E., Monteleone, E. & Ratti, S. (2001). Sensory profile of eight tomato cultivars (*Lycopersicon esculentum*) and its relationship to consumer preference. *Italian Journal of Food Science, 13*, 285-296.

Peng, Y., Zhang, Y. & Ye, J. (2008). Determination of phenolic compounds and ascorbic acid in different fractions of tomato by capillary electrophoresis with electrochemical detection. *Journal of Agricultural and Food Chemistry, 56*, 1838-1844.

Picha, D. (1986). Effect of harvest maturity on the final fruit composition of cherry and large-fruited tomato cultivars. *Journal of the American Society for Horticultural Science, 111*: 723-727.

Raffo, A., Leonardi, C., Fogliano, V., Ambrosino, P., Salucci, M., Gennaro, L., Bugianesi, R., Giuffrida, F. & Quaglia, G. (2002). Nutritional value of cherry tomatoes (Lycopersicon esculentum, Cv. Naomi F1) harvested at different ripening stages. *Journal of Agricultural and Food Chemistry, 50*, 6550-6556.

Seybold, C., Fröhlich, K., Bitsch, R., Otto, K. & Böhm, V. (2004). Changes in contents of carotenoids and vitamin E during tomato processing. *Journal of Agricultural and Food Chemistry*, *52*, 7005-7010.

Sharma, S. K. & Le Maguer, M. (1996). Lycopene in tomatoes and tomato pulp fractions. *Italian Journal of Food Science*, *8*, 107-113.

Shi, J., Le Maguer, M., Kakuda, Y., Liptay, A. & Niekamp, F. (1999). Lycopene degradation and isomerization in tomato dehydration. *Food Research International*, *32*, 15-21.

Siviero, P., Saccani, G. & Macchiavelli, L. (1999). Il pomodoro cherry cresce in Sicilia. *Informatore Agrario*, *20*, 37-43.

Slimestad, R., Fossen, T. & Verheul, M. J. (2008). The flavonoids of tomatoes. *Journal of Agricultural and Food Chemistry*, *56*, 2436-2441.

Societa` Italiana di Nutrizione Umana, 1996. Livelli di Assunzione Raccomandata di Energia e Nutrienti per la Popolazione Italiana. Revisione 1996. SINU, Roma.

Stacewicz-Sapuntzakis, M. & Bowen, P. E. (2005). Role of lycopene and tomato products in prostate health. *Biochimica et Biophysica Acta*, *1740*, 202-205.

Stahl, W. & Sies, H. (1992). Uptake of Lycopene and its geometrical isomers is greater from heat-processed than from unprocessed tomato juice in humans. *Journal of Nutrition*, *122*, 2161-2166.

Stewart, A., Bozonnet, S., Mullen, W., Jenkins, G. I., Lean, M. E. J. & Crozier, A. (2000). Occurrence of flavonols in tomatoes and tomato-based products. *Journal of Agricultural and Food Chemistry*, *48*, 2663-2669.

Sugarman, C. (2001). Attack of the grape tomatoes. How a tiny fruit took over the produce aisles. *Washington Post*, September 12. Available from: URL: http://www.washingtonpost.com/ac2/wp-dyn/A12414-2001Sep11?language=printer

Tonucci, L.H., Holden, J. M., Beecher, G. R., Khachik, F., Davis, C. S. & Mulokozi, G. (1995). Carotenoid content of thermally processed tomato-based food products. *Journal of Agricultural and Food Chemistry*, *43*, 579-586.

Toor, R. K. & Savage, G. P. (2005). Antioxidant activity in different fractions of tomatoes. *Food Research International*, *38*, 487-494.

Turrini, A., Saba, A., Perrone, D., Cialfa, E. & D'Amicis, A. (2001). Food consumption patterns in Italy: the INN-CA study 1994–1996. *European Journal of Clinical Nutrition*, *55*, 571-588.

In: Encyclopedia of Vitamin Research
Editor: Joshua T. Mayer

ISBN 978-1-61761-928-1
© 2011 Nova Science Publishers, Inc.

Chapter 36

Seafood: A Natural Source of Carotenoids[*]

Ana Rodríguez-Bernaldo de Quirós[†] and Julia López-Hernández
Analytical Chemistry, Nutrition and Bromatology Department,
Pharmacy Faculty, Campus Sur s/n, University of Santiago de Compostela,
15782 Santiago de Compostela (La Coruña), Spain

Abstract

Carotenoids are natural pigments associated with the lipidic fractions widely distributed in nature. They are responsible for the yellow, orange and red colours of many biological systems. Some of these compounds, in addition to provitamin A activity, are involved in other physiological functions such as immune response and cell communication.

Moreover, some carotenoids have been shown to be effective against certain types of cancer, cardiovascular diseases and age-related macular degeneration.

A large number of structures—more than 600—have been isolated and characterized from natural sources. Although the main sources of carotenoids are plants and fruits, the study of sea products as a new source of these substances has attracted the attention of scientists in recent years.

In the present contribution, a couple of examples for human consumption are analyzed and discussed: sea urchin *Paracentrotus lividus* L.—a marine invertebrate of the phylum Echinodermata—and red and brown algae.

---

[*] A version of this chapter was also published in *Beta Carotene: Dietary Sources, Cancer and Cognition,* *edited by Leiv Haugen and Terje Bjornson* published by Nova Science Publishers, Inc. It was submitted for appropriate modifications in an effort to encourage wider dissemination of research.
[†] Corresponding author. E-mail: ana.rodriguez.bernaldo@usc.es

Introduction

Carotenoids are natural lipid-soluble pigments widely distributed in nature. These substances are responsible for the red, orange and yellow colour of many plants, animals and food products. Animals are not able to synthesize carotenoids, so they obtain them through the food chain. The growing interest that these compounds have received from the scientific community in the past years is mainly due to their healthful effects. Besides provitamin A activity, carotenoids are involved in different biological functions such as immune response and cell communication. Moreover, these natural antioxidants have been shown to be effective against certain types of cancer, cardiovascular diseases and age-related macular degeneration [1, 2].

A large number of structures—more than 600—have been isolated and characterized from natural sources [3, 4]. Chemically, they are isoprenoid polyenes and can be classified into two main groups: (1) carotene hydrocarbons containing only carbon and hydrogen atoms, and (2) their oxygenated derivatives, xanthophylls, which carry at least one oxygen function—for instance hydroxy, methoxy, carboxy, oxo, and epoxy. Carotenes are soluble in non-polar solvents such as hexane and petroleum ether, whereas xanthophylls show a high solubility in polar solvents such as methanol and ethanol. Structurally, the carotenoids are characterized by a conjugated double bond system that confers to this class of compounds special spectroscopic properties [5] .

The extraction procedure is generally a critical step in the analysis. Due to the complex structure of carotenoids and wide distribution there is no standard procedure. The methods commonly used to extract carotenoids from food samples involve treatment with solvents, such as methanol, acetone, hexane, tetrahydrofuran or mixtures of different solvents such as acetone-petroleum ether (1:1v/v), tetrahydrofuran-methanol (1:1v/v), hexane-acetone-ethanol (50:25:25 v/v/v), etc. followed by a filtration. This process is repeated until the residue is colourless. After that, the carotenoid extract is evaporated and the residue is dissolved in an appropriate solvent. Sometimes, before the chromatographic analysis, a saponification step is necessary in order to remove undesirable lipids and chlorophylls. However, it has been reported that certain carotenoids are sensitive to alkaline treatments, so when the sample contains this type of carotenoids the saponification step should be avoided. Since carotenoids are sensitive to heat, light and oxygen, special care should be taken when handling. These methods are time-consuming, laborious, and often require large amounts of solvents. With the aim to overcome these drawbacks in the past years, supercritical fluid extraction has appeared as a promising alternative with excellent advantages: the method is rapid, easy to automate, and non-toxic solvents are required. Some examples and applications of this technique are detailed in two reviews [6, 7].

Regarding carotenoid analysis, the technique most frequently used is high-performance liquid chromatography in combination with UV or diode array detectors (DAD), although the lack of suitable standards makes the use of mass spectrometry coupled to liquid chromatographic systems necessary in many cases in order to identify the carotenoids. Successfully applications of liquid chromatography coupled to mass spectrometry for the characterization of carotenoids in natural products have been reported in the literature [8, 9].

Carotenoids in Sea Urchin and Algae

Marine organisms are an important source of carotenoid pigments. The carotenoid content of sea urchin and algae is discussed in this section.

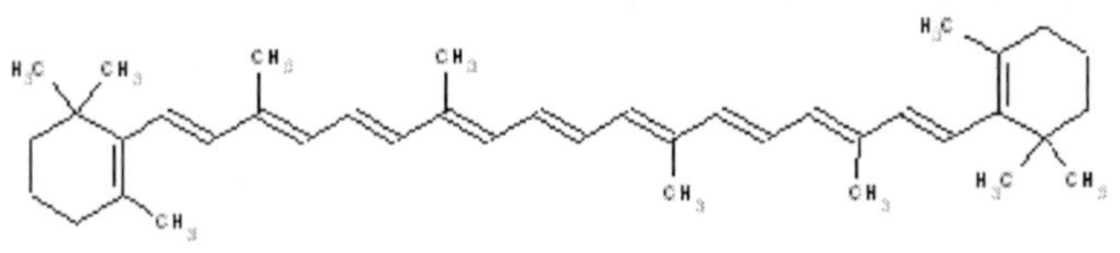

β-Carotene

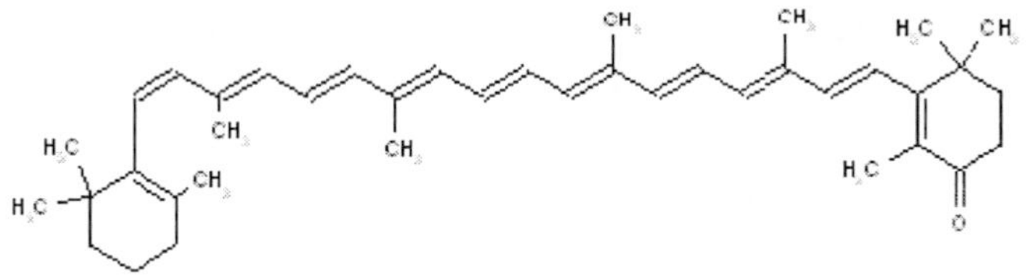

β-Echinenone

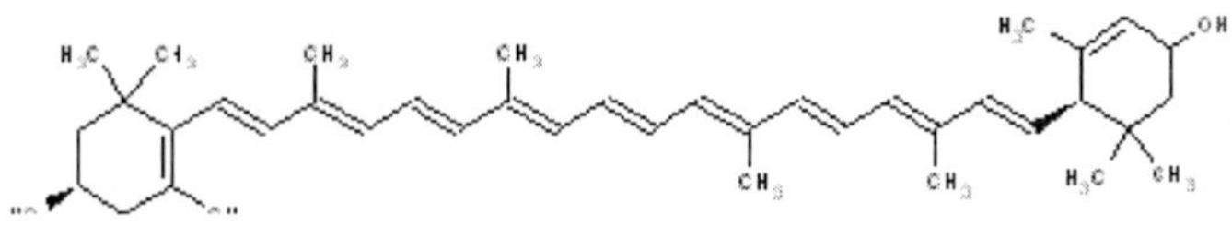

Lutein

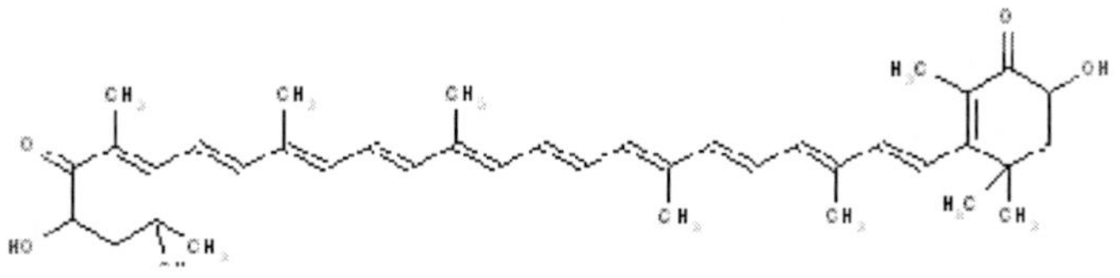

Astaxanthin

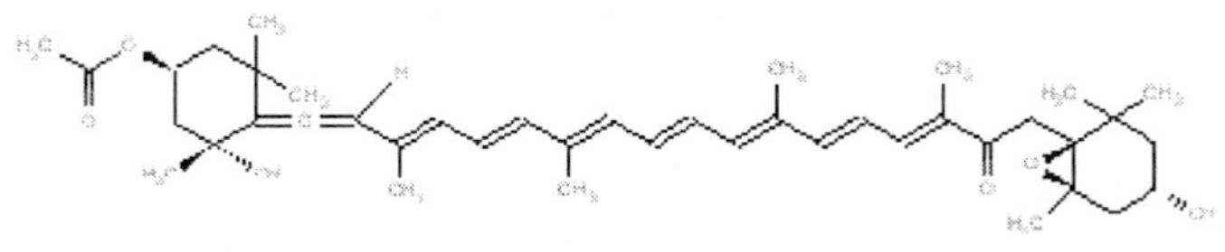

Fucoxanthin

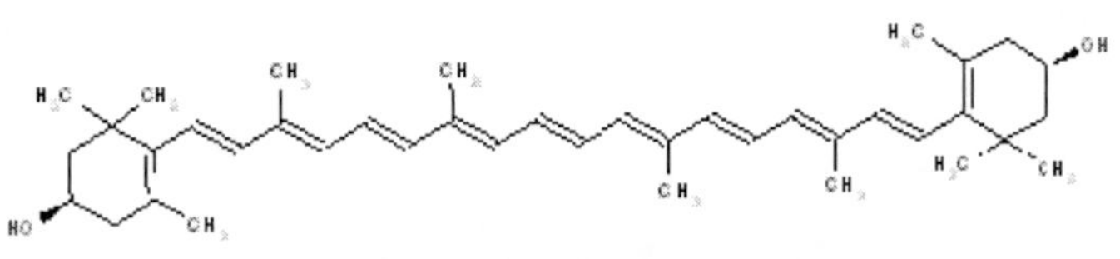

Zeaxanthin

Figure 1. Structures of carotenoids identified in different sea urchin species and seaweeds.

Sea urchins are marine invertebrates of the phylum Echinodermata. More than 750 species of sea urchins have been identified. Among them, *Paracentrotus lividus* is one of the most appreciated as food. From the morphological point of view, they have a globose shell (the test) covered with numerous sharp spines. The edible tissues are the gonads [10, 11].

Marine invertebrates, particularly echinoderms, are rich sources of carotenoids. Different carotenoid pigments have been isolated and identified in sea urchins, such as, β-carotene, α-carotene, β-echinenone, zeaxanthin, lutein, astaxanthin, cantaxanthin, β-isocryptoxanthin, fucoxanthin, etc. among them β-echinenone appears as the major pigment [12, 13]. The carotenoid composition in sea urchin is mainly determined by the diet. In echinoderms, the carotenoids are presented in the form of free pigments or bound to proteins in the form of complexes known as carotenoproteins [14].

In the work conducted in our laboratory [15] we observed that treatments such as heating appear to favour the release of carotenoids from the carotenoproteins. This fact could explain the higher content in β-echinenone that was detected in sea urchin gonads after a sterilization process (which involves heating to 112°C for 50 min) when compared with the contents of fresh gonads.

Some structures of the carotenoids identified in sea urchins and seaweeds are shown in Figure 1.

Seaweeds are excellent sources of bioactive compounds and nutritional components, so they could be considered a new functional food. However, their use as food is only widespread in Asia. Among the substances with biological activity present in macroalgae, the antioxidants have attracted the interest of the scientists because of their beneficial effects on health. Carotenoids are one of the compounds responsible for the antioxidant activity in algae.

α-, β-carotene, lutein and zeaxanthin have been identified in red seaweeds (Rhodophytes), while in brown seaweeds fucoxanthin—a powerful antioxidant—is the main carotenoid. A recent review [16] published the fucoxanthin content in different species of brown seaweeds in which the values ranged from 0.24 mg/g to 2.67 mg/g for *Laminaria religiosa* (young tallus) and *Undaria pinnatifida* (male gametophyte), respectively. The carotenoid levels in seaweeds depend on several factors such as UV irradiation exposure [17]. Several studies have shown the antitumor activity of fucoxanthin [16].

Conclusion

Although plants and fruits are the most common sources of carotenoids, several studies have demonstrated that marine organisms, particularly echinoderms and seaweeds, contain significant levels of carotenoids, so they could be considered an excellent source of these natural antioxidants.

References

[1]   Machlin, LJ. Critical assessment of epidemiological data concerning the impact of antioxidant nutrients on cancer and cardiovascular disease. *Critical Reviews in Food Science and Nutrition*, 1995, 35, 41-50.

[2] Bone, RA; Landrum, JT; Dixon, Z; Chen, Y; Llerena, CM. Lutein and zeaxanthin in the eyes, serum and diet of human subjects. *Experimental Eye Research*, 2000, 71, 239-245.

[3] Pfander, H. Key to Carotenoids. Basel: Birkhäuser Verlag; 1987.

[4] Carotenature (the carotenoids page), 2000. World Wide Web: http://www.carotenature. com.

[5] Nollet, LML. Food Analysis by HPLC. Second Edition. New York: Marcel Dekker, Inc; 2000.

[6] Oliver, J; Palou, A. Chromatographic determination of carotenoids in foods. *Journal of Chromatography A*, 2000, 881, 543-555.

[7] Rodríguez-Bernaldo de Quirós, A; S. Costa, H. Analysis of carotenoids in vegetable and plasma samples: A review. *Journal of Food Composition and Analysis*, 2006, 19, 97-111.

[8] Careri, M; Elviri, L; Mangia, A. Liquid chromatography electrospray mass spectrometry of β-carotene and xanthophylls: validation of the analytical method. *Journal of Chromatography A*, 1999, 854, 233-244.

[9] Weller, P; Breithaupt, DE. Identification and quantification of zeaxanthin esters in plants using liquid chromatography-mass spectrometry. *Journal of Agricultural and Food Chemistry*, 2003, 51, 7044-7049.

[10] Gabin-Sánchez, C; Lorenzo de Dios, F. El erizo de mar un recurso con futuro. Spain: Aula del Mar, Fundación Caixa Galicia; 1993.

[11] Campbell, AC. (Ed.), Guía de la flora y fauna de las costas de España y Europa. Barcelona: Omega; 1989.

[12] Shpigel, M; Schlosser, SC; Ben-Amotz, A; Lawrence, AL; Lawrence, JM. Effects of dietary carotenoid on the gut and the gonad of the sea urchin Paracentrotus *lividus.* *Aquaculture*, 2006, 261, 1269-1280.

[13] Kawakami, T; Tsushima, M; Katabami, Y; Mine, M; Ishida, A; Matsuno T. Effect of β,β-carotene, β-echinenone, astaxanthin fucoxanthin, vitamin A and vitamin E on the biological defense of the sea urchin *Pseudocentrotus depressus.* *Journal of Experimental Marine Biology and Ecology*, 1998, 226, 165-174.

[14] Zagalsky, PF. Invertebrate carotenoproteins. *Methods in Enzymology*, 1985, 111, 216-247.

[15] Rodríguez-Bernaldo de Quirós, A; López-Hernández, J; Simal-Lozano, J. Determination of carotenoids and liposoluble vitamins in sea urchin (*Paracentrotus lividus*) by high performance liquid chromatography. *European Food Research and Technology*, 2001, 212, 687-690.

[16] Kumar, CS; Ganesan, P; Suresh, PV; Bhaskar, N. Seaweeds as a source of nutritionally beneficial compounds—A review. *Journal of Food Science and Technology*, 2008, 45, 1-13.

[17] Yuan, YV. Antioxidants from edible seaweeds. *ACS Symposium Series*, 2007, 956, 268-301.

[18] Reviewed by Dr. M. José Oruna-Concha, School of Food Biosciences, Reading University, RG6 6AP, Reading, UK.

In: Encyclopedia of Vitamin Research
Editor: Joshua T. Mayer

ISBN: 978-1-61761-928-1
© 2011 Nova Science Publishers, Inc.

Chapter 37

In Vitro Antioxidant Activity of Synthetic β-carotene and Natural Carotenoid Extracts against the Oxidative Degradation of Food-Related Oil-in-Water Emulsions[*]

Sotirios Kiokias, Charikleia Dimakou and Vassiliki Oreopoulou
Laboratory of Food Chemistry and Technology, School of Chemical Engineering,
National Technical University of Athens, Polytechnioupoli Zografou,
Iroon Polytechniou 9, 15780, Athens, Greece

Abstract

In literature, carotenoids have been reported to act as chain-breaking antioxidants under specific conditions in vitro or in vivo. The antioxidant potential of certain carotenoids has been summarized by several authors. Though the in vivo antioxidant activity of dietary carotenoids (e.g., β-carotene and lycopene) has been widely investigated, so far there is still controversial scientific evidence regarding the factors that modulate their in vitro properties in oil-based systems. It should be noted that although the carotenoids have been repeatedly examined in bulk oil systems, there is limited evidence regarding the factors modulating their activity in dispersed systems.

This chapter examines the antioxidant potential of β-carotene as the main reference carotene, and of several natural carotenoid pigments, such as annatto (rich in bixin and norbixin), paprika (rich in capsanthin and capsorubin), marigold (rich in lutein isomers) and tomato (rich in lycopene and carotenes) extracts in various systems. Mechanisms and

---

[*] A version of this chapter was also published in *Beta Carotene: Dietary Sources, Cancer and Cognition, edited by Leiv Haugen and Terje Bjornson* published by Nova Science Publishers, Inc. It was submitted for appropriate modifications in an effort to encourage wider dissemination of research.

parameters affecting both the antioxidant and prooxidant activity of the carotenoids are discussed. Furthermore, the effect in the following model oil-in-water (o/w) emulsions is extensively investigated: (a) azo-initiated oxidation with AAPH (2, 2'- azobis - amidinopropane dihydrochloride) as a water soluble initiator in the water phase of simple 10% o/w emulsions emulsified by Tween 20 (0.1%) (as AAPH oxidation proceeds rapidly under low oxygen pressure, it mimics in vivo conditions in human tissues); (b) autoxidation of Tween-stabilized emulsions at 30°C, which offers a more realistic model reflecting oxidative changes of the product during storage; and (c) thermal accelerated autoxidation (60°C) of more concentrated homogenised 30% o/w emulsions stabilised by protein (sodium caseinate 1%). Finally the influence of other natural antioxidants (e.g., isomers of tocopherols, ascorbic acid, olive oil phenolics) on the carotenoid activity is discussed.

The understanding and optimisation of the carotenoid antioxidant character in novel emulsion systems can offer a basis for their more systematic use by the food industry as functional ingredients, which could protect the related food products from sensory and nutritional oxidative deterioration.

1. Introduction

The replacement of synthetic antioxidants by "safer natural mixtures" has been increasingly advocated up to the present by the food industry. This trend has been imposed by the worldwide preference of consumers for the use of natural antioxidants, some of which may exist inherently in foods or as intentional additives during processing (Kritchevski, 1999).

Among these, carotenoids comprise a widespread class of natural pigments, which are primarily used by industry as colorants in various manufactured food and drinks (Grobush et al., 2000). The best-documented function of carotenoids is their provitamin A activity, especially that of β-carotene and, to a lesser extent, of β-cryptoxanthin and lutein (Van de Berg et al., 2000). Although close to 600 carotenoids have been identified in nature, only 50 possess provitamin A activity and about 40 are present in a typical human diet that provides 1000–4000 μg of carotenoids daily (Mangels et al., 1993; Ribayamercado et al., 2000).

Most carotenoids are 40-carbon terpenoids having isoprene as their basic structural unit. General subdivisions are the following: (i) "carotenes", which are strictly hydrocarbons (α- and β-carotene, lycopene); and (ii) "xanthophylls" (lutein, bixin, capsanthin, etc.), which contain polar end groups reflecting an oxidative step in their formation (Faure et al., 1999; Kovary et al., 2001).

Though the in vivo antioxidant activity of dietary carotenoids (e.g., β-carotene and lycopene) has been widely investigated and well established (Kiokias et al., 2008), there is still controversial scientific evidence regarding the factors that influence their in vitro properties in oil-based systems (Pryor et al., 2000). For instance, in the presence of a sufficiently high concentration of other antioxidants (tocopherols or ascorbic acid), carotenoids may behave as antioxidants, even though they may present a prooxidant character in the absence of other additives (Palozza, 1998). It should be noted that, although the carotenoids have been repeatedly examined in bulk oil systems as protecting efficiently against photooxidation (Lee & Min, 1990), there is limited evidence regarding their activity in dispersed systems.

So far, little research on the antioxidant activity of carotenoids in multicomponent systems has been reported in the literature (Heinonen et al., 1997; Kiokias & Gordon 2003a). Investigation of factors that influence the oxidative stability of food emulsions are of great scientific interest given the increased importance of these systems in many industrial applications (margarines, dressings, sauces etc.). Moreover, apart from their technological importance, emulsion systems generally mimic the amphiphilic nature and the basic structural characteristics of important biological membranes, which are also prone to in vivo oxidative degradation when attacked by singlet oxygen and free radicals (Halliwell & Gutteridge, 1995; Rice Evans, 2000). In that aspect, in vitro research on the oxidative stability and antioxidation of model emulsions could provide with useful information of nutritional interest and thereby serve as pilot studies for in vivo clinical trials.

The present chapter examines the antioxidant activity of β-carotene as compared to several carotenoid-rich plant extracts (such as tomato, marigold, paprika and annatto extracts), particularly in food related emulsion systems. Simple, Tween-stabilised, dilute (10% o/w) emulsions, subjected to auto-oxidation or azo-initiated oxidation, are initially examined to distinguish the effect of concentration and structure on the antioxidant potential of carotenoids. Subsequently, the effect of carotenoids in more concentrated (30% o/w) protein-stabilised emulsions is presented. The latter systems are close to the structure and formulation of recently developed industrial products (fresh cheese types, coffee cream, etc.)

By elucidating the antioxidant capacity of carotenoids in novel food emulsion systems, new strategies for the improvement of oxidative stability (and thereby delay of quality deterioration) of many related products could be developed in the near future.

2. Composition of Natural Carotenoid Extracts

Natural extracts can be used as carotenoid sources to protect lipid food from oxidation. Raw materials rich in carotenoids include tomato, paprika, marigold, and annatto. High Performance Liquid Chromatography (HPLC) of the extracts (Hart & Scott, 1995) indicated that marigold extract contained mainly all-trans lutein as well as traces of zeaxanthin and 13-*cis* lutein. In paprika extract, capsanthin is the major compound followed by capsorubin, while β-carotene was also present in traces. The lipid soluble annatto extract contains bixin, while the water soluble preparation contains mainly norbixin (~93%) and traces of bixin. In the tomato extract, lycopene is by far the major component (~85%) but α- and β-carotenes are also present.

The "total active carotenoid concentration" of each tested extract, expressed as a percentage of the major identified carotenoid, estimated by visible absorption spectroscopy, using absorptivity values reported in the literature (Scott et al., 1996), is presented in Table 1, where also a summary of HPLC analysis is given together with the structure of the major carotenoid pigment in each extract.

3. Mechanisms and Parameters Affecting the Radical Scavenging Activity of Carotenoids

A large body of scientific evidence suggests that carotenoids scavenge and deactivate free radicals both in vitro (Kiokias & Gordon, 2003a) and in vivo (Bub et al., 2000; Matos et al., 2000; Kiokias & Gordon, 2003b). It has been reported that their antioxidant action is determined by:

Table 1. Composition of the tested carotenoid preparations in this study. The % of the identified carotenoids in their mixture was calculated by HPLC. The active carotenoid concentration of each extract was calculated by UV spectroscopy (at the λ max of their major carotenoid).

Tested carotenoids	Identified carotenoids by HPLC analysis	Structure of the main carotenoid in the extract
Marigold extract (55% activ.carot) at λ_{max} = 445	all-trans lutein (~83%) zeaxanthin (~12%) 13-cis lutein (~5%).	all-trans Lutein
Parika extract (9% activ.carot) at λ_{max} = 471	capsanthin, (~60%) capsorubin (~30%) β-carotene (~10%)	Capsanthin
Tomato extract (10.6% activ.carot) at λ_{max} = 472	lycopene (~85%) β-carotene (~11 %) α-carotene (~ 4%)	Lycopene
Lipid-soluble annatto extract (91% activ.carot) at λ_{max} = 458	Bixin (~100%)	Bixin
Water -soluble annatto extract (75% activ.carot) at λ_{max} = 435	Norbixin (~93%) Bixin (~7%)	Norbixin
Synthetic β-carotene at λ_{max} = 452	β-carotene (~100%)	β-carotene

- electron transfer reactions and the stability of the antioxidant free radical,
- the interplay with other antioxidants, and
- carotenoid structure and oxygen pressure of the tested system (Khachik et al., 1995).

Moreover, the antioxidant activity of carotenoids is characterized by literature data for - their relative rate of oxidation by a range of free radicals, and their capacity to inhibit lipid peroxidation in multilamellar liposomes (Bast et al., 1998).

The antioxidant activity of carotenoids is a direct consequence of the chemistry of their long polyene chain: a highly reactive, electron-rich system of conjugated double bonds susceptible to attack by electrophilic reagents, and forming stabilized radicals (Burton, 1988).

Burton and Ingold (1984) decsribed the mechanism by which β-carotene acts as a chain breaking antioxidant. The addition of a peroxyl radical (ROO˙) to a suitable double bond of the carotenoids should be the first step in the scavenging of a peroxyl radical (Reaction 3.1, also shown in Figure 1). The resulting carbon centered radical (ROO-CAR˙) reacts rapidly and reversibly with oxygen to form a new, chain-carrying peroxyl radical (ROO-CAR-OO˙, Reaction 3.2). The carbon centered radical is resonance stabilized to such an extent, that when the oxygen pressure is lowered, the equilibrium of this reaction shifts sufficiently to the left, to effectively lower the concentration of peroxyl radicals and hence reduce the amount of autoxidation in the system (Britton, 1995). Furthermore, the carotene radical adduct can also undergo termination by reaction with another peroxyl radical (Reaction 3.3).

Reactions

$$CAR + ROO˙ \rightarrow ROO\text{-}CAR˙ \tag{3.1}$$

$$ROO\text{-}CAR˙ + O_2 \leftrightarrow ROO\text{-}CAR\text{-}OO˙ \tag{3.2}$$

$$ROO\text{-}CAR˙ + ROO˙ \rightarrow \text{inactive products} \tag{3.3}$$

Reaction 3.3 is thought to take place at low oxygen pressures (such as <150 Torr) so that peroxyl radicals would be eventually consumed to allow carotenoids to act as chain breaking antioxidants. A strong effect of partial oxygen pressure on β-carotene antioxidant capacity has been reported in the literature (Kasaikina et al., 1998; Stocker et al., 1994).

The structure of carotenoids may also modulate their radical scavenging properties (Liebler & Kennedy, 1992). A difference in the reactivity of carotenoids against free radicals can be partly attributed to varying electron distribution along the polyene chain due to different chromophores, which would alter the susceptibility of free radical addition to the conjugated double bond (Woodall et al., 1997). Substitution of hydrogen atoms with a carbonyl group, at the 4 position of the carotenoid molecule, increases the overall peroxyl radical trapping ability due to the electron withdrawing character of the carbonyl oxygen atoms substantially reducing the unpaired electron density of the carbon centered radical and thereby its reactivity with oxygen (Mortensen et al., 1997).

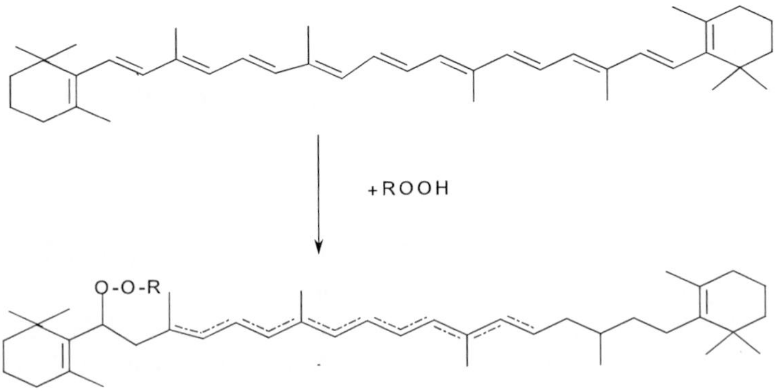

Figure 1. Addition of a peroxyl radical to the carotenoid molecule (formation of a resonance stabilized carbon centered radical). (Kiokias, 2002, PhD thesis.).

Table 2. Effect of carotenoids (1 g l⁻¹) on the oxidative stability of bulk olive oil at 60°C.

Treatment	[1]Peroxide values (PV, meq kg⁻¹) at 30 days of storage	[2]Protection factor (PF) (based on time to PV = 50 meq kg⁻¹)
Control	$101.8^b \pm 6.3$	$1.00^b \pm 0.00$
Marigold (Lutein)	$113.4^a \pm 7.0$	$0.86^c \pm 0.05$
Tomato (Lycopene)	$110.5^a \pm 7.9$	$0.88^c \pm 0.04$
Annatto (Norbixin)	$56.2^c \pm 3.4$	$1.56^a \pm 0.06$
Paprika	$97.3^b \pm 7.9$	$1.08^b \pm 0.08$

[1] PV results are expressed as mean (n=6) ± SD; significant differences from ANOVA test (p<0.05) indicated by superscripts. (order of antioxidant activity: a< b <c).

[2] Protection factors (PF) are given by: time for the antioxidant treatment / time for the control, to reach the oxidation level of PV= 50 meq kg⁻¹ (PF>1: antioxidant effect, PF<1: prooxidant effect, order of antioxidant activity: a>b>c).

Canthaxanthin, astaxanthin, and other carotenoids containing oxo-groups in the 4 position of the β-ionone ring, were reported to be more effective antioxidants than β-carotene on the free radical oxidation of methyl linoleate in solution (Terao, 1990; Mortensen & Skibsted, 1997). Similarly, annatto extracts containing bixin as the major component were found to inhibit the autoxidation of triglycerides, whereas lutein and lycopene were prooxidants (Haila et al., 1997). Paprika extracts containing mainly capsanthin exhibited a strong antioxidant effect against the production of methyl linoleate hydroperoxides (Matsufuji et al., 1998).

The antioxidant activity of carotenoid extracts (1 g l⁻¹) in bulk olive oil stored at 60°C is summarized in Table 2. As shown there, the water soluble (and more hydrophilic) annatto was a clear antioxidant, while between the lipid soluble preparations, paprika (containing carotenoids with carbonyl end groups) had a tendency for an antioxidant effect though it did not differ statistically from the control. Interestingly, the marigold and tomato extracts (rich in more hydrophobic carotenoids, such as lutein and lycopene respectively) were prooxidative by even promoting rather than inhibiting the formation of lipid hydroperoxides.

The protection factors (PF), calculated from the times required for the PV of each sample to reach a value of 50 meq kg⁻¹ (considering that this is a sufficient level of oil oxidative deterioration) indicated the following antioxidant hierarchy: annatto (1.56) > paprika (1.08) = control (1.00) > marigold (0.86) = tomato (0.88). Therefore, as regards the behavior of each treatment, there is a general consistency between the PF measurements and findings based on peroxide values at the end point of oxidation.

As a general conclusion, hydrophilic extracts seem to work much more effectively against oxidation of bulk olive oil, than the lipid soluble (hydrophobic) carotenoid preparations, a finding closer to the so-called "polar paradox", a theory first introduced by Frankel (1996).

Haila et al. (1997) also showed that β-carotene, lutein and lycopene increased hydroperoxide formation in autoxidised rapeseed oil triglycerides, both in the dark and light. Interestingly, in the same study, annatto was the only carotenoid that exerted an antioxidant effect, a conclusion that was partly observed here (Table 2) as norbixin extract (not bixin, though) inhibited significantly the formation of hydroperoxides. Henry et al. (1998) observed that both β-carotene and lycopene (at concentrations greater than 500 ppm) acted as prooxidants during the heat catalysed oxidation (75°C) of safflower oil. As mentioned there, lycopene and β-carotene are potentially radical forming compounds and therefore could propagate the reaction when the radicals are present at high concentrations. Therefore, the concentration of carotenoid in a system could play an important role in determining whether the carotenoid will act as an antioxidant or a prooxidant or have no effect.

However, the effects of carotenoids are sensitive to oxidation conditions. In photo-oxidation studies carotenoids have been shown to maintain the oxidative stability of olive oil (Kiritsakis, 1998; Fakourelis & Min, 1987). In addition, Jorgensen and Skibsted (1993) found that carotenoids in food storage experiments provided some protection against oxidative rancidity, while Pokorny and Reblova (1999) reported that oxidation of frying oil is inhibited by carotenoids.

To understand the mechanism of antioxidant activity of carotenoids it is also important to analyze the oxidation products that are formed during their reaction with lipid radicals (Yamauchi et al., 1993). Some work in the area has focused on the reactions of carotenoids with peroxyl radicals, generated mainly by thermal decomposition of azo-initiators that leads to a variety of products, mainly apocarotenals and apocarotenones (Palozza & Krinsky, 1992).

A relationship between product-forming oxidation reactions to carotenoid antioxidant effects has been additionally proposed. According to Liebler and McClure (1996) the epoxide forming reaction (homolytic cleavage) releases an alkoxyl radical and would not be expected to produce an antioxidant effect. However, heterolytic cleavage would lead to carbonyl fragments and a dialkyl peroxide and other non-radical products, so that β-carotene oxidation by this pathway results in consumption of two peroxyl radicals and an antioxidant effect (Figure 2).

4. Prooxidant Activity of Carotenoids in Lipid Systems: Effect of Oxygen Partial Pressure

In certain cases, and generally depending on the experimental conditions, carotenoids may loose their radical scavenging activity and even shift to a prooxidant character instead. This is affected by several factors such as oxygen partial pressure, concentration, etc. (Liebler, 1993).

At high oxygen levels, a carotenoid intermediate radical ($CAR^•$) might add oxygen to form a carotenoid peroxyl radical such as $CAR\text{-}OO^•$. Such an intermediate species could act as a prooxidant, initiating for example the process of lipid peroxidation:

Reactions

$$CAR\text{-}OO^• + RH \rightarrow CAR\text{-}OOH + R^• \qquad (4.1)$$
$$R^• + O_2 \rightarrow R\text{-}OO^• \qquad (4.2)$$

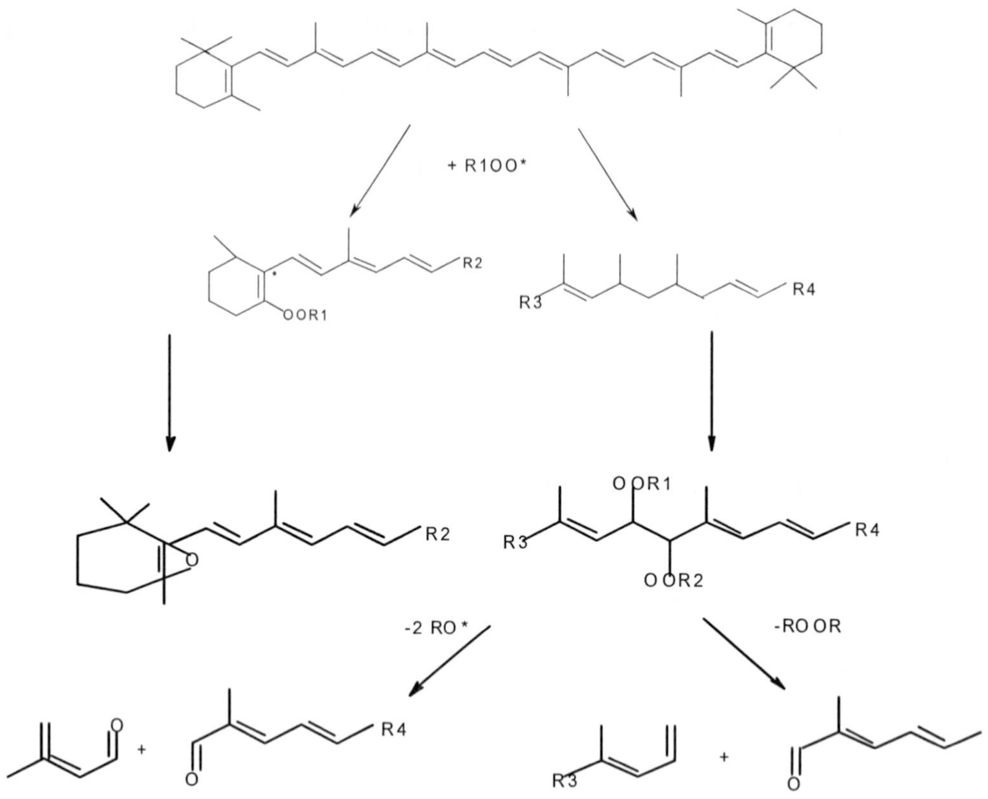

Figure 2. Oxidation of β-carotene by a peroxyl radical and relation of oxidation products to carotenoid activity (I) *Homolytic* (no antioxidant effect) (II) *Heterolytic* (antioxidant effect). (*Kiokias,2002, PhD thesis.*).

The loss in antioxidant efficiency of β-carotene at high pO_2 is due to the β-carotene being consumed by autoxidation without scavenging peroxyl radicals (Kennedy & Liebler, 1992).

β-carotene was found to act more efficiently as an antioxidant in the absence of oxygen (inhibiting 70% of lipid oxidation) and this effect decreased rapidly to about 50% inhibition, on increasing the partial pressure of oxygen to 8 mm Hg (Niki et al., 1995). Stocker et al. (1994) compared the effect of O_2 at both 20 and 2% concentration on the antioxidant activity of β-carotene and bilirubin, and reported that both additives were better antioxidants at low oxygen pressure. Similarly, Jorgensen and Skibsted (1993) found that carotenoid antioxidant activity increased substantially at lower oxygen concentrations (e.g., about 4-fold better antioxidant efficiency for β-carotene at 0.01 atm of oxygen).

In our laboratory (NTUA University), the effect of β-carotene at 0.5 g l^{-1} (level at which no carotenoid effect was observed) was compared with that of α-tocopherol (as a reference antioxidant compound) under both normal and reduced partial pressures. The statistical analysis of the results (Table 3), at normal oxygen pressure, (100% O_2) revealed that no antioxidant effect could be attributed to either β-carotene or α-tocopherol. However, under reduced oxygen pressure 5% O_2, the β-carotene exerted a significant antioxidant effect in contrast to α-tocopherol, which, as previously, did not present any significant inhibitory activity against lipid oxidation at this concentration level. The enhanced antioxidant activity of β-carotene under reduced oxygen pressure as observed in this experiment is consistent with the results of a similar study by Vile and Winterburn (1988). They observed that at pO_2: 0-4 mm Hg β-carotene was a stronger antioxidant than α-tocopherol and only at pO_2 >8 mm Hg did α-tocopherol become more efficient. However, Liebler et al., (1997) concluded that β-carotene was less effective than α-tocopherol, during AAPH-induced oxidation of rat liver microsomes, both under normal air pressure and 3.8 torr O_2.

Palozza et al. (1998) reported a prooxidant character (increase of lipid peroxidation products) at 760 mm Hg in rat liver microsomes exposed to AAPH radicals. On the contrary, Liebler (1993) reported that in a liposome model, β-carotene provided essentially equal antioxidant protection under an air atmosphere (150 torr O_2) or under a 15 torr O_2, atmosphere, which is similar to the oxygen tension in many tissues.

Table 3. Comparison between α-tocopherol (0.1 mM) and β-carotene (1 mM) during AAPH initiated oxidation of 10% sunflower o/w emulsions at 60°C operated under normal or reduced oxygen pressure (95% N_2).

(a) Normal pO_2	Reduced pO_2 (95% N_2)
Treatment [1,2] R values	Treatment [1,2] R values
Control 1.00 [a] ± 0.00	Control 1.00 [a] ± 0.00
α-tocopherol 1.14 [a] ± 0.12	α-tocopherol 1.16 [a] ± 0.12
β-carotene 0.85 [a] ± 0.09	β-carotene 1.46 [b] ± 0.09

$R = (t_{CAR} / t_{CNT})$,

where, t_{CAR}: time (h) for the carotenoid containing emulsion to reach the absorbance value (A_{233}) of 0.80 and

t_{CNT}: time (h) for the control emulsion to undergo the same level of oxidative deterioration in terms of conjugated dienes production

Results are expressed as means (n=3) ± SD; ANOVA test (p<0.05) (order of antioxidant activity: a< b).

Further to the oxygen pressure of the system, the carotene concentration may also have an effect on its function, with high concentrations of carotenes (such as >5mM) exerting generally a prooxidant rather than antioxidant character (Zhang & Omaye, 2000; Farombi & Britton, 1999). During the heat catalyzed oxidation of safflower seed oil, at concentrations >500 ppm both β-carotene and lycopene acted as prooxidants (Henry et al., 1998). Furthermore, carotenoid oxidation products may have an influence on the stability of edible oils. Oxidation products of β-carotene acted as prooxidants in soybean oils containing 3 ppm chlorophyll leading to higher peroxide values under storage in light (Kiokias & Gordon, 2004).

5. Activity of Carotenoids against the Photoxidative Degradation of Oil-Based Systems

Singlet molecular oxygen ($^1O_2$) participates in photoxidation of vegetables oils and oil-containing foods, and various chromophoric impurities such as chlorophylls are believed to act as photosensitizers generating this state of oxygen by transfer of excitation energy (Terao, 1990).

The discovery that carotenoids deactivate singlet molecular oxygen was an important advance in understanding their technological and biological effects. Addition of various carotenoids to foods containing unsaturated oils was found to improve their shelflife, by a mechanism that appears to depend largely on physical quenching (Di Mascio et al., 1992) and can be summarized as follows:

In the presence of β-carotene, singlet oxygen will preferentially transfer exchange energy to produce the triplet state carotene, while oxygen comes back to its ground energy state, and therefore is inactivated (Reaction 5.1). The transfer of energy from singlet oxygen to carotenoid takes place through an electron transfer exchange mechanism (Reische et al., 1997). Triplet state β-carotene releases energy in the form of heat, and the carotenoid returns to its normal energy state (Reaction 5.2). In this way, carotenoids act so effectively, that one carotenoid molecule is able to quench up to 1000 molecules of singlet oxygen (Halliwell & Gutteridge, 1995).

Reactions

$$^1O_2 + \beta\text{-carotene} \rightarrow {}^3\beta\text{-carotene}^* + {}^3O_2 \qquad\qquad (5.1)$$

$$^3\beta\text{-carotene}^* \rightarrow \beta\text{-carotene} + heat \qquad\qquad (5.2)$$

Increasing β-carotene concentration inhibited peroxide formation in high oleic and conventional canola oil (Goulson & Wartensen, 1999) or purified olive oil under photooxidative conditions (Fakourelis & Min, 1987). During chlorophyll sensitized photoxidation of soybean oil, the carotenoid antioxidant effect increased with an increasing concentration and number of double bonds (Lee & Min, 1990).

Researchers have reported that capsanthin which contains 11 conjugated double bonds, a conjugated keto- group and a cyclopentane ring, had higher antiphotooxidative activity than β-carotene, which has the same number of double bonds but neither of the functional groups (Nielsen et al., 1997).

6. Effect of Carotenoids in Azo-Initiated Oxidation of Sunlfower Oil-in-Water Emulsions

6.1. Activity of Natural Carotenoids against Oil Oxidative Degradation and Formation of Volatile Aldehydes

Experimental work with various carotenoids was conducted in 10% sunflower oil-in-water emulsions. The tocopherol content of sunflower oil had been removed with open column chromatography to accelerate the rate of oil deterioration. Tween 20 (1g/100g emulsion) was used as emulsifier and 1% of AAPH as a chemical initiator. It is known that azo-initiators form radicals that lose nitrogen and subsequently combine with oxygen to form peroxy-radicals (Liegeois et al., 2000). Oxidation was induced at 60°C in a shaking water bath.

The effect of the addition of various carotenoid extracts at a concentration of 2% in the oil phase of the emulsion is presented in Figure 3, in terms of increase of absorbance at 233 nm. The control emulsion presented a faster increase of absorbance at 233 nm, in comparison to the carotenoid-containing emulsions. Therefore, the tested carotenoids seem to inhibit the AAPH-initiated oxidation and exert an antioxidant character. It is known that at constant temperature of 60°C, the thermal decomposition of the AAPH initiator generates free radicals, which then react with oxygen to produce the corresponding peroxyl radicals. Under these conditions, carotenoid molecules compete with the linoleyl group of triglycerides (linoleic acid is the major fatty acid of sunflower oil) for reaction with the azo peroxyl radicals. Interestingly, probably due to the fact that the rate of reaction of carotenoids and linoleyl TGs with the radical species is sufficiently large from the beginning, no lag phase was observed in all oxidation experiments.

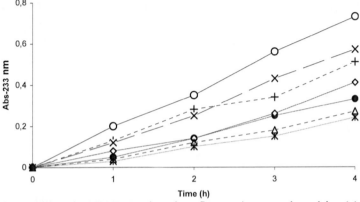

Figure 3. Oxidative stability of a 10% Tween based sunflower o/w, control emulsion (o), compared with emulsions containing tomato extract (×), β-carotene (+), lutein-rich extract (◊), paprika extract (●), bixin-extract (Δ) and norbixin (*) at 2g l^{-1} (AAPH-initiated oxidation at 60°C)

As the AAPH radical combines very fast with oxygen (pre-existing in the headspace of the sample vial), it is likely to reduce the oxygen content of the solution enhancing the antioxidant character of carotenoids, which is thereby favoured under these relatively low oxygen pressure conditions.

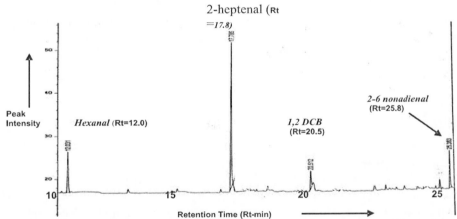

Figure 4. Chromatogram of the major volatile aldehydes formed by decomposition of linoleyl-hydroperoxides during AAPH initiated oxidation of 10% Tween based sunflower o/w emulsions at 60°C (GC-Static-Headspace Analysis).

As oxidation proceeds, some decomposition of hydroperoxides takes place. The static headspace solid phase microextraction (SPME) method has been widely accepted in recent years as a useful analytical tool to measure volatile components, having the advantages of being a relatively quick, one step method of extracting volatiles from the headspace that does not require solvents or costly equipment (Song et al., 1997; Zabaras & Wyllie, 2002).

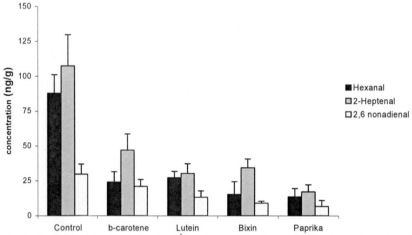

Figure 5. Effect of carotenoid extracts (at 1 g l^{-1} in oil) on volatile aldehydes formation after 4 hrs of AAPH-initiated oxidation of 10% Tween-based sunflower o/w emulsions at 60°C.

In the AAPH-initiated oxidation of emulsions, it was found that hexanal, 2-heptenal and 2,6-nonadienal were the major volatiles present in the oxidized emulsion samples (Figure 4). The finding generally agrees with similar studies identifying these certain aldehydes among the main products of linoleic acid hydroperoxide decomposition (Snyder et al., 1985).

All the carotenoid extracts (at 1 g l^{-1}) inhibited markedly the formation of the volatile aldehydes when compared with the control. As shown in Figure 5, the paprika extract was the most effective in reducing formation of volatile aldehydes followed by bixin and lutein, a finding which is partly consistent with their effectiveness in inhibiting conjugated dienes formation. There is no evidence in the literature about the effect of carotenoids in inhibiting the formation of volatiles in azo-initiated oxidation. Heinonen et al. (1997) did not observe any significant inhibitory effect of β-carotene by measuring the formation of hexanal and 2-heptenal in emulsions. However, Warner and Frankel (1987) reported that twice as much 2-heptenal was formed in the control sample compared to soybean oil containing 200 ppm of β-carotene, a conclusion closer to the finding of the present study.

6.2. Effect of Structure on Carotenoid Actioxidant Activity

There are relatively few studies on the antioxidant activity of natural carotenoid-rich extracts in food or biological systems. Matsufuji et al. (1998) found that paprika extracts, containing mainly capsanthin, exhibited a strong antioxidant effect against the production of methyl linoleate hydroperoxides, and Chen et al. (1997) observed an antioxidant effect of capsanthin on photoxidation of soyabean oil. Extracts from marigold flowers are useful as food colorants, and they can also inhibit oxidation of LDL in vitro (Chopra et al., 1996). The protective action of annatto extracts against lipid peroxidation has been demonstrated by several researchers. Haila et al. (1997) found that annatto, containing bixin as the major component, inhibited the autoxidation of triglycerides, whereas lutein and lycopene acted as prooxidants.

The statistical analysis (one-way ANOVA, p<0.05) of the results presented in 6.1 concluded evident differences in the antioxidant activity of the various carotenoids, with the following antioxidant hierarchy:

annatto extracts[e] > paprika extract[d]> marigold extract [c] > all-trans pure β-carotene [b] = tomato extract [b] > control [a]

(order of antioxidant activity: e>d>c>b>a).

The annatto extracts (rich in bixin or norbixin) were the strongest antioxidants with similar order of activity, followed by paprika extract (rich in capsanthin and capsorubin). Interestingly these extracts, (containing the above-mentioned polar carotenoids with carboxylic acid and esters groups) were stronger antioxidants than the marigold extract containing the lutein with 2-OH groups. Between the natural preparations, the tomato extract (mainly rich in lycopene but also containing α- and β-carotenes, all hydrophobic carotenoids lacking polar substitutes) was the least effective carotenoid with an activity similar to that of the reference β-carotene, though both exerted a clear antioxidant effect when compared to the control. This tendency reveals an association between structure and carotenoid activity, which somehow depends on the nature of the end group. It seems that the antioxidant potential of carotenoids against AAPH-derived radicals is enhanced with increasing polarity in the carotenoid molecule.

Several researchers (Woodall et al., 1997; Mortensen et al., 1997) have supported that the different reactivity of carotenoids against free radicals can be partly attributed to variations in the electron distribution along the polyene chain of different chromophores, which would alter the susceptibility of free radical addition to the conjugated double bond system. Therefore, the polyene chain is the structural feature, which is mainly responsible for the chemical reactivity of carotenoids towards oxidizing agents and free radicals, and consequently, for any antioxidant role.

Substitution of the hydrogens in the carotenoid molecule with polar oxo-groups (such as in bixin and norbixin) was found to increase the overall peroxyl radical trapping ability. This may happen due to the electron withdrawing character of the oxygen atoms, which substantially reduces the unpaired electron density of the carbon centred radical and thereby its reactivity with AAPH-derived radicals, leading to a more evident antioxidant character of the very polar carotenoids.

An alternative hypothesis, for the superior effect of polar carotenoids, refers to their distribution in an emulsion system. β-Carotene is likely to be homogeneously dispersed in the oil droplets, whereas the more polar xanthophylls (lutein, and annatto carotenoids) may be located near the oil-water interface, where free radical attack from AAPH-derived radicals first occurs. Therefore, if the more polar carotenoids are preferentially distributed at the droplet's surface they may exert a higher antioxidant activity (compared to the hydrophobic carotenoids β-carotene and lycopene) in the emulsions, since they can react more effectively with AAPH-radicals generated in the aqueous phase.

6.3. Effect of Concentration on Carotenoid Antioxidant Activity

The effect of carotenoid concentration (in the range of 0.5–5 g l^{-1} in oil) on their antioxidant activity is given in Figure 6, expressed in terms of a protective factor (R), which was calculated as following:

$$R = (t_{CAR} / t_{CNT}),$$

where, t_{CAR}: time (h) for the carotenoid containing emulsion to reach the absorbance value (A$_{233}$) of 0.80 (which represented a 200–300% increase of the initial absorbance), and t_{CNT}: time (h) for the control emulsion to undergo the same level of deterioration.

β-Carotene showed a clear increase in antioxidant activity with concentration up to 1 g l^{-1} (1.9 x 10^{-3} M) whereas a smaller but still clear change occurred in the whole tested range above this value. Bixin showed no significant increase in activity above 1 g l^{-1} carotenoid in oil (2.6 x 10^{-3} M). The same results were observed for paprika extract. For the marigold extract, the activity increased significantly with concentration up to 3 g l^{-1} (5.3 x 10^{-3} M) and then stabilized. The relatively high activity of xanthophylls (bixin, paprika, lutein) at low concentrations with no marked increase in activity above a certain level may reflect the increased concentration of these carotenoids at the oil-water interface as well as their more effective radical scavenging ability. The lack of an increase in antioxidant activity with higher concentrations of bixin and paprika may simply be due to the fact that the oxidation has already been strongly inhibited by lower concentrations of each carotenoid, so that a significant difference in the absorbance value with an increase in concentration cannot be detected. An alternative explanation is that the carotenoid molecules are only effective at inhibiting (AAPH) lipid oxidation if they are close to the oil water interface.

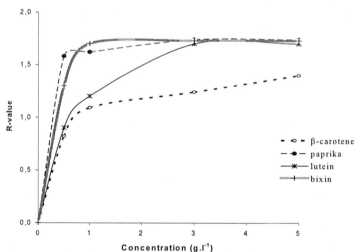

Figure 6. Effect of concentration (0.5–5 g l^{-1}) on the antioxidant activity (expressed by R-value) of several carotenoids during the AAPH-initiated oxidation of 10% Tween-based sunflower o/w emulsions at 60°C.

R = (t$_{CAR}$ / t$_{CNT}$), where,
t$_{CAR}$: time (h) for the carotenoid containing emulsion to reach the absorbance value (A$_{233}$) of 0.80 and
t$_{CNT}$: time (h) for the control emulsion to undergo the same level of oxidative deterioration in terms of conjugated dienes production.

6.4. Oxidative Degradation of Carotenoids

Understanding the fundamental chemistry of the reactions of carotenoids with oxidising agents is essential in order to assess their real value as protective antioxidants. In literature, relatively low activation energy for the oxidation of β-carotene has been reported, indicating that the carotenoid reaction with free radicals is quite fast as compared, for instance, to the autoxidation reaction of linoleic acid (Mortensen et al., 1997). This difference in reactivity can be attributed to the greater stability of the allylic radical produced from the β-carotene molecule, which is stabilised over 11 double bonds, compared with 2 double bonds in the linoleic acid.

Both spontaneous and radical-initiated oxidation of carotenoids can be followed by observing the loss of colour (or bleaching) in the visible spectrum, as oxidation proceeds. According to Miller et al. (1995) the bleaching is accompanied by loss of carotenoids with time and the reaction rate increases with temperature.

This hypothesis was checked in the AAPH-initiated oxidation of emulsions by measuring the absorbance at λ-max of the major carotenoid of each extract, which slightly differs between the pigments as following: β-carotene = 450nm, capsanthin = 471nm, lutein = 445nm, bixin = 458nm, norbixin = 435nm, lycopene = 472nm.

Results were expressed as % loss of absorbance at λ-max after 4 h of oxidation, expressed as DA(%):

$$DA\ (\%) = [A_{start} - A_{fin}] * 100 / A_{start}.$$

The mean values were found in the following order:

bixin[d] (45.8 ± 1.3) = norbixin[d] (49.6 ± 1.2) > paprika extract [c] (39.5 ± 0.5) = marigold extract[c] (31.9± 1.1) > all-trans pure β-carotene [b] (18.5 ± 2.6) = tomato extract [b] (21.5 ± 2.5) > control [a] (0.13 [a] ± 0.02), (where d>b>c>a).

It was interesting that all carotenoids showed a steady decrease as oxidation proceeded with time, reflecting a partial disruption of their polyene chromophore, during the reaction of the compounds with the produced radical species. It must be stressed that annatto carotenoids (which were previously mentioned as the most effective antioxidants) were the most rapidly consumed followed by lutein, whereas the carotene extracts were the most stable with time. It is therefore clear that the higher the rate of carotenoid degradation, the faster the carotenoids react with AAPH-derived peroxy radicals and consequently the more effectively they act as antioxidants under these conditions.

7. Carotenoids against The Autoxidative Degradation of Tween-Based Emulsion Systems

7.1. Activity of Natural Carotenoid Extracts on Autoxidation of Sunflower oil-in-water Emulsions

Sunflower o/w emulsions (10%) were used in order to investigate the carotenoid activity (at a concentration of 2 g l^{-1}) during their storage at 30°C. This is a more realistic oxidation model, which is closer to the conditions of use (or in even mistreatment, in certain cases) of related food products by distributors or consumers.

Statistical analysis of both conjugated dienes (CD) and peroxide values (PV) of carotenoid emulsions (in comparison with the control) after two months of oxidation, (Table 4) showed no inhibitory effect of carotenoids in retarding lipid oxidation of the emulsion samples. Actually, emulsions containing carotenoids reached even higher values of these oxidative markers than the control, although the ANOVA test showed no significant difference between the means of the control and the different carotenoid treatments.

Therefore, it was clear that the various carotenoid extracts did not present any antioxidant effects under these conditions. The absence of carotenoid antioxidant activity in this experiment, which was carried out under normal oxygen pressure conditions, is consistent with other reports in literature. In a similar study, Azuma et al. (1999) did not observe any antioxidant effect of β-carotene on oxidation of linoleic acid emulsions at 37°C, in the dark. Heinonen et al. (1997) observed a prooxidant character of β-carotene on autoxidation of 10% oil in water emulsions of rapeseed oil triglycerols, though much a lower carotenoid concentration (20 ppm), was used in that study.

In fact, as explained in previous sections, the extensive system of conjugated double bonds in carotenoid molecules makes them very susceptible to attack by free radical species, and at atmospheric oxygen pressures, relative alkoxy and peroxy radicals can be formed from the carotenoid. Apart from oxygen pressure, a high concentration of carotenoids has been also proposed to induce a prooxidant character (Lominsky et al., 1997). The prooxidant potency of high carotenoid concentrations could be due mainly to a more increased formation of carotene-peroxyl radicals, which promotes the propagation of autoxidation.

The formation of volatile aldehydes was also measured initially and at the end of the oxidation, to examine any effect on the secondary oxidation products. As characterised by flavour thresholds, these so-called "off-flavour" compounds can affect the sensory properties and thereby the quality of oil and fat containing foods (Akoh & Min, 1997). In particular, volatile aldehydes have a great importance as oxidative indicators due to their considerable contribution to the aroma and flavour deterioration of the final products.

Table 4. Effect of various natural carotenoids (2 g l[-1]) on the formation of hydroperoxides after 2 months of autoxidation of 10% Tween based sunflower o/w emulsions at 30°C. (CD and PV results are expressed as means, n=3 ± SD).

Treatment	Conjugated dienes (g kg-1)	Peroxide values (meq kg-1)
Control	5.5 ± 0.2	46.57 ± 1.75
β-Carotene	6.4 ± 0.3	47.13 ± 1.23
Tomato (lycopene)	6.6 ± 0.1	51.15 ± 1.20
Paprika	6.3 ± 0.1	45.60 ± 1.57
Marigold (lutein)	6.8 ± 0.2	46.95 ± 1.78
Annato (bixin)	6.0 ± 0.2	49.24 ± 1.35

Hexanal, 2-heptenal, pentanal and nonenal were the major volatile products, as confirmed by GC-MS analysis, after two months of autoxidation. According to recent literature evidence (Beltran et al., 2005), the same aldehydes were identified as the main volatiles during the oxidation of lipids via linoleic acid-13 hydroperoxides. The inhibitory effect of each tested carotenoid extract on the final amount of the identified volatiles at the end point of oxidation is summarised in Table 5. Interestingly, though all carotenoids generally inhibited the formation of volatile aldehydes, the more hydrophilic carotenoid preparations (paprika and annatto extracts) generally exerted a stronger inhibitory effect, as compared with the less polar ones (β-carotene, lutein or lycopene rich extracts).

Table 5. Effect of various natural carotenoids ($2 \ g \ l^{-1}$) on the formation of volatile aldehydes after two months of autoxidation of 10% Tween-based sunflower o/w emulsions at 30°C.

Concentration ($\mu g \ g^{-1}$) after two months of autoxidation				
Treatment	Pentanal	Hexanal	2-Heptanal	Nonanal
Control	$0.34^{a} \pm 0.00$	$0.65^{a} \pm 0.08$	$0.77^{a} \pm 0.01$	$0.80^{a} \pm 0.01$
β-carotene	$0.05^{b} \pm 0.00$	$0.62^{a} \pm 0.07$	$0.44^{b} \pm 0.01$	$0.68^{b} \pm 0.01$
lycopene	$0.06^{b} \pm 0.00$	$0.59^{a} \pm 0.07$	$0.35^{b} \pm 0.00$	$0.53^{b} \pm 0.00$
lutein	$0.08^{b} \pm 0.00$	$0.55^{a} \pm 0.07$	$0.48^{b} \pm 0.01$	$0.65^{b} \pm 0.01$
paprika	$0.03^{b} \pm 0.00$	$0.22^{b} \pm 0.00$	$0.20^{c} \pm 0.00$	$0.26^{c} \pm 0.00$
bixin	$0.03^{b} \pm 0.00$	$0.27^{b} \pm 0.00$	$0.23^{c} \pm 0.00$	$0.32^{c} \pm 0.00$
norbixin	$0.03^{b} \pm 0.00$	$0.32^{b} \pm 0.00$	$0.23^{c} \pm 0.01$	$0.35^{c} \pm 0.01$

Results are expressed as means (n=3) ± SD; significant differences from ANOVA test ($p<0.05$) indicated by superscripts (order of antioxidant activity: a< b <c).

The ability of carotenoids to decrease volatile aldehydes may seem to be in contradiction with the absence of their antioxidant character in inhibiting hydroperoxides formation in the same experiments. However, other antioxidants have similarly shown to exert a variable effect between the different stages of lipid oxidation. For instance, α-tocopherol was previously found to possess a prooxidant activity in oil-in-water emulsions, on the basis of hydroperoxide formation, but to inhibit hexanal formation with increasing concentrations under the same experimental conditions (Frankel et al., 1994). Frankel (1996) proposed that in the evaluation of antioxidants, it is important to distinguish between their effects at different stages of lipid oxidation. Therefore, such a contradictory picture was also observed for carotenoids under the present experimental conditions.

**Table 6. Effect of carotenoids (1 g l⁻¹) on the autoxidation of 10%
Tween-based olive o/w emulsions at 60°C.**

Treatment	[1]Conjugated dienes (CD) in g 100g⁻¹ at 30 days of storage	Protection factor (PF) (based on time to CD = 0.3 g 100g⁻¹)
Control	$0.33^b \pm 0.02$	$1.00^b \pm 0.00$
Tomato (Lycopene)	$0.46^a \pm 0.03$	$0.65^c \pm 0.03$
Marigold (Lutein)	$0.41^a \pm 0.01$	$0.64^c \pm 0.03$
Paprika	$0.34^b \pm 0.03$	$1.07^b \pm 0.03$
Annatto (Norbixin)	$0.22^c \pm 0.02$	$1.21^a \pm 0.03$

[1] CD results are expressed as mean (n=6) ± SD; significant differences from ANOVA test ($p<0.05$) indicated by superscripts (order of antioxidant activity: a< b <c).

[2] Protection factors (PF) are given by: time for the antioxidant treatment / time for the control, to reach the oxidation level of CD = 0.3 g 100 g⁻¹ (PF>1: antioxidant effect, PF<1: prooxidant effect, order of antioxidant activity: a>b>c)

7.2. Effect of Carotenoid Extracts on Autoxidation of Olive Oil-in-water Emulsions

The same natural carotenoid extracts added in 10% olive oil-in-water emulsions presented the results indicated in Table 6. Norbixin (water-soluble annatto) was again the only carotenoid that presented an antioxidant action, while marigold and tomato extracts acted as prooxidants by even increasing the production of conjugated dienes. Protective factors (PF) were calculated by the times required for conjugated dienes to reach a level of CD: 0.3 g/100g. As shown in Table 6, the results for PF values were in line with the above mentioned conclusions at the end of oxidation period.

8. Effect of Carotenoids During The Storage Autoxidation of Homogenised (Protein-Stabilised) Emulsions

High-pressure homogenization is an important process used in the preparation or stabilization of emulsions and suspensions, resulting in a decrease of the average droplet diameter and an increased interfacial area. The net result, from a practical point of view, is a much reduced tendency for creaming, contributing to an enhanced physical stability of the homogenized emulsions (Dimakou et al., 2007).

During the last years, milk proteins (e.g., caseins and whey proteins) are increasingly used as emulsifiers due to their property to facilitate both the formation and stability of food emulsions (Bot et al., 2003). More specifically, caseins and whey proteins are well known for their ability to prepare stable emulsions, by adsorbing at the interface, and creating thick stabilizing layers that protect oil droplets against flocculation and coalescence (Dickinson, 2001). A body of recent research has focused on homogenized, protein-stabilized oil-in-water emulsions, by elucidating their susceptibility at temperature-related microstructural irregularities (Kiokias et al., 2004; Kiokias and Bot, 2006; Kiokias et al., 2007). Concentrated protein-stabilised emulsions are structurally similar to relevant food emulsions (e.g., yoghurt, dairy cream or fresh cheese type of products).

Experimental results of carotenoids addition at an active concentration of $1g\,L^{-1}$ to emulsions composed of 30% sunflower oil and 2% of emulsifier mixture (sodium caseinate and Tween 20, 50/50) are presented in Table 7.

According to the results the hydrophobic carotenoids (β-carotene, lycopene) did not inhibit significantly ($p<0.05$) the production of conjugated diene hydroperoxides when compared with the control. On the contrary, the extracts containing mainly substituted carotenoids behaved as clear antioxidants, with the following hierarchy of activity (with c>b>a):

paprika extract[c] = bixin[c] (lipid soluble annatto extract) > lutein[b] (marigold-extract) > lycopene[a] (tomato-extract) = all-trans pure β-carotene[a] = control[a].

Table 7. Effect of various natural carotenoids ($1\,g\,l^{-1}$) against the production of primary and secondary oxidation products from the autoxidation of 30% sunflower protein based o/w emulsions at 60°C.

Treatment	Conjugated dienes-CD ($g\,kg^{-1}$) after 27 days of oxidation	Thiobarbituric acid related substances-TBARs ($mmol\,kg^{-1}$ oil) after 34 days of oxidation
Control	$7.18^a \pm 0.88$	$0.05^a \pm 0.01$
β-Carotene	$6.39^a \pm 0.29$	$0.04^a \pm 0.01$
Tomato (lycopene)	$6.46^a \pm 0.26$	$0.05^a \pm 0.01$
Paprika	$2.70^c \pm 0.14$	$0.02^b \pm 0.01$
Marigold (lutein	$4.59^b \pm 0.24$	$0.02^b \pm 0.00$
Annato (bixin)	$3.02^c \pm 0.28$	$0.02^b \pm 0.00$

CD and TBARs results are expressed as means (n=3) ± SD; significant differences from ANOVA test ($p<0.05$) indicated by superscripts (order of antioxidant activity: a< b <c).

Therefore, paprika containing mainly capsanthin and capsorubin (carotenoids with carbonyl end groups) and annatto (rich in bixin with carboxylic acid and ester groups) were the strongest radical scavengers in terms of conjugated diene hydroperoxides formation. The marigold extract containing mainly lutein isomers (with OH-groups at the ends of their polyene chain) still exerted an inhibitory effect against the production of conjugated hydroperoxides while the emulsions containing pure β-carotene or tomato extract (with non-substituted compounds: lycopene, α, β-carotene) did not differ significantly from the control. The above mentioned tendency therefore reveals a strong relationship between carotenoid structure and antioxidant potential in concentrated, homogenized emulsions.

The carotenoid extracts exerted a similar action against the formation of thiobarbituric-acid related substances (TBARs), produced through the breakdown of intermediate oxidation compounds. TBARs correlate well with the threshold values of undesirable "off flavours" (Hawrysh, 1990). The control emulsion and the emulsions containing hydrophobic carotenoids (β-carotene and lycopene) were not significantly different ($p<0.05$) and oxidised faster than the emulsions containing polar carotenoids (Table 7). Polar carotenoids (lutein, paprika extract, bixin) acted as clear antioxidants against the production of secondary oxidation products. Although lutein seems to offer less oxidative stability than paprika and bixin, statistical analysis revealed no significant differences between polar carotenoids.

Terao (1989) found that during the azo‐2, 2'‐azobis [2, 4 dimethylvalero nitrile] (AMVN) induced oxidation of methyl linoleate, canthaxanthin and astaxanthin (both having oxo-groups at the 4, 4' position of the β-ionone ring) were more effective antioxidants than β-carotene. Terao's results (though referred to synthetic and pure carotenoid substances) can associate themselves to the conclusions of our study, in which natural extracts rich in carotenoids with keto or carboxyl groups (paprika and annatto carotenoids) exhibited the strongest antioxidant character within the tested compounds. Moreover, in Terao's study, substitution of the hydrogen by a –OH group (zeaxanthin) did not increase the radical trapping ability. Our experimental results revealed that the marigold extract (containing mainly *all-trans* lutein with 2–OH groups in the molecule) was found to exert a lower antioxidant effect than the more polar carotenoid extracts but still a clear radical scavenging activity as compared to the control emulsion.

Calculations in previous studies (Britton, 1995) have shown that the electron density in the carotenoid polyene chain is greater towards the end of the carotenoid chromophore. Reactivity was found to be dependent on the nature of the end groups as these electron rich sites are likely to be preferred for reactions with free radical species. This theory seems to be confirmed by the enhanced antioxidant character of the polar xanthophylls (e.g., bixin, paprika, lutein, etc.) as compared to extracts containing mainly hydrophobic carotenoids (such as α, β-carotene and lycopene).

Interestingly, certain polar carotenoids (paprika, lutein) presented a clear antioxidant activity in homogenized emulsions, though in the ultrasonicated Tween-based emulsions, they did not exert any antioxidant effect when added individually. It could be that the experimental conditions may modulate the carotenoid activity. Therefore, the enhanced antioxidant activity of the more polar carotenoids in the protein-based emulsions could be explained by a favourable effect of homogenisation. The process of homogenisation under high pressure (e.g., 300 bars) may facilitate a better dispersion of the carotenoids in the oil phase of the emulsion resulting in their more efficient absorption at the oil water interface (as compared to the application of ultrasonication). Moreover, in the homogenised protein emulsions, an emulsifying mixture containing 50% of sodium caseinate has been recently found to exert an inhibitory effect on the emulsion oxidation as compared to Tween alone (Kiokias et al., 2006). Therefore, a synergistic effect of polar carotenoids with sodium caseinate in the interface could not be excluded as an alternative hypothesis for their strong radical scavenging character in the protein stabilised emulsions. Such a favourable interaction may not be observed in case of β-carotene or lycopene, which as hydrophobic carotenoids are expected to be located in the core of the oil droplets.

9. Combined Effect of Carotenoids in Mixtures with Other Natural Antioxidants

The most effective antioxidant systems for foods contain various antioxidants with different mechanisms of action and/or physical properties (Palozza, 1998). Components of mixed antioxidant systems can contribute to the inhibition of oxidation with the resulting antioxidant activity reflecting either additive or synergistic effects of the components (Kiokias et al., 2008). The use of synergistic mixtures of antioxidants was found to increase the antioxidant effectiveness as compared with the activity of each separate compound (Abdalla & Roozen, 1999; Kiokias & Gordon, 2004).

In case of carotenoids, a synergistic effect of lutein mixed with lycopene, against the oxidative damage of multilamellar liposomes has been reported (Stahl & Sies, 1997). In addition, combinations of various carotenoids have been reported to interact significantly in vivo (Chopra et al., 1996; Johnson et al., 1995) as well as to act efficiently against the azo-inititiated oxidation of sunflower based o/w emulsions (Kiokias, 2002).

It has been reported that carotenoids may play a role in recycling phenolic antioxidants, e.g., tocopherols (Tan & Saley, 1991). According to Bohm et al. (1997), a synergistic effect, observed in cell protection by β-carotene and vitamin E, may be related to the fact that β-carotene is not only quenching oxy-radicals but is also repairing the α-tocopheroxyl radicals (Reaction 9.1). Such a synergistic mechanism requires that the CAR$^{\bullet}$ is reconverted to CAR (Palozza & Krinsky, 1992).

$$CAR + TO^{\bullet} \Rightarrow CAR^{\bullet} + TOH \qquad\qquad (9.1)$$

Indeed, Palozza and Krinsky (1992) found that a combination of β-carotene with α-tocopherol inhibited lipid peroxidation significantly better than the sum of the effects of the individual antioxidants. Similarly, Henry et al. (1998) found that a mixture of β-carotene with α- or δ-tocopherol exhibited a stronger antioxidant effect than each single compound did. Palozza et al. (1995) reported that carotenoids exerted their radical trapping activity more efficiently when acting cooperatively with tocopherols in microsomal membranes.

Other photolysis studies demonstrated that carotenoid radicals are reduced by α- or β-tocopherols by an electron transfer mechanism as shown in Reaction 9.2 (Bohm et al., 1998). Tocopherols quench radicals directly, retard the formation of the carotenoid radical and inhibit its further degradation.

$$CAR^{\bullet} + TOH \rightarrow CAR + TO \qquad\qquad (9.2)$$

Lievonen (1996) reported that mixtures of γ-tocopherol with lutein (but not with α-carotene) were strongly antioxidative against the oxidation of a purified triglyceride fraction of rapeseed oil. Haila et al. (1997) observed that a combination of lutein and γ-tocopherol was more efficient than lutein alone. In vivo synergistic effects between tocopherols and carotenoids have been also reported in literature (Fuhrman et al., 2000).

Several in vitro studies have investigated for any interaction effect between carotenoids and vitamin C. Bohm et al. (1997) found that ascorbic acid can indeed reduce the carotenoid radical cations according to the Reaction 9.3 and thereby reinforce its antioxidant activity:

$$CAR^{\bullet +} + AscH_2 \rightarrow CAR + AscH^{\bullet} + H^{+} \qquad\qquad (9.3)$$

In a biological environment carotenoid radical cations would most probably orientate within the cell membrane so that the charge is near the polar interface and thus it is accessible to ascorbic acid in the aqueous phase (Jorgensen & Skibsted, 1993). The mechanism of carotenoids antioxidant action by interaction with ascorbic acid in a membrane system could be described as follows (Kiokias, 2002): Carotenoids with a 4-carbonyl group (such as astaxanthin) can trap an alkoxyl radical in the central hydrophobic region of the bilayer so that the conjugated polyene structure transports the unpaired electron to the lipid-water interphase, where the resonance-stabilised carotenoid reacts with ascorbic acid (water soluble reductant). The reaction yields non-radical products in the lipid phase and an ascorbyl radical in the aqueous phase.

According to Kanner (1977), the presence of an ascorbic acid-cupric ion couple at relatively high concentration inhibits carotene degradation in a β-carotene linoleate model system and thereby reinforces the antioxidant activity of the carotenoid. Besides, the stability of carotenoids during the storage of mago pulp, in the presence of ascorbic acid, has been observed by Sudhakar and Maini (1994).

A tendency of increased carotenoid antioxidant activity in presence of ascorbic acid was also reported during the azo-initiated oxidation of sunflower-based emulsions (Kiokias, 2002). In such a dispersed system, the ascorbic acid in the aqueous phase is likely to interact directly with azo-peroxy radicals and a reduction in the azo-peroxy radicals concentration before their subsequent reaction with lipid molecules appears to be the dominant effect of the ascorbic acid.

Mortensen and Skibsted (1998) proposed that dietary carotenoids react with a wide range of radical species to produce radical cations by electron transfer, which in turn react with vitamin C resulting in the regeneration of the carotenoid.

Norbixin was examined in mixtures with other common natural antioxidants (α-, and δ-, tocopherols, ascorbic acid and ascorbyl palmitate) in olive oil and 10% olive oil-in-water emulsions, which were left to autoxidise in an oven at constant temperature (60°C). All additives showed antioxidant activity in bulk oil, when oil deterioration was assessed by the peroxide value (Table 8), and the order of activity was: ascorbic acid > ascorbyl palmitate = δ-tocopherol = norbixin > α-tocopherol. The effect of the antioxidants was confirmed by analysis of the volatiles produced during lipid oxidation. Hexanal and 2-heptenal peaks were detected consistently in the samples, and these were produced from decomposition of linoleate hydroperoxides (13- and 9-OOH respectively). Other aldehydes such as octanal (form oleic acid 8-OOH), nonanal, 2-nonenal, 2 decenal (from oleic acid-9-OOH) formed during decomposition of oleate hydroperoxides, were also detected in the oxidized oil substrate. According to the results, expressed as total volatiles (Table 8), ascorbic acid was again being very effective while α-tocopherol did not inhibit the formation of volatiles. Combinations of norbixin with the natural antioxidants were strong antioxidants against the production of volatile aldehydes.

When the antioxidants added at the same concentration (0.1 mM) to oil-in-water emulsions, they also retarded the formation of hydroperoxides, but with a different order of antioxidant activity such as: norbixin = δ-tocopherol > ascorbyl palmitate = α-tocopherol > ascorbic acid (Table 9).

The change in activity of ascorbic acid from being the strongest antioxidant in oil to the weakest in the emulsion has been previously reported (Frankel et al., 1994) and the change in order of activity is consistent with the "polar paradox" theory. According the polar paradox, hydrophilic antioxidants are more active in oil whereas lipophilic antioxidants such as tocopherols and ascorbyl palmitate are more effective in the emulsion system, since they are concentrated at the oil-water interface where they are effective in quenching radicals generated in the aqueous phase. Norbixin molecules are soluble in water, mainly as aggregates, and insoluble in oil but the carotenoid is probably oriented at the oil - water interface in the emulsion due to its extensive hydrocarbon backbone. This would allow it to show the strong antioxidant activity observed in the emulsion system.

Table 8. Effect of norbixin (2mM) and mixtures compared with antioxidants (0.1 mM) on the oxidative stability of bulk olive oil at 60° after 40 days of storage.

Treatment	[1]Peroxide values (meq kg^{-1})	[2]Protection factors (PF)	[1]Volatile aldehydes (mg kg^{-1})		Synergy (%)
			Hexanal	Total volatiles	
Control	76.9^d ± 4.2	1.00	0.83^e ± 0.09	2.59^e ± 0.35	-------
Norbixin	55.6^b ± 3.1	1.26	0.73^d ± 0.06	2.26^d ± 0.15	------
α-tocopherol (AT)	60.7^c ± 3.3	1.15	0.89^e ± 0.06	2.82^e ± 0.17	------
δ-tocopherol (DT)	53.5^b ± 2.7	1.27	0.75^d ± 0.04	2.34^d ± 0.21	------
ascorbic acid (AS)	40.4^a ± 2.1	1.62	0.16^b ± 0.03	0.74^c ± 0.14	------
ascor-palmitate (AP)	47.7^b ± 2.2	1.42	0.32^c ± 0.04	0.85^c ± 0.21	------
Norbixin + AT	39.9^a ± 1.2	1.73	0.12^b ± 0.02	0.53^b ± 0.07	-27.4
Norbixin + DT	44.5^a ± 2.8	2.93	0.10^b ± 0.03	0.45^b ± 0.05	-13.3
Norbixin + AS	49.3^b ± 2.4	3.33	0.04^a ± 0.01	0.19^a ± 0.04	-17.6
Norbixin + AP	51.4^b ± 3.4	3.47	0.06^a ± 0.02	0.16^a ± 0.04	-50.8

[1] Mean (n=6) ± SD; Significant differences from ANOVA test (p<0.05) indicated by superscripts (order of antioxidant activity for both PV and volatiles: a>b>c>d>e)

[2] Protection factors (PF) are given by the ratio: time for the antioxidant treatment / time for the control, to reach the oxidation level of PV= 50 meq kg^{-1} (PF>1: antioxidant effect, PF<1: prooxidant effect, order of antioxidant activity: a>b>c)

In refined olive oil, combinations of norbixin with α- and δ-tocopherol showed enhanced activity compared with each antioxidant, although the effects were additive rather than synergistic. Synergism between the various carotenoid and vitamins (tocopherols or ascorbic acid) was evaluated by the following equation:

% Synergism = [IP mixture –(IP vitamin + IP carotenoid)]*100/(IP vitamin +IP carotenoid)

where IP= induction period, calculated here as the time required for samples to reach a PV=5 meq kg^{-1} (low level indicating that oxidation has not proceeded yet).

In every case, negative values for % synergism were obtained for each mixture of carotenoid with tocopherols. Combinations of norbixin with ascorbic acid or ascorbyl palmitate did not lead to increased protection against lipid autoxidation compared with the individual additives when oil deterioration was assessed by peroxide values (Table 8).

In the emulsion system, combinations of norbixin with the other additives reduced the oxidative deterioration of the samples to a greater extent than the individual additives The protective effect, calculated by induction times to conjugated diene values of 0.5 g/100g, was synergistic for each combination (Table 9) with synergy being greatest between norbixin and ascorbic acid (23.5%).

Table 9. Antioxidant effects of norbixin (2 mM) and mixtures compared with other antioxidants (0.1 mM) on the oxidative stability of 10% olive oil-in-water emulsions at 60° after 40 days of storage.

Treatment	[1]Conjugated dienes (g 100g^{-1})	Protection factors (PF)	Synergism (%)
Control	2.41^d ± 0.02	1.00	-------
Norbixin	1.49^a ± 0.03	1.33	------
α-tocopherol (AT)	1.94^b ± 0.05	1.14	------
δ-tocopherol (DT)	1.48^a ± 0.03	1.37	------
ascorbic acid (AS)	2.08^c ± 0.05	1.17	------
ascor-palmitate (AP)	1.98^b ± 0.07	1.33	------
Norbixin + AT	1.31^b ± 0.04	1.73	+ 8.3
Norbixin + DT	0.91^a ± 0.03	2.93	+13.5
Norbixin + AS	1.23^b ± 0.04	2.33	+ 23.5
Norbixin + AP	0.92^a ± 0.03	2.97	+ 21.4

[1] CD results are expressed as mean (n=6) ± SD; significant differences from ANOVA test (p<0.05) indicated by superscripts (order of antioxidant activity: a> b >c>d).

[2] Protection factors (PF) are given by: time for the antioxidant treatment / time for the control, to reach the oxidation level of CD= 0.5 g 100 g^{-1} (PF>1: antioxidant effect, PF<1: prooxidant effect, order of antioxidant activity: a>b>c)

Table 10. Effect of carotenoids (1 g l^{-1}) mixed with olive oil polar extract (0.2 g l^{-1}) on the oxidative stability of bulk olive oil and 10% Tween-based olive o/w emulsions at 60°C.

Treatment	[1]Peroxide values (PV, meq kg^{-1}) of olive oil at 30 days of storage	[2]Conjugated dienes (CD g 100g^{-1}) of olive oil-in-water emulsions at 30 days of storage
Control	101.8^a ± 6.3	0.33^b ± 0.02
Olive oil extract (OE)	89.4^b ± 5.2	0.20^c ± 0.02
Paprika + OE	60.5^d ± 4.5	0.28^b ± 0.02
Tomato (Lycopene) + OE	80.5^c ± 7.3	0.29^b ± 0.02
Annatto (Norbixin) + OE	51.4^d ± 3.3	0.18^c ± 0.02
Marigold (Lutein) + OE	92.5^b ± 6.8	0.27^b ± 0.03

[1] PV results are expressed as mean (n=6) ± SD; significant differences from ANOVA test (p<0.05) indicated by superscripts (order of antioxidant activity: a< b <c< d).

[2] CD results are expressed as mean (n=6) ± SD; significant differences from ANOVA test (p<0.05) indicated by superscripts (order of antioxidant activity: a< b).

The interaction of carotenoids with the phenolic extracts from olive oil was also examined in both bulk olive oil and olive oil-in-water emulsions (Table 10). Phenyl alcohols (3,4-dihydroxyphenylethanol, and p-hydroxyphenylethanol) and phenyl acids (caffeic acid, p-coumaric acid, ferulic, syringic and vanillic acid), are present in the olive oil extract and contribute to its clear antioxidant efficiency (Blekas et al., 1995; Satue et al., 1995). In any combination, it was observed that antioxidant mixtures significantly reduced peroxide values compared with the control during oxidation of bulk olive oil, and generally had a better activity than the phenolic extract itself (Table 10). In olive oil-in-water emulsions, norbixin mixtures with olive oil extract presented a clear antioxidant action, , while mixtures of marigold and tomato and paprika extracts were not significant different from the control considering the production of conjugated dienes. However, in contrast with the experiment in bulk oil where all the antioxidant mixtures had a strong effect, here only the norbixin-olive oil extract mixture reduced significantly the oxidation rate.

Data in the literature suggest that the presence of other antioxidants, such as phenolic compounds, may modify the involvement of carotenoids in the oxidative process. In the presence of a sufficiently high concentration of other antioxidants, carotenoids may behave as antioxidants, even though they presented a prooxidant character in the absence of other additives (Palozza, 1998). There is little research evidence about carotenoid interactions with olive oil extracts, but a few studies have proposed a synergistic effect when olive oil polar phenolics are associated with tocopherols (Salvador et al., 1999).

Conclusion

The antioxidant activity of carotenoids is mainly due to their radical scavenging ability. However, in certain cases, depending on the different experimental conditions, they may even act as prooxidants. This is affected by several factors, such as oxygen partial pressure, concentration, structure, presence of light, etc. In a series of experiments, β-carotene and several natural carotenoid extracts (such as tomato, marigold, paprika and annatto extracts) were tested in vitro in different food-related emulsion systems. The carotenoid preparations were found to be strong antioxidants during the AAPH-initiated oxidation of sunflower oil-in-water emulsions, while they also inhibited significantly the production of secondary oxidation products in autoxidised model Tween emulsions. Considering the homogenised protein-based emulsions only, the most polar preparations exerted an enhanced antioxidant character.

Carotenoids can also be combined in mixtures with other natural antioxidants having different mechanisms of action. Components of mixed antioxidant systems may contribute to the inhibition of oxidation, reflecting either additive or synergistic effects of the components. The mixtures of carotenoids with other natural antioxidants (tocopherols, ascorbic acid and olive oil phenolics) showed, in certain cases, a better antioxidant activity than that of the the individual preparations, exhibiting a kind of synegism against the oxidative deterioration of food emulsions.

The understanding of the parameters and mechanisms of action that modulated the antioxidant action of carotenoids will lead to optimisation of their activity in novel emulsion systems. This could offer a basis for their more systematic use by the food industry as functional ingredients, which could protect the related food products against their sensory and nutritional oxidative deterioration.

References

Abdalla, E. A. & Roozen, P. J. (1999). Effect of plant extracts on the oxidative stability of sunflower oil and emulsion. *Food Chemistry, 64*, 323-329.

Akoh, C. C. & Min, B. D. (1997). *Food Lipid Chemistry, Nutrition and Biotechnology*. New York: Marcel Dekker.

Azuma, K., Ippoushi, K., Ilto, H., Higashio, H. & Terao, J. (1999). Evaluation of antioxidative activity of vegetable extracts in linoleic acid emulsion and phospholipid bilayers. *Journal of the Science of Food and Agriculture, 79*, 2010-2016.

Bast, A., Haanen, G. R. & VandenBerg, H. (1998). Antioxidant effects of carotenoids. *International Journal for Vitamin and Nutrition Research, 68*, 399-403.

Beltran, G., Aguilera, M. P. & Gordon, M. H. (2005). Solid phase microextraction of volatile oxidation compounds in oil-in-water emulsion. *Food Chemistry, 92*, 401-406.

Blekas, G., Tsimidu, M. & Bosku, D. (1995). Contribution of α-tocopherol to olive oil stability. *Food Chemistry, 52*, 289-294.

Bohm, F., Edge, R., Lange, L. & Truscott, T. G. (1998). Enhanced protection of human cells against ultraviolet antioxidant combinations involving dietary carotenoids. *Journal of Photochemistry and Photobiology, 44*, 211-215.

Bohm, F., Edge, R., Lange, L., McGarvey, J. & Truscott, T. G. (1997). Carotenoids enhance vitamin E antioxidant activity. *American Chemical Society, 119*, 621-622.

Bot, A., Kiokias, S., van Maurik, S., Hoos, P. B. & Reszka, A. A. (2003). Droplet size measurements in heat-treated acidified protein stabilised oil-in-water emulsions using static light scattering and low-field NMR. *Food Structure and Rheology, 3*, 353-357.

Britton, G. (1995). Structure and properties of carotenes in relation to function. *The Journal of the Federation of American Societies for Experimental Biology, 9*, 1551-1558.

Bub, A., Waltz, B., Abrahamse, Z., Adam, S., Wever, J., Muller, H. S. & Rechenmmer, G. (2000). Moderate intervention with carotenoid rich vegetable products reduces lipid peroxidation in men. *American Society for Nutritional Sciences, 130*, 2200-2206.

Burton, W. G. & Ingold, K. U. (1984). Beta carotene: An unusual type of lipid antioxidant. *Science, 224*, 569-573.

Burton, W. G. (1988). Antioxidant action of carotenoids. *British Journal of Nutrition, 119*, 109-111.

Chen, J. H., Lee, T. C. & Ho, C. T. (1997). Antioxidant effect and kinetics study of capsanthin on the chlorophyll-sensitized photooxidation of soybean oil and selected flavor compounds. *ACS Symposium Series, 660*, 188-198.

Chopra, M., Thurhan, D. J. & Wilson, R. L. (1996). Free radical scavenging of lutein in vitro. *Annals of the New York Academy of Sciences, 1*, 246-249.

Di Mascio, P., Sundquist, A. R, Devasagayam, T. P. A. & Sies, H. (1992). Assay of lycopene and other carotenoids as singlet oxygen quenchers. *Methods in Enzymology, 213*, 429-438.

Dickinson, E. (2001). Milk protein interfacial layers and the relationship to emulsion stability and rheology. *Colloids and Surfaces B: Biointerfaces, 20*, 197-210.

Dimakou, C., Kiokias, S., Tsaprouni, I. & Oreopoulou, V. (2007). Effect of processing and storage parameters on oxidative deterioration of oil-in-water emulsions. *Food Biophysics, 2*, 38-45.

Fakourelis, E. C. & Min, B. D. (1987). Effects of chlorophyll and β-carotene on the oxidative stability of olive oil. *Journal of Food Science, 52*, 234-235.

Farombi, E. O. & Britton, G. (1999). Antioxidant activity of palm oil carotenes in organic solution-effect of structural and chemical reactivity. Food Chemistry, *64*, 315-321.

Faure, H., Galabert, G., Le Moel, G. & Nabet, F. (1999). Carotenoids: metabolism and physiology. *Annales de Biologie Clinique, 57*, 169-183.

Frankel, E. N. (1996). Antioxidants in lipid foods and their impact on food quality. *Food Chemistry, 57,* 51-56.

Frankel, E. N., Huang, W., Kanner, J. & German, B. (1994). Interfacial phenomena in the evaluation of antioxidants: bulk oils vs emulsions. *Journal of Agricultural and Food Chemistry, 42,* 1054-1059.

Fuhrman, B., Volkova, N., Rosenhalt, M. & Aviram, M. (2000). Lycopene synergistically inhibits LDL oxidation in combination with vitamin E, rosmarinic acid, carnosic acid, or garlic. *Antioxidant & Redox Signalling, 2,* 491-506.

Goulson, M. J. & Wartensen, I. J. (1999). Stability and antioxidant activity of β-carotene in conventional and high oleic canola oil. *Journal of Food Science, 64,* 996-999.

Grobush, K., Lanner, L. J., Geleinjinse, J. M., Boeing, H., Hofman, A. & Witteman, J. C. (2000). Serum carotenoids and atherosclerosis. The Roterdam Study. *Atherosclerosis, 148,* 49-56.

Haila, K. M., Nielsen, B. R., Heinonen, M. I. & Skibsted, L. H. (1997). Carotenoid reaction with free radicals in acetone and toluene at different oxygen partial pressures. *Zeitschrift fur Lebbensmitteln, 204,* 81-87.

Halliwell, B. & Gutteridge, J. Free radicals in Biology and Medicine. 2nd Edition. Oxford: Clavenendon Preis; 1995.

Hart, J. D. & Scott, K., (1995). Development and evaluation of HPLC methods for the analysis of carotenoids in foods and the measurement of carotenoid content of vegetables commonly consumed in UK. *Food Chemistry, 54,* 101-111.

Hawrysh, J. Z. (1990). Title: Stability of conola oil. In: Shahidi, F, editor. *Title: Canola & rapeseed oil. Production, chemistry, nutrition, and processing.* New York: Van Nortland Reinhlod; 99-122.

Heinonen, M., Haila. K., Lampi, M. & Piironen, V. (1997). Inhibition of oxidation in 10% oil in water emulsions by β-carotene with α-, γ-, and δ- tocopherols. *Journal of the American Oil Chemists' Society, 74,* 1047-1051.

Henry, L. K., Gatignani, G. L. & Scwharz, S. (1998). The influence of carotenoids and tocopherols on the stability of safflower seed oil during heat-catalysed oxidation. *Journal of the American Oil Chemists' Society, 75,* 1399-1402.

Johnson, E., Suter, M. P., Sahum, N., Ribayo-Mercado, R. & Russell, M. R. (1995). Interaction between β-carotene intake and plasma concentrations of carotenoid and retinoids. *American Journal of Clinical Nutrition, 62,* 598-603.

Jorgensen, K. & Skibsted, L. H. (1993). Carotenoid scavenging of radicals-effect of carotenoid structure and oxygen partial pressure on antioxidative activity. *Zeitshrift fur lebensmitteln, 196,* 423-429.

Kanner, J. (1977). Prooxidant and antioxidant effects of ascorbic acid and metal salts in α- and β-carotene linoleate model system. *Journal of Food Sci*ence, *42,* 60-64.

Kasaikina, O. T., Kartaseva, Z. S., Lobanova, T. V. & Sirota, T. V. (1998). Effect of environmental factors on the β-carotene reactivity toward oxygen and free radicals. *Biologiche Membrany, 15,* 168-176.

Kennedy, T. A. & Liebler, D. C. (1992). Peroxyl radical scavenging by β-carotene in lipid bilayers. *Journal of Biological Chemistry, 267,* 4658-4662.

Khachik, F., Beecher, G. R. & Smith, J. C. (1995). Lutein, lycopene, and their oxidative metabolites in chemoprevention of cancer. *Journal of Cellular Biochemistry*, *22*, 236-246.

Kiokias, S. & Bot, A. (2006). Temperature cycling stability of pre-heated acidified whey protein-stabilised o/w emulsion gels in relation to the internal surface area of the emulsion, *Food Hydrocolloids*, *20*, 246-252.

Kiokias, S. & Gordon M. (2004). Properties of carotenoids in *vitro* and in *vivo*. *Food Reviews International*, *20*, 99-121.

Kiokias, S. & Gordon, M. (2003a). Antioxidant properties of annatto carotenoids. *Food Chemistry*, *83*, 523-529.

Kiokias, S. & Gordon, M. (2003b). Dietary supplementation with a natural carotenoid mixture decreases oxidative stress. *European Journal of Clinical Nutrition*, *57*, 1135-1140.

Kiokias, S. (2002). In *vitro* and in *vivo* antioxidant properties of natural carotenoid mixtures. PhD Thesis. School of Food Biosciences, The University of Reading.

Kiokias, S., Dimakou, C. & Oreopoulou,V. (2007). Effect of heat treatment and droplet size on the oxidative stability of whey protein emulsions. *Food Chemistry*, *105*, 94-100.

Kiokias, S., Dimakou, C., Tsaprouni, I. & Oreopoulou,V. (2006). Effect of compositional factors against the thermal oxidative deterioration of novel food emulsions. *Food Biophysics*, *1*, 115-123.

Kiokias, S., Reiffers-Magnani, C. & Arjen Bot. (2004). Stability of whey-protein stabilized oil in water emulsions during chilled storage and temperature cycling. *Journal of Agricultural and Food Chemistry*, *52*, 3823- 3830.

Kiokias, S., Varzakas, T. & Oreopoulou, V. (2008). In vitro activity of vitamins, flavonoids, and natural phenolic antioxidants against the oxidative deterioration of oil-based systems. *Critical Reviews in Food Science and Nutrition*, *48*, 78-93.

Kiritsakis, A. Olive oil-from tree to the table. 2nd Edition. Trumbull: Food and Nutrition Press; 1998.

Kovary, K., Lourain, T., Silva, C., Albano, F., Pires, M. B., Lage, S. L. & Felzenswalb, I. (2001). Biochemical behavior of norbixin during in vitro DNA damage induced by reactive oxygen species. *British Journal of Nutrition*, *85*, 431-440.

Kritchevski, S. B. (1999). β-carotene, carotenoids and the prevention of coronary heart disease. *The Journal of Nutrition*, *129*, 5-8.

Lee, H. S. & Min, B. D. (1990) Effects, quenching mechanisms, and kinetics of carotenoids in chlorophyll-sensitized photo-oxidation of soyabean oil. *Journal of Agricultural and Food Chemistry*, *38*, 1630-1634.

Liebler, D. C. & Kennedy, T. A. (1992). Epoxide products of β-carotene antioxidant reactions. *Methods in Enzymology*, *213*, 472-479.

Liebler, D. C. & McClure, T. D. (1996). Antioxidant reactions of β-carotene: Identification of carotenoid-radical adducts. *Chemical Research in Toxicology*, *9*, 8-11.

Liebler, D. C., Stratton, S. P. & Kaysen, K. L. (1997). Antioxidant actions of β-carotene in liposomal and microsomal membranes: role of carotenoid-membrane incorporation and α-tocopherol. *Archives of Biochemistry and Biophysics*, *338*, 244-250.

Liebler, D. C. (1993). Antioxidant reaction of carotenoids. *Annals of the New York Academy of Sciences*, *691*, 20-31.

Liegeois, C., Lernseau, G. & Collins, S. (2000). Measuring antioxidant efficiency of wort, malt, and hops against the 2,2,-azobis (2-qmidinopropane) dihydrochloride-induced oxidation of an aqueous dispersion of linoleic acid. *Journal of Agricultural and Food Chemistry*, 48, 1129-1134.

Lievonen, S. (1996). The effects of carotenoids on lipid oxidation. PhD Thesis. Food Department of University of Elsinky.

Lominsky, S., Grossman, S. & Bergaman, H. (1997). In vitro and *in vivo* effects of β-carotene in rat epidermal lipoxygenase. *International Journal for Vitamin and Nutrition Research*, 67, 407-414.

Mangels, G. A., Holden, M. J., Beecher, G. R. & Lanza, E. (1993). The carotenoid content of fruits and vegetables on evaluation of analytical data. *Journal of the American Dietetic Association*, 93, 284-296.

Matos, H. R., Di Mascio, P. & Medeiroc, M. H. G. (2000). Protective effect of lycopene on lipid peroxidation and oxidative damage in cell culture. *Archives of Biochemictry and Biophysics*, 383, 56-59.

Matsufuji, H., Nakamura, H., Chino, M. & Takeda, M. (1998). Antioxidant activity of capsanthin and the fatty acid esters in paprika. *Journal of Agricultural and Food Chemistry*, 46, 3468-3472.

Miller, N. G., Pagagna, G., Wiseman, S., Van Nielen, W. & Rice-Evans, C. A. (1995). Total antioxidant capacity in LDL and the relationship with α-tocopherol. *Letters*, 365, 164-166.

Mortensen, A. & Skibsted, L. H. (1997). Importance of carotenoid structure in radical-scavenging reactions. *Journal of Agricultural and Food Chemistry*, 45, 2970-2977.

Mortensen, A. & Skibsted, L.H. (1998). Reactivity of β-carotene towards peroxyl radicals studied by later flash state photolysis. *Federation of European Biochemical Societies Letters*, 426, 392-396.

Mortensen, A., Skibsted, L. H., Sampson, J. & Everett, A. S. (1997). Comparative mechanisms and rates of free radical scavenging by carotenoid antioxidants. *Federation of European Biochemical Societies Letters*, 418, 91-97.

Nielsen, B. R., Mortensen, A., Jorgenesen, K. & Skibsted, L. H. (1997). Singlet versus triplet reactivity in photodegradation of C40 carotenoids. *Journal of Agricultural and Food Chemistry*, 44, 2106-2113.

Niki, E., Noguchi, N., Tsuchihashi, H. & Goton, N. (1995). Interactions among vitamin E, vitamin C, and β-carotene. *American Journal of Clinical Nutrition*, 62, 1322s-1326s.

Palozza, P. & Krinsky, N. I. (1992). Antioxidant effects of carotenoids in *vitro* and *in vivo*. An overview. *Methods in Enzymology*, 213, 403-420.

Palozza, P. (1998). Pro-oxidant actions of carotenoids in biological systems. *Nutrition Reviews*, 56, 257-265.

Palozza, P., Calvello, G. & Bartoli, G. M. (1995). Prooxidant activity of β-carotene under 100% oxygen pressure in rat liver microsomes. *Free Radical Biology and Medicine*, 19, 887-892.

Pokorny, J. & Reblova, Z. (1999). Effect of food components on changes in frying oil. *Food Technology and Biotechnology*, 37, 139-143.

Pryor, W. A., Stahl, W. & Rock, C. L. (2000). Beta-carotene: From biochemistry to clinical trials. *Nutrition Reviews*, 58, 39-53.

rao, J. (1989). Antioxidant activity of β-carotene-related carotenoids in solution. *Lipids, 24,* 659-663.

Reische, WD., Dorris, A. & Eitenmiller, R. (1997). Title: Antioxidants. In: Akoh, CC. & Min, BD, editors. *Title: Food Lipid Chemistry, Nutrition and Biotechnology*; New York: Marcel Dekker; 489-516.

Ribayamercado, J. D., Solon, S. F., Tang, G., Cabal-Borza, M., Perfecto, S. C. & Russel, R. M. (2000). Bionconversion of plant carotenoids to Vit-A in Filipino school-aged children varies inversely with Vit-A status. *American Journal of Clinical Nutrition, 72,* 455-465.

Rice Evans, A. C. (2000). Measurement of total antioxidant action as a marker of antioxidant status *in vivo*. Proceedings and limitations, *Free Radical Research, 33,* 59-68.

Salvador, M. D., Arande, F. & Fregapane, C. (1999). Contribution of chemical components of virgin olive oils to oxidative stability. *Journal of the American Oil Chemists' Society, 76,* 427-431.

Satue, T., Hung, S. W. & Frankel, E. N. (1995). Effect of natural antioxidants in virgin olive oil, on oxidative stability of refined, bleached and deodorized olive oil. *Journal of the American Oil Chemists' Society, 72,* 1131-1137.

Scott J. K., Finglas, P., Seale, R., Hart, D. & Gortz, I. (1996). Interlaboratory studies of HPLC procedures for the analysis of carotenoids in foods. *Food Chemistry, 57,* 85-90.

Snyder, J. M., Frankel, E. N. & Selke, E. (1985). Capillary gas chromatographic analysis of headspace volatiles from vegetable oils. *Journal of the American Oil Chemists' Society, 62,* 1675-1679.

Song, J., Gardner, B. D., Holland, F. J. & Beudry M. R. (1997). Rapid analysis of volatile flavour compounds in apple fruits using SPME and GC/Time-of-flight Mass Spectrometry. *Journal of Agricultural and Food Chemistry, 45,* 1801-1807.

Stahl, V. & Sies, H. (1997). Antioxidant defense: Vitamins E, C and carotenoids. *Diabetes, 46s,* 14-18.

Stocker, R., Yamamoto, Y., Mc Dough, A. F., Glazer, A. N. & Ames, B. N. (1994). Bilirubin is an antioxidant of possible physiological importance. *Science, 235,* 1043- 1044.

Sudhakar, D. V. & Maini, S. B. (1994). Stability of carotenoids during the storage of mago pulp. *Journal of Food Science and Technology, 31,* 228-230.

Tan, B. & Saley, M. H. (1991). Antioxidant activities of tocopherols and tocotrienols on plant color carotenes. *American Chemical Society, 202,* 39.

Terao, J. (1990). Inhibitory effects of carotenoids on singlet oxygen-initiated photooxidation of methyl-linolate and soybean oil. *Journal of Food Processing and Preservation, 4,* 79-93.

Van den Berg, H., Faulks, R., Granado, F., Hirscheberg, J., Olmedilla, B., Sandmann, G., Southon, S. & Stahl, W. (2000). The potential for the improvement of carotenoid levels in foods and the likely systematic effects. *Journal of the Science of Food and Agriculture, 80,* 880-912.

Vile, G. F. & Winterburn, C. C. (1988). Inhibition of microsomal lipid peroxidation by β-carotene, α-tocopherol and retinal at high and low oxygen pressures. *Federation of European Biochemical Societies Letters, 38,* 353-356.

Warner, K. & Frankel, E. N. (1987). Effects of β-carotene on light stability of soyabean oil. *Journal of the American Oil Chemists' Society, 64,* 213-218.

Woodall, A. A., Britton, G. & Jackson, M. J. (1997). Carotenoids and protection of phospholipids in solute or in liposomes against oxidation by peroxyl radicals. Relationship between structure and protective ability. *Biochimica et Biophysica Acta Subjects, 1336*, 575-586.

Yamauchi, R., Miyake, N. & Kato, K. (1993). Products formed by peroxyl radical mediated initiated oxidation of canthaxanthin, in benzene and in methyl linoleate. *Journal of Agricultural and Food Chemistry, 41*, 708-713.

Zabaras, D. & Wyllie, S. G. (2002). Rearrangement of p-menthane terpenes by Carboxen during HS-SPME. *Journal of Separation Science, 25*, 685-690.

Zhang, P. & Omaye, S. T. (2000). β-Carotene and protein oxidation: Effects of ascorbic acid and α-tocopherol. *Toxicology, 146*, 37-47.99

In: Encyclopedia of Vitamin Research
Editor: Joshua T. Mayer

ISBN: 978-1-61761-928-1
© 2011 Nova Science Publishers, Inc.

Chapter 38

Bioavailability and Metabolism of Dietary Flavonoids – Much Known – Much More to Discover[*]

David E. Stevenson[†1], Arjan Scheepens[2] and Roger D. Hurst[1]
[1]The New Zealand Institute for Plant and Food Research Limited,
Private Bag 3123, Waikato Mail Centre, Hamilton 3240, New Zealand
[2]The New Zealand Institute for Plant and Food Research Limited,
Private Bag 92-169, Mt Albert, Auckland, New Zealand

Abstract

There have been many epidemiological studies linking flavonoid intake to health benefits and many *in vitro* studies demonstrating various biological effects of flavonoids that should be reflected by health benefits. It has been widely assumed that these observations are linked and dietary flavonoids are readily absorbed into the circulation and influence many regulatory and signalling pathways in tissues. More recently, it has become apparent that only a small proportion of dietary flavonoid intake is actually absorbed directly and measured relative absorption varies about 2 orders of magnitude between different compounds.

It is also apparent that most of the dietary load of flavonoids finds its way to the colon where the numerous and varied microflora metabolise them into simpler but much more bioavailable compounds. Further complications to the bioavailability of flavonoids are added by human Phase II conjugative metabolism, which is thought to convert most absorbed flavonoids into polar conjugates.

---

[*] A version of this chapter was also published in *Flavonoids: Biosynthesis, Biological Effects and Dietary Sources, edited by Raymond B. Keller* published by Nova Science Publishers, Inc. It was submitted for appropriate modifications in an effort to encourage wider dissemination of research.
[†] Correspondence: Dr. David E Stevenson. Tel: +64 7 959 4485. Fax: +64 7 959 4431, E-Mail: dstevenson@ hortresearch.co.nz

There is no doubt that some unconjugated flavonoids do get into the circulation at low concentrations, but they are quantitatively swamped by the bulk of flavonoid conjugates and colonic metabolites.

In contrast with the much-studied metabolism of flavonoids, relatively little is known about the biological activities of their conjugates and metabolites, although what is known comes from a predominance of *in vitro* studies and suggests that the metabolites do have numerous and significant biological activities. Hence we actually know very little about the real and mostly indirect benefits and mechanisms of action of dietary flavonoids.

In this review, we discuss the current state of knowledge in this area, with the aim of stimulating further research (especially by intervention studies) to aid greater understanding.

Introduction

Numerous epidemiological trials have associated dietary flavonoid intake with health benefits, such as reductions in incidence of cardiovascular disease, stroke, diabetes and some types of cancer [1-12].

In addition, numerous *in vitro* studies have linked flavonoids to biological effects that could reasonably underlie the observed health benefits [13]. Although it is very tempting to assume a simple relationship between the two observations, decades of research into the absorption, distribution, metabolism and excretion (ADME) of flavonoids strongly contradicts this simplistic idea.

Research into this field started in the 1950s and was so prolific that in 1991, Scheline was able to include over 100 studies (mostly in animals) on flavonoid metabolism in his comprehensive "Handbook of mammalian metabolism of plant compounds" [14]. The main conclusion from all this work was that, unlike pharmaceutical compounds, which are mainly found relatively intact, as glucuronide derivatives in plasma or urine, flavonoids were much more extensively metabolised.

In addition to glucuronides, sulphates and methyl conjugates, the main urinary metabolites found were phenolic acids of the type also found to be produced by biotransformation using intestinal bacteria. A few studies using, ^{14}C-labelled flavonoids, found significant or even extensive degradation into simple compounds such as acetate, butyrate and carbon dioxide.

It appeared that the major part of the dietary flavonoid intake was not absorbed directly, but found its way into the colon where the extensive and varied microflora metabolised the flavonoids into simpler and apparently more bioavailable compounds. Examples of structures of the major compound classes discussed here are shown in Figure 1 (common flavonoids) and Figure 2 (common metabolites).

In recent years, much more detail has been added and we now have a relatively good understanding of flavonoid ADME. It appears that only a tiny proportion (approx 1-2%) of most dietary flavonoids is actually available to tissues and cells.

Most is metabolised by colonic microflora and most of the remainder that is absorbed through the gut is conjugated, mainly by glucuronidation, but also by sulphation and methylation.

The distribution of flavonoids is made more complex by factors like binding of flavonoids to serum proteins, such as albumin and the activities of cellular efflux pumps expressed by some cell types.

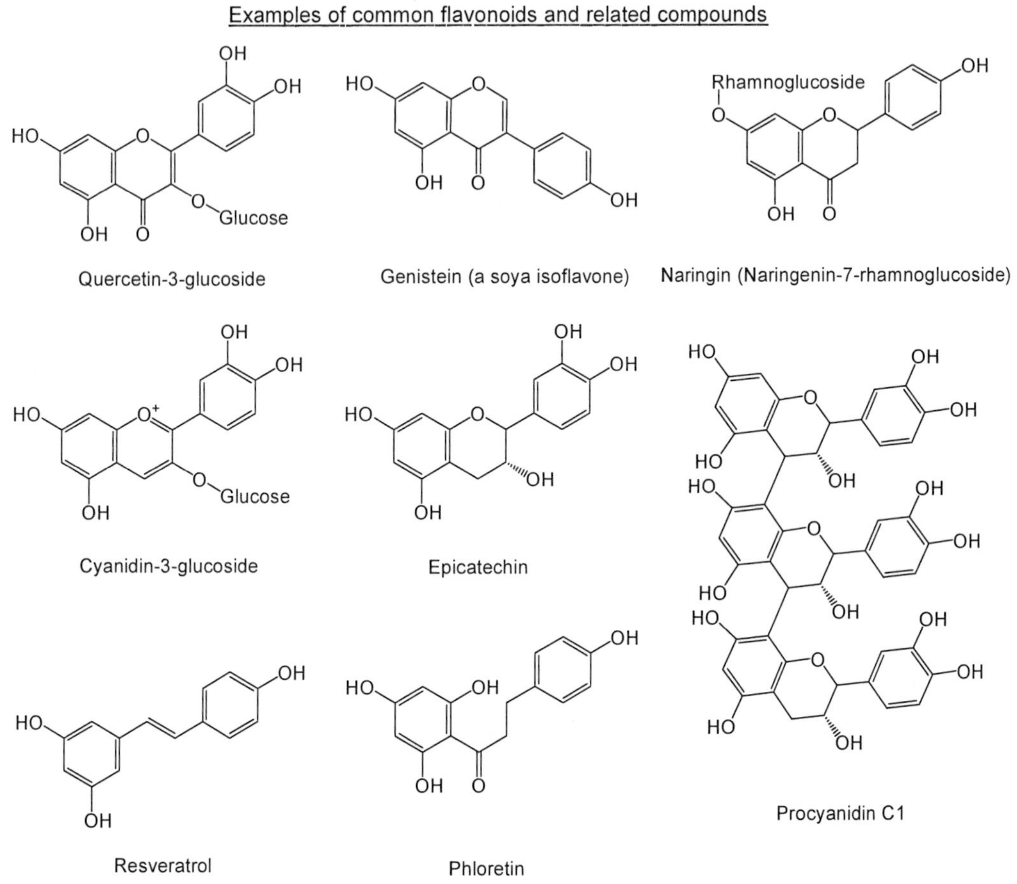

Examples of common flavonoids and related compounds

Figure 1. Structures of common flavonoids. Most flavonoids occur in plants predominantly as glycosides, with the exception of catechins and procyanidins. Resveratrol, a stilbene, is often found as its glucoside (piceid) and phloretin, a chalcone, as its glucoside (phloridzin).

There have been many excellent reviews discussing various aspects of these findings [15-30], but it is only relatively recently that serious attention has been given to determination of the biological activities of flavonoid metabolites and comparison with the parent compounds.

In contrast to the many hundreds of published studies on the biological effects of the quantitatively very minor species absorbed *in vivo*, i.e., flavonoid aglycones, published studies on metabolites only number around 50 at the time of writing.

We still, therefore, have little idea of the actual, as opposed to potential, relative contributions to health of flavonoid aglycones, flavonoid conjugates and colonic metabolites.

We have attempted to bring together all available information to date, to stimulate further research into the biology of flavonoid metabolites.

Our overall understanding of flavonoid ADME is summarised in Figure 3 and the chapter is organised to follow flavonoids through the various stages of digestion, absorption, distribution and metabolism and cover what is known about each stage.

The last section describes what we currently understand about the biological activities of the metabolites.

Examples of mammalian conjugates of flavonoids and colonic metabolites

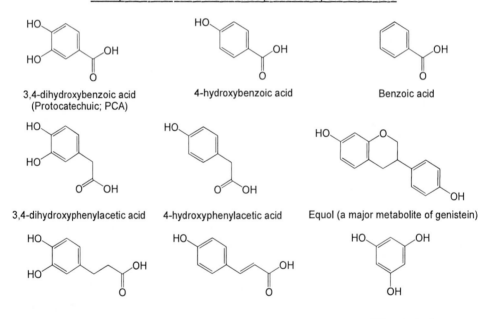

| Quercetin-7-glucuronide | Hippuric acid (benzoyl glycine) | Quercetin-7-sulphate |

Examples of Flavonoid metabolites produced by the colon flora

3,4-dihydroxybenzoic acid   4-hydroxybenzoic acid   Benzoic acid
(Protocatechuic; PCA)

3,4-dihydroxyphenylacetic acid   4-hydroxyphenylacetic acid   Equol (a major metabolite of genistein)

3,4-dihydroxyphenylpropionic acid   4-hydroxycinnamic acid (p-coumaric acid)   Phloroglucinol

Figure 2. Structures of some flavonoid conjugates and colon flora-derived metabolites. Many other isomers of the phenolic acids have been detected, e.g., 2-, 3-, and 4-hydroxybenzoic acid and also O-methylated metabolites.

It is important to note that, although hundreds of different flavonoids are produced by plants, in thousands of differently glycosylated forms, only a small proportion occurs commonly in human foods.

The majority of scientific studies to date have focussed on the major human dietary flavonoids and the information obtained does not necessarily apply to the majority of flavonoids.

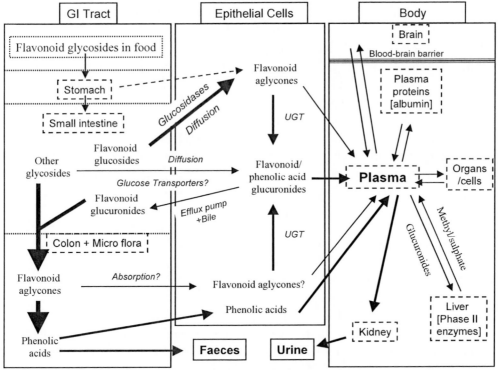

Figure 3. Summary of the great complexity of flavonoid metabolism, as currently understood. Thickness of arrows is an indication of relative quantitative significance of flows. UGT = Uridine diphosphoglucuronyl transferase. It has been estimated that dietary intake of flavonoids is ~100-200 mg/day [16, 31]; ~5% of this intake is absorbed via the intestine, ~95% passes into the colon [16].

Flavonoid Absorption and Metabolism in the Gastrointestinal Tract

The Oral Cavity

Human saliva was found to have significant, but highly variable hydrolytic activity [32], and hence hydrolysis of flavonoid glucosides may start in the oral cavity. It was not clear whether detached epithelial cells or bacteria, or both are the source of glucosidases. The resulting aglycones may be absorbed from the stomach, most likely by passive transport, whereas glycosides appear only to be absorbed by the intestine [33].

The Stomach

It is unclear whether procyanidins are metabolised in the stomach. In one study under simulated stomach acid conditions, procyanidins (epicatechin polymers, trimers to hexamers) have been found to be partially broken down, primarily to monomers and dimers [34]. This would be expected to enhance both bioavailability via intestinal absorption and colonic metabolism. In contrast, however, another study found that procyanidins were stable in the stomach [35], suggesting that they should be predominantly available to colonic flora.

Quercetin was absorbed in the rat stomach whereas its glycosides were not [33]. This suggests absorption by passive diffusion and the probable relative absence of suitable transporters or glycosidases. This result is the opposite of what is generally found in the intestine (see below). Anthocyanins at the very high concentration of 750 μM were absorbed directly from rat stomach to the extent of ~20% of the administered dose over 30 minutes [36]. The stomach is therefore clearly capable of anthocyanin absorption, but the physiological relevance of the high concentration used is questionable. Investigation of raspberry fruit extracts in an *in vitro* digestion model [37] suggested that anthocyanins and other flavonoids bind reversibly to other food components (protein, polysaccharides etc) and that this may increase their stability. This binding to polymers appears to modify the absorption and excretion of anthocyanins, but not their metabolism in rats [38], or pigs [39].

The Small Intestine

Manach *et al* [20] provided an excellent overview of the bioavailability of various flavonoids (aglycones and conjugates) and other relevant information obtained from a collection of human studies. Pharmacokinetic behaviour from these studies was very diverse, for example, the time to maximum plasma concentration ranged from 1-6 hours after dosing and elimination half-life from 1.5 hours to as long as nearly 20 hours. The percentage of dose excreted in the urine also varied from ~40% for isoflavone glycosides to under 1% for epigallocatechin gallate (EGCG), anthocyanins and rutin (quercetin rutinoside). Maximum reported plasma concentrations (C_{max}) also varied widely from 1-2 μM for isoflavones, quercetin glucosides and epigallocatechin (EGC), to 0.5 μM for naringin, 0.2 μM for rutin, 0.12 μM for EGCG and 0.03 μM for anthocyanins. Given that many studies have demonstrated that conjugates predominate in plasma, these results suggest that the concentrations of individual flavonoid aglycones are likely to be sub-micromolar [16, 18].

Table 1 summarises the main outcomes of human and animal studies, mostly carried out since the Manach *et al* review. In general, the results are very similar, but one recent development has been longer-term feeding studies to augment the more commonly studied single-dose trials. Resveratrol is a stilbene that has been relatively well-studied and its ADME appears similar to that of flavonoids, so some studies on resveratrol have also been included.

Table 2 summarises the main outcomes of *in vitro* cell-based studies, mostly using Caco-2 (human colon carcinoma) cell monolayers, a well-established system to measure parameters like permeability of the gut cell wall [40, 41]. The cells are grown to confluency on a semi-porous membrane, the upper or "apical" side corresponding to the intestinal lumen side and the lower or "basolateral" side corresponding to the "tissue" side of the intestinal wall. Samples are added to the apical medium and may or may not be detected in the basolateral medium, after passing through the cells. Caco-2 cells also express both functional Phase II conjugative enzymes and multi-drug resistance (MDR) efflux pumps, such as P-glycoprotein and breast cancer resistance protein (BCRP). Flavonoid conjugates have been detected in both the apical and basolateral medium, indicating that a compound has been taken up by the cells, conjugated and pumped back out [42]. This suggests that efflux pumps can limit bioavailability by returning flavonoid conjugates to the apical side/lumen, but cannot completely prevent some material from reaching the basolateral side/circulation.

The overall picture that emerges from the numerous bioavailability/metabolism studies is that there are essentially three groups of flavonoids with distinctively different behaviour, anthocyanins, procyanidins/catechins and "everything else". The aglycone forms of common flavonoids, such as quercetin, naringenin, or daidzein (and probably less common but structurally similar flavonoids) have been tested in many studies and are consistently the best-absorbed. These flavonoids are generally both more hydrophobic and more stable than anthocyanins or catechins and this may account for their higher observed plasma concentrations. Single doses routinely give plasma C_{max} values in the low micromolar range in humans (Table 1). Long-term dosing of pigs with quercetin gave similar results to single doses (~1 µM) [43], but in rats, plasma concentrations were over 20 µM, suggesting that pigs are probably a better model of human physiology [44]. Flavonoid aglycones, however, are rare in plant foods, glycosides usually being the only form found, with the exception of the relatively polar catechins, which are rarely glycosylated but, nevertheless, apparently much less bioavailable than hydrophobic compounds like quercetin. Where flavonoid aglycones are found in foods (specifically quercetin in onion skin), they appear to be more bioavailable than even glucoside derivatives [45].

The nature of glycosylation has an important influence on absorption. A number of studies have demonstrated the abundance of β-glucosidase, but the absence of other glycosidase activities in the GI tract and its tissues. Two β-glucosidases capable of hydrolysing flavonoid glycosides were found in human small intestinal mucosa. Lactase-phloridzin hydrolase (LPH) was localized in the apical membrane of gut epithelial cells while β-glucosidase was found in the cytosol [46]. This suggests that LPH can facilitate absorption by deglycosylating flavonoids and promoting passive diffusion, whereas the cytosolic enzyme can only act after absorption of the glucoside. Ovine lactase phloridzin hydrolase, a β-glucosidase found on the brush border of the mammalian small intestine, was readily able to hydrolyse glucosides of quercetin, genistein and daidzein [47]. Intestinal and liver β-glucosidases readily cleaved flavonoid glucosides, but not other glycosides [48]. There is some evidence from the studies in Table 2, that quercetin glucosides and maybe other flavonoid glucosides, can be transported intact by glucose transporters, but the main mechanism of glucoside absorption appears to be deglycosylation by membrane-bound β-glucosidase, followed by relatively rapid diffusion of the aglycone across the cell membrane [49-51]. Other glycosides may diffuse slowly across cell membranes [52-55], but the major proportion appears to pass into the colon, where microflora expressing various glycosidases can liberate the aglycones for absorption. It appears, for example, that a relatively high proportion of quercetin from the glucoside is absorbed from the intestine, as its plasma concentration peaks in 1-2 hours and it is predominantly cleared in 5-6 hours. In contrast, Rutin is absorbed much more slowly [56], to a much lower C_{max}, but most is deglycosylated in and absorbed from the colon as quercetin, giving a low but more sustained plasma level of quercetin conjugates that can last more than 24 hours.

Intestinal epithelial cells have high glucuronyl transferase activity and appear to glucuronidate ~95% of flavonoids before transfer into the bloodstream, or efflux back into the lumen [57-60].

Table 1. Summary of recent published studies involving determination of plasma/tissue bioavailability (C_{max}) from oral ingestion of flavonoids or flavonoid-rich foods and /or identification of major detected metabolites

Flavonoid/Source	Species	Bioavailability in plasma/tissues; Metabolites detected	Reference
Acylated anthocyanins from purple sweet potato	Human	Study on anthocyanins acylated with benzoic or cinnamic acids; plasma Cmax 2.5 μM after 1.5 hours; urinary excretion 0.01-0.03%; suggests absorption and plasma half-life much longer than non-acylated anthocyanins.	[76]
Anthocyanins from blackberry	Rat	Anthocyanins and methylated and/or glucuronidated metabolites detected in plasma, liver, kidney and brain (~0.25 μM); 0.2% of dose in urine.	[77]
Anthocyanins from Blood orange (fed 12 days)	Rat	~20% of dose absorbed from stomach, but only ~0.1% excreted in urine. Metabolites detected were methylated intact anthocyanins, plus un-metabolised anthocyanins.	[74]
Anthocyanins from grape	Rat/gastric intubation	~0.5 μM anthocyanins in plasma and brain after 10 min.	[78]
Apigenin, luteolin, oral/200 mg/kg	Rat	Peak plasma concentrations/% excreted in urine: Apigenin 50 μM/16%, Luteolin 15μM/6%; total recoveries ~40%, suggesting metabolism to simpler compounds in colon.	[79]
Apple juice	Ileostomised humans	Variable extent of metabolism of some unabsorbed flavonoids: Phloretin glycosides partially converted to phloretin and its 2-glucuronide; 90% of procyanidins recovered intact.	[60]
Apple juice, blueberries	Ileostomised humans	<33% of apple polyphenolics passed into collection bags, but up to 85% of those from blueberry. Suggests that berry phenolics are much more available for colonic metabolism.	[80]
Baicalein	Perfused rat intestine and Caco-2 monolayer	Extensive glucuronidation in both systems and efflux of glucuronide apically and basolaterally. Glucuronidation reduced proportionally at higher loadings of flavonoid.	[57]
Baicalin (plant-derived glucuronide of the flavone baicalein.	Rat	Baicalin readily absorbed in small intestine, to yield plasma baicalin. Baicalin poorly absorbed, but apparently readily de-glucuronidated by colonic flora, absorbed and then re-glucuronidated.	[81]
Bilberry extract, oral/400 mg/kg	Rat	Plasma anthocyanin C_{max} 1.2 μM after 15 minutes, 30% of dose excreted in urine.	[82]
Blackcurrant juice or whole fruit	Human	0.05% of anthocyanins excreted intact with ~5% of dose excreted in the form of hippuric acid and its 3- and 4-hydroxyl derivatives.	[71]
Blueberries up to 4% of diet	Pig	No anthocyanins in plasma or urine, but traces detected in all tissues tested.	[83]
Blueberry extract, 2% of diet/10 weeks	Aged rat	Anthocyanins detected in brain of treatment but not control group.	[84]

Table 1. (Continued)

Flavonoid/Source	Species	Bioavailability in plasma/tissues; Metabolites detected	Reference
Breviscapine (plant extract; 85% scutellarin)	Rat	11 glucuronides, methyl-glucuronides and sulpho-glucuronides.	[85]
Catechin epicatechin,	Isolated rat intestine	O-methylated (~30%), glucuronidated (~45%) conjugates (~20% with both) detected in the isolated jejunum after perfusion; 5 fold more flavanols overall, were detected in the isolated ileum after perfusion, predominantly unconjugated.	[86]
Catechins from tea	Human	Plasma C_{max} 1 μM catechins, after enzymic de-conjugation.	[87]
Catechins from tea	Rat foetal organs	Approx. 1 nM concentrations of catechins detected in foetal organs between 0.5-1 hour after dosing of mother	[88]
Cyanidin-3-glucoside (a common anthocyanin)	Isolated rat intestine	Cyanidin glucoside absorption was inhibited by quercetin glucoside, suggesting the involvement of active transport in absorption of anthocyanin glucosides	[89]
EGCG, Radio-labelled (^{3}H-aromatic protons)	Mouse	Widely distributed in mouse organs and tissues, indicating ability of EGCG or its metabolites to access all tissues. Excretion was 6% in urine and 35% in faeces. It appears likely that the remainder was lost as water vapour, following complete degradation by colon flora.	[90]
Chokeberry extract	Human	Peak of ~0.5 μM total anthocyanins in serum, Intact anthocyanins and conjugates, trace of protocatechuic acid (PCA) in plasma and urine.	[91]
Cyanidin glucoside orally; 400 mg/kg	Rat	Plasma C_{max} ~0.3 μM cyanidin glucoside and ~2.5μM protocatechuic acid (PCA).	[92]
Daidzein or daidzin (glucoside) 1mg/kg	Human (7 men)	C_{max}/T_{max} (intact and conjugated) 2.5 μM/10 hours from daidzin, 0.5 μM/8 hours from daidzein; main metabolites equol (one subject), dihydrodaidzein, O-desmethylangolensin.	[93]
Delphinidin glucoside	Rat	Main plasma metabolite 4'-O-methyl derivative; suggests that methylation is a major metabolic pathway for compounds with pyrogallol moiety (1, 2, 3-trihydroxyphenyl).	[94]
Dihydrocaffeic acid/18 mg/Kg (3,4-dihydroxypropionic acid; a putative colonic metabolite of flavonoids)	Rat	Rapid absorption, plasma T_{max} 30 min; 1% of dose excreted un metabolised in urine, along with methyl, glucuronide and sulphate conjugates.	[95]
Elderberry extract	Elderly women	Peak of ~0.16 μM total anthocyanins in serum, only intact anthocyanins observed in plasma and urine.	[96]
Genistein, hesperetin	Perfused rat intestine	Significant proportion of absorbed flavonoid glucuronidated and excreted back into lumen/perfusate.	[58]

Table 1. (Continued)

Flavonoid/Source	Species	Bioavailability in plasma/tissues; Metabolites detected	Reference
Glabridin 10 mg/kg	Rat	Peak plasma concentration of ~0.1 µM; un-metabolised material, conjugates not detected: monocyte chemo-attractant protein-1 secretion reduced in dosed rats.	[97]
Grapefruit extract	Dog	Plasma C_{max} 0.3-0.4 µM, primarily naringin, with small proportions of naringenin and its glucuronide.	[98]
Hesperetin, naringenin (aglycones) 135 mg each	Human	Plasma Max concentrations 3 and 7 µM respectively, mostly as conjugated forms. Phenolic acid metabolites also detected.	[99]
Isoflavones (glucosides of genistein and daidzein)	Human	Intact isoflavones are absorbed in 2 "peaks"; apparently the first from direct intestinal absorption and the second from the colon after microbial metabolism.	[100]
Kaempferol (a flavonol, like quercetin)	Human	Even a low dose (9 mg) resulted in a peak plasma concentration of 0.1 µM and urinary excretion of 2% of dose. Suggests that bioavailability higher than quercetin.	[101]
Luteolin and related permethylated flavone, Nobiletin	Rat	Nobiletin much better absorbed and widely distributed in tissues. Major metabolites were 3 mono-demethylated and 2 di-demethylated forms.	[64]
Naringenin and its glucoside	Rat	Orally, ~10% of both compounds absorbed and mainly recovered as glucuronide. Intravenously, glucoside recovered largely unchanged. Glucoside readily cleaved and glucuronidated during intestinal absorption.	[102]
Naringenin, hesperetin glycosides from Blood orange juice	Human	Peak plasma concentrations reached after 5 hours of ~0.1-0.2 µM. 95% detected as conjugates.	[103]
Normal diet	Human	Thirteen polyphenols and metabolites were found suitable as biomarkers of polyphenol intake; cinnamic acids: chlorogenic acid, caffeic acid, m-coumaric acid, gallic acid, 4-O-methylgallic acid; flavonoids: quercetin, isorhamnetin, kaempferol, hesperetin, naringenin, phloretin; lignans: enterolactone, enterodiol. Suggests that cinnamic acids, hydrophobic flavonoids and lignans are the most bioavailable phenolics.	[104]
Pelargonidin aglycone by oral gavage	Rat	18% of dose absorbed after 2 hours and detected in liver, kidney, brain, lung but not heart, spleen. Main metabolites glucuronide and 4-hydroxybenzoic acid.	[73]
Phloretin, quercetin and their glucosides	Rat intestine in situ	Perfusion of glucosides or aglycones generated same mixture of conjugates in blood. Glucosylation increased quercetin absorption, but reduced phloretin absorption.	[105]
Polymethoxylated flavone mixture isolated from Chinese herb	Rat	Plasma metabolites all glucuronides of parent compound or demethylated forms.	[106]

Table 1. (Continued)

Flavonoid/Source	Species	Bioavailability in plasma/tissues; Metabolites detected	Reference
Procyanidin dimers	Isolated rat intestine	95% absorbed as unconjugated epicatechin, i.e., the dimers were cleaved into monomers by the intestinal cells.	[107]
Procyanidin-rich chocolate	Human	Plasma Cmax of epicatechin range from 0.13–0.35 μM.	[108]
Procyanidins and catechins from oral grape seed extract	Rat	Conjugates of catechins only, no evidence of absorption or degradation of procyanidins.	[109]
Procyanidins and catechins from oral grape seed extract	Rat	No evidence of procyanidin absorption, only gallic acid and catechin monomers detected.	[110]
Puerarin (daidzein-8-C-glucoside)	Rat	Un-metabolised puerarin plasma conc 6 μM after 4 hours, detected in brain extracts. Metabolites detected: hydroxylated and reduced forms including equol.	[111]
Quercetin	Rat intestine	Quercetin rapidly absorbed, but ~ half glucuronidated and excreted back in to lumen.	[59]
Quercetin	Rat	Quercetin conjugates (no aglycone) appeared in lymphatic fluid, with the maximum concentration at 30 minutes.	[112]
Quercetin aglycone from Shallot skin, quercetin glucosides (shallot flesh/1.4 mg/kg total quercetin	Human	Cmax 1μM from flesh and 4μM from skin; suggests that food matrix increases aglycone solubility/absorption compared with pure compound.	[45]
Quercetin and its glucoside	Isolated rat intestine	Glucoside absorbed faster than aglycone, via hexose transporter, but deglycosylated during or after absorption. Only aglycone and glucuronides found in mucosal tissue.	[49]
Quercetin glycosides	Rat intestine	Deglycosylation and absorption of quercetin aglycone was much higher from glucosides than other glycosides.	[50]
Quercetin glycosides from onions	Human	Quercetin-3-glucuronide, 3'-methyl-quercetin-3-glucuronide and quercetin-3'-sulfate, no source glycosides detected.	[113, 114]
Quercetin glycosides from onions	Human	Five isomeric quercetin glucuronides.	[115]
Quercetin in diet	Pig	Single dose of 25 mg/kg (50 mg/kg/day/4 weeks) resulted in μM concentrations of: plasma 1.6 (0.8), liver 0.03 (0.15), muscle 0.3 nM (both), brain (0.07 nM).	[43]
Quercetin mono- and di-glucoside from fried onions	Human	Sub-micromolar maximum concentrations of intestinal conjugates (glucuronide, sulphate) after~40 min and peak of liver metabolite (sulpho-glucuronide) after 2.5 hours. Considerable differences between plasma and urinary conjugate profiles. Total urinary excretion 4.7%.	[116]

Table 1. (Continued)

Flavonoid/Source	Species	Bioavailability in plasma/tissues; Metabolites detected	Reference
Quercetin, catechin, red wine polyphenols, orally	Rat	Only quercetin could be detected in plasma, as conjugates. None of the supplements reduced lipid peroxidation markers.	[117]
Quercetin, long-term dietary supplementation	Rat, Pig	Rats, 0.1% quercetin in diet/11 weeks resulted in ~20 µM total quercetin (inc. conjugates) in plasma and 0-4 µM in organs; pigs, 500mg/kg in diet/3 days resulted in 1.25 µM in plasma, 6 µM in liver and 2.5 µM in kidney.	[44]
Quercetin, oral/6 weeks	Rat	11 different conjugates after absorption, major one a methyl, sulpho, glucuronide.	[70]
Quercetin-3- and -4'-glucosides	Isolated rat intestine	Quercetin from 3-glucoside was only absorbed after hydrolysis by lactase phloridzin hydrolase in lumen; 4-glucoside was absorbed both after hydrolysis and directly by SGLT1. (Note contrast with [51], this table, below]).	[118]
Quercetin glycosides from apple or onion	Human	Bioavailability of quercetin from apples and of pure quercetin rutinoside both 30% relative to onions. Plasma Cmax at~40 min after ingestion of onions, 2.5 h after apples and 9 h after the rutinoside. Half-lives of elimination were 28 h for onions and 23 h for apples.	[56]
Quercetin supplement, 500 mg/3 times daily/7 days	Human	Plasma concentration >0.6 µM for 8 hours after last dose, Cmax 1.1 µM, 94.5% present as conjugates.	[119]
Red wine whole/de-alcoholised	Rat intestinal preparation	Absorption of quercetin (3-fold) and its 3-glucoside (1.5-fold) was increased in the presence of alcohol, compared with de-alcoholised wine.	[120]
Resveratrol	Isolated rat intestine	Predominantly glucuronide found in mucosal tissue.	[121]
Resveratrol, catechin, quercetin	Human	Proportion of compound present in plasma as conjugates/proportion of dose excreted in urine/: Resveratrol – 98%/17%, catechin – 97%/2%, quercetin – 80%/5%.	[122]
Resveratrol; radio-labelled (14C)	Rat	Apparently predominantly intact resveratrol conjugates predominated and were distributed throughout tissues.	[123]
Scutellarin (plant-derived 7-glucuronide of flavone scutellarein)	Human	Peak plasma concentration ~0.3 µM, urinary metabolites were 6-glucuronide, 2 sulpho-glucuronides and methyl scutellarin, scutellarein.	[124]
Semi-synthetic diet	Rat	Numerous flavonoid conjugates and colonic metabolites detected in intestinal mucosa, plasma and caecal contents.	[125]
Various flavonoids and glucosides	Isolated rat intestine	Glucosides except quercetin-3-glucoside (absorbed directly) deglycosylated during absorption and extensively glucuronidated.	[51]
Vitexin-rhamnoside (flavone derivative)	Isolated rat intestine	Good permeability by passive diffusion, increased by P-glycoprotein inhibitors; suggests P-glycoprotein involved in luminal efflux.	[62]

Table 2. Summary of recent published studies involving determination of absorption/bioavailability using Caco-2 and/or other gut epithelial cell cultures

Test compound	Outcome	Reference
Apigenin	At low apical concentrations main conjugate formed is sulphate, which is mainly effluxed apically. At higher concentrations, glucuronidation predominates and is mostly effluxed basolaterallly. Enteric recycling apparently limited by low efflux pump capacity.	[42]
Benzoic acid, p-coumaric acid, gallic acid, mono-hydroxybenzoic acids	Indication that observed rapid transport is mediated by a mono-carboxylic acid-specific carrier.	[126-129]
Blackcurrant anthocyanins	~11% apparently absorbed by cells, no basolateral efflux.	[130]
Catechins from tea	Catechins inhibit drug efflux by multidrug resistance P-glycoprotein . This effect may potentially enhance absorption of other flavonoids by inhibiting efflux.	[131]
Catechins from tea	Catechins inhibit mono-carboxylic acid transporter (MCT) but are absorbed by paracellular diffusion and also effluxed apically.	[132, 133]
Diosmin, hesperidin, naringin (rutinosides of flavones) and algycones	Aglycones had measurable permeabilities, rutinosides did not. Supports low absorption of glycosides other than glucosides.	[52]
Flavonoid aglycones	The human organic anion transporter OAT1 is inhibited by flavonoids and may be involved in their cellular absorption.	[134]
Galangin (5,7-dimethoxy flavone), mono- and di-methyl derivatives.	Methylated forms 5-8 times more permeable and more resistant to metabolism in Caco-2 cells and hepatocytes. Suggests that methylation should greatly increase oral bioavailability of flavonoids.	[135, 136]
Genistein, apigenin with siRNA treatment	Determination of which glucuronyl transferase (UGT) iso-forms expressed by Caco-2 cells.	[137]
Glabridin (isoflavan from liquorice)	Extensive glucuronidation observed and apical efflux appears to be meditated by P-glycoprotein and MDR1.	[61]
Hesperetin	Apically applied hesperetin slowly diffused basolaterallly, but most conjugates formed were transported back to the apical medium; addition of efflux pump inhibitors suggested the main pump operating was breast cancer resistance protein (BCRP).	[53]
Hesperetin, hesperidin (hesperetin-7-rutinoside)	Hesperidin absorbed by proton-coupled active transport, apparently by MCT transporter; hesperidin is not and is likely only bioavailable after deglycosylation by micro flora.	[54, 55]
Hydroxy tyrosol (3,4-dihydroxyphenylethanol)	Absorption is by passive diffusion and a methylated metabolite was detected.	[138]
Luteolin and its permethylated derivative, Nobiletin	Nobiletin, but not luteolin, preferentially accumulated in the Caco-2 cell monolayer, suggesting much higher bioavailability.	[139]
Quercetin and 3-glucoside	Glucoside absorbed unchanged and as aglycone, aglycone absorbed better.	[140]
Quercetin-3-glucoside	Absorption by Caco-2 and Chinese hamster ovary cells facilitated by sodium-dependent glucose co-transporter (SGLT1).	[141]
Quercetin-3-glucoside	Basolateral efflux from cells appears to be mediated by GLUT2 glucose transporter.	[142]

Various efflux pumps have been implicated in the return of glucuronidated flavonoids to the lumen [61, 62]. The material returned to the lumen is thought to pass into the colon and to subsequently become available for microbial metabolism. The positional isomer distribution of absorbed glucuronides may be influenced not only by the positional selectivity of intestinal epithelial cell glucuronyl transferase iso-forms, but also by selective efflux back into the lumen. The MRP2 efflux pump shows selectivity between quercetin glucuronide isomers [63] and this may contribute to the observed isomer distribution in the circulation. Some flavonoids, primarily from citrus fruits (e.g., Nobiletin, Sinensetin, Tangeretin) are permethylated, i.e., they have O-methyl groups in place of phenolic hydroxyl groups. Other flavonoids can also be easily methylated chemically and permethylated flavonoids have considerably different ADME properties from other flavonoids [64-68]. Methylation increases hydrophobicity and therefore intestinal absorption. Blocking of all potential conjugation sites (i.e., phenols) by methylation inhibits Phase II conjugative metabolism, requiring Phase I, cytochrome P_{450}-mediated demethylation before conjugation is possible [66]. These findings suggest an approach to counteract the issue of low flavonoid bioavailability for health studies (assuming that it is desirable), and also highlight the effectiveness of mammalian cell metabolism at limiting the absorption of flavonoids.

The array of flavonoid conjugates from gut cell metabolism appears to be further expanded by the liver, which appears to accumulate higher concentrations of flavonoids than any other organ [44]. Liver β-glucuronidase can apparently remove glucuronidation added by the intestinal cells and sulpho-transferase and catechol O-methyl transferase (COMT) can substitute (or add) sulphation and/or methylation. For example, quercetin is primarily glucuronidated by intestinal cells, before passage into the bloodstream. When cultured hepatocytes were treated with purified quercetin glucuronides to investigate potential further metabolism in the liver, three major processes were observed. Firstly, methylation of the quercetin moiety of the glucuronides by COMT was noted before removal of glucuronyl residues by β-glucuronidase, followed by sulphation [69]. The potential for a complex conjugate mixture resulting from conjugation by both intestine and liver was highlighted by a rat study with quercetin [70]. Eleven conjugates were detected, the most abundant having all 3 conjugate groups, i.e., methyl, glucuronide and sulphate, in the same molecule.

Anthocyanins are very unstable compared with other flavonoids, particularly at neutral or alkaline pH. The anthocyanin content of a wide variety of processed blackcurrant products was only 0.05-10% of that in fresh fruit. Although they should be relatively stable in the acidic environment of the stomach, degradation in the neutral small intestine may be very rapid [71]. Bioavailability studies on anthocyanins consistently find barely detectable concentrations in plasma (<0.05 μM) with only a tiny proportion of the dose (often <0.1%) excreted in urine (Tables 1, 4). This low urinary excretion compares with up to ~20% for some other flavonoids (see below). Elevated levels of phenolic acid metabolites can account for only a low percentage of intake (Tables 1, 4). It is becoming clear from the numerous bioavailability studies on anthocyanins that 60-90% of the dietary load disappears from the GI tract within 4 hours of a meal [72]. It is not clear, however, what happens to them. Possibilities are that they are degraded/structurally rearranged into as-yet unidentified derivatives, or covalently bound to proteins or other polymers (i.e., resistant to extraction/detection), either in the intestinal lumen, plasma, or inside cells. Anthocyanin detection is commonly achieved using very sensitive techniques such as liquid chromatography-mass spectroscopy (LC-MS). However, recoveries from anthocyanin extraction procedures performed from plasma are often very low (less than 20%) and hence it is possible that the apparently low bioavailability of anthocyanins is partly due to a lack of robust techniques to enable complete extraction and detection.

Anthocyanins are unusual in that, unlike other flavonoids, the predominant forms detected in plasma and urine are intact, un-metabolised glycosides, rather than aglycones or conjugates. They may be very unstable under physiological conditions after deglycosylation, because, apart from the strawberry anthocyanin, pelargonidin [73], there is very little evidence of significant deglycosylation or conjugation of anthocyanins. Although it may appear that anthocyanins probably do not have significant biological activities because of their apparently low bioavailability, there is some evidence that absorption from the stomach [74] and the jejunum [75], may be both rapid and relatively high. Particularly rapid degradation after absorption, however, appears to severely limit the duration of significant anthocyanin plasma concentrations, in normal circumstances. Only traces survive long enough to be detected in the urine. Localised biological effects of anthocyanins immediately after absorption, or direct effects on the gastrointestinal tract or its microflora are possible, however.

The Colon and Microflora

Colonic microflora display an extensive capability to metabolise flavonoids that reach the colon either directly, or after intestinal epithelial cell metabolism and apical efflux of glucuronides, biliary excretion etc. Numerous studies (Table 3) have demonstrated the ability of isolated cultures, faecal slurries, etc, to remove glycosylation that is resistant to endogenous mammalian β-glucosidases and cleave flavonoids into simpler compounds. As with the published bioavailability studies, quercetin is the most studied and best understood. It appears that quercetin glucosides, for example, are relatively well absorbed in the small intestine (see above discussion), whereas the glucosidase-resistant rutin reaches the colon mostly intact where it can be deglycosylated by microflora making it potentially available for both absorption by colonic epithelial cells and degradation into simpler compounds. One report proposed a mechanism to explain the observed degradation of quercetin by pig caecum microflora, predominantly into phloroglucinol and 3,4-dihydroxyphenylacetic acid [143]. These degradation products appear to accumulate in the colon to concentrations 1-2 orders of magnitude higher than the flavonoid aglycones [144]. There is evidence from urinary studies [145-148], that the phenolic acid degradation products, particularly benzoic acid, a likely final product of these degradation pathways, are well absorbed and increased urinary excretion correlates with consumption of flavonoid-rich foods. Hippuric acid (benzoylglycine) is regularly detected at high concentrations in urine, following consumption of flavonoid-rich foods and is known to be the major human conjugate of benzoic acid [146]. Studies *in vitro* using Caco-2 and other gut epithelial cells (Table 2) have demonstrated that these low molecular weight acids are efficiently transported, possibly by a mono-carboxylic acid transporter present in the colonic epithelia and so rapid absorption through the gut wall is not unexpected. One recent study found various small aromatic compounds in urine resulting from quercetin consumption and in addition reported for the first time, mercapturic acid conjugates of phenolic acids in the urine, apparently derived from colonic breakdown of glutathione conjugates of quercetin that had been detected in the plasma [149].

Table 3. Summary of published studies of the biotransformation of flavonoids using microbial cultures

Flavonoid	Culture	Metabolites Found	Reference
Anthocyanins	Human faecal flora	Rapid conversion into phenolic acids; major products were: protocatechuic acid from cyanidin; syringic acid from malvidin; vanillic acid from peonidin; 4-hydroxybenzoic acid from pelargonidin.	[165]
Biochanin A, formononetin, glycitein (methylated isoflavones	Eubacterium limosum (human intestinal strict anaerobe	Demethylated isoflavones.	[166]
Catechin, epicatechin	Human faecal flora	Main metabolites from both catechins were 3-hydroxyphenyl-propionic acid and phenylpropionic acid; 3,4-dihydroxyphenylacetic acid and 3-hydroxyphenylacetic acid were not detected.	[167]
Catechins from tea (EGCG etc)	Human, rat faecal flora	15 compounds to be confirmed.	[168]
Catechins from tea (EGCG etc)	Eubacterium sp. strain SDG-2	Removal of esterified gallate and cleavage of flavanols to 1,3-diphenylpropan-2-ol derivatives.	[169]
Daidzein	Rat faecal flora	Daidzein, dihydrodaidzein, but no equol detected.	[170]
Flavonoid aglycones	Pig caecum micro flora	Major metabolites: 3-(4-hydroxyphenyl)-propionic acid, 3-phenylpropionic acid from naringenin; phloroglucinol, 3,4-dihydroxyphenylacetic acid, 3,4-dihydroxytoluene from quercetin; 3-(3-hydroxyphenyl)-propionic acid, phloroglucinol from hesperetin.	[171]
Flavonoids from tea, citrus and soy	In vitro colon model	3-methoxy-4-hydroxyphenylacetic acid, 4-hydroxyphenyl acetic acid, 3,4-dihydroxyphenylacetic acid, 3-(3-hydroxyphenyl) propionic acid, 2,4,6-trihydroxybenzoic acid, 3-(4-hydroxy-3-methoxyphenyl) propionic acid, 3-hydroxyphenyl acetic acid, hippuric acid.	[172]
Genistein, daidzein	Mouse intestinal isolate	Equol, 5-hydroxyequol.	[173]
Genistein, daidzein and their glycosides	Eubacterium ramulus	6'-hydroxy-O-desmethylangolensin, 2-(4-hydroxyphenyl)-propionic acid.	[174]
Procyanidins (epicatechin polymers)	Human colonic flora	Mainly mono-hydroxylated phenylacetic, phenylpropionic and phenylvaleric acids.	[175]
Quercetin glucoside	2 human isolates	Removal and metabolism of glucoside group by Enterococcus casseliflavus, degradation of flavonol moiety to 3,4-dihydroxyphenylacetic acid, acetate and butyrate by Eubacterium ramulus.	[176]

Table 3. (Continued)

Flavonoid	Culture	Metabolites Found	Reference
Quercetin glycosides	Human faecal flora	3,4-dihydroxyphenylacetic acid, 3-hydroxyphenylacetic acid.	[177]
Quercetin, hesperetin, naringenin and their rutinosides	Human faecal flora	Rutinosides readily deglycosylated, accumulating hesperetin, naringenin, but not quercetin. Aglycones metabolised to phenolic acids.	[178]
Quercetin, luteolin	Eubacterium ramulus	Intermediate formation of taxifolin (quercetin) and eriodyctiol (luteolin), final conversion to 3,4-dihydroxyphenylacetic acid and 3-(3,4-dihydroxyphenyl)propionic acid.	[179]
Quercetin, Rutin	Pig caecum micro flora	3,4-dihydroxyphenylacetic acid, phloroglucinol.	[143]
Quercetin, taxifolin; luteolin, eriodictyol, apigenin, naringenin, phloretin and glycosides	Clostridium orbiscindens	No glycoside cleavage, but conversion of aglycones to 3,4-dihydroxyphenylacetic acid, 3-(3,4-dihydroxyphenyl)propionic acid, 3-(4-hydroxyphenyl)propionic acid.	[180]
Quercetin-3-glucoside	Germ free rats with/without, Enterococcus casseliflavus	Germ-free, urine, faeces contained quercetin and isorhamnetin (methylated quercetin). Colonised with bacteria, main metabolite found was 3,4-dihydroxyphenylacetic acid.	[181]
Unrestricted diet	Human faecal water	Compounds detected (micromolar concentrations): Naringenin (1.20); quercetin (0.63); other flavonoids (<= 0.17); phenylacetic acid (479); 3-phenylpropionic acid (166); 3-(4-hydroxy)-phenylpropionic acid (68); 3,4-dihydroxycinnamic (caffeic) acid (52); benzoic acid (51); 3-hydroxylphenylacetic acid (46); 4-hydroxyphenylacetic acid (19).	[144]
Various flavonoid aglycones and glycosides	Eubacterium ramulus	Luteolin-7-glucoside, rutin, quercetin, kaempferol, luteolin, eriodictyol, naringenin, taxifolin (dihydroquercetin), phloretin, were degraded to phenolic acids. Luteolin-5-glucoside, diosmetin-7-rutinoside, naringenin-7-neohesperidoside, (+)-catechin, (−)-epicatechin were not degraded.	[182]
Various flavonoid glycosides	Pig caecum micro flora	Deglycosylation was fastest for mono-glycosides, slower for di- or tri-saccharide glycosides; aglycones degraded to primarily 3,4-dihydroxyphenylacetic acid, 4-hydroxyphenylacetic acid, phloroglucinol.	[183]

It was proposed that the glutathione conjugates arose from a reaction between a quinone form of quercetin (resulting from oxidation) and glutathione. This is thought to occur both spontaneously and catalysed by glutathione-S-transferase.

Although it is clear that flavonoids can be degraded into phenolic acids, there are alternative dietary sources which make the picture more complicated. Blueberry fruits in particular (and presumably plant foods in general), contain large amounts of phenolic acid compounds bound to insoluble polymeric plant cell wall material, i.e., "fibre". Simple esters between phenolic acids and other compounds, including, for example, caffeic-quinic acid esters (chlorogenic acid) are common in apples and coffee. p-Coumaric-tartaric acid esters (coutaric acid) are found at reasonable levels in grapes. Unbound acids are a relatively small proportion of the total phenolic acids present in the edible parts of plants. The bound or conjugated acids are predominantly hydroxy-benzoic and hydroxy-cinnamic acids and 12 were detected in hydrolysed blueberry fruit fibre [150]. When this insoluble fraction of blueberry was incubated with human faecal slurry, over 20 phenolic acids were detected, some clearly liberated unchanged from the fruit fibre, others, (phenylacetic acids in particular), apparently transformed by the faecal bacteria. An alternative source of phenolic acids may have been transformation of residual flavonoids. A widely occurring hydroxycinnamic acid, caffeic acid, can be metabolised by human faecal flora into similar compounds to those derived from flavonoids, i.e., 4-hydroxyphenylpropionic acid and benzoic acid [151]. Gut microbe-derived cinnamoyl esterases have been shown to be primarily responsible for the liberation of free phenolic acids from phenolic acid esters in the colon [152], whilst endogenous mammalian esterase activity can be found throughout the gastro-intestinal tract [153]. Since there are apparently three potential source materials for the phenolic acids generated by the colon flora, flavonoids, fibre and cinnamic acids, care must be taken linking particular phenolic acid metabolites and flavonoids, using animal or human studies, unless pure flavonoids are administered.

The occurrence of small phenolic acids in plants is also a complicating factor. It has been claimed that protocatechuic acid (PCA) is the major metabolite of cyanidin glycosides in humans, based on a trial involving the consumption of blood orange juice (BOJ). PCA was the main plasma and urinary metabolite detected and a relatively high (compared with other anthocyanin studies) proportion of anthocyanins (1.2%) were detected in urine [154]. It was claimed that the PCA came primarily from intestinal microbial metabolism of cyanidin. This assumption was based on the finding of PCA as a major metabolite of purified anthocyanins in rats [73, 92]. The former finding is not conclusive, however, because the T_{max} (time after dosing at which C_{max} is attained) of PCA was relatively short, at 2 hours (suggesting direct absorption). BOJ contains a small amount of PCA and its flavanone content (which may also be metabolised to PCA) is similar to its anthocyanin content [155]. BOJ consumption clearly results in significant amounts of absorbed PCA, but it does not necessarily derive from cyanidin.

Beer, unsurprisingly for a fermented product, is a good direct dietary source of small phenolic acids. Phenolic acids from beer (some of which are the same compounds as colonic metabolite acids) were readily absorbed in human subjects and the degree of conjugation varied considerably [156]. 4-Hydroxyphenylacetic acid reached much higher plasma concentrations (~1 μM) than cinnamic acids, such as ferulic or caffeic acids and was predominantly non-conjugated. This suggests that simple phenolic acids, both as produced by colonic microflora and in the diet, would be readily absorbed and may be conjugated to a much lesser extent than flavonoids. Similarly, consumed free p-coumaric acid is rapidly and extensively absorbed through the stomach wall and upper intestine using both passive diffusion and the mono-carboxylic transporter, reaching plasma levels of 165 μM, albeit with a very short plasma half-life of 10 minutes [157]. *In vitro* studies using these acids would have more physiological relevance than those on unconjugated flavonoids because of their higher bioavailability in relatively unaltered states.

It also appears that most of the flavonoids studied so far are not absorbed directly by the small intestine, based on total urinary excretion of conjugates of the intact flavonoid. The highest reported proportion of a dose of flavonoid excreted in urine was 20%, for phloridzin-derived phloretin [158].

Another study reported 10% from phloridzin or phloretin itself [159]. This implies that at least 80-90% would have passed on to the colon and been available for microfloral breakdown (or direct absorption contributing to percentage excreted in urine). Commonly reported percentages of urinary excretion of intact flavonoids are in single figures and those for anthocyanins rarely exceed 0.1% (Tables 1, 4).

There is some evidence that anthocyanins may be rapidly and relatively well absorbed from large doses, but their (presumed) instability under physiological conditions results in very little surviving to be excreted in the urine. It seems unlikely that the absorbed proportion could often exceed that for phloretin, so the major proportion of dietary anthocyanins would be potentially able to reach the colon. As discussed above, however, losses to as-yet unknown destinations or forms, appear to be extensive although a study in rats shows that at least part of the dietary intake of intact anthocyanins can reach the colon and undergo metabolism by faecal flora [160].

High-anthocyanin berryfruit extracts (2.5-5% of diet) were fed for 14 weeks. Recoveries of different individual anthocyanins from faeces were very variable (6-25%). Interestingly, it was noted that anthocyanin degradation in faecal samples stored at -18°C was rapid unless these were pasteurised before storage, suggesting that faecal bacteria were still active during storage.

An exception to the extensive degradation of flavonoids to phenolic acids are the soy isoflavones, which are metabolised to modified, but intact flavonoids such as equol or angolensin [161]. The isoflavones, (as discussed below), are also the best example of alternative flavonoid metabolism end products produced by individuals with different populations of gut microflora, where some individual's flora can produce equol, whereas others cannot [162].

Limited evidence suggests that the consumption of flavonoids in the diet can modify the composition of the colonic flora. This can in turn, modify the metabolism of the flavonoids by the microflora. Soy isoflavone metabolism was compared in children, who had been, or were being fed either soy- or cows-milk based infant formula. Those currently or recently consuming infant formula showed differences in metabolism depending on the type of formula consumed, but there was no difference in older children [163]. This suggests that dietary flavonoids can influence the composition of the colonic microflora that metabolise them, but the effect is not long-lasting.

Tea polyphenolics and their colonic metabolites were recently tested for their effects on the growth of human colonic microfloral cultures [164]. The phenolics and metabolites generally inhibited bacterial growth, and pathogenic strains were much more severely affected than commensal strains. This also suggests that dietary flavonoids can beneficially influence the composition of the colonic microflora.

Table 4. Summary of published studies on urinary metabolites of flavonoids

Flavonoid/source	Species	Excretion Level/Metabolites Found	Reference
Apple cider (phloretin, quercetin epicatechin and glycosides)	Human	Only phloretin (20% of dose) detected in urine directly, but 3-fold increase in hippuric acid.	[158]
Berry anthocyanins	Human, rat	Only un-metabolised anthocyanins detected in urine.	[184]
Biochanin A. quercetin, EGCG	Rat	Biochanin A absorption increased and clearance decreased, when co-administered with quercetin and EGCG; may be due to inhibition of efflux pumps.	[185]
Black tea	Human	Hippuric acid was the major excretion product and accounted for nearly all of the polyphenolic intake from the tea.	[146, 147]
Blackcurrant juice	Human	Essentially similar to above study.	[186]
Boysemberry extract	Human	Intact anthocyanins and glucuronides detected.	[187]
Chocolate	Human	Increased urinary extraction of 3-hydroxyphenylpropionic acid, ferulic acid, 3,4-dihydroxyphenylacetic acid, 3-hydroxyphenylacetic acid, vanillic acid, and 3-hydroxybenzoic acid.	[148]
Chokeberry, blackcurrant, elderberry, marionberry	Weanling pigs	0.1–0.2% urinary excretion of intact anthocyanins, glucuronides and methyl derivatives; colonic metabolites not analysed.	[188, 189]
Cocoa powder or epicatechin	Rat	Similar composition and concentration of urinary metabolites from cocoa procyanidins and epicatechin administration.	[190]
Cocoa procyanidins	Human	Epicatechin conjugate excretion increased relative to controls. Milk had no effect on apparent bioavailability.	[191, 192]
Daidzein, genistein	Human	Tetrahydrodaidzein, dihydrogenistein, 6'-hydroxy-O-demethylangolensin, 2-dehydro-O-demethylangolensin, equol, dehydrodaidzein, O-demethyl-angolensin, daidzein, genistein, glycitein, enterolactone.	[161]
Dried cranberry juice	Human	Main metabolites hippuric and 2-hydroxy hippuric acids, PCA, gentisic acid (methylated PCA) and quercetin conjugates. The juice contained PCA and other phenolic acids, so not all were necessarily flavonoid metabolites.	[193]
EGCG	Human, rat, mouse	0.1% of dose as EGCG, dimethylated EGCG, up to 16% as hydroxyphenyl-γ-valerolactone derivatives	[194]
Elderberry juice 400 ml	Human	~0.04% of anthocyanin dose excreted unchanged.	[195]
Epicatechin	Human, rat	Glucuronides and methyl glucuronides.	[196]
Flavonoid-rich meal	Human	Traces (<1 mg) of flavonoid and hydroxycinnamic acid conjugates, moderate amounts (1-20 mg) of glucuronides of 3-hydroxyphenylacetic, homovanillic, vanillic, isoferulic acids, 3-(3-methoxy-4-hydroxyphenyl)-propionic, 3-(3-hydroxyphenyl)-propionic acid, and 3-hydroxyhippuric acid, very large amounts (3–400 mg) of hippuric acid.	[145]
Genistein	Rat	Genistein glucuronide, dihydrogenistein glucuronide, genistein sulphate, dihydrogenistein, 4-hydroxyphenyl-2-propionic acid.	[197]
Green Tea	Human	(-)-5-(3',4',5'-Trihydroxyphenyl)-γ-valerolactone, (-)-5-(3',4'-dihydroxyphenyl)-γ-valerolactone.	[198]

Table 4. (Continued)

Flavonoid/source	Species	Excretion Level/Metabolites Found	Reference
Naringenin	Rat	Glucuronides and 3-(4-hydroxyphenyl) propionic acid.	[199]
Normal diet	Human	Flavonoids sufficiently measurable to act as biomarkers for polyphenol-rich food intake were quercetin, isorhamnetin, kaempferol, hesperetin, naringenin, phloretin (all relatively hydrophobic) suggesting they are more bioavailable than more polar flavonoids, e.g. catechins.	[200]
Oral blackberry anthocyanins	Rat	Unchanged anthocyanidin glycosides (<1% of dose) detected in urine, no aglycones or conjugates.	[201]
Oral elderberry anthocyanins	Human	Unchanged anthocyanidin glycosides detected in urine (~0.1% of dose), no aglycones, but traces of conjugates.	[202, 203]
Phloretin, phloridzin	Rat	Both compounds led to ~10% urinary excretion of phloretin metabolites (glucuronides, sulphates). Phloridzin appears to be deglycosylated completely during absorption.	[159]
Procyanidins from apple, 1000mg/kg, oral	Rat	Plasma T_{max} 2 hours, C_{max} ~40 μM catechin equivalents; still present after 24 hours. The physiological relevance of this extreme dose is uncertain.	[204]
Quercetin	Human	3,4-Dihydroxyphenylacetic acid, 3-hydroxyphenylacetic acid, and homovanillic acid.	[205]
Quercetin/cooked onions	Human	First report of glutathione conjugates, in addition to glucuronides, sulphates. Also colonic metabolites, dihydroxytoluene, dihydroxybenzaldehyde, dihydroxyphenylacetic acid, dihydroxycinnamic acid, dihydroxyphenylpropionic acid and mercapturic acid conjugates of the colonic metabolites, presumably from microbial degradation of quercetin glutathione conjugates.	[149]
Radio labelled (^{3}H) catechin, epicatechin	Rat	Intravenous administration led to ~1/3 urinary and 2/3 faecal excretion. Oral administration led to ~5% urinary excretion and exchange of label with plasma water, suggesting that most radiolabel was transferred to water during metabolism by colon flora.	[206]
Radiolabelled EGCG	Rat	Plasma radioactivity peaked at 24 hours post dosing and 32% appeared in urine. Antibiotic-treated rats excreted <1% of radioactivity in urine. Implies that only EGCG colonic metabolites are bioavailable. Major identified metabolites; 5-(5'-hydroxyphenyl)-γ-valerolactone 3'-O-glucuronide (urine), 5-(3',5'-dihydroxyphenyl)-γ-valerolactone (faeces).	[207]
Red clover extract (methylated isoflavones)	Human	Demethylated, hydroxylated and reduced intact isoflavones.	[208, 209]
Red wine, grape juice, 400 ml	Human	~0.2% of anthocyanin dose excreted in urine.	[210]
Strawberries (pelargonidin-3-glucoside, a relatively non-polar anthocyanin)	Human	Relatively high proportion of anthocyanidin (~1.8%) detected in urine, as glucoside, aglycone, 3 glucuronides and one sulpho-glucuronide.	[211]
Strawberries, 200g (source of pelargonidin-3-glucoside)	Human	C_{max} 0.27 μM at T_{max} of 1.1 hours for main metabolite pelargonidin-glucuronide. Total urinary excretion of pelargonidin 1%.	[212]
Tea polyphenolics	Human, normal or with colostomy	Normal subjects produced large amounts of hippuric acid and ~20 other phenolic acids. (primarily phenylacetic and benzoic acid derivatives) Colostomy subjects produced almost no phenolic acids.	[213]

Distribution of Flavonoid Metabolites
Round the Body

Blood proteins and lipoproteins appear to have a potentially major influence on the plasma transport, stability and biological activity of flavonoids. The main role of the major blood protein, serum albumin, appears to be regulation of the binding of lipophilic hormones to their receptors [214]. It has been proposed that one of many functions of flavonoids in plants is endocrine disruption of herbivores [215, 216]. Baker [214] has also suggested that albumin has evolved in mammals to inhibit the endocrine-disrupting effects of flavonoids, phytoestrogens in particular, by holding them in the plasma and reducing availability to cellular receptors. This system is complementary to conjugative metabolism, which probably evolved for similar reasons. A number of studies on albumin have produced evidence consistent with this hypothesis.

Considerable differences were found when quercetin and its metabolites were compared for their capacity to inhibit Copper(II)-induced LDL oxidation and their binding strength to serum albumin [217]. Quercetin and its glucuronides were much better inhibitors of LDL oxidation than its sulphate or methyl/glucuronide conjugates. Albumin binding was strongest for quercetin and its sulphate and up to 5-fold weaker for glucuronides. Furthermore, different isomers of quercetin glucuronides showed differences in albumin binding behaviour. A spectroscopic study of quercetin binding to bovine serum albumin in equimolar mixtures of the two found maximal binding at 10 μM and that bound quercetin was much more resistant to oxygen-dependent degradation [218]. Given that the human serum concentration of albumin is ~350-500 μM, ~100-fold higher than observed for any flavonoid, it was estimated that plasma flavonoids are probably predominantly albumin bound. A similar study found a relative binding affinity order of quercetin>rutin=(epi)catechin [219]. Flavonoid aglycones showed moderate affinity for bovine albumin, with binding constants of $1\text{-}15 \times 10^4 \text{ M}^{-1}$, whereas conjugates had binding constants ~10 times lower. It was again estimated that, given realistic plasma concentrations, even conjugates of flavonoids like quercetin would be predominantly bound to albumin *in vivo* [220]. Resveratrol uptake by liver hepatocytes appears to be a combination of passive diffusion and carrier-mediated transport and is inhibited by competitive binding to serum albumin [221]. It is well known that human serum albumin has a major influence on drug pharmacokinetics [222], and hence the influence of serum albumin on flavonoid distribution and biological activity in the body could be similarly important.

Multi-drug resistance (MDR) efflux transporters/pumps in cells other than intestinal cells may also significantly modulate flavonoid distribution in the body. Absorption of EGCG by cultured cells expressing high levels of drug efflux pump proteins was increased around 10-fold in the presence of specific synthetic pump inhibitors [223]. Flavonoids have been demonstrated to inhibit transport of model substrates by p-Glycoprotein and organic anion transporters [131, 134]. It was not clear whether the flavonoids were inhibitors of the pumps, or competitive substrates. This suggests that MDR efflux pumps may significantly reduce net cellular absorption of flavonoids or their metabolites and that flavonoids may influence each other's transport. These findings also raise the interesting notion that pharmaceutical drug absorption into tissues for therapeutic activity and efficacy may be improved by a diet rich in isoflavones.

Flavonoid Bioavailability to the Central Nervous System

It appears to be difficult for flavonoid metabolites to get into organs and tissues in general, but the central nervous system is a particular challenge. This is because of the relative impermeability of the interface between blood and brain – the blood-brain barrier (BBB), which is comprised of highly specialised cerebral endothelial cells which express a complex array of tight junction proteins and numerous MDR efflux transporters. Paradoxically, flavonoids have about the right hydrophobicity to cross the BBB, but glucuronidation and or sulphation greatly reduces their permeability, by greatly reducing their hydrophobicity. Flavonoid permeability into the brain has not been well investigated.

When evaluating *in vivo* organ bioavailability studies, it is important to consider whether the tissues were thoroughly perfused in order to remove circulating blood prior to tissue collection and analysis. This is especially important in studies evaluating brain bioavailability as there is generally a much larger difference between brain and blood content of specific compounds, than there is between the blood and other organs, because of the presence of the BBB. Practically, this is usually achieved by transcardial perfusion with saline or a similar physiological buffer at the time of euthanasia, but it can be technically difficult to remove all the blood, especially from brain blood vessels. Many variables can affect the quality of perfusion, including; the pressure applied to the perfusion apparatus, placement of the infusion needles, temperature and formulation of the perfusate, time taken and volume of perfusate used. It is generally recommended to fine-tune these procedures for any given study and a measure of haemoglobin content in the resulting organ homogenates can be used an indication of the quality of the perfusion. Given the extremely limited ability of any polyphenolic compound to enter the brain, if even 1-2% of the blood circulating in the brain (or other target organs) at the time of death is not washed away then spurious, variable and inaccurate measures will result. Some authors have used a correction method, where the amount of blood contamination is estimated in organ homogenates and the resulting blood-borne phytochemical content is then subtracted from the total found in organ homogenates [44]. This method may be especially useful if the compounds of interest are easily degraded and consequently the time between death and compound analysis is crucial.

In a study using an *in vitro* BBB cell monolayer model [224], hesperetin and naringenin aglycones had high permeabilities and were detected basolaterally (i.e., having crossed the cell monolayer) within 30 minutes, but their glycosides and glucuronide metabolites had much lower permeabilities, as did anthocyanins and these findings correlate well with their respective hydrophobicity. The latter were detected basolaterally only after incubation for 18 hours. Epicatechin, its glucuronides and 3 typical phenolic acid colonic metabolites had no detectable basolateral permeability, but accumulated within the cell monolayer [225]. In another study, however, when epicatechin was fed to rats at the extreme dose of 100 mg/kg, (equating to over 10 L of green tea in a single consumption in humans), epicatechin glucuronide and 3'-O-methyl epicatechin glucuronide were detected in the brain at 0.4 nmol/g brain tissue whilst plasma levels approximately 100-fold higher at 40 μM were detected [226].

The central nervous system also effectively limits anthocyanin access. In a study by Kalt *et al* [83], pigs which were fed a 1,2 or 4% blueberry fruit diet for 4 weeks and then fasted for a day before sacrifice and analysis had 11 anthocyanin moieties at detectable levels within the cerebral cortex and cerebellum, whereas none were detected in plasma. The total amount of anthocyanins detected was in the order of 0.7 to 0.9 pmol/g brain tissue and included the un-metabolised compounds: arabinose, galactose and glucose glycosides of cyanidin, delphinidin, malvidin and peonidin. This experimental method, where the phytochemical-containing diet is removed from the animals for 24 hours prior to euthanasia, thus allowing phytochemical clearance from blood, is a convenient way to prevent blood-borne phytochemical contamination of organs. Similar low levels of anthocyanins (0.25nmol/g brain tissue) were found in the brains of rats after 14 days of a blackberry fruit supplemented diet [77]. In this study the anthocyanins consisted primarily of un-metabolised anthocyanins, except for a methylated peonidin 3-glucoside. In another study where rats were administered red grape anthocyanins directly into the stomach, the authors found brain levels of intact anthocyanins of up to 192 ng/g (~0.6 μM) after only 10 minutes, unfortunately the tissues were not perfused and the unusually high levels of anthocyanins measured were therefore likely of both brain and blood origin [78].

The BBB has an extensive expression of MDR efflux transporter pumps which remove many xenobiotics, phytochemicals and drugs from the BBB endothelial cell layer and thereby prevent access to the brain proper. The most well characterised and possibly most relevant to the export of phytochemicals from the brain is P-glycoprotein (P-gp), an ATP-driven efflux pump which has a preference for lipophilic compounds (reviewed in detail in [225]). *In vitro* BBB models can be used to elucidate which of the efflux pumps might be responsible for the export of specific compounds, for example, Youdim *et al* [227] showed that both quercetin and naringenin have some level of central nervous system access which is limited by the activity of BBB efflux pumps. Pre-treatment with a specific P-gp inhibitor demonstrated some specificity, inhibiting the efflux of naringenin but not quercetin. When their system was pre-treated with a P-gp inhibitor which also blocks the action of the breast cancer resistance protein (BCRP) efflux pump, quercetin efflux was also severely limited. These results indicate that the naringenin is primarily exported by P-gp whereas quercetin is preferentially exported by the BCRP efflux pump [227].

It is not clear whether the primary mode by which flavonoids cross the BBB is diffusion or carrier-mediated transport, but whatever the process, they are apparently very susceptible to export via efflux pumps with some specificity for individual compounds. This efflux system is, however, not completely effective, as indicated by *in vivo* studies showing the retention of flavonoids within brain tissue at the picomolar to low nanomolar range. It is, therefore, important that *in vitro* studies evaluating the action of phytochemicals on brain cell cultures make use of physiologically relevant doses within this low concentration range.

Biological Activity of Flavonoid Metabolites

The majority of *in vitro* studies of flavonoid biological activity have been carried out on aglycones, so their physiological relevance is questionable. Recently, however, increasing attention has been paid to determining the biological activity of known conjugates or putative colonic metabolites (Table 5).

Table 5. Summary of *in vitro* studies of biological activity of flavonoid metabolites

Compounds tested	Assay	Outcome	Reference
Quercetin (a flavonol), catechin (a flavanol) and their glucuronides, sulphates and methyl ethers, extracted from plasma of rats fed the algycones	Blood monocyte adhesion to cultured human aortic endothelial cells, or reactive oxygen species (ROS) formation stimulated by interleukin-1β (IL-1β) or hydrogen peroxide (H_2O_2).	Quercetin aglycone or catechin conjugates inhibited monocyte adhesion. Catechin or its conjugates inhibited H_2O_2-induced ROS and only catechin conjugates inhibited IL-1β-induced ROS.	[228]
Quercetin and several likely colonic microbial metabolites	Chemical and cell-based antioxidant assays, inhibition of cholesterol biosynthesis in hepatocytes	Quercetin was active in all three assays and other *ortho* diphenols were equally effective in the chemical antioxidant assay. Of the metabolites, only 3,4-diydroxy toluene was active in the cell-based antioxidant assays.	[229]
Quercetin glucuronide	Lipid peroxidation	Effective inhibitor.	[230]
Quercetin and its 3-glucuronide	Generation of H_2O_2-induced ROS in mouse 3T3 fibroblasts	Only glucuronide inhibited ROS generation, after 4 hours pre-treatment, apparently because quercetin was methylated to isorhamnetin. When applied simultaneously with H_2O_2, both were active, but quercetin was better.	[231]
Quercetin and its 3-glucuronide	Inhibition of angiotensin II-induced vascular smooth-muscle cell hypertrophy in a cell culture model	Both were effective, possibly by inhibition of c-Jun N-terminal kinase activation.	[232]
Quercetin conjugates (glucuronide, sulphate, O-methyl)	COX-2 gene expression	Reduced expression *in vitro* by Caco-2 gut epithelial cells.	[233]
Quercetin, isorhamnetin quercetin-3-glucuronide and quercetin-3-sulphate	Superoxide generation in aqueous buffer and inhibition of blood vessel vasodilatory activity of nitric oxide (NO)	Glucuronide inactive in all assays; quercetin active against NO; quercetin isorhamnetin and sulphate generated superoxide.	[234]
Quercetin	Neutrophil-mediated LDL oxidation	Inhibited LDL oxidation at 1 μM apparently by inhibiting myeloperoxidase (IC50 1μM) and radical-induced LDL oxidation (IC50 1.5 μM). 3'-methylation and 3-glucuronidation moderately weakened this activity, but both together, or 3-sulphation greatly reduced it.	[235]

Table 5. (Continued)

Compounds tested	Assay	Outcome	Reference
Quercetin, Isorhamnetin	Neurotoxicity in cell culture	Active, apparently through inhibition of survival signalling/induction of apoptosis but only at supra-physiological levels not attained in the brain *in vivo*. Isorhamnetin had lower toxicity; quercetin glucuronide was non-toxic.	[236]
Quercetin glucuronide isomers	Xanthine oxidase and lipoxygenase inhibition	All isomers active.	[237]
Quercetin glucuronide isomers	Inhibition of acetylation of carcinogen 2-amino fluorene by HL-60 leukaemia cells	All isomers were inhibitors and all exhibited cytotoxicity..	[238]
Quercetin and conjugates	Chromosomal damage in cultured lymphoblastoid cells	Quercetin caused damage, apparently through generation of H_2O_2, 3-sulphate and isorhamnetin did not. All reduced damage by added H_2O_2, in the order quercetin>isorhamnetin>3-sulphate.	[239]
Quercetin disulphate (potential but un-reported human metabolite)	Pig platelet aggregation; prevention may be of value in CVD	Effective inhibitor.	[240]
Morin (another flavonol)	Macrophage function	Conjugates modulated macrophage function.	[241, 242]
Quercetin	Inhibition of MDR efflux pumps	Quercetin conjugates as good as or better than quercetin.	[243]
Protocatechuic acid (PCA)	Oxidative stress in rat hepatocytes	PCA had cytoprotective effects, but only at very high concentrations.	[244]
PCA	Human leukaemia cells	Promoted apoptosis at 2 mM concentration.	[245]
PCA	Cultured hepatocytes treated with t-butylhydroperoxide (t-BH)	Reduced oxidative stress markers in hepatocytes and administered orally, protected rats from liver damage by oral t-BH, according to several biochemical parameters.	[246]
PCA and other isolated colonic metabolites	Antiproliferative activity on prostate and colon cancer cells	Only PCA showed activity.	[172]
PCA, cyanidin, cyanidin glucoside	Protection of cultured neuronal cells from H2O2-induced oxidative stress	All 3 compounds were effective at the membrane level, but only PCA and cyanidin operated at the cytosolic (i.e., intracellular) level, suggesting ability to enter cells.	[247]

Table 5. (Continued)

Compounds tested	Assay	Outcome	Reference
Tea catechins and synthetic glucuronides	Scavenging of free radicals and inhibition of arachidonic acid release from HT-29 gut epithelial cells	Some synthetic tea catechin glucuronides retained similar activity to their aglycones.	[248]
Epicatechin and metabolites	Protection of cultured cells from H2O2-induced cytotoxicity	Epicatechin and a methylated metabolite had high protective capacity; glucuronides had almost none. The protection appears to arise from inhibition of the apoptotic associated enzyme, caspase-3.	[249, 250]
Mono- and di-demethylated metabolites of Nobiletin (hexamethoxyflavone)	Inhibition of bacterial lipopolysaccharide (LPS)-induced NO production and inducible nitric oxide synthase (iNOS), (COX-2) protein expression in RAW264.7 macrophages	The metabolites had stronger anti-inflammatory effects than nobiletin itself.	[251]
Quercetin, catechin, epicatechin, phloretin, phloridzin and corresponding mixtures of isomeric mono-glucuronides	Cytoprotection capacity for Jurkat T cells stressed with H2O2	All compounds reduced cell death, but glucuronide mixtures were less potent (IC50 1-16 µM) than aglycones (IC50 <0.5 µM).	[252]
Polyphenolic aglycones, glycosides and mammalian conjugates	Superoxide scavenging capacity	Flavonoid sophoroside, rhamnoglucoside and glucuronide derivatives had the highest capacity; sulphates and aglycones had much lower capacity. Cinnamic acids (caffeic and ferulic acids) were ineffective.	[253]
Hesperetin and glucuronides	UV-A-induced necrotic cell death	Hesperetin glucuronides were protective against cell death; the aglycone was not.	[254]

In addition to the numerous *in vitro* studies listed in Table 5, there have been a number of studies, often *in vivo,* combining investigation of metabolism and determination of biological activities of the metabolites.

Quercetin/Flavonols

Spencer *et al* investigated the uptake, metabolism and protection from oxidative stress of quercetin and its major metabolites (3'-O-methyl quercetin, 4'-O-methyl quercetin and quercetin 7-O-beta-D-glucuronide) in dermal fibroblasts [255]. Uptake and oxidative stress protection was highest with quercetin itself and lower with methyl derivatives. The glucuronide was not taken up by the cells and conferred no protection. In that study, quercetin appeared to be metabolised by the cells to a glutathione conjugate and a quinine derivative. Quercetin conjugates (glucuronide, sulphate, O-methyl) reduced COX-2 gene expression in *ex vivo* human lymphocytes, but a single feeding of human subjects with onions (containing 163.9 mg quercetin 3, 4'-diglucoside, 140.6 mg quercetin 4'-glucoside, and 2.4 mg quercetin aglycone) had no effect. Plasma quercetin metabolites attained a C_{max} of 4 µM [256].

Quercetin has been implicated in the anti-depressant effects of St John's Wort (SJW). When tested on rats using a forced swimming test, SJW extract, rutin and the quercetin metabolite isorhamnetin (3'-methyl quercetin) all exhibited anti-depressant activity after administration for 9 days; Isorhamnetin being most effective [257]. After eight days administration of SJW extract, concentrations in plasma and the central nervous system were 9.6 and 1.3 µM for quercetin and conjugates and 7.4 and 2 µM for methylated quercetin and conjugates.

High acute doses of quercetin glucopyranoside (Isoquercitrin; 100 mg/kg) achieved quercetin C_{max} in the plasma and central nervous system of 16.5 and 2.9 µM, respectively. Unfortunately, in this study the brains were not perfused prior to analysis and the brain levels of these compounds are likely overstated due to contamination from blood circulating in the brain at the time of death. The corresponding C_{max} values for methylated quercetin and conjugates were 10.7 and 2.7 µM. Human subjects fed a soup high in quercetin exhibited higher plasma quercetin conjugate concentrations and reduced collagen-stimulated platelet aggregation than controls on low quercetin soup [258].

Antibody staining of quercetin-3-glucuronide showed that it preferentially accumulated in macrophage-derived foam cells, abundant in human aortic atherosclerotic lesions, but not normal aorta, where foam cells are rare.

In addition, the glucuronide was taken up by murine macrophages and de-conjugated to quercetin aglycone. The aglycone suppressed expression of genes involved in foam cell formation, suggesting that quercetin conjugates may inhibit atherosclerosis [259]. Conjugation, therefore, appears to have the potential to considerably modify the *in vivo* biological activity of absorbed flavonoids.

The picture that emerges from the many studies on quercetin is that the aglycone and its conjugates share many activities, although often with considerably different efficacy. In addition, some conjugates lose activities or exhibit activities that the aglycone does not. It is clearly not valid to assume any relationship between *in vitro* activities of flavonoid aglycones and *in vivo* effects from that compound in the diet. In addition, positive results *in vitro*, even from verified conjugates, do not necessarily translate into *in vivo* effects following an acute dose.

Isoflavones

Some individuals produce equol, as a major metabolite of daidzein, whereas others do not produce detectable equol [162], presumably because of differences in colonic microflora composition and isoflavone metabolism. Equol has well characterised cardiovascular benefits [260]. It also inhibits neoplastic cell transformation *in vitro*, a potential mechanism for the anti-cancer effect attributed to daidzein [261]. With regard to cancer therapy genistein and daidzein glucuronides were oestrogenic, but ~10-fold weaker than their aglycones and weakly activated natural killer (NK) cells against cancer cells [262]. Microarray analysis of the effects of soy isoflavones on gene expression uncovered a relationship between the ability to produce equol and a greater expression in oestrogen-responsive genes [263]. Equol appears to affect gene expression more than daidzein. Dietary equol attenuated weight gain in ovariectomised rats, but did not prevent bone-loss and had an undesirable uterotrophic effect [264, 265]. In contrast, a similar study found that equol did prevent bone loss, but the other major daidzein metabolite, O-desmethylangolensin, did not [266]. In a study on menopausal women, 135 mg/day for one week of soy isoflavones only improved menopausal symptoms in individuals who were equol producers. Equol appears to be primarily responsible for the health benefits of dietary soy isoflavones. High-dose oral equol (400 mg/kg) in ovariectomised rats produced a mammotropic (stimulatory) effect, suggesting that equol is weakly oestrogenic [267].

Catechins

A human intervention trial suggested that the increase in flow-mediated arterial dilation resulting from tea consumption is inversely related to an individual's ability to methylate tea flavonoids [6], i.e., methylation decreases biological activity.

Other Flavonoids

Anthocyanins and their suspected colonic phenolic acid metabolites were tested for their ability to inhibit platelet activation *in vitro* [268], an ability thought to be beneficial in the prevention of coronary vascular disease (CVD). Significant inhibition was observed with 1 μM anthocyanins or 10 μM of most of the phenolic acids tested. Notable exceptions, showing no activity, were hippuric acid and homovanillic acid. A mixture of all the tested compounds, (probably more representative of the *in vivo* situation), was the most effective, even at 1 μM total concentration. Although the phenolic acids required a higher concentration, they are likely to be present individually at much higher concentrations than anthocyanins in the body. The "simulated metabolite mixture" of both individually active and inactive compounds exhibited a strong synergy, although which of the components were synergistic was not determined.

Some flavonoid conjugates demonstrate anti-inflammatory activity. Myricetin glucuronide had an anti-inflammatory effect in a carrageenan-induced rat model of inflammation and showed inhibitory activity for 5-lipoxygenase and cyclo-oxygenase (COX)-1 and COX-2 and [269]. Oral administration to rats of 100 mg/Kg of astilbin (a flavanone rhamnoside) resulted in low micromolar concentrations in plasma of astilbin and a methylated metabolite, plus a glucuronide in bile only [270]. The methylated metabolite and astilbin had similar anti-inflammatory effects when injected intra-peritoneally into mice, i.e., ~halving picryl chloride-induced ear swelling and nearly normalising elevated levels of tumour necrosis factor α (TNF) and Interferon-γ (IFN-).

Apple juice phenolic extracts, fermented anaerobically by human faecal flora, had 30-50% of the Trolox equivalent antioxidant capacity (TEAC) of the unfermented extracts, but in Caco-2 cell-based antioxidant assays, the fermented extract was significantly better at inhibiting ROS formation induced by t-BH [271]. The main identified constituent of the fermented extract were 3,4-dihydroxy- and 4-hydroxy-phenylpropionic acid, phloroglucinol and 3,4-dihydroxyphenylacetic acid. These data indicate that inhibition of ROS formation by phenolics is not likely the result of their chemical antioxidant activity but rather, induction of endogenous cytoprotective mechanisms.

The plant-derived glucuronide baicalin (bicalein-7-glucuronide) is both the major natural form and the major human conjugate of the flavonoid baicalein [81]. The glucuronide was able to induce apoptosis in cultured prostate cancer cells [272] and Jurkat leukemic T lymphocytes [273]. In the latter case, it appeared to act by caspase activation via the mitochondrial pathway but cytotoxicity for normal peripheral blood mononuclear cells was much lower. The intestinal absorption of this compound is much lower than its aglycone [81] but these results demonstrate the biological activity of a flavonoid glucuronide.

Conclusion

Although there is considerable quantitative variation between different studies, even of the same compound, as to the proportions absorbed, excreted, degraded, or metabolised by different means, some generalisations can be made. It is clear that net intestinal absorption of a few individual flavonoids may be as high as 10-20% of intake, under experimental conditions, but under normal circumstances, figures of 1-2% appear more likely and some compounds may be lower still. The more hydrophobic flavonoids, when consumed as glucosides, appear to be the best absorbed, usually via enzymic deglycosylation, followed by diffusion of the aglycone across intestinal cell membranes. More polar compounds, such as catechins, are relatively poorly absorbed and glycosides other than glucosides are resistant to deglycosylation and are slowly absorbed, by diffusion or possibly sugar transporters. Anthocyanins appear to be hardly absorbed at all, based on urinary excretion measurements, but newer evidence suggests that their absorption may be both relatively extensive and rapid, but counterbalanced by very rapid degradation and a consequent very short plasma half-life. The plasma typically appears to contain only traces of most flavonoid aglycones or their original glycosidic forms; a very high, but somewhat variable, percentage is in the form of the polar conjugates, glucuronides and sulphates. The flavonoids in plasma appear to be predominantly bound to serum albumin and maybe other proteins and this, combined with cellular MDR efflux pumps, limits organ bioavailability, particularly to the brain. The only apparent exception is the liver, which may actively take up flavonoid glucuronides, to relatively high concentrations and appears to modify their conjugation. The intestine appears to predominantly glucuronidate flavonoids, whereas the liver may de-glucuronidate them and/or add sulphate and/or methyl groups.

It appears that ~90% of the dietary intake of most flavonoids passes into the colon, either directly, after absorption and MDR-mediated efflux by intestinal cells, or biliary excretion. The colonic microflora can deglycosylate most flavonoid glycosides, thus potentially increasing bioavailability, but can also further degrade the aglycones into phenolic acids and further into simple compounds like benzoic acid, acetic acid and carbon dioxide. The phenolic acids appear to be generally very well absorbed and may make a significant indirect contribution to any health benefits attributed to the flavonoid they were derived from.

Hence, although bioavailability and metabolism studies of flavonoids have discovered a great deal, the information is very fragmented and contradictory. We still have minimal ability to predict or model the expected intracellular concentrations of the numerous metabolites of even one flavonoid. The complex metabolite mixture arising from the numerous flavonoids in a typical diet may not be amenable to modelling in the foreseeable future.

Although the quantitative significance of the biological activities of flavonoid aglycones *in vivo* is doubtful, there are many examples of similarly potent *in vitro* activities of their metabolites, in many different biological aspects. The critical observation, however, is that the activity of the metabolites is, more often than not, considerably different in type of response or magnitude of biological effect, from the original flavonoid. There is one example (see above) in which a combination of weakly active phenolic acid metabolites showed a strong synergy [268], suggesting that a combination of *in vivo* metabolites may have greater health benefits than any of the individual compounds.

Theoretically, a detailed knowledge of flavonoid metabolism, combined with extensive *in vitro* testing of the metabolites, individually and in combination, could elucidate their specific health benefits, to the extent that health benefits could be attributed to individual compounds. However, the permutations of many metabolites and assays may be too numerous and complex for this to ever be a practical proposition. There is also at least one example of the failure of this approach [256]. In this study, an *in vitro* bioassay of identified metabolites of quercetin reduced COX-2 gene-expression but a human trial of quercetin failed to replicate the result.

An alternative approach has recently been proposed [274] that has potential to evaluate real *in vivo* activities of flavonoids, without the necessity to gather huge amounts of ADME data. This involves human subjects consuming the compound or food of interest and the application of their serum to cell cultures. The cells should thus be treated with a truly representative mixture of flavonoid metabolites, at physiologically relevant concentrations, along with any endogenous signalling molecules that they induce. In this particular study, it was found that endothelial cell cultures produced completely different responses in expression of CVD biomarker genes when treated with serum from red-wine drinkers or red wine itself. It is likely that better results could have been obtained from treating the cells with a simulated red-wine polyphenol metabolite mixture, but determining the composition of such a mixture would be a huge undertaking and probably impractical for the hundreds of foods that need to be tested. Another recent study detected anti-inflammatory effects from pomegranate phenolic extract using this approach on rabbits [275]. More work is needed to confirm the validity of this novel approach, but if it is proved successful, it would be a major step towards simplifying the whole area of flavonoid biological activity determination. This approach may be very useful to assist with interpretation of complex ADME data.

References

[1] Heiss, C.; Finis, D.; Kleinbongard, P.; Hoffmann, A.; Rassaf, T.; Kelm, M.; and Sies, H. (2007). Sustained increase in flow-mediated dilation after daily intake of high-flavanol cocoa drink over 1 week. *Journal of Cardiovascular Pharmacology and Therapeutics, 49,* 74-80.

[2] Tavani, A.; Spertini, L.; Bosetti, C.; Parpinel, M.; Gnagnarella, P.; Bravi, F.; Peterson, J.; Dwyer, J.; Lagiou, P.; Negri, E.; and La Vecchia, C. (2006). Intake of specific flavonoids and risk of acute myocardial infarction in Italy. *Public Health Nutrition, 9,* 369-374.

[3] Mink, P. J.; Scrafford, C. G.; Barraj, L. M.; Harnack, L.; Hong, C.-P.; Nettleton, J. A.; and Jacobs, D. R., Jr. (2007). Flavonoid intake and cardiovascular disease mortality: a prospective study in postmenopausal women. *American Journal of Clinical Nutrition, 85,* 895-909.

[4] Naissides, M.; Pal, S.; Mamo, J. C. L.; James, A. P.; and Dhaliwal, S. (2006). The effect of chronic consumption of red wine polyphenols on vascular function in postmenopausal women. *European Journal of Clinical Nutrition, 60,* 740-745.

[5] Bayard, V.; Chamorro, F.; Motta, J.; and Hollenberg, N. K. (2007). Does flavanol intake influence mortality from nitric oxide-dependent processes? Ischemic heart disease, stroke, diabetes mellitus, and cancer in Panama. *International Journal of Medical Sciences, 4,* 53-58.

[6] Hodgson, J. M.; Puddey, I. B.; Burke, V.; and Croft, K. D. (2006). Is reversal of endothelial dysfunction by tea related to flavonoid metabolism? *British Journal of Nutrition, 95,* 14-17.

[7] Neuhouser, M. L. (2004). Dietary flavonoids and cancer risk: Evidence from human population studies. *Nutrition and Cancer, 50,* 1-7.

[8] Hertog, M. G. L.; Feskens, E. J. M.; Hollman, P. C. H.; Katan, M. B.; and Kromhout, D. (1994). Dietary flavonoids and cancer risk in the Zutphen Elderly Study. *Nutrition and Cancer-an International Journal, 22,* 175.

[9] Hertog, M. G. L.; Feskens, E. J. M.; Hollman, P. C. H.; Katan, M. B.; and Kromhout, D. (1993). Dietary antioxidant Ffonoids and risk of coronary heart-disease - the Zutphen Elderly Study. *Lancet, 342,* 1007.

[10] Bosetti, C.; Rossi, M.; McLaughlin, J. K.; Negri, E.; Talamini, R.; Lagiou, P.; Montella, M.; Ramazzotti, V.; Franceschi, S.; and LaVecchia, C. (2007). Flavonoids and the risk of renal cell carcinoma. *Cancer Epidemiology Biomarkers and Prevention, 16,* 98-101.

[11] Cui, Y.; Morgenstern, H.; Greenland, S.; Tashkin, D. P.; Mao, J. T.; Cai, L.; Cozen, W.; Mack, T. M.; Lu, Q.-Y.; and Zhang, Z.-F. (2008). Dietary flavonoid intake and lung cancer - A population-based case-control study. *Cancer, 112,* 2241-2248.

[12] Hooper, L.; Kroon, P. A.; Rimm, E. B.; Cohn, J. S.; Harvey, I.; Le Cornu, K. A.; Ryder, J. J.; Hall, W. L.; and Cassidy, A. (2008). Flavonoids, flavonoid-rich foods, and cardiovascular risk: a meta-analysis of randomized controlled trials. *American Journal of Clinical Nutrition, 88,* 38-50.

[13] Stevenson, D. E.; and Hurst, R. D. (2007). Polyphenolic phytochemicals - just antioxidants or much more? *Cellular and Molecular Life Sciences, 64,* 2900-2916.

[14] Scheline, R. R. (1991). *Handbook of mammalian metabolism of plant compounds*. Boca Raton: CRC Press.

[15] Aura, A.-M. (2008). Microbial metabolism of dietary phenolic compounds in the colon. *Phytochemistry Reviews, 7,* 407-429.

[16] Clifford, M. N. (2004). Diet-derived Phenols in plasma and tissues and their implications for health. *Planta Medica, 70,* 1103-1114.

[17] Kroon, P.; and Williamson, G. (2005). Polyphenols: dietary components with established benefits to health? *Journal of the Science of Food and Agriculture, 85,* 1239-1240.

[18] Kroon, P. A.; Clifford, M. N.; Crozier, A.; Day, A. J.; Donovan, J. L.; Manach, C.; and Williamson, G. (2004). How should we assess the effects of exposure to dietary polyphenols in vitro? *American Journal of Clinical Nutrition, 80,* 15-21.

[19] Manach, C.; and Donovan, J. L. (2004). Pharmacokinetics and metabolism of dietary flavonoids in humans. *Free Radical Research, 38,* 771-785.

[20] Manach, C.; Williamson, G.; Morand, C.; Scalbert, A.; and Remesy, C. (2005). Bioavailability and bioefficacy of polyphenols in humans. I. Review of 97 bioavailability studies. *American Journal of Clinical Nutrition, 81,* 230S-242S.

[21] Walle, T. (2004). Absorption and metabolism of flavonoids. *Free Radical Biology and Medicine, 36,* 829-837.

[22] Williamson, G. (2002). The use of flavonoid aglycones in in vitro systems to test biological activities: based on bioavailability data, is this a valid approach? *Phytochemistry Reviews, V1,* 215-222.

[23] Williamson, G.; and Manach, C. (2005). Bioavailability and bioefficacy of polyphenols in humans. II. Review of 93 intervention studies. *American Journal of Clinical Nutrition, 81,* 243S-255S.

[24] Scalbert, A.; Morand, C.; Manach, C.; and Remesy, C. (2002). Absorption and metabolism of polyphenols in the gut and impact on health. *Biomedicine and Pharmacotherapy, 56,* 276-282.

[25] Karakaya, S. (2004). Bioavailability of phenolic compounds. *Critical Reviews in Food Science and Nutrition, 44,* 453-464.

[26] Clifford, M. N.; and Brown, J. E. (2006). Dietary flavonoids and health - broadening the perspective. In O. M. Andersen; and K. R. Markham (Eds.), *Flavonoids: Chemistry, Biochemistry and Applications* (pp. 319-370). Boca Raton: CRC Press.

[27] Kay, C. D. (2006). Aspects of anthocyanin absorption, metabolism and pharmacokinetics in humans. *Nutrition Research Reviews, 19,* 137-146.

[28] McGhie, T. K.; and Walton, M. C. (2007). The bioavailability and absorption of anthocyanins: Towards a better understanding. *Molecular Nutrition and Food Research, 51,* 702-713.

[29] Zhang, L.; Zuo, Z.; and Lin, G. (2007). Intestinal and hepatic glucuronidation of flavonoids. *Molecular Pharmaceutics, 4,* 833-845.

[30] Larkin, T.; Price, W. E.; and Astheimer, L. (2008). The key importance of soy isoflavone bioavailability to understanding health benefits. *Critical Reviews in Food Science and Nutrition, 48,* 538-552.

[31] Mullie, P.; Clarys, P.; Deriemaeker, P.; and Hebbelinck, M. (2008). Estimation of daily human intake of food flavonoids. *International Journal of Food Sciences and Nutrition, 59,* 291-298.

[32] Walle, T.; Browning, A. M.; Steed, L. L.; Reed, S. G.; and Walle, U. K. (2005). Flavonoid glucosides are hydrolyzed and thus activated in the oral cavity in humans. *Journal of Nutrition*, *135*, 48-52.

[33] Crespy, V.; Morand, C.; Besson, C.; Manach, C.; Demigne, C.; and Remesy, C. (2002). Quercetin, but not its glycosides, is absorbed from the rat stomach. *Journal of Agricultural and Food Chemistry*, *50*, 618-621.

[34] Spencer, J. P. E.; Chaudry, F.; Pannala, A. S.; Srai, S. K.; Debnam, E.; and Rice-Evans, C. (2000). Decomposition of cocoa procyanidins in the gastric milieu. *Biochemical and Biophysical Research Communications*, *272*, 236-241.

[35] Rios, L. Y.; Bennett, R. N.; Lazarus, S. A.; Remesy, C.; Scalbert, A.; and Williamson, G. (2002). Cocoa procyanidins are stable during gastric transit in humans'. *American Journal of Clinical Nutrition*, *76*, 1106-1110.

[36] Talavera, S.; Felgines, C.; Texier, O.; Besson, C.; Lamaison, J. L.; and Remesy, C. (2003). Anthocyanins are efficiently absorbed from the stomach in anesthetized rats. *Journal of Nutrition*, *133*, 4178-4182.

[37] McDougall, G. J.; Dobson, P.; Smith, P.; Blake, A.; and Stewart, D. (2005). Assessing potential bioavailability of raspberry anthocyanins using an in vitro digestion system. *Journal of Agricultural and Food Chemistry*, *53*, 5896-5904.

[38] Walton, M. C.; Hendriks, W. H.; Broomfield, A. M.; and McGhie, T. (2009). A viscous food matrix influences absorption and excretion but not metabolism of blackcurrant anthocyanins in rats. *Journal of Food Science*, *74, H22-H29*.

[39] Walton, M. C.; Lentle, R. G.; Reynolds, G. W.; Kruger, M. C.; and McGhie, T. K. (2006). Anthocyanin absorption and antioxidant status in pigs. *Journal of Agricultural and Food Chemistry*, *54*, 7940-7946.

[40] Sergent, T.; Ribonnet, L.; Kolosova, A.; Garsou, S.; Schaut, A.; De Saeger, S.; Van Peteghem, C.; Larondelle, Y.; Pussemier, L.; and Schneider, Y. J. (2008). Molecular and cellular effects of food contaminants and secondary plant components and their plausible interactions at the intestinal level. *Food and Chemical Toxicology*, *46*, 813-841.

[41] Shah, P.; Jogani, V.; Bagchi, T.; and Misra, A. (2006). Role of Caco-2 cell monolayers in prediction of intestinal drug absorption. *Biotechnology Progress*, *22*, 186-198.

[42] Hu, M.; Chen, J.; and Lin, H. M. (2003). Metabolism of flavonoids via enteric recycling: Mechanistic studies of disposition of apigenin in the Caco-2 cell culture model. *Journal of Pharmacology and Experimental Therapeutics*, *307*, 314-321.

[43] Bieger, J.; Cermak, R.; Blank, R.; de Boer, V. C. J.; Hollman, P. C. H.; Kamphues, J.; and Wolffram, S. (2008). Tissue distribution of quercetin in pigs after long-term dietary supplementation. *Journal of Nutrition*, *138*, 1417-1420.

[44] de Boer, V. C. J.; Dihal, A. A.; van der Woude, H.; Arts, I. C. W.; Wolffram, S.; Alink, G. M.; Rietjens, I. M. C. M.; Keijer, J.; and Hollman, P. C. H. (2005). Tissue distribution of quercetin in rats and pigs. *Journal of Nutrition*, *135*, 1718-1725.

[45] Wiczkowski, W.; Romaszko, J.; Bucinski, A.; Szawara-Nowak, D.; Honke, J.; Zielinski, H.; and Piskula, M. K. (2008). Quercetin from shallots (Allium cepa L. var. aggregatum) is more bioavailable than its glucosides. *Journal of Nutrition*, *138*, 885-888.

[46] Nemeth, K.; Plumb, G. W.; Berrin, J.-G.; Juge, N.; Jacob, R.; Naim, H. Y.; Williamson, G.; Swallow, D. M.; and Kroon, P. A. (2003). Deglycosylation by small intestinal

epithelial cell beta-glucosidases is a critical step in the absorption and metabolism of dietary flavonoid glycosides in humans. *European Journal of Nutrition*, *42*, 29-42.

[47] Day, A. J.; Canada, F. J.; Diaz, J. C.; Kroon, P. A.; McLauchlan, R.; Faulds, C. B.; Plumb, G. W.; Morgan, M. R. A.; and Williamson, G. (2000). Dietary flavonoid and isoflavone glycosides are hydrolysed by the lactase site of lactase phlorizin hydrolase. *FEBS Letters*, *468*, 166-170.

[48] Day, A. J.; DuPont, M. S.; Ridley, S.; Rhodes, M.; Rhodes, M. J. C.; Morgan, M. R. A.; and Williamson, G. (1998). Deglycosylation of flavonoid and isoflavonoid glycosides by human small intestine and liver beta-glucosidase activity. *FEBS Letters*, *436*, 71-75.

[49] Gee, J. M.; DuPont, M. S.; Day, A. J.; Plumb, G. W.; Williamson, G.; and Johnson, I. T. (2000). Intestinal transport of quercetin glycosides in rats involves both deglycosylation and interaction with the hexose transport pathway. *Journal of Nutrition*, *130*, 2765-2771.

[50] Arts, I. C. W.; Sesink, A. L. A.; Faassen-Peters, M.; and Hollman, P. C. H. (2004). The type of sugar moiety is a major determinant of the small intestinal uptake and subsequent biliary excretion of dietary quercetin glycosides. *British Journal of Nutrition*, *91*, 841-847.

[51] Spencer, J. P. E.; Chowrimootoo, G.; Choudhury, R.; Debnam, E. S.; Srai, S. K.; and Rice-Evans, C. (1999). The small intestine can both absorb and glucuronidate luminal flavonoids. *FEBS Letters*, *458*, 224-230.

[52] Serra, H.; Mendes, T.; Bronze, M. R.; and Simplicio, A. L. (2008). Prediction of intestinal absorption and metabolism of pharmacologically active flavones and flavanones. *Bioorganic and Medicinal Chemistry*, *16*, 4009-4018.

[53] Brand, W.; van der Wel, P. A. I.; Rein, M. J.; Barron, D.; Williamson, G.; van Bladeren, P. J.; and Rietjens, I. (2008). Metabolism and transport of the citrus flavonoid hesperetin in Caco-2 cell monolayers. *Drug Metabolism and Disposition*, *36*, 1794-1802.

[54] Kobayashi, S.; and Konishi, Y. (2008). Transepithelial transport of flavanone in intestinal Caco-2 cell monolayers. *Biochemical and Biophysical Research Communications*, *368*, 23-29.

[55] Kobayashi, S.; Tanabe, S.; Sugiyama, M.; and Konishi, Y. (2008). Transepithelial transport of hesperetin and hesperidin in intestinal Caco-2 cell monolayers. *Biochimica et Biophysica Acta-Biomembranes*, *1778*, 33-41.

[56] Hollman, P. C. H.; Van Trijp, J. M. P.; Buysman, M. N. C. P.; V.d. Gaag, M. S.; Mengelers, M. J. B.; De Vries, J. H. M.; and Katan, M. B. (1997). Relative bioavailability of the antioxidant flavonoid quercetin from various foods in man. *FEBS Letters*, *418*, 152-156.

[57] Zhang, L.; Lin, G.; Chang, Q.; and Zuo, Z. (2005). Role of intestinal first-pass metabolism of baicalein in its absorption process. *Pharmaceutical Research*, *22*, 1050-1058.

[58] Silberberg, M.; Morand, C.; Mathevon, T.; Besson, C.; Manach, C.; Scalbert, A.; and Remesy, C. (2005). The bioavailability of polyphenols is highly governed by the capacity of the intestine and of the liver to secrete conjugated metabolites. *European Journal of Nutrition*, *45*, 88-96.

[59] Crespy, V.; Morand, C.; Manach, C.; Besson, C.; Demigne, C.; and Remesy, C. (1999). Part of quercetin absorbed in the small intestine is conjugated and further secreted in

the intestinal lumen. *American Journal of Physiology-Gastrointestinal and Liver Physiology, 277*, G120-G126.

[60] Kahle, K.; Huemmer, W.; Kempf, M.; Scheppach, W.; Erk, T.; and Richling, E. (2007). Polyphenols are intensively metabolized in the human gastrointestinal tract after apple juice consumption. *Journal of Agricultural and Food Chemistry, 55*, 10605-10614.

[61] Cao, J.; Chen, X.; Liang, J.; Yu, X. Q.; Xu, A. L.; Chan, E.; Duan, W.; Huang, M.; Wen, J. Y.; Yu, X. Y.; Li, X. T.; Sheu, F. S.; and Zhou, S. F. (2007). Role of P-glycoprotein in the intestinal absorption of glabridin, an active flavonoid from the root of Glycyrrhiza glabra. *Drug Metabolism and Disposition, 35*, 539-553.

[62] Xu, Y. A.; Fan, G. R.; Gao, S.; and Hong, Z. Y. (2008). Assessment of intestinal absorption of vitexin-2"-O-rhamnoside in hawthorn leaves flavonoids in rat using in situ and in vitro absorption models. *Drug Development and Industrial Pharmacy, 34*, 164-170.

[63] Williamson, G.; Aeberli, I.; Miguet, L.; Zhang, Z.; Sanchez, M. B.; Crespy, V.; Barron, D.; Needs, P.; Kroon, P. A.; Glavinas, H.; Krajcsi, P.; and Grigorov, M. (2007). Interaction of positional isomers of quercetin glucuronides with the transporter ABCC2 (cMOAT, MRP2). *Drug Metabolism and Disposition, 35*, 1262-1268.

[64] Murakami, A.; Ohigashi, H.; Koshimizu, K.; Kawahara, S.; Matsuoka, Y.; Kuwahara, S.; Kuki, W.; Takahashi, Y.; and Hosotani, K. (2002). Characteristic rat tissue accumulation of nobiletin, a chemopreventive polymethoxyflavonoid, in comparison with luteolin. *BioFactors, 16*, 73-82.

[65] Walle, T. (2007). Methylation of dietary flavones greatly improves their hepatic metabolic stability and intestinal absorption. *Molecular Pharmaceutics, 4*, 826-832.

[66] Walle, T. (2007). Methoxylated flavones, a superior cancer chemopreventive flavonoid subclass? *Seminars in Cancer Biology, 17*, 354-362.

[67] Walle, T.; Wen, X.; and Walle, U. K. (2007). Improving metabolic stability of cancer chemoprotective polyphenols. *Expert Opinion on Drug Metabolism and Toxicology, 3*, 379-388.

[68] Walle, U. K.; and Walle, T. (2007). Bioavailable flavonoids: Cytochrome P450-mediated metabolism of methoxyflavones. *Drug Metabolism and Disposition, 35*, 1985-1989.

[69] O'Leary, K. A.; Day, A. J.; Needs, P. W.; Mellon, F. A.; O'Brien, N. M.; and Williamson, G. (2003). Metabolism of quercetin-7-and quercetin-3-glucuronides by an in vitro hepatic model: the role of human beta-glucuronidase, sulfotransferase, catechol-O-methyltransferase and multi-resistant protein 2 (MRP2) in flavonoid metabolism. *Biochemical Pharmacology, 65*, 479-491.

[70] Graf, B. A.; Ameho, C.; Dolnikowski, G. G.; Milbury, P. E.; Chen, C.-Y.; and Blumberg, J. B. (2006). Rat gastrointestinal tissues metabolize quercetin. *Journal of Nutrition, 136*, 39-44.

[71] Hollands, W.; Brett, G. M.; Radreau, P.; Saha, S.; Teucher, B.; Bennett, R. N.; and Kroon, P. A. (2008). Processing blackcurrants dramatically reduces the content and does not enhance the urinary yield of anthocyanins in human subjects. *Food Chemistry, 108*, 869-878.

[72] Prior, R. L.; and Wu, X. L. (2006). Anthocyanins: Structural characteristics that result in unique metabolic patterns and biological activities. *Free Radical Research, 40*, 1014-1028.

[73] El Mohsen, M. A.; Marks, J.; Kuhnle, G.; Moore, K.; Debnam, E.; Srai, S. K.; Rice-Evans, C.; and Spencer, J. P. E. (2006). Absorption, tissue distribution and excretion of pelargonidin and its metabolites following oral administration to rats. *British Journal of Nutrition, 95*.

[74] Felgines, C.; Talavera, S.; Texier, O.; Besson, C.; Fogliano, V.; Lamaison, J.-L.; Fauci, L. l.; Galvano, G.; Remesy, C.; and Galvano, F. (2006). Absorption and metabolism of red orange juice anthocyanins in rats. . *British Journal of Nutrition, 95*, 898-904.

[75] Matuschek, M. C.; Hendriks, W. H.; McGhie, T. K.; and Reynolds, G. W. (2006). The jejunum is the main site of absorption for anthocyanins in mice. *Journal of Nutritional Biochemistry, 17*, 31-36.

[76] Harada, K.; Kano, M.; Takayanagi, T.; Yamakawa, O.; and Ishikawa, F. (2004). Absorption of acylated anthocyanins in rats and humans after ingesting an extract of Ipomoea batatas purple sweet potato tuber. *Bioscience Biotechnology and Biochemistry, 68*, 1500-1507.

[77] Talavéra, S.; Felgines, C.; Texier, O.; Lamaison, J.-L.; Besson, C.; Gil-Izquierdo, A.; and Réme?sy, C. (2005). Anthocyanin metabolism in rats and their distribution to digestive area, kidney, and brain. *Journal of Agricultural and Food Chemistry, 53*, 3902-3908.

[78] Passamonti, S.; Vrhovsek, U.; Vanzo, A.; and Mattivi, F. (2005). Fast access of some grape pigments to the brain. *Journal of Agricultural and Food Chemistry, 53*, 7029-7034.

[79] Chen, T.; Li, L. P.; Lu, X. Y.; Jiang, H. D.; and Zeng, S. (2007). Absorption and excretion of luteolin and apigenin in rats after oral administration of Chrysanthemum morifolium extract. *Journal of Agricultural and Food Chemistry, 55*, 273-277.

[80] Kahle, K.; Kraus, M.; Scheppach, W.; Ackermann, M.; Ridder, F.; and Richling, E. (2006). Studies on apple and blueberry fruit constituents: Do the polyphenols reach the colon after ingestion? *Molecular Nutrition and Food Research, 50*, 418-423.

[81] Akao, T.; Kawabata, K.; Yanagisawa, E.; Ishihara, K.; Mizuhara, Y.; Wakui, Y.; Sakashita, Y.; and Kobashi, K. (2000). Balicalin, the predominant flavone glucuronide of scutellariae radix, is absorbed from the rat gastrointestinal tract as the aglycone and restored to its original form. *Journal of Pharmacy and Pharmacology, 52*, 1563.

[82] Ichiyanagi, T.; Shida, Y.; Rahman, M. M.; Hatano, Y.; and Konishi, T. (2006). Bioavailability and Tissue Distribution of Anthocyanins in Bilberry (Vaccinium myrtillus L.) Extract in Rats. *Journal of Agricultural and Food Chemistry, 54*, 6578-6587.

[83] Kalt, W.; Blumberg, J. B.; McDonald, J. E.; Vinqvist-Tymchuk, M. R.; Fillmore, S. A. E.; Graf, B. A.; O'Leary, J. M.; and Milbury, P. E. (2008). Identification of anthocyanins in the liver, eye, and brain of blueberry-fed pigs. *Journal of Agricultural and Food Chemistry, 56*, 705-712.

[84] Andres-Lacueva, C.; Shukitt-Hale, B.; Galli, R. L.; Jauregui, O.; Lamuela-Raventos, R. M.; and Joseph, J. A. (2005). Anthocyanins in aged blueberry-fed rats are found centrally and may enhance memory. *Nutritional Neuroscience, 8*, 111 - 120.

[85] Xia, H. J.; Qiu, F.; Zhu, S.; Zhang, T. Y.; Qu, G. X.; and Yao, X. S. (2007). Isolation and identification of ten metabolites of breviscapine in rat urine. *Biological and Pharmaceutical Bulletin, 30*, 1308-1316.

[86]   Kuhnle, G.; Spencer, J. P. E.; Schroeter, H.; Shenoy, B.; Debnam, E. S.; Srai, S. K. S.; Rice-Evans, C.; and Hahn, U. (2000). Epicatechin and catechin are O-methylated and glucuronidated in the small intestine. *Biochemical and Biophysical Research Communications*, *277*, 507-512.

[87]   Yang, C. S.; Chen, L. S.; Lee, M. J.; Balentine, D.; Kuo, M. C.; and Schantz, S. P. (1998). Blood and urine levels of tea catechins after ingestion of different amounts of green tea by human volunteers. *Cancer Epidemiology Biomarkers and Prevention*, *7*, 351-354.

[88]   Chu, K. O.; Wang, C. C.; Chu, C. Y.; Choy, K. W.; Pang, C. P.; and Rogers, M. S. (2006). Uptake and distribution of catechins in fetal organs following in utero exposure in rats. *Human Reproduction*, *22*, 280-287.

[89]   Walton, M. C.; McGhie, T. K.; Reynolds, G. W.; and Hendriks, W. H. (2006). The flavonol quercetin-3-glucoside inhibits cyanidin-3-glucoside absorption in vitro. *Journal of Agricultural and Food Chemistry*, *54*, 4913-4920.

[90]   Suganuma, M.; Okabe, S.; Oniyama, M.; Tada, Y.; Ito, H.; and Fujiki, H. (1998). Wide distribution of H-3 (-)-epigallocatechin gallate, a cancer preventive tea polyphenol, in mouse tissue. *Carcinogenesis*, *19*, 1771-1776.

[91]   Kay, C. D.; Mazza, G.; Holub, B. J.; and Wang, J. (2004). Anthocyanin metabolites in human urine and serum. *British Journal of Nutrition*, *91*, 933-942.

[92]   Tsuda, T.; Horio, F.; and Osawa, T. (1999). Absorption and metabolism of cyanidin 3-O-[beta]-glucoside in rats. *FEBS Letters*, *449*, 179-182.

[93]   Ruefer, C. E.; Bub, A.; Moeseneder, J.; Winterhalter, P.; Stuertz, M.; and Kulling, S. E. (2008). Pharmacokinetics of the soybean isoflavone daidzein in its aglycone and glucoside form: a randomized, double-blind, crossover study. *American Journal of Clinical Nutrition*, *87*, 1314-1323.

[94]   Ichiyanagi, T.; Rahman, M. M.; Kashiwada, Y.; Ikeshiro, Y.; Shida, Y.; Hatano, Y.; Matsumoto, H.; Hirayama, M.; Tsuda, T.; and Konishi, T. (2004). Absorption and metabolism of delphinidin 3-O-[beta]-glucopyranoside in rats. *Free Radical Biology and Medicine*, *36*, 930-937.

[95]   Poquet, L.; Clifford, M. N.; and Williamson, G. (2008). Investigation of the metabolic fate of dihydrocaffeic acid. *Biochemical Pharmacology*, *75*, 1218-1229.

[96]   Cao, G.; Muccitelli, H. U.; Sanchez-Moreno, C.; and Prior, R. L. (2001). Anthocyanins are absorbed in glycated forms in elderly women: a pharmacokinetic study. *American Journal of Clinical Nutrition*, *73*, 920-926.

[97]   Ito, C.; Oi, N.; Hashimoto, T.; Nakabayashi, H.; Aoki, F.; Tominaga, Y.; Yokota, S.; Hosoe, K.; and Kanazawa, K. (2007). Absorption of dietary licorice isoflavan glabridin to blood circulation in rats. *Journal of Nutritional Science and Vitaminology*, *53*, 358-365.

[98]   Mata-Bilbao, M. D.; Andres-Lacueva, C.; Roura, E.; Jaduregui, O.; Escriban, E.; Torre, C.; and Lamuela-Raventos, R. M. (2007). Absorption and pharmacokinetics of grapefruit flavanones in beagles. *British Journal of Nutrition*, *98*, 86-92.

[99]   Kanaze, F. I.; Bounartzi, M. I.; Georgarakis, M.; and Niopas, I. (2007). Pharmacokinetics of the citrus flavanone aglycones hesperetin and naringenin after single oral administration in human subjects. *European Journal of Clinical Nutrition*, *61*, 472-477.

[100] Franke, A. A.; Custer, L. J.; and Hundahl, S. A. (2004). Determinants for urinary and plasma isoflavones in humans after soy intake. *Nutrition and Cancer, 50*, 141-154.

[101] DuPont, M. S.; Day, A. J.; Bennett, R. N.; Mellon, F. A.; and Kroon, P. A. (2004). Absorption of kaempferol from endive, a source of kaempferol-3-glucuronide, in humans. *European Journal of Clinical Nutrition, 58*, 947.

[102] Choudhury, R.; Chowrimootoo, G.; Srai, K.; Debnam, E.; and Rice-Evans, C. A. (1999). Interactions of the flavonoid naringenin in the gastrointestinal tract and the influence of glycosylation. *Biochemical and Biophysical Research Communications, 265*, 410-415.

[103] Gardana, C.; Guarnieri, S.; Riso, P.; Simonetti, P.; and Porrini, M. (2007). Flavanone plasma pharmacokinetics from blood orange juice in human subjects. *British Journal of Nutrition, 98*, 165-172.

[104] Mennen, L. I.; Sapinho, D.; Ito, H.; Galan, P.; Hercberg, S.; and Scalbert, A. (2008). Urinary excretion of 13 dietary flavonoids and phenolic acids in free-living healthy subjects variability and possible use as biomarkers of polyphenol intake. *European Journal of Clinical Nutrition, 62*, 519-525.

[105] Crespy, V.; Morand, C.; Besson, C.; Manach, C.; Demigne, C.; and Remesy, C. (2001). Comparison of the intestinal absorption of quercetin, phloretin and their glucosides in rats. *Journal of Nutrition, 131*, 2109-2114.

[106] Zhou, D. Y.; Xing, R.; Xu, Q.; Xue, X. Y.; Zhang, F. F.; and Liang, X. M. (2008). Polymethoxylated flavones metabolites in rat plasma after the consumption of Fructus aurantii extract: Analysis by liquid chromatography/electrospray ion trap mass spectrometry. *Journal of Pharmaceutical and Biomedical Analysis, 46*, 543-549.

[107] Spencer, J. P. E.; Schroeter, H.; Shenoy, B.; Srai, S. K. S.; Debnam, E. S.; and Rice-Evans, C. (2001). Epicatechin is the primary bioavailable form of the procyanidin dimers B2 and B5 after transfer across the small intestine. *Biochemical and Biophysical Research Communications, 285*, 588-593.

[108] Wang, J. F.; Schramm, D. D.; Holt, R. R.; Ensunsa, J. L.; Fraga, C. G.; Schmitz, H. H.; and Keen, C. L. (2000). A dose-response effect from chocolate consumption on plasma epicatechin and oxidative damage. *Journal of Nutrition, 130*, 2115S-2119S.

[109] Donovan, J. L.; Manach, C.; Rios, L.; Morand, C.; Scalbert, A.; and Remesy, C. (2002). Procyanidins are not bioavailable in rats fed a single meal containing a grapeseed extract or the procyanidin dimer B-3. *British Journal of Nutrition, 87*, 299-306.

[110] Nakamura, Y.; and Tonogai, Y. (2003). Metabolism of grape seed polyphenol in the rat. *Journal of Agricultural and Food Chemistry, 51*, 7215 -7225.

[111] Prasain, J. K.; Jones, K.; Brissie, N.; Moore, R.; Wyss, J. M.; and Barnes, S. (2004). Identification of Puerarin and Its Metabolites in Rats by Liquid Chromatography-Tandem Mass Spectrometry. *Journal of Agricultural and Food Chemistry, 52*, 3708-3712.

[112] Murota, K.; and Terao, J. (2005). Quercetin appears in the lymph of unanesthetized rats as its phase II metabolites after administered into the stomach. *FEBS Letters, 579*, 5343-5346.

[113] Day, A. J.; Mellon, F.; Barron, D.; Sarrazin, G.; Morgan, M. R. A.; and Williamson, G. (2001). Human metabolism of dietary flavonoids: Identification of plasma metabolites of quercetin. *Free Radical Research, 35*, 941-952.

[114] Graefe, E. U.; Wittig, J.; Mueller, S.; Riethling, A. K.; Uehleke, B.; Drewelow, B.; Pforte, H.; Jacobasch, G.; Derendorf, H.; and Veit, M. (2001). Pharmacokinetics and bioavailability of quercetin glycosides in humans. *Journal of Clinical Pharmacology*, *41*, 492-499.

[115] Wittig, J.; Herderich, M.; Graefe, E. U.; and Veit, M. (2001). Identification of quercetin glucuronides in human plasma by high-performance liquid chromatography-tandem mass spectrometry. *Journal of Chromatography B*, *753*, 237-243.

[116] Mullen, W.; Edwards, C. A.; and Crozier, A. (2006). Absorption, excretion and metabolite profiling of methyl-, glucuronyl-, glucosyl- and sulpho-conjugates of quercetin in human plasma and urine after ingestion of onions. *British Journal of Nutrition*, *96*, 107-116.

[117] Benito, S.; Mitjavila, M. T.; and Buxaderas, S. (2004). Flavonoid metabolites and susceptibility of rat lipoproteins to oxidation. *American Journal of Physiology - Heart and Circulatory Physiology*, *287*.

[118] Day, A. J.; Gee, J. M.; DuPont, M. S.; Johnson, I. T.; and Williamson, G. (2003). Absorption of quercetin-3-glucoside and quercetin-4 '-glucoside in the rat small intestine: the role of lactase phlorizin hydrolase and the sodium-dependent glucose transporter. *Biochemical Pharmacology*, *65*, 1199-1206.

[119] Moon, Y. J.; Wang, L.; DiCenzo, R.; and Morris, M. E. (2008). Quercetin pharmacokinetics in humans. *Biopharmaceutics and Drug Disposition*, *29*, 205-217.

[120] Dragoni, S.; Gee, J.; Bennett, R.; Valoti, M.; and Sgaragli, G. (2006). Red wine alcohol promotes quercetin absorption and directs its metabolism towards isorhamnetin and tamarixetin in rat intestine in vitro. *British Journal of Pharmacology*, *147*, 765-771.

[121] Kuhnle, G.; Spencer, J. P. E.; Chowrimootoo, G.; Schroeter, H.; Debnam, E. S.; Srai, S. K. S.; Rice-Evans, C.; and Hahn, U. (2000). Resveratrol is absorbed in the small intestine as resveratrol glucuronide. *Biochemical and Biophysical Research Communications*, *272*, 212-217.

[122] Goldberg, D. A.; Yan, J.; and Soleas, G. J. (2003). Absorption of three wine-related polyphenols in three different matrices by healthy subjects. *Clinical Biochemistry*, *36*, 79-87.

[123] Vitrac, X.; Desmouliere, A.; Brouillaud, B.; Krisa, S.; Deffieux, G.; Barthe, N.; Rosenbaum, J.; and Merillon, J. M. (2003). Distribution of C-14 -trans-resveratrol, a cancer chemopreventive polyphenol, in mouse tissues after oral administration. *Life Sciences*, *72*, 2219-2233.

[124] Chen, X. Y.; Cui, L.; Duan, X. T.; Ma, B.; and Zhong, D. F. (2006). Pharmacokinetics and metabolism of the flavonoid scutellarin in humans after a single oral administration. *Drug Metabolism and Disposition*, *34*, 1345.

[125] Gee, J. M.; Wroblewska, M. A.; Bennett, R. N.; Mellon, F. A.; and Johnson, I. T. (2004). Absorption and twenty-four-hour metabolism time-course of quercetin-3-O-glucoside in rats, in vivo. *Journal of the Science of Food and Agriculture*, *84*, 1341-1348.

[126] Tsuji, A.; Takanaga, H.; Tamai, I.; and Terasaki, T. (1994). Transcellular Transport of Benzoic Acid Across Caco-2 Cells by a pH-Dependent and Carrier-Mediated Transport Mechanism. *Pharmaceutical Research*, *11*, 30-37.

[127] Tamai, I.; Takanaga, H.; Maeda, H.; Yabuuchi, H.; Sai, Y.; Suzuki, Y.; and Tsuji, A. (1997). Intestinal brush-border membrane transport of monocarboxylic acids mediated

by proton-coupled transport and anion antiport mechanisms. *Journal of Pharmacy and Pharmacology*, *49*, 108-112.

[128] Konishi, Y.; Kobayashi, S.; and Shimizu, M. (2003). Transepithelial transport of p-coumaric acid and gallic acid in caco-2 cell monolayers. *Bioscience Biotechnology and Biochemistry*, *67*, 2317-2324.

[129] Haughton, E.; Clifford, M. N.; and Sharp, P. (2007). Monocarboxylate transporter expression is associated with the absorption of benzoic acid in human intestinal epithelial cells. *Journal of the Science of Food and Agriculture*, *87*, 239-244.

[130] Steinert, R. E.; Ditscheid, B.; Netzel, M.; and Jahreis, G. (2008). Absorption of black currant anthocyanins by monolayers of human intestinal epithelial Caco-2 cells mounted in using type chambers. *Journal of Agricultural and Food Chemistry*, *56*, 4995-5001.

[131] Jodoin, J.; Demeule, M.; and Beliveau, R. (2002). Inhibition of the multidrug resistance P-glycoprotein activity by green tea polyphenols. *Biochimica et Biophysica Acta-Molecular Cell Research*, *1542*, 149-159.

[132] Konishi, Y.; Kobayashi, S.; and Shimizu, M. (2003). Tea polyphenols inhibit the transport of dietary phenolic acids mediated by the monocarboxylic acid transporter (MCT) in intestinal Caco-2 cell monolayers. *Journal of Agricultural and Food Chemistry*, *51*, 7296-7302.

[133] Konishi, Y.; Kubo, K.; and Shimizu, M. (2003). Structural effects of phenolic acids on the transepithelial transport of fluorescein in Caco-2 cell monolayers. *Bioscience Biotechnology and Biochemistry*, *67*, 2014-2017.

[134] Hong, S. S.; Seo, K.; Lim, S. C.; and Han, H. K. (2007). Interaction characteristics of flavonoids with human organic anion transporter 1 (hOAT1) and 3 (hOAT3). *Pharmacological Research*, *56*, 468-473.

[135] Wen, X.; and Walle, T. (2006). Methylation protects dietary flavonoids from rapid hepatic metabolism. *Xenobiotica*, *36*, 387-397.

[136] Wen, X.; and Walle, T. (2006). Methylated flavonoids have greatly improved intestinal absorption and metabolic stability. *Drug Metabolism and Disposition*, *34*, 1786-1792.

[137] Liu, X.; Tam, V. H.; and Hu, M. (2007). Disposition of flavonoids via enteric recycling: Determination of the UDP-Glucuronosyltransferase Isoforms responsible for the metabolism of flavonoids in intact caco-2 TC7 cells using siRNA. *Molecular Pharmaceutics*, *4*, 873-882.

[138] Manna, C.; Galletti, P.; Maisto, G.; Cucciolla, V.; D'Angelo, S.; and Zappia, V. (2000). Transport mechanism and metabolism of olive oil hydroxytyrosol in Caco-2 cells. *FEBS Letters*, *470*, 341-344.

[139] Murakami, A.; Koshimizu, K.; Kuwahara, S.; Takahashi, Y.; Ito, C.; Furukawa, H.; Ju-Ichi, M.; and Ohigashi, H. (2001). In vitro absorption and metabolism of nobiletin, a chemopreventive polymethoxyflavonoid in citrus fruits. *Bioscience, Biotechnology and Biochemistry*, *65*, 194-197.

[140] Boyer, J.; Brown, D.; and Rui, H. L. (2004). Uptake of quercetin and quercetin 3-glucoside from whole onion and apple peel extracts by Caco-2 cell monolayers. *Journal of Agricultural and Food Chemistry*, *52*, 7172-7179.

[141] Walgren, R. A.; Lin, J.-T.; Kinne, R. K. H.; and Walle, T. (2000). Cellular uptake of dietary flavonoid quercetin 4'-beta -glucoside by sodium-dependent glucose transporter SGLT1. *Journal of Pharmacology and Experimental Therapeutics*, *294*, 837-843.

[142] Chen, C. H.; Hsu, H. J.; Huang, Y. J.; and Lin, C. J. (2007). Interaction of flavonoids and intestinal facilitated glucose transporters. *Planta Medica, 73,* 348-354.

[143] Keppler, K.; Hein, E. M.; and Humpf, H. U. (2006). Metabolism of quercetin and rutin by the pig caecal microflora prepared by freeze-preservation. *Molecular Nutrition and Food Research, 50,* 686-695.

[144] Jenner, A. M.; Rafter, J.; and Halliwell, B. (2005). Human fecal water content of phenolics: The extent of colonic exposure to aromatic compounds. *Free Radical Biology and Medicine, 38,* 763-772.

[145] Rechner, A. R.; Kuhnle, G.; Bremner, P.; Hubbard, G. P.; Moore, K. P.; and Rice-Evans, C. A. (2002). The metabolic fate of dietary polyphenols in humans. *Free Radical Biology and Medicine, 33,* 220-235.

[146] Clifford, M. N.; Copeland, E. L.; Bloxsidge, J. P.; and Mitchell, L. A. (2000). Hippuric acid as a major excretion product associated with black tea consumption. *Xenobiotica, 30,* 317-326.

[147] Mulder, T. P.; Rietveld, A. G.; and van Amelsvoort, J. M. (2005). Consumption of both black tea and green tea results in an increase in the excretion of hippuric acid into urine. *American Journal of Clinical Nutrition, 81,* 256S-260S.

[148] Rios, L. Y.; Gonthier, M. P.; Remesy, C.; Mila, L.; Lapierre, C.; Lazarus, S. A.; Williamson, G.; and Scalbert, A. (2003). Chocolate intake increases urinary excretion of polyphenol-derived phenolic acids in healthy human subjects. *American Journal of Clinical Nutrition, 77,* 912-918.

[149] Hong, Y. J.; and Mitchell, A. E. (2006). Identification of glutathione-related quercetin metabolites in humans. *Chemical Research in Toxicology, 19,* 1525-1532.

[150] Russell, W. R.; Labat, A.; Scobbie, L.; and Duncan, S. H. (2007). Availability of blueberry phenolics for microbial metabolism in the colon and the potential inflammatory implications. *Molecular Nutrition and Food Research, 51,* 726-731.

[151] Gonthier, M. P.; Remesy, C.; Scalbert, A.; Cheynier, V.; Souquet, J. M.; Poutanen, K.; and Aura, A. M. (2006). Microbial metabolism of caffeic acid and its esters chlorogenic and caftaric acids by human faecal microbiota in vitro. *Biomedicine and Pharmacotherapy, 60,* 536-540.

[152] Gonthier, M.-P.; Verny, M.-A.; Besson, C.; Remesy, C.; and Scalbert, A. (2003). Chlorogenic acid bioavailability largely depends on its metabolism by the gut microflora in rats. *Journal of Nutrition, 133,* 1853-1859.

[153] Andreasen, M. F.; Kroon, P. A.; Williamson, G.; and Garcia-Conesa, M. T. (2001). Intestinal release and uptake of phenolic antioxidant diferulic acids. *Free Radical Biology and Medicine, 31,* 304-314.

[154] Vitaglione, P.; Donnarumma, G.; Napolitano, A.; Galvano, F.; Gallo, A.; Scalfi, L.; and Fogliano, V. (2007). Protocatechuic acid is the major human metabolite of cyanidin-glucosides. *Journal of Nutrition, 137,* 2043-2048.

[155] Kelebek, H.; Canbas, A.; and Selli, S. (2008). Determination of phenolic composition and antioxidant capacity of blood orange juices obtained from cvs. Moro and Sanguinello (Citrus sinensis (L.) Osbeck) grown in Turkey. *Food Chemistry, 107,* 1710-1716.

[156] Nardini, M.; Natella, F.; Scaccini, C.; and Ghiselli, A. (2006). Phenolic acids from beer are absorbed and extensively metabolized in humans. *Journal of Nutritional Biochemistry, 17,* 14-22.

[157] Konishi, Y.; Hitomi, Y.; and Yoshioka, E. (2004). Intestinal absorption of p-coumaric and gallic acids in rats after oral administration. *Journal of Agricultural and Food Chemistry*, *52*, 2527-2532.

[158] DuPont, M. S.; Bennett, R. N.; Mellon, F. A.; and Williamson, G. (2002). Polyphenols from alcoholic apple cider are absorbed, metabolized and excreted by humans. *Journal of Nutrition*, *132*, 172-175.

[159] Crespy, V.; Aprikian, O.; Morand, C.; Besson, C.; Manach, C.; Demigne, C.; and Remesy, C. (2001). Bioavailability of phloretin and phloridzin in rats. *Journal of Nutrition*, *131*, 3227-3230.

[160] He, J.; Magnuson, B. A.; and Giusti, M. M. (2005). Analysis of Anthocyanins in Rat Intestinal Contents-Impact of Anthocyanin Chemical Structure on Fecal Excretion. *Journal of Agricultural and Food Chemistry*, *53*, 2859-2866.

[161] Joannou, G. E.; Kelly, G. E.; Reeder, A. Y.; Waring, M.; and Nelson, C. (1995). A urinary profile study of dietary phytoestrogens. The identification and mode of metabolism of new isoflavonoids. *The Journal of Steroid Biochemistry and Molecular Biology*, *54*, 167-184.

[162] Yuan, J. P.; Wang, J. H.; and Liu, X. (2007). Metabolism of dietary soy isoflavones to equol by human intestinal microflora - implications for health. *Molecular Nutrition and Food Research*, *51*, 765-781.

[163] Hoey, L.; Rowland, I. R.; Lloyd, A. S.; Clarke, D. B.; and Wiseman, H. (2004). Influence of soya-based infant formula consumption on isoflavone and gut microflora metabolite concentrations in urine and on faecal microflora composition and metabolic activity in infants and children. *British Journal of Nutrition*, *91*, 607-616.

[164] Lee, H. C.; Jenner, A. M.; Low, C. S.; and Lee, Y. K. (2006). Effect of tea phenolics and their aromatic fecal bacterial metabolites on intestinal microbiota. *Research in Microbiology*, *157*, 876-884.

[165] Fleschhut, J.; Kratzer, F.; Rechkemmer, G.; and Kulling, S. E. (2006). Stability and biotransformation of various dietary anthocyanins in vitro. *European Journal of Nutrition*, *45*, 7-18.

[166] Hor-Gil Hur, F. R. (2000). Biotransformation of the isoflavonoids biochanin A, formononetin, and glycitein by Eubacterium limosum. *FEMS Microbiology Letters*, *192*, 21-25.

[167] Aura, A.-M.; Mattila, I.; Seppänen-Laakso, T.; Miettinen, J.; Oksman-Caldentey, K.-M.; and Oresic, M. (2008). Microbial metabolism of catechin stereoisomers by human faecal microbiota: Comparison of targeted analysis and a non-targeted metabolomics method. *Phytochemistry Letters*, *1*, 18-22.

[168] Meselhy, M. R.; Nakamura, N.; and Hattori, M. (1997). Biotransformation of (-)-epicatechin 3-O-gallate by human intestinal bacteria. *Chemical and Pharmaceutical Bulletin*, *45*, 888-893.

[169] Wang, L.-Q.; Meselhy, M. R.; Li, Y.; Nakamura, N.; Min, B.-S.; Qin, G.-W.; and Hattori, M. (2001). The Heterocyclic Ring Fission and Dehydroxylation of Catechins and Related Compounds by Eubacterium sp. Strain SDG-2, a Human Intestinal Bacterium. *Chemical and Pharmaceutical Bulletin*, *49*, 1640-1643.

[170] Rafii, F.; Jackson, L. D.; Ross, I.; Heinze, T. M.; Lewis, S. M.; Aidoo, A.; Lyn-Cook, L.; and Manjanathas, M. (2007). Metabolism of daidzein by fecal bacteria in rats. *Comparative Medicine*, *57*, 282-286.

[171] Labib, S.; Erb, A.; Kraus, M.; Wickert, T.; and Richling, E. (2004). The pig caecum model: A suitable tool to study the intestinal metabolism of flavonoids. *Molecular Nutrition and Food Research*, *48*, 326-332.

[172] Gao, K.; Xu, A. L.; Krul, C.; Venema, K.; Liu, Y.; Niu, Y. T.; Lu, J. X.; Bensoussan, L.; Seeram, N. P.; Heber, D.; and Henning, S. M. (2006). Of the major phenolic acids formed during human microbial fermentation of tea, citrus, and soy flavonoid supplements, only 3,4-dihydroxyphenylacetic acid has antiproliferative activity. *Journal of Nutrition*, *136*, 52-57.

[173] Matthies, A.; Clavel, T.; Gutschow, M.; Engst, W.; Haller, D.; Blaut, M.; and Braune, A. (2008). Conversion of daidzein and genistein by an anaerobic bacterium newly isolated from the mouse intestine. *Applied and Environmental Microbiology*, *74*, 4847-4852.

[174] Schoefer, L.; Mohan, R.; Braune, A.; Birringer, M.; and Blaut, M. (2002). Anaerobic C-ring cleavage of genistein and daidzein by Eubacterium ramulus. *FEMS Microbiology Letters*, *208*, 197-202.

[175] Deprez, S.; Brezillon, C.; Rabot, S.; Philippe, C.; Mila, I.; Lapierre, C.; and Scalbert, A. (2000). Polymeric Proanthocyanidins Are Catabolized by Human Colonic Microflora into Low-Molecular-Weight Phenolic Acids. *Journal of Nutrition*, *130*, 2733-2738.

[176] Schneider, H.; Schwiertz, A.; Collins, M. D.; and Blaut, M. (1999). Anaerobic transformation of quercetin-3-glucoside by bacteria from the human intestinal tract. *Archives of Microbiology*, *171*, 81-91.

[177] Aura, A. M.; O'Leary, K. A.; Williamson, G.; Ojala, M.; Bailey, M.; Puupponen-Pimia, R.; Nuutila, A. M.; Oksman-Caldentey, K. M.; and Poutanen, K. (2002). Quercetin derivatives are deconjugated and converted to hydroxyphenylacetic acids but not methylated by human fecal flora in vitro. *Journal of Agricultural and Food Chemistry*, *50*, 1725-1730.

[178] Justesen, U.; Arrigoni, E.; Larsen, B. R.; and Amado, R. (2000). Degradation of flavonoid glycosides and aglycones during in vitro fermentation with human faecal flora. *Lebensmittel-Wissenschaft und-Technologie*, *33*, 424-430.

[179] Braune, A.; Gutschow, M.; Engst, W.; and Blaut, M. (2001). Degradation of quercetin and luteolin by Eubacterium ramulus. *Applied and Environmental Microbiology*, *67*, 5558-5567.

[180] Schoefer, L.; Mohan, R.; Schwiertz, A.; Braune, A.; and Blaut, M. (2003). Anaerobic degradation of flavonoids by Clostridium orbiscindens. *Applied and Environmental Microbiology*, *69*, 5849-5854.

[181] Schneider, H.; Simmering, R.; Hartmann, L.; Pforte, H.; and Blaut, M. (2000). Degradation of quercetin-3-glucoside in gnotobiotic rats associated with human intestinal bacteria. *Journal of Applied Microbiology*, *89*, 1027-1037.

[182] Schneider, H.; and Blaut, M. (2000). Anaerobic degradation of flavonoids by Eubacterium ramulus. *Archives of Microbiology*, *173*, 71-75.

[183] Hein, E. M.; Rose, K.; Van't Slot, G.; Friedrich, A. W.; and Humpf, H. U. (2008). Deconjugation and degradation of flavonol glycosides by pig cecal microbiota characterized by fluorescence in situ hybridization (FISH). *Journal of Agricultural and Food Chemistry*, *56*, 2281-2290.

[184] McGhie, T. K.; Ainge, G. D.; Barnett, L. E.; Cooney, J. M.; and Jensen, D. J. (2003). Anthocyanin Glycosides from Berry Fruit Are Absorbed and Excreted Unmetabolized

by Both Humans and Rats. *Journal of Agricultural and Food Chemistry*, *51*, 4539 - 4548.

[185] Moon, Y. J.; and Morris, M. E. (2007). Pharmacokinetics and bioavailability of the bioflavonoid biochanin A: Effects of quercetin and EGCG on biochanin A disposition in rats. *Molecular Pharmaceutics*, *4*, 865-872.

[186] Rechner, A. R.; Kuhnle, G.; Hu, H. L.; Roedig-Penman, A.; van den Braak, M. H.; Moore, K. P.; and Rice-Evans, C. A. (2002). The metabolism of dietary polyphenols and the relevance to circulating levels of conjugated metabolites. *Free Radical Research*, *36*, 1229-1241.

[187] Cooney, J. M.; Jensen, D. J.; and McGhie, T. K. (2004). LC-MS identification of anthocyanins in boysenberry extract and anthocyanin metabolites in human urine following dosing. *Journal of the Science of Food and Agriculture*, *84*, 237-245.

[188] Wu, X.; Pittman, H. E., III; McKay, S.; and Prior, R. L. (2005). Aglycones and sugar moieties alter anthocyanin absorption and metabolism after berry consumption in weanling pigs. *Journal of Nutrition*, *135*, 2417-2424.

[189] Wu, X.; Pittman, H. E., III; and Prior, R. L. (2004). Pelargonidin is absorbed and metabolized differently than cyanidin after marionberry consumption in pigs. *Journal of Nutrition*, *134*, 2603-2610.

[190] Baba, S.; Osakabe, N.; Natsume, M.; Muto, Y.; Takizawa, T.; and Terao, J. (2001). Absorption and urinary excretion of (-)-epicatechin after administration of different levels of cocoa powder or (-)-epicatechin in rats. *Journal of Agricultural and Food Chemistry*, *49*, 6050-6056.

[191] Roura, E.; Almajano, M. P.; Bilbao, M. L. M.; Andres-Lacueva, C.; Estruch, R.; and Lamuela-Raventos, R. M. (2007). Human urine: Epicatechin metabolites and antioxidant activity after cocoa beverage intake. *Free Radical Research*, *41*, 943-949.

[192] Roura, E.; Andres-Lacueva, C.; Estruch, R.; Mata-Bilbao, M. L.; Izquierdo-Pulido, M.; Waterhouse, A. L.; and Lamuela-Raventos, R. M. (2007). Milk does not affect the bioavailability of cocoa powder flavonoid in healthy human. *Annals of Nutrition and Metabolism*, *51*, 493-498.

[193] Valentova, K.; Stejskal, D.; Bednar, P.; Vostalova, J.; Cihalik, C.; Vecerova, R.; Koukalova, D.; Kolar, M.; Reichenbach, R.; Sknouril, L.; Ulrichova, J.; and Simanek, V. (2007). Biosafety, antioxidant status, and metabolites in urine after consumption of dried cranberry juice in healthy women: A pilot double-blind placebo-controlled trial. *Journal of Agricultural and Food Chemistry*, *55*, 3217-3224.

[194] Meng, X.; Sang, S.; Zhu, N.; Lu, H.; Sheng, S.; Lee, M. J.; Ho, C. T.; and Yang, C. S. (2002). Identification and Characterization of Methylated and Ring-Fission Metabolites of Tea Catechins Formed in Humans, Mice, and Rats. *Chemical Research in Toxicology*, *15*, 1042-1050.

[195] Netzel, M.; Strass, G.; Bitsch, R.; Dietrich, H.; Herbst, M.; Bitsch, I.; and Frank, T. (2005). The excretion and biological antioxidant activity of elderberry antioxidants in healthy humans. *Food Research International*, *38*, 905-910.

[196] Natsume, M.; Osakabe, N.; Oyama, M.; Sasaki, M.; Baba, S.; Nakamura, Y.; Osawa, T.; and Terao, J. (2003). Structures of (-)-epicatechin glucuronide identified from plasma and urine after oral ingestion of (-)-epicatechin: differences between human and rat. *Free Radical Biology and Medicine*, *34*, 840-849.

[197] Coldham, N. G.; Howells, L. C.; Santi, A.; Montesissa, C.; Langlais, C.; King, L. J.; Macpherson, D. D.; and Sauer, M. J. (1999). Biotransformation of genistein in the rat: elucidation of metabolite structure by product ion mass fragmentologyn. *The Journal of Steroid Biochemistry and Molecular Biology, 70,* 169-184.

[198] Li, C.; Lee, M. J.; Sheng, S.; Meng, X.; Prabhu, S.; Winnik, B.; Huang, B.; Chung, J. Y.; Yan, S.; Ho, C. T.; and Yang, C. S. (2000). Structural identification of two metabolites of catechins and their kinetics in human urine and blood after tea ingestion. *Chemical Research in Toxicology, 13,* 177-184.

[199] Abd El Mohsen, M.; Marks, J.; Kuhnle, G.; Rice-Evans, C.; Moore, K.; Gibson, G.; Debnam, E.; and Srai, S. K. (2004). The differential tissue distribution of the citrus flavanone naringenin following gastric instillation. *Free Radical Research, 38,* 1329-1340.

[200] Mennen, L. I.; Sapinho, D.; Ito, H.; Bertrais, S.; Galan, P.; Hercberg, S.; and Scalbert, A. (2007). Urinary flavonoids and phenolic acids as biomarkers of intake for polyphenol-rich foods. *British Journal of Nutrition, 96,* 191-198.

[201] Felgines, C.; Texier, O.; Besson, C.; Fraisse, D.; Lamaison, J.-L.; and Remesy, C. (2002). Blackberry anthocyanins are slightly bioavailable in rats. *Journal of Nutrition, 132,* 1249-1253.

[202] Milbury, P. E.; Cao, G.; Prior, R. L.; and Blumberg, J. (2002). Bioavailablility of elderberry anthocyanins. *Mechanisms of Ageing and Development, 123,* 997-1006.

[203] Wu, X.; Cao, G.; and Prior, R. L. (2002). Absorption and metabolism of anthocyanins in elderly women after consumption of elderberry or blueberry. *Journal of Nutrition, 132,* 1865-1871.

[204] Shoji, T.; Masumoto, S.; Moriichi, N.; Akiyama, H.; Kanda, T.; Ohtake, Y.; and Goda, Y. (2006). Apple procyanidin oligomers absorption in rats after oral administration: Analysis of procyanidins in plasma using the porter method and high-performance liquid chromatography/tandem mass spectrometry. *Journal of Agricultural and Food Chemistry, 54,* 884-892.

[205] Gross, M.; Pfeiffer, M.; Martini, M.; Campbell, D.; Slavin, J.; and Potter, J. (1996). The quantitation of metabolites of quercetin flavonols in human urine. *Cancer Epidemiology Biomarkers and Prevention, 5,* 711-720.

[206] Catterall, F.; King, L. J.; Clifford, M. N.; and Ioannides, C. (2003). Bioavailability of dietary doses of H-3-labelled tea antioxidants (+)-catechin and (-)-epicatechin in rat. *Xenobiotica, 33,* 743-753.

[207] Toshiyuki, K.; Natsuki, M.; Mana, Y.; Masayuki, S.; Fumio, N.; Yukihiko, H.; and Naoto, O. (2001). Metabolic fate of (-)-[4-3H]epigallocatechin gallate in rats after oral administration. *Journal of Agricultural and Food Chemistry, 49,* 4102 -4112.

[208] Heinonen, S. M.; Wahala, K.; and Adlercreutz, H. (2004). Identification of urinary metabolites of the red clover isoflavones formononetin and biochanin A in human subjects. *Journal of Agricultural and Food Chemistry, 52,* 6802-6809.

[209] Heinonen, S. M.; Wahala, K.; Liukkonen, K. H.; Aura, A. M.; Poutanen, K.; and Adlercreutz, H. (2004). Studies of the in vitro intestinal metabolism of isoflavones aid in the identification of their urinary metabolites. *Journal of Agricultural and Food Chemistry, 52,* 2640-2646.

[210] Bitsch, R.; Netzel, M.; Strass, G.; Frank, T.; and Bitsch, I. (2004). Bioavailability and biokinetics of anthocyanins from red grape juice and red wine. *Journal of Biomedicine and Biotechnology, 2004*, 293-298.

[211] Felgines, C.; Talavera, S.; Gonthier, M.-P.; Texier, O.; Scalbert, A.; Lamaison, J.-L.; and Remesy, C. (2003). Strawberry anthocyanins are recovered in urine as glucuro- and sulfoconjugates in humans. *Journal of Nutr*ition *133*, 1296-1301.

[212] Mullen, W.; Edwards, C. A.; Serafini, M.; and Crozier, A. (2008). Bioavailability of pelargonidin-3-O-glucoside and its metabolites in humans following the ingestion of strawberries with and without cream. *Journal of Agricultural and Food Chemistry, 56*, 713-719.

[213] Olthof, M. R.; Hollman, P. C. H.; Buijsman, M. N. C. P.; Amelsvoort, J. M. M. v.; and Katan, M. B. (2003). Chlorogenic acid, quercetin-3-rutinoside and black tea phenols are extensively metabolized in humans. *The Journal of Nutrition, 133*, 1806-1814.

[214] Baker, M. E. (2002). Albumin, steroid hormones and the origin of vertebrates. *Journal of Endocrinology, 175*, 121-127.

[215] Ames, B. N.; and Gold, L. S. (1997). Environmental pollution, pesticides, and the prevention of cancer: Misconceptions. *Faseb Journal, 11*, 1041-1052.

[216] Baker, M. E. (1995). Endocrine activity of plant-derived compounds - an evolutionary perspective. *Proceedings of the Society for Experimental Biology and Medicine, 208*, 131-138.

[217] Janisch, K. M.; Williamson, G.; Needs, P.; and Plumb, G. W. (2004). Properties of quercetin conjugates: Modulation of LDL oxidation and binding to human serum albumin. *Free Radical Research, 38*, 877-884.

[218] Kitson, T. M. (2004). Spectrophotometric and kinetic studies on the binding of the bioflavonoid quercetin to bovine serum albumin. *Bioscience Biotechnology and Biochemistry, 68*, 2165-2170.

[219] Papadopoulou, A.; Green, R. J.; and Frazier, R. A. (2005). Interaction of flavonoids with bovine serum albumin: A fluorescence quenching study. *Journal of Agricultural and Food Chemistry, 53*, 158-163.

[220] Dufour, C.; and Dangles, O. (2005). Flavonoid-serum albumin complexation: determination of binding constants and binding sites by fluorescence spectroscopy. *Biochimica et Biophysica Acta-General Subjects, 1721*, 164-173.

[221] Lancon, A.; Delmas, D.; Osman, H.; Thenot, J. P.; Jannin, B.; and Latruffe, N. (2004). Human hepatic cell uptake of resveratrol: involvement of both passive diffusion and carrier-mediated process. *Biochemical and Biophysical Research Communications, 316*, 1132-1137.

[222] Fasano, M.; Curry, S.; Terreno, E.; Galliano, M.; Fanali, G.; Narciso, P.; Notari, S.; and Ascenzi, P. (2005). The extraordinary ligand binding properties of human serum albumin. *Iubmb Life, 57*, 787-796.

[223] Hong, J.; Lambert, J. D.; Lee, S. H.; Sinko, P. J.; and Yang, C. S. (2003). Involvement of multidrug resistance-associated proteins in regulating cellular levels of (-)-epigallocatechin-3-gallate and its methyl metabolites. *Biochemical and Biophysical Research Communications, 310*, 222-227.

[224] Hurst, R. D.; and Fritz, I. B. (1996). Properties of an immortalised vascular endothelial glioma cell co-culture model of the blood-brain barrier. *Journal of Cellular Physiology, 167*, 81-88.

[225] Youdim, K. A.; Dobbie, M. S.; Kuhnle, G.; Proteggente, A. R.; Abbott, N. J.; and Rice-Evans, C. (2003). Interaction between flavonoids and the blood-brain barrier: in vitro studies. *Journal of Neurochemistry*, 85, 180-192.

[226] Abd El Mohsen, M. M.; Kuhnle, G.; Rechner, A. R.; Schroeter, H.; Rose, S.; Jenner, P.; and Rice-Evans, C. A. (2002). Uptake and metabolism of epicatechin and its access to the brain after oral ingestion. *Free Radical Biology and Medicine*, 33, 1693-1702.

[227] Youdim, K. A.; Qaiser, M. Z.; Begley, D. J.; Rice-Evans, C. A.; and Abbott, N. J. (2004). Flavonoid permeability across an in situ model of the blood-brain barrier. *Free Radical Biology and Medicine*, 36, 592-604.

[228] Koga, T.; and Meydani, M. (2001). Effect of plasma metabolites of (+)-catechin and quercetin on monocyte adhesion to human aortic endothelial cells. *American Journal of Clinical Nutrition*, 73, 941-948.

[229] Gläßer, G.; Graefe, E. U.; Struck, F.; Veit, M.; and Gebhardt, R. (2002). Comparison of antioxidative capacities and inhibitory effects on cholesterol biosynthesis of quercetin and potential metabolites. *Phytomedicine*, 9, 33-40.

[230] Shirai, M.; Moon, J. H.; Tsushida, T.; and Terao, J. (2001). Inhibitory effect of a quercetin metabolite, quercetin 3-O-beta-D-Glucuronide, on lipid peroxidation in liposomal membranes. *Journal of Agricultural and Food Chemistry*, 49, 5602-5608.

[231] Shirai, M.; Yamanishi, R.; Moon, J. H.; Murota, K.; and Terao, J. (2002). Effect of quercetin and its conjugated metabolite on the hydrogen peroxide-induced intracellular production of reactive oxygen species in mouse fibroblasts. *Bioscience Biotechnology and Biochemistry*, 66, 1015-1021.

[232] Yoshizumi, M.; Tsuchiya, K.; Suzaki, Y.; Kirima, K.; Kyaw, M.; Moon, J.-H.; Terao, J.; and Tamaki, T. (2002). Quercetin glucuronide prevents VSMC hypertrophy by angiotensin II via the inhibition of JNK and AP-1 signaling pathway. *Biochemical and Biophysical Research Communications*, 293, 1458-1465.

[233] O'Leary, K. A.; Pascual-Tereasa, S. d.; Needs, P. W.; Bao, Y.-P.; O'Brien, N. M.; and Williamson, G. (2004). Effect of flavonoids and Vitamin E on cyclooxygenase-2 (COX-2) transcription. *Mutation Research/Fundamental and Molecular Mechanisms of Mutagenesis*, 551, 245-254.

[234] Lodi, F.; Jimenez, R.; Menendez, C.; Needs, P. W.; Duarte, J.; and Perez-Vizcaino, F. (2008). Glucuronidated metabolites of the flavonoid quercetin do not auto-oxidise, do not generate free radicals and do not decrease nitric oxide bioavailability. *Planta Medica*, 74, 741-746.

[235] Loke, W. M.; Proudfoot, J. M.; McKinley, A. J.; Needs, P. W.; Kroon, P. A.; Hodgson, J. M.; and Croft, K. D. (2008). Quercetin and its in vivo metabolites inhibit neutrophil-mediated low-density lipoprotein oxidation. *Journal of Agricultural and Food Chemistry*, 56, 3609-3615.

[236] Spencer, J. P. E.; Rice-Evans, C.; and Williams, R. J. (2003). Modulation of pro-survival Akt/Protein Kinase B and ERK1/2 signaling cascades by quercetin and Its in vivo metabolites underlie their action on neuronal viability. *Journal of Biological Chemistry*, 278, 34783-34793.

[237] Day, A. J.; Bao, Y.; Morgan, M. R. A.; and Williamson, G. (2000). Conjugation position of quercetin glucuronides and effect on biological activity. *Free Radical Biology and Medicine*, 29, 1234-1243.

[238] Kuo, H. M.; Ho, H. J.; Chao, P. D. L.; and Chung, J. G. (2002). Quercetin glucuronides inhibited 2-aminofluorene acetylation in human acute myeloid HL-60 leukemia cells. *Phytomedicine*, *9*, 625-631.

[239] Saito, A.; Sugisawa, A.; Umegaki, K.; and Sunagawa, H. (2004). Protective Effects of Quercetin and Its Metabolites on H2O2-Induced Chromosomal Damage to WIL2-NS Cells. *Bioscience, Biotechnology, and Biochemistry*, *68*, 271-276.

[240] Liu, W.; and Liang, N. (2000). Inhibitory effect of disodium qurecetin-7, 4'-disulfate on aggregation of pig platelets induced by thrombin and its mechanism. *Acta Pharmacologica Sinica*, *21*, 737-741.

[241] Fang, S.-H.; Hou, Y.-C.; Chang, W.-C.; Hsiu, S.-L.; Lee Chao, P.-D.; and Chiang, B.-L. (2003). Morin sulfates/glucuronides exert anti-inflammatory activity on activated macrophages and decreased the incidence of septic shock. *Life Sciences*, *74*, 743-756.

[242] Hsieh, C.-L.; Chao, P. D. L.; and Fang, S. H. (2005). Morin sulphates/glucuronides enhance macrophage function in microgravity culture system. *European Journal of Clinical Investigation*, *35*, 591-596.

[243] van Zanden, J. J.; van der Woude, H.; Vaessen, J.; Usta, M.; Wortelboer, H. M.; Cnubben, N. H. P.; and Rietjens, I. (2007). The effect of quercetin phase II metabolism on its MRP1 and MRP2 inhibiting potential. *Biochemical Pharmacology*, *74*, 345-351.

[244] Tseng, T.-H.; Wang, C.-J.; Kao, E.-S.; and Chu, h.-Y. (1996). Hibiscus protocatechuic acid protects against oxidative damage induced by tert-butylhydroperoxide in rat primary hepatocytes. *Chemico-Biological Interactions*, *101*, 137-148.

[245] Tseng, T.-H.; Kao, T.-W.; Chu, C.-Y.; Chou, F.-P.; Lin, W.-L.; and Wang, C.-J. (2000). Induction of apoptosis by Hibiscus protocatechuic acid in human leukemia cells via reduction of retinoblastoma (RB) phosphorylation and Bcl-2 expression. *Biochemical Pharmacology*, *60*, 307-315.

[246] Liu, C.-L.; Wang, J.-M.; Chu, C.-Y.; Cheng, M.-T.; and Tseng, T.-H. (2002). In vivo protective effect of protocatechuic acid on tert-butyl hydroperoxide-induced rat hepatotoxicity. *Food and Chemical Toxicology*, *40*, 635-641.

[247] Tarozzi, A.; Morroni, F.; Hrelia, S.; Angeloni, C.; Marchesi, A.; Cantelli-Forti, G.; and Hrelia, P. (2007). Neuroprotective effects of anthocyanins and their in vivo metabolites in SH-SY5Y cells. *Neuroscience Letters*, *424*, 36-40.

[248] Lu, H.; Meng, X.; Li, C.; Sang, S.; Patten, C.; Sheng, S.; Hong, J.; Bai, N.; Winnik, B.; Ho, C.-T.; and Yang, C. S. (2003). Glucuronides of Tea Catechins: Enzymology of Biosynthesis and Biological Activities. *Drug Metabolism and Disposition*, *31*, 452-461.

[249] Spencer, J. P. E.; Schroeter, H.; Crossthwaithe, A. J.; Kuhnle, G.; Williams, R. J.; and Rice-Evans, C. (2001). Contrasting influences of glucuronidation and O-methylation of epicatechin on hydrogen peroxide-induced cell death in neurons and fibroblasts. *Free Radical Biology and Medicine*, *31*, 1139-1146.

[250] Spencer, J. P. E.; Schroeter, H.; Kuhnle, G.; Srai, S. K. S.; Tyrrell, R. M.; Hahn, U.; and Rice-Evans, C. (2001). Epicatechin and its in vivo metabolite, 3'-O-methyl epicatechin, protect human fibroblasts from oxidative-stress-induced cell death involving caspase-3 activation. *Biochemical Journal*, *354*, 493-500.

[251] Li, S. M.; Sang, S. M.; Pan, M. H.; Lai, C. S.; Lo, C. Y.; Yang, C. S.; and Ho, C. T. (2007). Anti-inflammatory property of the urinary metabolites of nobiletin in mouse. *Bioorganic and Medicinal Chemistry Letters*, *17*, 5177-5181.

[252] Stevenson, D.; Cooney, J.; Jensen, D.; Wibisono, R.; Adaim, A.; Skinner, M.; and Zhang, J. (2008). Comparison of enzymically glucuronidated flavonoids with flavonoid aglycones in an in vitro cellular model of oxidative stress protection. *In Vitro Cellular and Developmental Biology - Animal, 44*, 73-80.

[253] Cano, A.; Arnao, M. B.; Williamson, G.; and Garcia-Conesa, M. T. (2002). Superoxide scavenging by polyphenols: effect of conjugation and dimerization. *Redox Report, 7*, 379-383.

[254] Proteggente, A. R.; Basu-Modak, S.; Kuhnle, G.; Gordon, M. J.; Youdim, K.; Tyrrell, R.; and Rice-Evans, C. A. (2003). Hesperetin glucuronide, a photoprotective agent arising from Ffavonoid metabolism in human skin fibroblasts and para. *Photochemistry and Photobiology, 78*, 256-261.

[255] Spencer, J. P. E.; Kuhnle, G. G. C.; Williams, R. J.; and Rice-Evans, C. (2003). Intracellular metabolism and bioactivity of quercetin and its in vivo metabolites. *Biochemical Journal, 372*, 173-181.

[256] de Pascual-Teresa, S.; Johnston, K. L.; DuPont, M. S.; O'Leary, K. A.; Needs, P. W.; Morgan, L. M.; Clifford, M. N.; Bao, Y. P.; and Williamson, G. (2004). Quercetin metabolites downregulate cyclooxygenase-2 transcription in human lymphocytes ex vivo but not in vivo. *Journal of Nutrition, 134*, 552-557.

[257] Paulke, A.; Noldner, M.; Schubert-Zslavecz, M.; and Wurglics, M. (2008). St. John's wort flavonolds and their metabolites show antidepressant activity and accumulate in brain after multiple oral doses. *Pharmazie, 63*, 296-302.

[258] Hubbard, G. P.; Wolffram, S.; de Vos, R.; Bovy, A.; Gibbins, J. M.; and Lovegrove, J. A. (2006). Ingestion of onion soup high in quercetin inhibits platelet aggregation and essential components of the collagen-stimulated platelet activation pathway in man: a pilot study. *British Journal of Nutrition, 96*, 482-488.

[259] Kawai, Y.; Nishikawa, T.; Shiba, Y.; Saito, S.; Murota, K.; Shibata, N.; Kobayashi, M.; Kanayama, M.; Uchida, K.; and Terao, J. (2008). Macrophage as a target of quercetin glucuronides in human atherosclerotic arteries - Implication in the anti-atherosclerotic mechanism of dietary flavonoids. *Journal of Biological Chemistry, 283*, 9424-9434.

[260] Jackman, K. A.; Woodman, O. L.; and Sobey, C. G. (2007). Isoflavones, equol and cardiovascular disease: Pharmacological and therapeutic insights. *Current Medicinal Chemistry, 14*, 2824-2830.

[261] Nam Joo, K.; Ki Won, L.; Rogozin, E. A.; Yong-Yeon, C.; Yong-Seok, H.; Bode, A. M.; Hyong Joo, L.; and Zigang, D. (2007). Equol, a metabolite of the soybean isoflavone daidzein, inhibits neoplastic cell transformation by targeting the MEK/ERK/p90RSK/activator protein-1 pathway. *Journal of Biological Chemistry, 282*, 32856-32866.

[262] Zhang, Y.; Song, T. T.; Cunnick, J. E.; Murphy, P. A.; and Hendrich, S. (1999). Daidzein and genistein glucuronides in vitro are weakly estrogenic and activate human natural killer cells at nutritionally relevant concentrations. *The Journal of Nutrition, 129*, 399-405.

[263] Niculescu, M. D.; Pop, E. A.; Fischer, L. M.; and Zeisel, S. H. (2007). Dietary isoflavones differentially induce gene expression changes in lymphocytes from postmenopausal women who form equol as compared with those who do not. *Journal of Nutritional Biochemistry, 18*, 380-390.

[264] Rachon, D.; Seidlova-Wuttke, D.; Vortherms, T.; and Wuttke, W. (2007). Effects of dietary equol administration on ovariectomy induced bone loss in Sprague-Dawley rats. *Maturitas, 58,* 308-315.

[265] Rachon, D.; Vortherms, T.; Seidlova-Wuttke, D.; and Wuttke, W. (2007). Effects of dietary equol on body weight gain, intra-abdominal fat accumulation, plasma lipids, and glucose tolerance in ovariectomized Sprague-Dawley rats. *Menopause-the Journal of the North American Menopause Society, 14,* 925-932.

[266] Ohtomo, T.; Uehara, M.; Penalvo, J. L.; Adlercreutz, H.; Katsumata, S.; Suzuki, K.; Takeda, K.; Masuyama, R.; and Ishimi, Y. (2008). Comparative activities of daidzein metabolites, equol and O-desmethylangolensin, on bone mineral density and lipid metabolism in ovariectomized mice and in osteoclast cell cultures. *European Journal of Nutrition, 47,* 273-279.

[267] Rachon, D.; Menche, A.; Vortherms, T.; Seidlova-Wuttke, D.; and Wuttke, W. (2008). Effects of dietary equol administration on the mammary gland in ovariectomized Sprague-Dawley rats. *Menopause-the Journal of the North American Menopause Society, 15,* 340-345.

[268] Rechner, A. R.; and Kroner, C. (2005). Anthocyanins and colonic metabolites of dietary polyphenols inhibit platelet function. *Thrombosis Research, 116,* 327-334.

[269] Hiermann, A.; Schramm, H. W.; and Laufer, S. (1998). Anti-inflammatory activity of myricetin-3-O-beta-D-glucuronide and related compounds. *Inflammation Research, 47,* 421-427.

[270] Guo, J. M.; Qian, F.; Li, J. X.; Xu, Q.; and Chen, T. (2007). Identification of a new metabolite of astilbin, 3 '-O-methylastilbin, and its immunosuppressive activity against contact dermatitis. *Clinical Chemistry, 53,* 465-471.

[271] Bellion, P.; Hofmann, T.; Pool-Zobel, B. L.; Will, F.; Dietrich, H.; Knaup, B.; Richling, E.; Baum, M.; Eisenbrand, G.; and Janzowski, C. (2008). Antioxidant effectiveness of phenolic apple juice extracts and their gut fermentation products in the human colon carcinoma cell line caco-2. *Journal of Agricultural and Food Chemistry, 56,* 6310-6317.

[272] Chan, F. L.; Choi, H. L.; Chen, Z. Y.; Chan, P. S. F.; and Huang, Y. (2000). Induction of apoptosis in prostate cancer cell lines by a flavonoid, baicalin. *Cancer Letters, 160,* 219-228.

[273] Ueda, S.; Nakamura, H.; Masutani, H.; Sasada, T.; Takabayashi, A.; Yamaoka, Y.; and Yodoi, J. (2002). Baicalin induces apoptosis via mitochondrial pathway as prooxidant. *Molecular Immunology, 38,* 781-791.

[274] Canali, R.; Ambra, R.; Stelitano, C.; Mattivi, F.; Scaccini, C.; and Virgili, F. (2007). A novel model to study the biological effects of red wine at the molecular level. *British Journal of Nutrition, 97,* 1053-1058.

[275] Shukla, M.; Gupta, K.; Rasheed, Z.; Khan, K.; and Haqqi, T. (2008). Bioavailable constituents/metabolites of pomegranate (Punica granatum L) preferentially inhibit COX2 activity ex vivo and IL-1beta-induced PGE2 production in human chondrocytes in vitro. *Journal of Inflammation, 5,* 9.

In: Encyclopedia of Vitamin Research
Editor: Joshua T. Mayer

ISBN: 978-1-61761-928-1
© 2011 Nova Science Publishers, Inc.

Chapter 39

Cytoprotective Activity of Flavonoids in Relation to Their Chemical Structures and Physicochemical Properties[*]

Jingli Zhang[†] and Margot A. Skinner

The New Zealand Institute for Plant and Food Research Ltd,
Auckland, New Zealand

Abstract

Flavonoids are widely distributed in fruit and vegetables and form part of the human diet. These compounds are thought to be a contributing factor to the health benefits of fruit and vegetables in part because of their antioxidant activities. Despite the extensive use of chemical antioxidant assays to assess the activity of flavonoids and other natural products that are safe to consume, their ability to predict an *in vivo* health benefit is debateable. Some are carried out at non-physiological pH and temperature, most take no account of partitioning between hydrophilic and lipophilic environments, and none of them takes into account bioavailability, uptake and metabolism of antioxidant compounds and the biological component that is targeted for protection. However, biological systems are far more complex and dietary antioxidants may function via multiple mechanisms. It is critical to consider moving from using 'the test tube' to employing cell-based assays for screening foods, phytochemicals and other consumed natural products for their potential biological activity. The question then remains as to which cell models to use. Human immortalized cell lines derived from many different cell types from a wide range of anatomical sites are available and are established well-characterized models.

---

[*] A version of this chapter was also published in *Flavonoids: Biosynthesis, Biological Effects and Dietary Sources, edited by Raymond B. Keller* published by Nova Science Publishers, Inc. It was submitted for appropriate modifications in an effort to encourage wider dissemination of research.

[†] Correspondence: Dr. Jingli Zhang. Tel: ++64 9 9257100, Fax: ++64 9 9257001, Email jzhang@hort research.co.nz

The cytoprotection assay was developed to be a more biologically relevant measurement than the chemically defined antioxidant activity assay because it uses human cells as a substrate and therefore accounts for some aspects of uptake, metabolism and location of flavonoids within cells. Knowledge of structure activity relationships in the cytoprotection assay may be helpful in assessing potential *in vivo* cellular protective effects of flavonoids. This chapter will discuss the cytoprotective properties of flavonoids and focuses on the relationship between their cytoprotective activity, physicochemical properties such as lipophilicity (log P) and bond dissociation enthalpies (BDE), and their chemical structures. The factors influencing the ability of flavonoids to protect human gut cells are discussed, and these support the contention that the partition coefficients of flavonoids as well as their rate of reaction with the relevant radicals help define the protective abilities in cellular environments. By comparing the geometries of several flavonoids, we were able to explain the structural dependency of the antioxidant action of these flavonoids.

Introduction

The flavonoids are among the most numerous and widespread natural products found in plants and have many diverse applications and properties. Over the years, a wide range of beneficial properties related to human health have been reported. These include effects related to cancer (Colic and Pavelic, 2000; Eastwood, 1999; Middleton *et al.*, 2000), cardiovascular diseases (Riemersma *et al.*, 2001), including coronary heart disease (Eastwood, 1999; Giugliano, 2000; Middleton *et al.*, 2000) and atherosclerosis (Wedworth and Lynch, 1995); anti-inflammatory effects (Manthey, 2000; Middleton *et al.*, 2000), and other diseases in which an increase in oxidative stress have been implicated (Diplock *et al.*, 1998; Harborne and Williams, 2000; Packer *et al.*, 1999). A number of studies have shown that consumption of fruits and vegetables can reduce the risk of cardiovascular diseases and cancer, potentially through the biological actions of the phenolic components such as flavonoids.

The precise mechanisms by which flavonoids may protect different cell populations from oxidative insults are currently unclear. However, potential mechanisms that involve their classical antioxidant properties, interactions with mitochondria, modulation of intracellular signalling cascades, and stimulation of adaptive responses have been proposed. The effects of a flavonoid in a cellular environment may well extend beyond conventional antioxidant actions. In the cellular environment, the coexistence of other factors such as the bioavailability of the compound, the effectiveness of the compound within the cell, and the effectiveness of the compound in the body must also be considered. Therefore, using a cell-based assay format, these compounds react with cells and provide information regarding the cellular response, taking into account some aspects of uptake, metabolism, location of antioxidant compounds within cells and intracellular effects on signalling pathways and enzyme activity. These effects are likely to be the result of differential modulation of cellular activities such as signalling pathways, enzyme activity, transport and bioavailability, rather than simply a result of free radical scavenging. Furthermore, as cells from different anatomical sites respond differently to both stressors and treatments, it is important to use the appropriate cell types to test a particular cellular response, rather than a chemically-defined system for the antioxidant activity. Here, we employed and established cell-based assays using gut-derived cultured human cell lines. The rationale to use cultured human cell lines over primary cells is that human primary cells are not readily available, but human immortalized cell lines derived from many different cell types from a wide range of anatomical sites are available and are established well-characterized models.

The multiple biological activities of flavonoids as well as their structural diversity make this class of compounds a rich source for modelling lead compounds with targeted biological properties. Different classes of flavonoids are not equally physiologically active, presumably because they are structurally different. Despite the enormous interest in flavonoids and other polyphenolic compounds as potential protective agents against the development of human diseases, the real contribution of such compounds to health maintenance and the mechanisms through which they act are still unclear. Structure activity relationships (SARs) represent an attempt to correlate physicochemical or structural descriptors of a set of structurally related compounds with their biological activities or physical properties. Molecular descriptors usually include parameters accounting for electronic properties, hydrophobicity, topology, and steric effects. Activities include chemical and biological measurements. Once developed, SARs provide predictive models of biological activity and allow the identification of those molecular parameters responsible for the biological and physicochemical properties. These may shed light on the mechanism of action.

SARs of flavonoids have been previously reported for scavenging of peroxynitrite, hydroxyl radical and superoxide, and protection against lipid peroxidation (Chen *et al.*, 2002; Choi *et al.*, 2002; Cos *et al.*, 1998), inhibition of LDL oxidation (van Acker *et al.*, 1996; Vaya *et al.*, 2003), and the influence of flavonoid structure on biological systems has also been investigated, e.g., induction of DNA degradation; growth and proliferation of certain malignant cells; acute toxicity in isolated rat hepatocytes, and inhibition of gastric H^+, K^+-ATPase (Agullo *et al.*, 1997; Moridani *et al.*, 2002; Murakami *et al.*, 1999; Sugihara *et al.*, 2003).

Chemical Structure of Flavonoids

The flavonoids are a group of phenolic compounds that share common structural features and physicochemical properties, which are important in determining their biological effects. Phenylpropanoid metabolism, which encompasses natural product metabolic pathways unique to plants, transforms phenylalanine into a variety of plant secondary metabolites, including lignins, sinapate esters, stilbenoids and flavonoids. Amongst these phenylpropanoids, flavonoids (C_6-C_3-C_6) have received significant attention in the past few decades because they appear to have diverse functions in plant defence systems and effects on human health such as antiallergic, anti-inflammatory, antithrombotic, anticancer, and antioxidant effects. Flavonoids constitute a relatively diverse family of aromatic molecules that are derived from phenylalanine via a *p*-coumaric acid (C_6-C_3) intermediate step (Figure 1) (Havsteen, 2002; Ververidis *et al.*, 2007; Winkel-Shirley, 2001). They account for a variety of colours in flowers, berries and fruits, from yellow to red and dark purple. The term "flavonoids" is generally used to describe a broad collection of natural products that include a C_6-C_3-C_6 carbon framework, which possess phenylbenzopyran functionality. Chalcones and dihydrochalcones are considered to be the primary C_6-C_3-C_6 precursors and constitute important intermediates in the synthesis of flavonoids. The nomenclature of flavonoids is with respect to the aromatic ring A condensed to the heterocyclic ring C and the aromatic ring B most often attached at the 2-position of the C-ring. The various attached substituents are listed first for the C-ring and A-ring and, as primed numbers, for the B-ring (Figure 1).

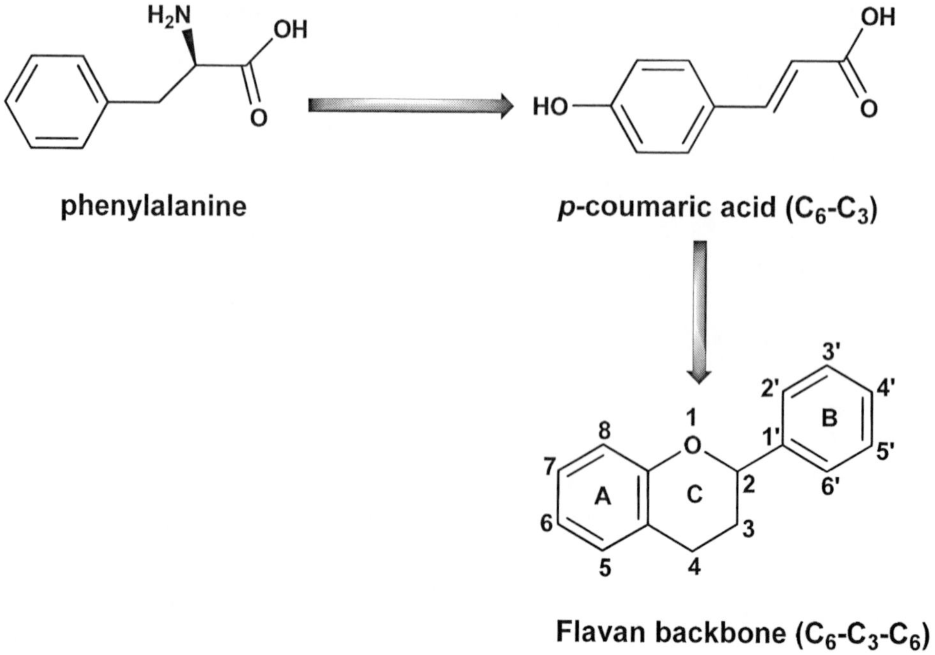

Figure 1. Diagram of biosynthetic formation of flavonoid backbone from phenylalanine. The basic flavonoid structure consists of the fused A and C-rings, with the phenyl B-ring attached through its 1'-position to the 2-position of the C-ring (numbered from the pyran oxygen).

Flavonoids differ in the arrangements of hydroxyl, methoxy, and glycosidic side groups, and in the configuration of the C-ring that joins the A- and B-rings. These give rise to a multitude of different compounds (Middleton *et al.*, 2000). In plants, the majority of the flavonoids are found as glycosides with different sugar groups linked to one or more of the hydroxyl groups. They are mainly found in the outer parts of the plants, such as leaves, flowers and fruits, whereas the content in stalks and roots is usually very limited. The flavonoids located in the upper surface of the leaf or in the epidermal cells have a role to play in the physiological survival of plants. They contribute to the disease resistance of the plant, either as constitutive antifungal agents or as induced phytoalexins (Harborne *et al.*, 2000). Multiple combinations of hydroxyl groups, sugars, oxygen atoms, and methyl groups attached to the basic ring structural skeleton create the various classes of flavonoids. According to the configuration of the C-ring, flavonoid can be classified as flavonol, flavonone, flavone, flavanol, anthocyanidin, chalcone, and isoflavone (Herrmann, 1976; Herrmann, 1989) as illustrated in Figure 2. It should be noted that chalcones contain an opened C-ring (Dziezak, 1986) and the numbering system for chalcones is reversed. Flavonoids comprise a large group of secondary plant metabolites. Presently more than 7000 individual compounds are known, which are based on very few core structures (Fossen and Andersen, 2006; Stack, 1997). Within each class, individual flavonoids may vary in the number and distribution of hydroxyl groups as well as in their degree of alkylation or glycosylation.

Flavones and flavonols occur as aglycones in foods. These compounds possess a double bond between C_2 and C_3. Flavones are a class of flavonoids based on the backbone of 2-phenylchromen-4-one, such as chrysin, apigenin, and luteolin. Flavones are lacking the 3-OH group on the backbone. Flavones are commonly found in fruit skins, celery, and parsley.

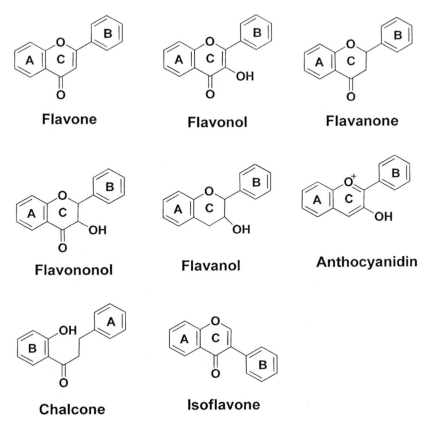

Figure 2. The basic ring structure of the subclasses of flavonoids.

Flavonols are a class of flavonoids that use the 3-hydroxyflavone backbone (3-hydroxy-2-phenylchromen-4-one (Figure 2). Flavonols are different from flavones in that they possess a hydroxyl group in the 3-position and can be regarded as 3-hydroxyflavones. The formation of flavonol and flavone glycosides depends on the action of light; therefore, they are found mainly in leaves and fruit skins with only trace amounts in parts of plants below the soil surface (Herrmann, 1976). In general, flavonols occur in the diet as glycosides (Hollman and Arts, 2000). Flavonols, such as galangin, kaempferol, quercetin, morin, rutin, myricetin, and isoquercetin, are found in plant-based foods, with onions, apples, berries, kale, and broccoli having the highest concentrations. Flavonols are present mainly as mono-, di- and triglycosides. The monoglycosides occur mainly as 3-O-glycosides. In the case of diglycosides, the two sugar moieties may be linked to the same or two different carbons.

Flavonones and flavononols are characterized by the presence of a saturated C_2–C_3 bond and an oxygen atom (carbonyl group) in the 4-position. Thus, flavonones may be referred to as dihydroflavones. Flavanones, such as hesperidin and naringin, have a more restricted distribution than other flavonoid compounds and are specific to citrus fruits. Naringin is the predominant flavanone in grapefruit (*Citrus paradisi*) (up to 10% of the dry weight) and is responsible for the bitterness of grapefruit juices. The flavonones in plants are often glycosylated in the 7-position with disaccharides rutinose and neohesperoside. Both of these disaccharides are made of rhamnose and glucose and differ only in their linkage type: 1→6 for rutinose and 1→2 for neohesperoside. It is worth noting that flavononol glycosides are good fungistatic and fungitoxic substances (Kefford and Chandler, 1970). Flavononols differ from flavanones by having a hydroxyl group in the 3-position and are often referred to as 3-hydroxyflavonones or dihydroflavonols, such as taxifolin. Flavonones have one centre of asymmetry in the 2-position, while flavononols possess a second centre of asymmetry in the 3-position.

Among flavonoids, anthocyanins and flavanols are known collectively as flavans because of lack of the carbonyl group in the 4-position. Flavanols are a class of flavonoids that use the 2-phenyl-3,4-dihydro-2H-chromen-3-ol skeleton. These compounds include catechin, epicatechin and its derivates. Flavanols are building blocks for proanthocyanidins. Proanthocyanidins consist of monomeric units of flavans linked through C-C and ether linkages. Fifteen subclasses of proanthocyanidins have been identified (Porter, 1993), however, only three appear to be prominent in human foods of plant origin, procyanidins (epicatechin or catechin polymers), prodelephinidins (epigallocatechin or gallocatechin polymers) and propelargonidins (epiafselechin or afselechin polymers) or their mixtures (Gu et al., 2003). These proanthocyanidins are soluble up to a molecular weight of approximately 7000, corresponding to ca. 20 flavan units. The name proanthocyanidins, previously called leucoanthocyanidins, implies that these are colorless precursors of anthocyanidins. On heating in acidic solutions, the C-C bond made during formation is cleaved and terminal flavan units are released from the oligomers as carbocations, which are then oxidized to colored anthocyanidins by atmospheric oxygen. Anthocyanidins are naturally colored compounds occurring in the form of glycosides (anthocyanins), the largest group of water-soluble pigments in the plant kingdom. They are responsible for most of the red, blue, and purple colors of fruits, vegetables, flowers, and other plant tissues (Harborne *et al.*, 2000). Anthocyanidins are characterized by having the basic flavylium cation structure and different substituents on ring B. The electron deficiency of their structure makes anthocyanidins highly reactive, and their stability is both pH and temperature dependent. Their glycosides are usually much more stable than the aglycons (Delgado-Vargas *et al.*, 2000). The anthocyanins are all based chemically on the structure of cyanidin, and all are derived from this base structure by the addition or subtraction of hydroxyl groups, by the degree of methylation of these hydroxyl groups, and by the nature and number of sugars and their position on the aglycon (Harborne, 1962; Harborne and Williams, 2001). In aqueous media, most of the natural anthocyanins behave as pH indicators, being red at low pH, bluish at intermediate pH, and colorless at high pH. The nature of the chemical structures that these anthocyanins can adopt upon changes in pH has been described (Briviba *et al.*, 1993; Brouillard, 1983).

Chalcones are flavonoids lacking a heterocyclic C-ring. The chalcone structure contains an aromatic ketone that forms the central core for a variety of important biological compounds. The most common chalcones found in apples and other fruit of the Rosaceae family are phloretin and phloretin-7-glycoside (phloridzin).

Physicochemical Properties of Flavonoids

The UV Absorption of Flavonoids

Studies on flavonoids by UV spectrophotometry have revealed flavonols exhibit two major absorption peaks in the region 240–400 nm, in which 300–380 nm (Band I) is considered to be associated with the absorption due to the B-ring cinnamoyl system, and 240–280 nm (Band II) with absorption involving the A-ring benzoyl system (Alonso-Salces et al., 2004; Cook and Samman, 1996; Rice-Evans et al., 1995). Functional groups attached to the flavonoid skeleton may cause a shift in absorption, such as from 367 nm in (3,5,7,4′-hydroxyl groups), to 371 nm in quercetin (3,5,7,3′,4′-hydroxyl groups), and to 374 nm in myricetin (3,5,7,3′,4′,5′-hydroxyl groups) (Cook et al., 1996). The absence of a 3-hydroxyl group in flavones distinguishes them from flavonols. Thus, Band I occurs at a wavelength shorter by 20–30 nm, such as the 337 nm exhibited for apigenin (Rice-Evans et al., 1995; Rice-Evans et al., 1996). Flavanones have a saturated heterocyclic C ring, with no conjugation between the A and B rings, as determined by their UV spectral characteristics (Rice-Evans et al., 1995). Flavanones and flavanonols exhibit a very strong Band II absorption maximum between 270 and 295 nm, namely 288 nm (naringenin) and 285 nm (taxifolin) and only a shoulder for Band I at 326 and 327 nm. As anthocyanins show distinctive Band I peaks in the 450–560-nm region due to the hydroxyl cinnamoyl system of the B-ring and Band II peaks in the 240–280-nm region due to the benzoyl system of the A-ring, the colour of the anthocyanins varies with the number and position of the hydroxyl groups (Wollenweber and Dietz, 1981).

Physical Properties of Flavonoids

Theoretical parameters employed to characterize radical scavenging activity of a flavonoid can be roughly grouped into the following classes: (1) indices reflecting O–H bond dissociation enthalpy (BDE), where a relatively low BDE value facilitates the H-abstraction reaction between antioxidant and radical (Dewar et al., 1985; van Acker et al., 1993; Zhang et al., 2003b); (2) parameters representing electron-donating ability, such as ionization potential (IP) or relative adiabatic ionization potential (van Acker et al., 1993), and enthalpy of single electron transfer (also defined as activation energy of the intermediate cation) (Vedernikova et al., 1999); (3) factors stabilizing the corresponding radical after hydrogen-abstraction (Vedernikova et al., 1999); (4) electrochemical properties, such as redox potentials (van Acker et al., 1996; Vedernikova et al., 1999); and (5) solubility, which controls the mobility of the antioxidant between lipid membranes (Gotoh et al., 1996; Noguchi et al., 1997), e.g. lipophilicity (logarithm of octanol/water partition coefficient).

Bond Dissociation Energy (BDE)

BDE is the measure of the energy change on bond making or bond breaking and is defined as the amount of energy required to break a given bond to produce two radical fragments when the molecule is in the gas phase at 25°C (298.15 °K) (McMurry, 1992).

$$A:B \xrightarrow{\text{BDE}} A^{\bullet} + B^{\bullet} \qquad\qquad [1]$$

Bond dissociation energies have long been considered to provide the best quantitative measure of the stabilities of the radicals formed (Bordwell and Zhang, 1993). Since the rate constants of this reaction depend largely on the strength of the ArO-H bond (ArOH represents flavonoid molecule), the BDE of flavonoids is defined by the following equation:

$$A_rOH \xrightarrow{\text{BDE}} A_rO^{\bullet} + H^{\bullet} \qquad\qquad [2]$$

BDE (ArO-H) can be obtained as:

$$BDE = H_{fr} + H_{fh} - H_{fp} \qquad\qquad [3]$$

where H_{fr} is the enthalpy for radicals generated after H abstraction, H_{fh} is the enthalpy for the hydrogen atom, -0.49792 hartrees, and H_{fp} is the enthalpy of the parent molecule (Zhang *et al.*, 2003a).

The properties of the A_rO-H bond appear to be essential to understanding the chemical and biochemical behaviour of flavonoids. The A_rO-H bond must be broken to generate the truly active species, i.e. the phenoxy radical, in order to exhibit its antioxidant activity. There are a number of studies, using a diversity of modern experimental and computational tools, on the determinations of the BDEs of phenolic derivatives (Bordwell *et al.*, 1993; Lucarini and Pedulli, 1994; van Acker *et al.*, 1996). Their aim was to understand how the strength of the phenolic bond is affected by nature, position, and number of substituents. BDE can be experimentally determined in the gas phase using approaches such as radical kinetics, gas-phase acidity cycles and photoionization mass spectrometry (Berkowitz *et al.*, 1994) and in solutions using techniques such as photoacoustic calorimetry (PAC) (Mulder *et al.*, 1988), electrochemical (EC) (Wayner and Parker, 1993), and other measurements (Mahoney and DaRooge, 1975). It should be noted that neither the EC technique nor the PAC method for measuring BDEs is a stand-alone method. Both techniques are dependent upon at least one gas-phase measurement (Wayner *et al.*, 1995). However, all the above-mentioned methods are limited especially for the larger organic compounds since most of them are not stable in the gas phase. Moreover, these measurements require very sophisticated instruments. For these reasons, the number of experimentally known BDEs for flavonoids is very small (Denisov and Khydyakov, 1987).

Besides these experimental studies, a number of theoretical investigations of varying degrees of sophistication have also been reported in order to understand the structural factors determining the stability of the O-H phenolic bond. Both experimental and theoretical results indicate that the change of the O-H bond strength due to a given substituent is approximately constant in the variously substituted phenols and that, for each substituent in the *ortho, meta,* and *para* positions, an additive contribution may be derived that can be used to estimate the bond BDE of polysubstituted phenols for which experimental data are lacking (Wright *et al.*, 1997; Wright *et al.*, 2001).

As a fundamental chemical parameter (Borges dos Santos and Simoes, 1998), there have been several types of theoretical methods to estimate O-H BDE (Chipman *et al.*, 1994). The first is through the additive rule (Wright *et al.*, 2001). Although this is convenient to estimate the O-H BDEs for monophenols (Brigati *et al.*, 2002; Lucarini *et al.*, 1996), it has not been demonstrated as generally effective for catechols (Zhang *et al.*, 2003a). The second is through semi-empirical quantum chemical calculations by means of intermediate neglect of differential overlap (INDO) (Pople *et al.*, 1968), modified neglect of diatomic overlap (MNDO) (Dewar and Thiel, 1977), the Austin Model 1 (AM1) (Dewar *et al.*, 1985), and the parameterization method 3 (PM3) (Stewart, 1989). The third is through density functional theory (DFT) (Qin and Wheeler, 1995; Ziegler, 1991) or *ab initio* molecular dynamics (Bakalbassis *et al.*, 2001; Car, 2002) calculations.

The parameterization method 3 (PM3) uses nearly the same equations as the AM1 method along with an improved set of parameters. PM3 predicts energies and bond lengths more accurately than AM1 (Yong, 2001). Several computer programs, such as Gaussian, Hyperchem, and MOPAC have been developed based on these theories. All these programs can be employed to perform the calculation of BDEs. In this chapter, in order to investigate the cytoprotective mechanism, the BDEs of selected flavonoids were calculated using the PM3 method using the MOPAC2002 program through Chem3D Ultra 2008 (http://www.camsoft.com/). In this chapter, the difference (ΔH_f) between the heat of formation of a parent molecule (H_{fp}) and that of its phenoxyl radical (H_{fr}) is used to represent the BDE. As stated above, the heat of formation of the H atom (H_{fh}) is treated as a constant in order to simplify the calculations (Zhang, 1998; Zhang *et al.*, 1999) and can be ignored. Thus, BDE can be expressed:

$$BDE \approx \Delta H_f = H_{fr} - H_{fp} \qquad\qquad [4]$$

Therefore, ΔH_f was used in this chapter to approximate BDE and these two terms are interchangeable.

Lipophilicity (Log P)

Lipophilicity of compounds of bioactive interest is an important parameter in the understanding of transport processes across biological barriers (Lipinski *et al.*, 1997). The lipophilic behaviour of an antioxidant is determined by its partition between phases differing in polarity. The forces of interaction between molecules that result from attraction of different functional groups can lead to different partition behaviour (Schwarz *et al.*, 1996). It is possible to quantify the degree to which an antioxidant's action is moderated by its ability to enter the locus of autoxidation (Castle and Perkins, 1986; Porter *et al.*, 1989). Uptake of most organic chemicals to the site of action is by passive diffusion and is best modelled by lipophilicity (MacFarland, 1970). Lipophilicity characterizes the tendency of molecules (or parts of molecules) to escape contact with water and to move into a lipophilic environment.

Since Hansch *et al.* (Hansch *et al.*, 1968) recognized that the partition coefficient of a molecule in the n-octanol/water solvent system mimics molecule transport across biological membranes, the basic quantity to measure lipophilicity has been the logarithm of the partition coefficient, log P. The partition coefficient (P) is defined according to the Nernst Partition Law as the ratio of the equilibrium concentrations (C) of a dissolved substance in a two-phase system consisting of two largely-immiscible solvents, e.g. *n*-octanol and water (Eadsforth and

Moser, 1983). The partition coefficient is therefore dimensionless, being the quotient of two concentrations, and it is customary to express them in logarithmic form to base ten, i.e., as log P because P values commonly range over many orders of magnitude (Fujita *et al.*, 1964). The logarithm of the partition coefficient, log P, has been successfully used as a hydrophobic parameter (Leo, 1991).

Pioneering work by Leo and Hansch (Leo *et al.*, 1971) has led to the use of log P in quantitative structure-activity relation methods (QSAR), as a general description of cell permeability. In the field of drug development, log P has become a standard property determined for potential drug molecules (Lipinski *et al.*, 1997). The lipophilicity of the flavonoids is an important parameter in chemical toxicology as it can indicate metabolic fate, biological transport properties and intrinsic biological activity (Hansch *et al.*, 2000). Lipophilicity is of central importance for biological potency as it plays a role in the interaction of flavonoids with many of the targets in a biological system. Log P probably can be considered the most informative and successful physicochemical property in biochemistry and medicinal chemistry (Leo, 1991). Since log P is an additive, constitutive molecular property, it is possible to estimate the log P value of a molecule from the sum of its component molecular fragment values (Masuda *et al.*, 1997). Many programs developed to do this are based on substructure approaches such as ClogP (Leo, 1991; Leo, 1993), KOWWIN (Meylan and Howard, 1995), AB/LogP (Japertas et al., 2002), ACD/LogP (Buchwald and Bodor, 1998; Osterberg and Norinder, 2001), and KLOGP (Klopman and Zhu, 2001). The substructure methods usually require a long calculation time because a large number of structural parameters need to be taken into account (Mannhold and Petrauskas, 2003). An alternative approach for the computation of log P is based on additive atomic contributions. The Ghose-Crippen approach is the most widely used atom-based method (Ghose and Crippen, 1987). The parameters used in the calculation of log P can be obtained by first classifying atoms into different types according to their topological environments, which contribute differently to the global log P value. Several computer programs are developed based on atomic contribution techniques such as XLOG P (Wang *et al.*, 1997) and SMILOGP (Convard *et al.*, 1994). Since the whole is more than the sum of its parts, any method of calculating log P of a molecule from its parts has limitations. Thus, other methods have been proposed based on calculated molecular properties. Fewer programs are based on a whole-molecule approach compared with a substructure approach. The most widely available one is SciLogP Ultra (Bodor *et al.*, 1989). From a theoretical perspective, it is difficult to judge the validity of any particular method since it depends on the methodology used in data analysis and algorithm derivation.

Health Effects of Flavonoids

One of the most widely publicized properties of flavonoids is their capability to scavenge reactive oxygen species (ROS). Although this has been known for some time, flavonoids are gaining more and more attention because of the impact of ROS on human (Guarnieri *et al.*, 2007) and plant metabolism and physiology (Reddy *et al.*, 2007). ROS such as singlet oxygen ($^1O_2$), super oxide ($O_2^{\cdot}$), hydrogen peroxide (H_2O_2) and hydroxyl radical ($HO^{\cdot}$) are implicated in membrane function and permeability, in oxidative degradation of proteins and DNA, in oxidation of pigments, in reduction of photosynthetic activity and respiration, and in senescence and cell death (Potapovich and Kostyuk, 2003; Williams *et al.*, 2004). It is well established that the ability that some the flavonoids and stilbenoids exert in inhibiting free-radical mediated events mainly depends on the arrangement of substituents in their structure. Such protective properties, particularly of flavonoids against oxidative stress, have been reported to be structure dependent (Barbouti *et al.*, 2002; Lien *et al.*, 1999; Rastija and Medic-Saric, 2008; Rice-Evans *et al.*, 1996; Zhang *et al.*, 2008; Zhang *et al.*, 2006a). The biochemical activities of flavonoids and their metabolites depend on their chemical structure and relative orientation of various moieties attached to the molecule. For a flavonoid to be defined as an antioxidant it should meet two basic criteria: first, when present in low concentrations, related to the substrate to be oxidized, it can delay, retard, or prevent the oxidation process (Halliwell, 1990); second, the resulting radical formed after scavenging should be stable (Shahidi and Wanasundara, 1992).

Usually inflammation is part of an immune response caused by bacterial infection, injury, trauma or UV light irradiation. As such, it is a necessary reaction of the body for protection from bacterial infection and to facilitate wound healing. Chronic inflammation on the other hand is associated with several degenerative diseases such as arthritis, atherosclerosis, heart disease, Alzheimer's disease and cancer (Brod, 2000; Kumazawa *et al.*, 2006; O'Byrne and Dalgleish, 2001). Formation of ROS and subsequent activation of the transcription factor nuclear factor-κB (NF-κB) plays a key role in triggering inflammation (Schreck *et al.*, 1991). Many of the naturally occurring anti-inflammatory substances are also antioxidants and/or inhibitors of the NF-κB signaling pathway. As mentioned previously, since most flavonoids are quickly metabolized to less potent antioxidants, their main mode of action may rather be their influence on cell signaling than their antioxidant properties (Williams *et al.*, 2004).

It is likely that the polyphenols that are the most common in the human diet are not necessarily the most active within the body, either because they have a lower intrinsic activity or because they are poorly absorbed from the intestine, highly metabolized, or rapidly eliminated. During metabolism, hydroxyl groups of flavonoids are added, methylated, sulphated or glucuronidated. In addition, the metabolites that are found in blood and target organs and that result from digestive or hepatic activity may differ from the native substances in terms of biological activity. Extensive knowledge of the bioavailability of polyphenols is thus essential if their health effects are to be understood. Metabolism of polyphenols occurs via a common pathway (Scalbert and Williamson, 2000). The aglycones can be absorbed from the small intestine. However, most polyphenols are present in food in the form of esters, glycosides, or polymers that cannot be absorbed in their native form. These compounds must be hydrolyzed by intestinal enzymes or by the colonic microflora before they can be absorbed. When the flora are involved, the efficiency of absorption is often reduced because the flora also degrade the aglycones that they release and produce various simple aromatic acids in the process.

During the course of absorption, polyphenols are conjugated in the small intestine and later in the liver. This process mainly includes methylation, sulphation, and glucuronidation (Spencer *et al.*, 2004; Spencer *et al.*, 2003). This is a metabolic detoxication process common to many xenobiotics that restricts their potential toxic effects and facilitates their biliary and urinary elimination by increasing their lipophilicity. The conjugation mechanisms are highly efficient, and aglycones are generally either absent in blood or present in low concentrations after consumption of nutritional doses. Circulating flavonoids are conjugated derivatives that are extensively bound to albumin. Flavonoids are able to penetrate tissues, particularly those in which they are metabolized, but their ability to accumulate within specific target tissues needs to be further investigated. Flavonoids and their derivatives are eliminated chiefly in urine and/or bile, and are secreted via the biliary route into the duodenum, where they are subjected to the action of bacterial enzymes, especially ß-glucuronidase, in the distal segments of the intestine, after which they may be reabsorbed. This enterohepatic recycling may lead to a longer presence of polyphenols within the body.

Anthocyanins can be absorbed intact as glycosides. The mechanism of absorption is not clear. However, it has been found that anthocyanins can serve as ligands for bilitranslocase, an organic anion membrane carrier found in the epithelial cells of gastric mucosa (Passamonti et al., 2002). This finding suggested that bilitranslocase could play a role in the bioavailability of anthocyanins. Considering the physiological implications, the interaction of anthocyanins with bilitranslocase suggests that, at the gastric level, it could promote the transport of these compounds from the lumen into the epithelial layers of the gastric mucosa, thus favoring their transfer to the portal blood, and then, at the hepatic level, from the portal blood into the liver cell. At this level, anthocyanins could also be transported by other organic anion carriers.

It has been reported that procyanidin dimmer (B2), epicatechin, and catechin were detected in the plasma of human subjects as early as 30 min (16, 2.61, 0.13 μM, respectively) after acute cococa consumption and reached maximal concentrations by 2 h (41, 5.92, and 0.16 μM, respectively) (Holt et al. 2002).

Cytoprotection Assay

Oxidative stress refers to the cytopathological consequences of an imbalance between the production of free radicals and the ability of the cell to neutralize them. Reactive oxygen species (ROS) have been suggested to be a major cause of neurodegenerative disorders, such as Alzheimer's disease, Parkinson's disease and Huntington's disease (Simonian and Coyle, 1996). Hydrogen peroxide (H_2O_2) can traverse membranes and exerts cytotoxic effects on cells in the proximity of those responsible for its production (Halliwell, 1992). Although H_2O_2 is not a free radical and has a limited reactivity, it is thought to be the major precursor of the highly reactive hydroxyl radical ($HO^{\bullet}$). Recent studies have shown a close association between H_2O_2 and neurodegenerative disease, and it has been suggested that H_2O_2 levels are increased during pathological conditions such as ischemia (Behl et al., 1994; Hyslop et al., 1995).

ROS such as H_2O_2 and $HO^{\bullet}$ readily damage biological molecules that can eventually lead to apoptotic or necrotic cell death (Gardner et al., 1997). Exposure of cells to oxidative stress induces a range of cellular events that can result in apoptosis or necrosis (Davies, 1999). Apoptotic cells can be evaluated based on the measurement of the loss of plasma membrane asymmetry (van Engeland et al., 1998). Under normal physiological conditions, a cell maintains a strictly asymmetric distribution of phospholipids in the two leaflets of the cellular membranes with phosphatidylserine (PS) facing the cytosolic side (Devaux, 1991). However, during early apoptosis this membrane asymmetry is rapidly lost without concomitant loss of membrane integrity (van Engeland et al., 1998). Cell surface exposure of PS, which precedes the loss of membrane integrity, can be detected by fluorescein isothiocyanate (FITC)-labelled annexin V, a reagent that has high affinity for PS residues in the presence of millimolar concentrations of calcium (Ca^{2+}) (Andree *et al.*, 1990). By simultaneous probing of membrane integrity by means of exclusion of the nuclear dye propidium iodide (PI), apoptotic cells can be discriminated from necrotic cells (Darzynkiewicz *et al.*, 1997). The importance of apoptosis in the regulation of cellular homeostasis has mandated the development of accurate assays capable of measuring this process. Apoptosis assays based on flow cytometry have proven particularly useful; they are rapid, quantitative, and provide an individual cell-based mode of analysis (rather than a bulk population).

In this chapter, the relationship between physicochemical properties, chemical structures and cytoprotective capacity of twenty-four different flavonoids was established using human colon adenocarcinoma (HT-29) cells.

Materials And Methods

Materials

4-[3-(4-iodophenyl)-2-(4-nitrophenyl)-2H-5-tetrazolio]-1, 3-benzene disulphonate (WST-1 reagent) was obtained from Roche (Basel, Switzerland). Hydrogen peroxide was obtained from BDH Chemicals (Poole, England). Annexin V-FITC and binding buffer were obtained from BD Biosciences (San Diego, CA). All other chemicals were obtained from Sigma (St. Louis, MO). All solvents were of HPLC grade. Deionized water (MilliQ) was used in all experiments. All cell culture media were obtained from Invitrogen-Life Technologies (Carlsbad, CA). Cultured human colon adenocarcinoma HT-29) were obtained from the ATCC (American Type Culture Collection; Manassas, VA).

Assessment of Cell Viability

Cell viability was assessed using the WST-1 assay. The WST-1 assay is based on the cleavage of the tetrazolium salt WST-1 by mitochondrial dehydrogenases to form dark red formazan, which absorbs at 450 nm. Cultured human cells were seeded in 96-well plates (in 0.1 ml medium) at a density of 5×10^5 cells/ml with various concentrations (0.25-20 μM) of testing compounds. Tested compounds were either dissolved in DMSO or deionised water depending on their solubility (the amount of DMSO in cell culture was limited to 0.1%). Equivalent amounts of the DMSO vehicle had no effect compared with results in control cells. After 24 h of incubation in a humidified 5% CO_2, 95% air atmosphere at 37°C, 10 μl WST-1 tetrazolium salt was added to each well and the cells were incubated for 2 h to allow the reaction between the mitochondrial dehydrogenase released from viable cells and the tetrazolium salt of the WST-1 reagent.

The absorbance was measured at 450 nm with a reference at 690 nm using a microplate reader (Synergy HT, BioTEK Instruments, Winooski, VT). The level of absorbance directly correlates to viable cell numbers. Each assay was performed in triplicate and the cell viability was expressed as a percentage of the absorbance of cells exposed to test samples compared with that of controls (cells only).

Culture and Treatment of HT-29 Cells

HT-29 cells were grown in McCoy's 5A medium (modified) supplemented with 10% fetal bovine serum (FBS) in the presence of 100 U/ml penicillin and 0.1 g/l streptomycin at 37°C in humidified air with 5% CO_2. Cultured HT-29 cells were plated in 24-well plates at a density of 5×10^5 cells/ml. A range of non-toxic concentrations (0-20 μM) of testing compounds were added together with 150 μM H_2O_2. Cells were incubated for 24 h at 37°C in humidified air with 5% CO_2.

Annexin V Staining and Flow Cytometric Analysis

Annexin V coupled with fluorescein isothiocyanate (FITC) is typically used in conjunction with a vital dye such as propidium iodide (PI) to identify different stages of apoptotic and necrotic cells using flow cytometry. This assay was performed according to the method described by Vermes and co-workers (Vermes *et al.*, 2000) with slight modifications. After 24 h of incubation, cells were harvested and stained with both annexin V and propidium iodide to identify different stages of apoptotic and necrotic cell death using flow cytometry.

Briefly, the washed cells were resuspended in 100 μl of 1X binding buffer containing Annexin V-FITC (5 μl per test according to the manufacturer's instruction) and incubated in the dark for 20 min. Then, another 400 μl binding buffer containing PI (5 μl per test from 1 mg/ml stock solution) was added and incubated for a further 10 min. Flow cytometric analysis was performed within 1 h using a Cytomics FC500 MPL (Beckman Coulter, Miami, FL). The total cell count was set to 35,000 cells per sample.

Calculation of Results

Cell Death Index (CDI)

The percentages of viable, early, late apoptotic and necrotic cells were determined as illustrated in the cytogram (Figure 3).

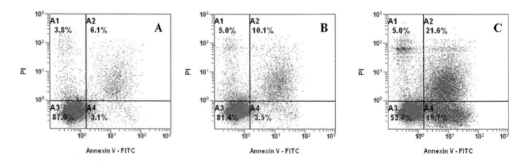

Figure 3. Cytograms of control (prior to incubation) (A), incubated control (B) and 150 μM H_2O_2 treated (C) human colon adenocarcinoma (HT-29) cells.

The viable cells are located in the lower left corner (negative in both annexin V-FITC and propidium iodide) (A3). Early apoptotic cells are in the lower right corner (annexin V-FITC positive only) (A4). Late apoptotic cells that show progressive cellular membrane and nuclear damage are in the upper right corner (both annexin V-FITC and PI positive) (A2). Necrotic cells are located in the upper left corner (PI positive only) (A1). The total percentage of damaged cells (both apoptotic and necrotic) was considered as (A1+A2+A4). The cell death index (CDI) was calculated based on the cytogram by the following equation (equation 1):

$$CDI = \frac{(A1+A2+A4)}{A3} \times 100 \qquad (5)$$

The CDI is the ratio of total damaged cells to viable cells and is used to remove inter-experimental variations in cell density. The net cell damage ($\boxed{}$) is derived by subtracting the CDI of incubated control cells (Figure 3B) from that of treated cells (Figure 3C) (equation 4-2).

$$\Delta CDI = (CDI_{Treated\ cells} - CDI_{Incubated\ control\ cells}) \qquad (6)$$

Calculation of 50% Reduction in Cell Death (EC$_{50}$)

The cytoprotective effects of test compounds were measured by the inhibition of the cytotoxic effects of H_2O_2 using both apoptosis and necrosis endpoints (approximately causing 50% total cell death). The percentage of inhibition of cell death was calculated by equation 7:

$$\% \text{ Inhibition of cell death} = \frac{\Delta CDI_{HP} - \Delta CDI_{Sample}}{\Delta CDI_{HP}} \times 100 \qquad (7)$$

where ΔCDI_{HP} and ΔCDI_{Sample} are the net cell damage caused by H_2O_2 and test sample, respectively. The EC$_{50}$ values were calculated from the dose-response relationship between the concentrations of antioxidant and % inhibition of cell death.

Quantum Chemical Calculations

Calculation of Heat of Formation

All geometry calculations of flavonoid were performed by using PM3 of the MOPAC2002 molecular package through Chem3D Ultra 2008 interface. The procedures were as follows. The molecular geometries were optimized by MM2 and then by the semiempirical quantum chemical method (PM3), and energies were minimized by using the EF algorithm. After the calculation of the heat of formation of the parent molecules (H_{fp}), the phenolic H was removed to get its free radical and a restricted Hartree-Fock optimization was performed on the phenoxyl radical. The differences in heat of formation was calculated by calculated by $\Delta H_f = H_{fr} - H_{fp}$.

Calculation of Log P

The log P of flavonoids was obtained by using ClogP in the Chem3D Ultra 2008 molecular package.

Results And Discussion

Cytotoxic Effects of H_2O_2

Hydrogen peroxide is known to be able to induce both apoptosis and necrosis in cells (Antunes and Cadenas, 2001; Barbouti *et al.*, 2002; Kim *et al.*, 2000), with the required concentrations and exposure time dependent on the cell type being investigated. The response of cultured human cells to H_2O_2 in terms of both concentration and exposure time was determined to calculate the dosage required to kill approximately half the cells. The CDI increased with increasing concentrations of H_2O_2 on HT-29 cells (Figure 4).

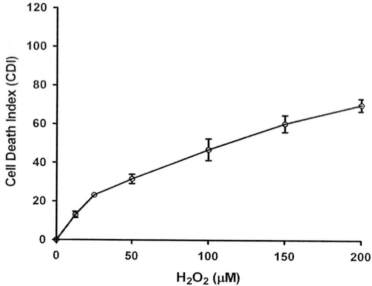

Figure 4. Cell death responses of cultured human HT-29 cells exposed to increasing concentrations of hydrogen peroxide (H_2O_2). HT-29 cells (5 x 10^5 cells per ml) were exposed to different concentrations of H_2O_2 and incubated at 37°C in humidified air with 5% CO_2 for 24 h. Bars indicate standard deviation from the mean of two separate determinations.

A concentration of 150 μM H_2O_2 was selected for the cytoprotection assay using HT-29 cells (CDI of 63.5 ± 2.7) with a 24-hour exposure to H_2O_2. These conditions were used in this assay to investigate the protective effects of antioxidants against H_2O_2-induced total cell death. Although H_2O_2 itself is a relatively unreactive species and easily scavenged by cellular catalase (Gille and Joenje, 1992), it can cause membrane damage by increasing the release of arachidonic acid from the cell membrane, which may account for the prolonged damage caused by H_2O_2 even after being scavenged (Cantoni *et al.*, 1989). Thus, even at low concentrations, H_2O_2 can cause damage to cultured cells. These facts demonstrate that the cytoprotection assay can be used to screen for and compare the protective effects of flavonoids in a biologically relevant cellular environment.

Cytotoxicity of Flavonoids

The cytotoxicities of Trolox, catechol, pyrogallol and selected flavonoids were tested on cultured human HT-29 cells at different concentrations for 24 h using the WST-1 assay (data not shown). None of the compounds tested affected the viability of HT-29 cells within the concentration range used (0–20.0 μM) in this study.

The Influence of Trolox on Cytotoxic Effects of H_2O_2

As described above, Trolox is a common compound used as a standard for most antioxidant assays. Trolox was co-incubated with cultured HT-29 cells at doses of 0, 0.25, 0.5, 1.0, 5.0, 10.0, 20.0 μM immediately prior to the addition of the H_2O_2. Trolox protected HT-29 cells against H_2O_2-induced cell death in a dose dependent manner (Figure 5).

The EC_{50} value (7.91 ± 0.22 μM) of Trolox was calculated from its dose-response curve. Trolox could thus be used as a standard antioxidant in this cytoprotection assay for comparison with other antioxidant compounds.

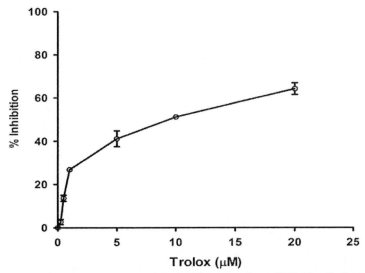

Figure 5. The concentration-response curve of Trolox for protection of HT-29 cells from 150 μM hydrogen peroxide. HT-29 cells (5 x 10^5 cells per well) were incubated at 37°C in humidified air with 5% CO_2 for 24 h. After incubation, cells were stained with both Annexin V-FITC and PI and analyzed by flow cytometry. Bars indicate standard deviation from the mean of two separate determinations.

Structural Related Cytoprotective Activity of Flavonoids

In the present Chapter, the cytoprotective activities (EC_{50}) of a range of structurally diverse flavonoids were measured (Table 1). Structural variations within the rings subdivide the flavonoids into several families (Figure 2). Measurement of the potential health effects of dietary-derived phenolic compounds needs to be undertaken at concentration ranges that are relevant to levels that might be achieved *in vivo*. Maximum plasma concentrations attained after a polyphenol-rich meal are thought to be in the range of 0.1–10 μM (Kroon *et al.*, 2004). In this work gut-derived cells were used but general bioavailability was taken into account. Hence, the 24 flavonoids, catechol and pyrogallol were added to HT-29 cells at doses of 0, 0.25, 0.5, 1.0, 5.0, 10.0, 20.0 μM immediately prior to the addition of the H_2O_2.

Table 1. Calculated differences of heat of formation (ΔH_f) between the parent flavonoid, catechol, and pyrogallol and each possible corresponding relative radical, the lipophilities (log P) and their cytoprotective activities

Compounds	EC$_{50}$ (μM)	Least OH ΔH_f (KJ/mol)	3-OH ΔH_f (KJ/mol)	3'-OH ΔH_f (KJ/mol)	4'-OH ΔH_f (KJ/mol)	5'-OH ΔH_f (KJ/mol)	Log P
Chrysin	15.42 ± 1.99	162.83					3.56
Apigenin	12.87 ± 0.94	149.84			149.84		2.91
Luteolin	4.05 ± 0.48	127.03		127.03	137.14		2.31
Galangin	16.64 ± 2.30	167.08	105.67				2.76
Kaempferol	10.98 ± 1.17	154.25	104.87		154.25		2.10
Quercetin	2.11 ± 0.40	125.80	103.06	125.80	138.53		1.50
Isoquercetin	2.72 ± 0.50	110.17		124.61	110.17		-0.34
Rutin	4.14 ± 0.40	109.91		109.91	137.32		-2.68
Morin	9.98 ± 1.07	154.18	104.29	154.18		158.51	1.43
Myricetin	4.47 ± 0.53	123.43	104.06	133.34	123.43	140.68	0.84
Naringenin	12.27 ± 0.87	149.91			149.91		2.44
Naringin	16.50 ± 2.25	158.11			158.11		-0.09
Hesperitin	6.86 ± 0.69	135.31		135.31			2.29
Hesperidin	7.73 ± 1.29	124.38		124.38			-0.29
Taxifolin	4.79 ± 0.22	124.86	210.59	139.16	124.86		0.77
Catechin	5.01 ± 0.47	123.12	211.65	124.65	123.12		0.53
Phloretin	7.26 ± 0.71	141.91	163.29		141.91		2.22
Phloridzin	9.57 ± 1.00	137.90	159.37		137.90		0.79
Cyanidin	5.48 ± 0.53	144.49		144.49	159.40		1.76
Idaein	6.36 ± 0.87	143.06		143.06	159.64		0.19
Keracyanin	9.63 ± 1.81	144.67	157.04	144.67	165.47		-0.84
Delphinidin	8.33 ± 0.98	140.03		146.39	140.03	158.62	1.10
Callistephin	18.69 ± 1.52	184.06	151.50		184.06		0.78
Pelargonidin	17.95 ± 2.11	182.16			182.16		2.36
Catechol	6.61 ± 0.78	126.93		126.93	126.93		0.88
Pyrogallol	3.22 ± 0.25	119.87		137.26	119.87	125.70	0.21

Notes: Structural optimization of each flavonoid and its radical was determined by calculating the minimum energy conformation by the MM2 method. MOPAC2002 in Chem3D Ultra was used to determine the final minimum energy conformation of the flavonoids and was calculated by applying the semi-empirical Hamiltonian PM3 calculation to obtain the final heat of formation of each compound. The lowest ΔH_f of chrysin and galangin were obtained from their hydroxyl groups in the A ring. All other flavonoids were calculated from their B ring hydroxyl groups.

Effects of Hydroxyl Groups in the B Ring

The manipulation of the hydroxyl substitutions in the B-ring in flavones (with the 2,3-double bond and 4-keto function in the C-ring, but no 3-OH group) allows the observation of the contribution of these hydroxyl groups to their cytoprotective activities. With the 3',4'-dihydroxyl group, the EC_{50} value of luteolin is 4.05 µM. Dehydroxylation at the 3'-position as in apigenin increases the value to 12.87 µM, making the cytoprotective activity of apigenin only one-third of luteolin (Figure 6). The EC_{50} value of chrysin is further increased because of the lack of any hydroxyl group in its B-ring. The cytoprotective activity of chrysin can be reasonably attributed to the 5,7-*meta*-dihydroxyl groups of its A-ring.

As a group of flavonols, galangin, quercetin, morin and myricetin have the same structures on the A and C-rings but the number of hydroxyl groups in the B-ring increases from zero to three (Figure 7).

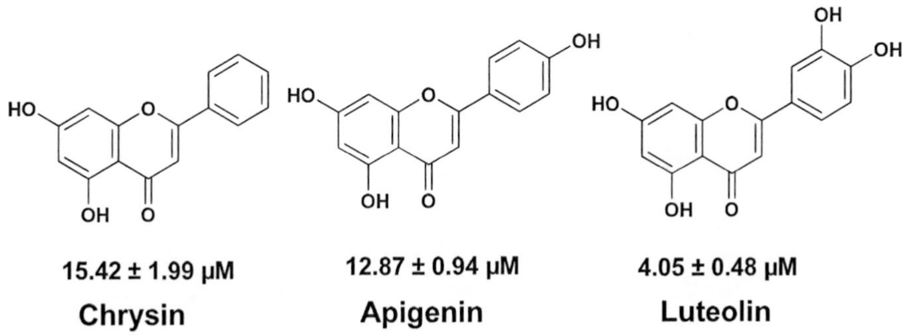

| 15.42 ± 1.99 µM | 12.87 ± 0.94 µM | 4.05 ± 0.48 µM |
| **Chrysin** | **Apigenin** | **Luteolin** |

Figure 6. The influences of hydroxylation in the B ring on the cytoprotective activity of the flavones.

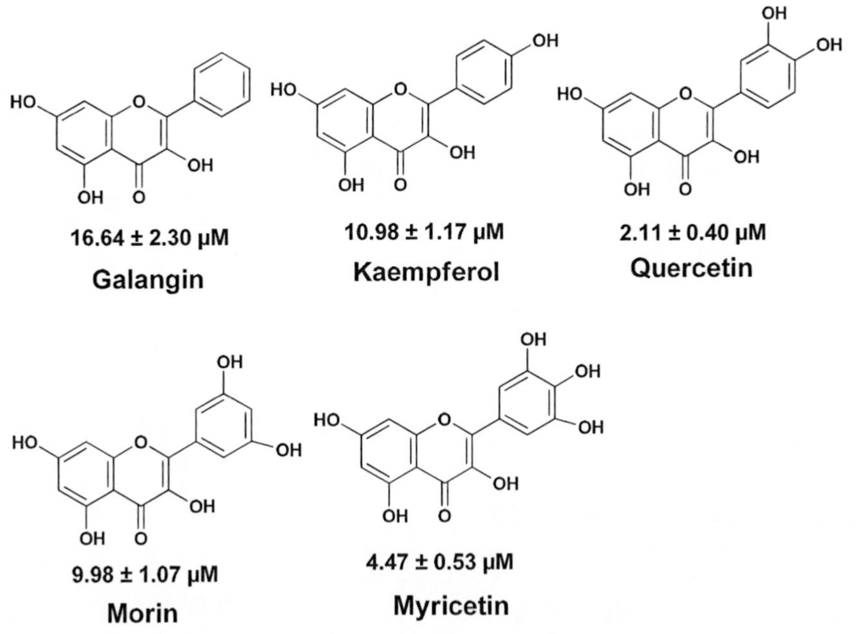

| 16.64 ± 2.30 µM | 10.98 ± 1.17 µM | 2.11 ± 0.40 µM |
| **Galangin** | **Kaempferol** | **Quercetin** |

9.98 ± 1.07 µM
Morin

4.47 ± 0.53 µM
Myricetin

Figure 7. The influences of hydroxylation in the B ring on the cytoprotective activity of the flavanols.

As the number of hydroxyl groups increases the EC_{50} value decreases except for quercetin, which is more active than myricetin. With morin, the dihydroxyl groups in the B-ring are arranged *meta* to each other. This significantly reduces its cytoprotective activity compared with quercetin (the EC_{50} value of morin was four times than that of quercetin). This result confirms that the presence of two adjacent hydroxyl groups in the B-ring plays a significant role in the high cytoprotective activity of flavonoids. Possibly, the two adjacent hydroxyl groups at position 3' and 4' in quercetin are more vulnerable to loss of a proton than the two hydroxyl groups at position 3' and 5' in morin. Myricetin, which possesses *ortho*-trihydroxyl (pyrogallol) groups in the B-ring, is much less active than quercetin. This suggests that the additional 5'-hydroxyl group has a negative impact on its cytoprotective activity. However, the cytoprotective activity of pyrogallol is much more active than that of catechol as illustrated in Figure 8. This may be the result of the rest of the quercetin structure (C- and A-rings) stabilizing the oxidation product (*o*-quninoe) as shown in Figure 9.

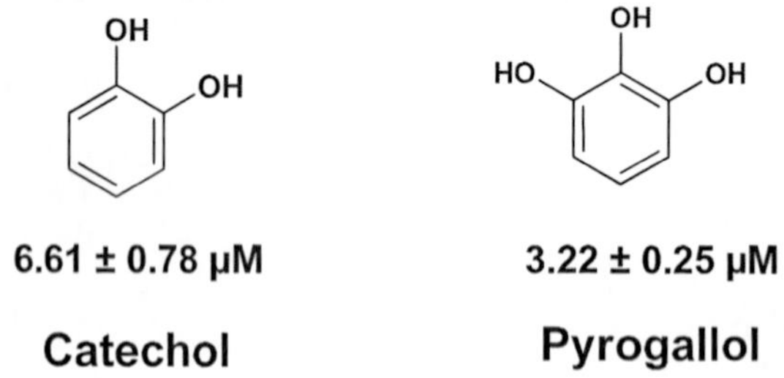

6.61 ± 0.78 µM   3.22 ± 0.25 µM

Catechol   **Pyrogallol**

Figure 8. The cytoprotective activity of catechol and pyrogallol.

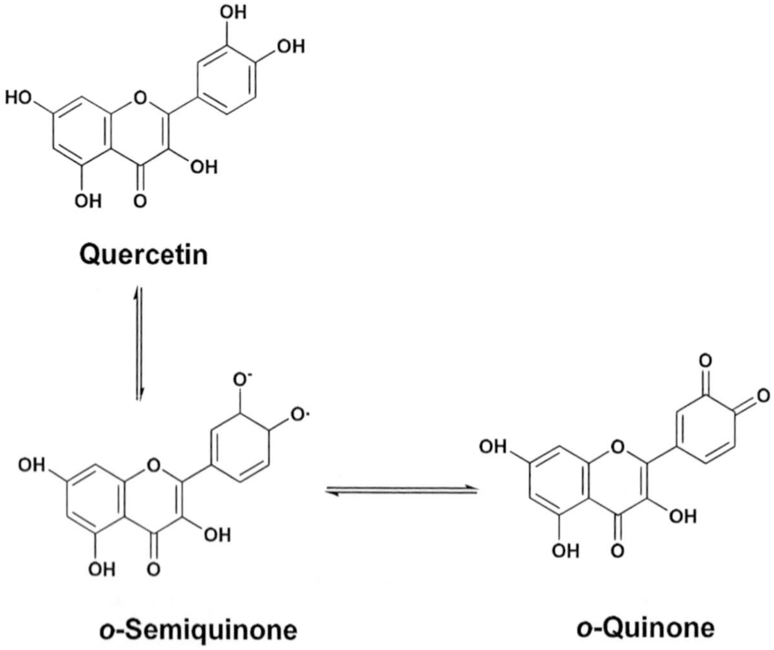

Quercetin

o-**Semiquinone**   *o*-**Quinone**

Figure 9. Quercetin oxidation and its possible consequences.

A fairly stable *ortho*-semiquinone radical can be formed by oxidation of a flavonoid on the B ring, when the 3'4'-catechol structure is present facilitating electron delocalization (Arora *et al.*, 1998; Mora *et al.*, 1990). The formation of flavonoid aroxyl radicals is an essential step after initial scavenging of an oxidizing radical (Bors *et al.*, 1990). The stability of aroxyl radicals strongly depends on their bimolecular disproportionation reaction and electron delocalization. For instance the oxidation of quercetin can form an *o*-semiquinone radical and then an *o*-quinone radical (Awad *et al.*, 2001; Awad *et al.*, 2003; Boersma *et al.*, 2000; Metodiewa *et al.*, 1999) as illustrated in Figure 9. However, with only one hydroxyl group in the B-ring the EC_{50} value of kaempferol was significantly increased. Without any hydroxyl substitutions in its B-ring, the cytoprotective activity of galangin was almost negligible like that of chrysin. The flavanone, naringenin, with only a single 4'-OH group in the B-ring has a EC_{50} value twice than that of hesperitin, which has an identical structure to naringenin except for the 3'-OH, 4'-methoxy substitution in the B-ring (Figure 10).

This finding suggested that methoxylation does not destroy cytoprotective activity. Repeated studies have shown that flavonoids having greater numbers of hydroxyl groups, or hydroxyl groups localized *ortho* to one another, are more effective antioxidants. The B-ring of most flavonoids is usually the initial target of oxidants, as it is more electron-rich than the A- and C-rings, whose electron densities are somewhat drained away by the carbonyl group.

These properties are consistent with the expected mechanisms of oxidation of phenols; electron-donating substitutes, such as hydroxyl groups, should lower the oxidation potential for a compound, and *ortho* hydroxylation should stabilize phenoxyl radicals.

The cytoprotective activity pattern of pelargonidin, cyanidin and delphinidin (Figure 11) shows a similar trend to that revealed by kaempferol, quercetin and myricetin (Figure 7). The EC_{50} value of cyanidin is much lower than that of delphinidin, and the cytoprotective activity of pelargonidin, which has a lone 4'-OH, is almost negligible. With the anthocyanin C-ring, the cytoprotective activity of cyanidin is only half of that of quercetin. The same trend also applies to delphinidin and myricetin.

The presence of a third OH group in the B-ring does not enhance the effectiveness against H_2O_2-induced cell death. This is also supported by the findings that myricetin was less active in protecting liposome oxidation (Zhang *et al.*, 2006b).

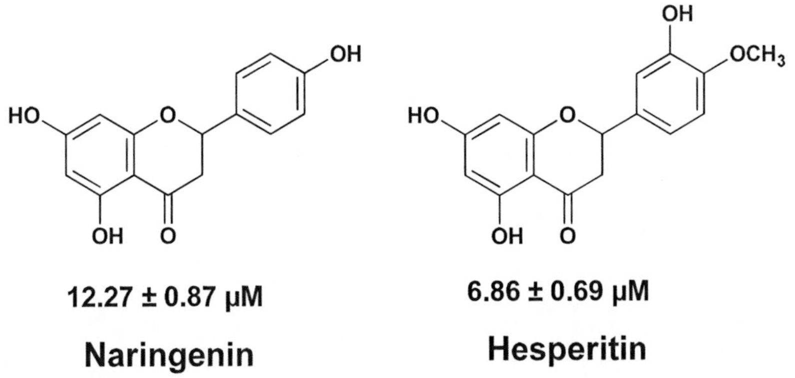

12.27 ± 0.87 µM

Naringenin

6.86 ± 0.69 µM

Hesperitin

Figure 10. The influences of hydroxylation and methoxylation in the B-ring on the cytoprotective activity of the flavanones.

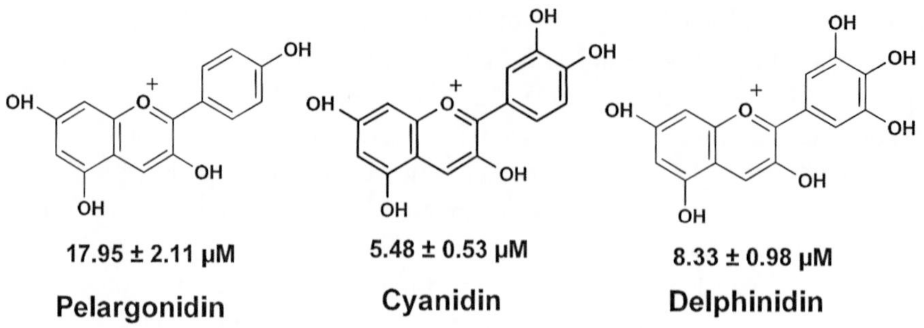

| 17.95 ± 2.11 µM | 5.48 ± 0.53 µM | 8.33 ± 0.98 µM |
| Pelargonidin | Cyanidin | Delphinidin |

Figure 11. The influences of hydroxylation in the B-ring on the cytoprotective activity of the anthocyanins.

In acidic or neutral media, four anthocyanin structures exist in equilibrium (Figure 12): the flavylium cation, the quinonoidal base, the carbinal pseudobase, and the chalcone (Borkowski *et al.*, 2005; Brouillard, 1983).

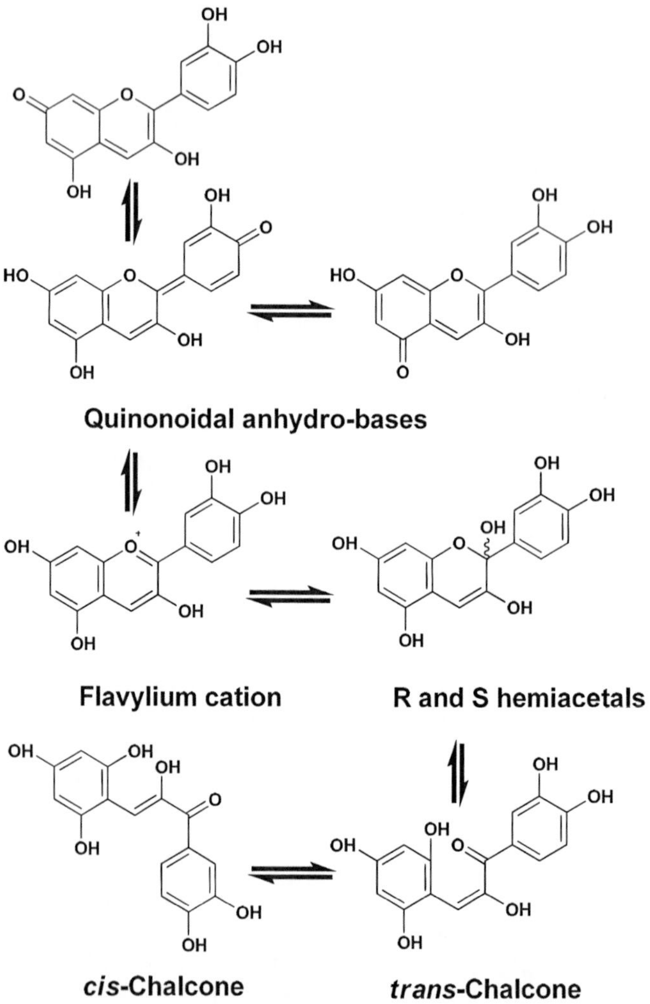

Quinonoidal anhydro-bases

Flavylium cation   **R and S hemiacetals**

cis-Chalcone   *trans*-Chalcone

Figure 12. Structural transformations of cyanidin in acidic to alkaline aqueous media.

The equilibrium among the four different structural conformations of anthocyanin is illustrated in Figure 12 (using cyanidin as an example).

At pH less than 2, the anthocyanin exists primarily in the form of the red (with a 3-O-sugar substitute) or yellow (with a 3-OH) flavylium cation. As the pH is raised, there is a rapid proton loss to yield the red or blue quinonoidal forms. At higher pH, hydration of the flavylium cation occurs to give the colorless carbinol or pseudobase. The relative amounts of flavylium cation, quinonoidal forms, pseudobases and chalcones at equilibrium vary with both pH and the structure of the anthocyanin. At pH 3.5-4.5, a mixture of the flavylium ion and the neutral quinonoidal anhydro-base is found. At pH 4.5-6.0, the concentration of the flavylium ion becomes vanishingly small, the quinonoidal anhydro-base increasingly predominates and there is a mixture of both the neutral and the ionized (blue anionic) quinonoidal anhydro-base forms present at pH 7.0 (around neutrality) (Brouillard and Dubois, 1977b). As their quinonoidal anhydro-base or as their flavylium cations, anthocyanins could be strongly stabilized by neutral salts such as magnesium chloride and sodium chloride in concentrated aqueous solutions. The anthocyanidin structural transformation path is very sensitive to the substitution pattern of the pyrilium ring, especially the C_3 position. The 3-OH substituted anthocyanidins are significantly shifted towards colorless pseudobase forms causing color instability (Timberlake and Bridle, 1967). In addition, an increase in the number of hydroxyl groups tends to deepen the color to a more bluish shade. The hydroxyl groups at C_5, C_7 on the A-ring and $C_{4'}$ on the B-ring of the flavylium cation can lose a proton at pH values close to equilibrium.

It must be emphasized that the interpretation of the cytoprotective properties of anthocyanins is complicated by the relatively complex pathway of reversible structural transformations of anthocyanins in aqueous solution (Brouillard and Delaporte, 1977a; Brouillard et al., 1977b), which not only includes proton transfer between coloured forms but also water addition to the pyrylium ring leading to colourless hemiacetal and chalcone forms. Hence, the EC_{50} values of anthocyanins measured here are actually a reflection of the cytoprotective properties of the transformed products, i.e. the quinonoidal anhydro-base (Hoshino, 1991; Hoshino and Goto, 1990; Hoshino et al., 1981).

Effect of the 3-OH Group, 2,3-Double Bond and 4-Keto Group

Without the 3-OH group in the C-ring, the EC_{50} values of apigenin and luteolin are increased compared with those of kaempferol and quercetin, respectively (Figure 13). However, the EC_{50} value is reduced for chrysin compared with that of galangin. The results presented in Figure 13 demonstrate that when the 3-hydroxyl group is absent, its contribution to electron dislocation is substantially reduced and so consequently is the flavonoid cytoprotective activity, although this reduction is smaller when the catechol structure is absent in the B ring. This fact indicated that 3-OH is required to stabilize the catechol structure in the B ring. A distinguishing feature among the flavonoid structural classes is the presence or absence of an unsaturated 2,3-double bond in conjugation with a 4-keto group.

Comparison of naringenin with apigenin shows that the 2,3-double bond in the C-ring has a slightly negative influence on the cytoprotective activity (Figure 13). On the other hand, the introduction of a 2,3-double bound and 4-keto group to catechin with the existing 3-hydroxyl group decreases the EC_{50} value as in quercetin. This fact indicates that the presence of the 3-hydroxyl group is an important factor in neutralizing the negative impact of the 2,3-double bond on the cytoprotective activity. This may also indicate that the combined effect of the 2,3-double bond in the C-ring and the *ortho*-hydroxyl groups in the B-ring have positive effect on cytoprotective activity as demonstrated by the comparison of apigenin and luteolin.

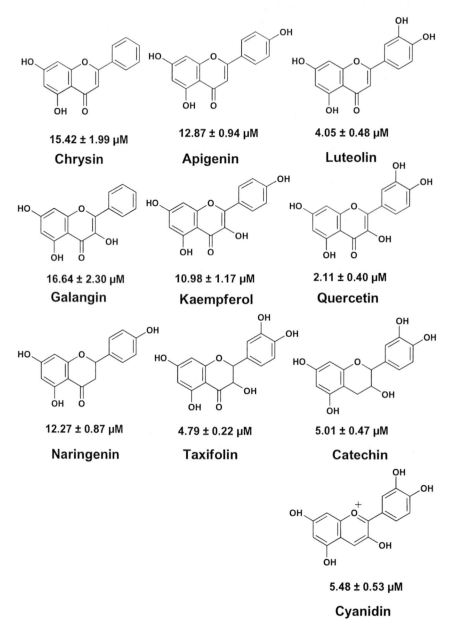

15.42 ± 1.99 µM

Chrysin

12.87 ± 0.94 µM

Apigenin

4.05 ± 0.48 µM

Luteolin

16.64 ± 2.30 µM

Galangin

10.98 ± 1.17 µM

Kaempferol

2.11 ± 0.40 µM

Quercetin

12.27 ± 0.87 µM

Naringenin

4.79 ± 0.22 µM

Taxifolin

5.01 ± 0.47 µM

Catechin

5.48 ± 0.53 µM

Cyanidin

Figure 13. Structure-cytoprotective activity comparisons of the 3-OH, 2,3-double bond and 4-keto group of flavonoids.

However, the presence of a 2,3-double bond when the 3-hydroxyl group is absent (apigenin and luteolin) does not significantly change the cytoprotective activity of flavonoids relative to those that do not contain this double bond (naringenin and taxifolin). When the 3-hydroxyl group is present (quercetin), it significantly enhances cytoprotective activity compared with those that do not contain this double bond (taxifolin). The loss of the 4-keto group at the C-ring and introduction of a positive charge decreases cytoprotective activities as seen in cyanidin and quercetin. As shown in Figure 13, quercetin, catechin and cyanidin have identical A- and B-rings, but quercetin is more than twice as cytoprotective as catechin and cyanidin. This observation indicates the important contribution of the 2,3-double bond and 4-keto group to the cytoprotective activity.

Effect of the Carbohydrate Moieties

Blocking the 3-hydroxyl group in the C-ring of quercetin as a glycoside (while retaining the 3',4'-dihydroxy structure in the B-ring) as in isoquercetin (quercetin-3-glucoside) decreases the cytoprotective activities. Replacement of the hydroxyl group at the C_3 position of quercetin by the disaccharide rutinose in rutin further decreases cytoprotective activity (Figure 14).

The presence of the 3-OH group on the C-ring double bond undoubtedly contributes to attack by free radicals. If the 3-OH is replaced by an O-sugar group (as in the glycoside rutin or isoquercetin, for example), reactivity is decreased by about a factor of 2-3 (Briviba et al., 1993; Tournaire et al., 1993). The results shown in Figure 14 also indicate that when the 3-hydroxyl group is substituted, the reduction in cytoprotective activity of the flavonoids depends on the nature of the substituted sugar group. This reduction can be smaller when this hydroxyl group is substituted (isoquercetin) than when it is just absent (luteolin).

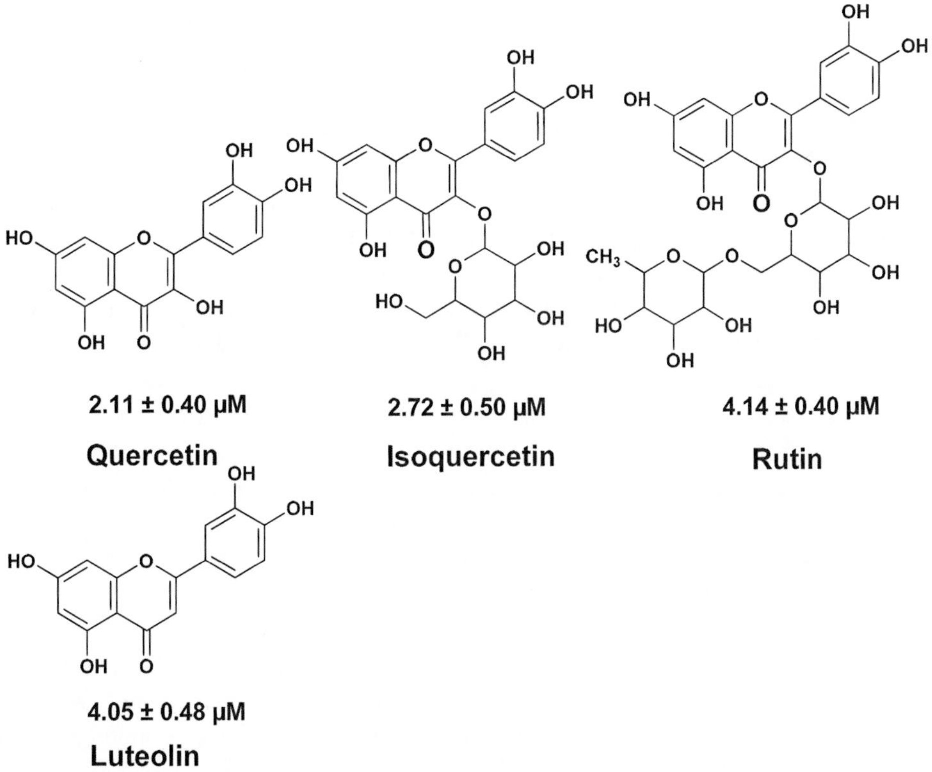

Figure 14. Influences of glycosylation of flavanols on their cytoprotective activity.

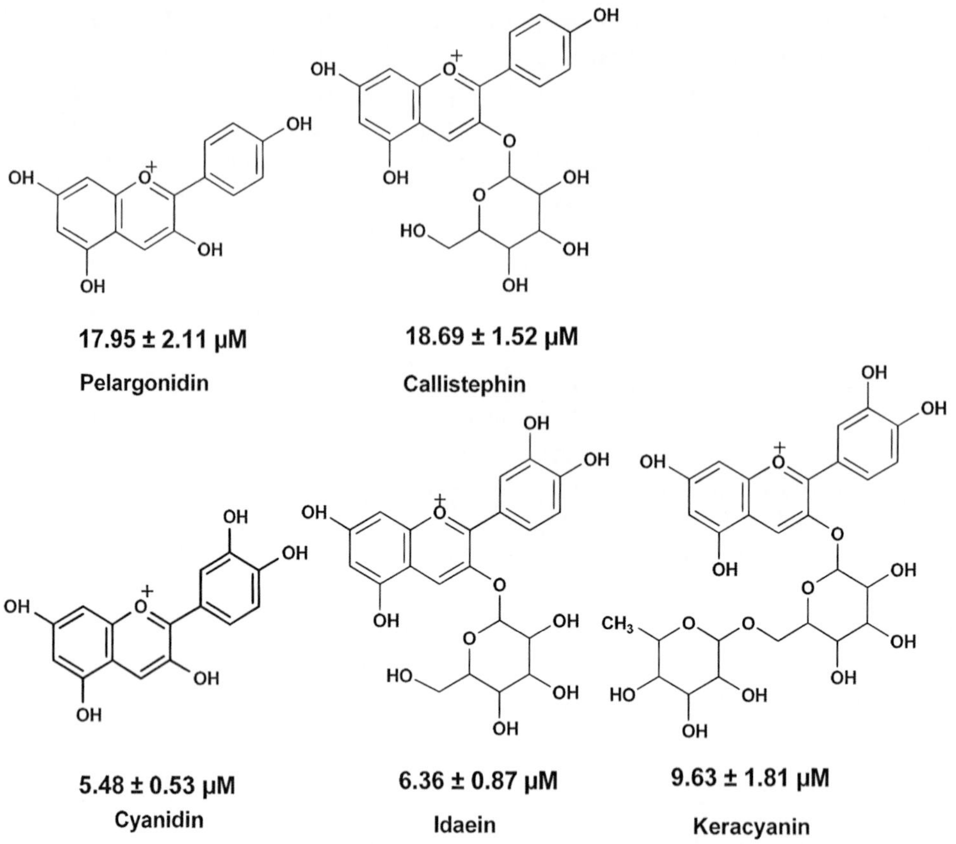

Figure 15. Influences of glycosylation of anthocyandins on their cytoprotective activity.

Similar effects are observed when cyanidin is compared with its 3-glucoside, idaein and its 3-rutinoside, keracyanin, and when pelargonidin is compared with its 3-glucoside, callistephin (Figure 15).

Comparison of naringenin with naringin shows that glycosylation of the 7-hydroxyl group in a structure with a saturated heterocyclic C-ring and with a single hydroxyl group on the B-ring has a significant negative impact on the EC_{50} values. Similar trends are observed with hesperitin when a 4'-hydroxyl group in the B-ring is replaced by a methoxy and 3'-hydroxyl group, in contrast to naringenin, compared with its rhamnoside, hesperidin, which has a glycosylated 7-hydroxyl group. However, hesperidin is much more cytoprotective than that of naringin because of its B-ring configuration (Figure 16).

The results presented in Figure 16 and 17 demonstrate that the presence of both 3- and 5-hydroxyl groups is also necessary to maximize cytoprotective activity of flavonoids.

The sugar moiety is reported to have a negative effect on the oxidizability of flavonoid glycosides (Hedrickson et al., 1994). The oxidation rate of compounds decreased as the substituent at the 3-position became a poorer leaving group. Disaccharides are a poorer leaving group than monosaccharides, thus rutin is less oxidizable than isoquercetin (Hopia and Heinonen, 1999). This observation may explain why rutin displays a lower cytoprotective activity than quercetin and isoquercetin.

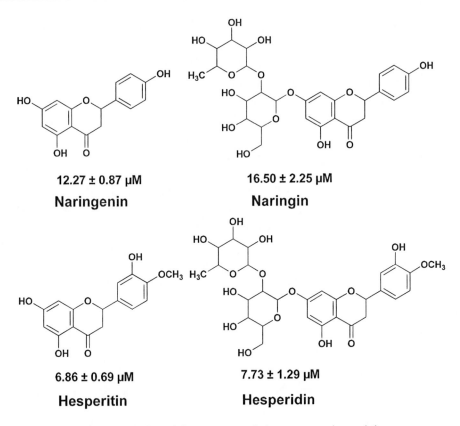

Figure 16. Influences of glycosylation of flavanones on their cytoprotective activity.

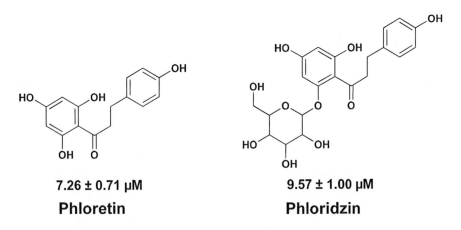

Figure 17. Influences of glycosylation of chalcones on their cytoprotective activity.

The structural criteria for the very high cytoprotective activity by flavonoids can be summarized as: 1) the o-dihydroxy (catechol) structure in the B-ring; 2) the 2,3-double bond in conjugation with the 4-keto group in the C-ring; and 3) the 3-hydroxyl group in the C-ring. Thus, quercetin, for example, satisfies all the above-mentioned determinants and has the highest cytoprotective activities among 24 flavonoids tested.

Cytoprotective Activities and Physicochemical Properties of Flavonoids

Correlation between O-H Bond Dissociation Enthalpy (BDE) and Cytoprotective Activity (EC_{50}) of Flavonoids

Possible explanations of the cytoprotective capacity of flavonoids obtained from cell-based assay could be derived by calculating the heat of formation differences (ΔH_f) between radicals and their parent molecules (bond dissociation energy approximation) of flavonoids. Quantum chemical calculations of the geometry of the flavonoids and their corresponding radicals give their heat of formation. The ΔH_f calculated between each flavonoid and its corresponding radicals provides an estimation of the ease with which radicals may be formed (Lien *et al.*, 1999). The ΔH_f of a given compound represents the difference between the parent compound and the appropriate radical, which was constructed by an abstraction of a hydrogen atom from assigned hydroxyl moiety (Zhang, 1998). This value may represent the relative stability of a radical with respect to its parent compound, and it enables a comparison to be made between the stabilization achieved by hydrogen abstraction (toward radical formation) (Sun *et al.*, 2002; Zhang, 1998; Zhang *et al.*, 2002a; Zhang and Wang, 2002b). Generally speaking , the smaller the ΔH_f, the more stable the phenoxyl radical and the weaker the O-H bond in the molecule, so the more active is the flavonoid (van Acker *et al.*, 1993).

A summary of calculated ΔH_f for the H-abstraction from hydroxyl groups (in the B ring and 3-OH) in all the flavonoids tested is shown in Table 1. All heat of formations were calculated or selected by the PM3 semi-empirical method, for energy-optimized species as described in the method section.

The ΔH_f of chrysin and galangin were calculated from the hydroxyl groups in their A-ring because there are no hydroxyl groups in their B-ring. The calculated ΔH_f shows that the least energy required for abstracting a hydrogen atom is from the 3-OH, when the C-ring contains the 2,3-double bond and the 4-keto group (flavonols). In the absence of flavonol structure, the most favored position for donating a hydrogen atom is from the two adjacent hydroxyls in the B-ring, with 3'-OH preferred over 4'-OH. In myricetin and delphinidin, in which 4'-OH is adjacent to two hydroxyl groups (3'-OH and 5'-OH), the donation of a hydrogen atom from 4'-OH is favored over 3'-OH or 5'-OH. The calculated ΔH_f of 5'-OH is larger than that of 3'-OH (Table 1). However, the 3-hydroxyl group is not the determining factor for the cytoprotective activity of flavonoids and this is better demonstrated by galangin, which showed a very weak cytoprotective activity. The ΔH_f of flavonols (galangin, kaempferol, quercetin, morin and myricetin) is almost identical regardless of their cytoprotective activities. Therefore, the least ΔH_f of flavonoids was obtained from their hydroxyl groups in the B ring, and then the A ring.

As shown in previous work, flavonoids with a catechol group in the B ring are the most active free radical scavengers (Zhang *et al.*, 2006b). It appears that the rest of the hydroxyl groups of the flavonoid are of little importance to the antioxidant activity, except for quercetin and its derivatives, in which the combination of the catechol moiety with a 2,3-double bond at the C-ring and a 3-hydroxyl group results in an extremely active scavenger. Therefore, the ΔH_f values were calculated from the O-H bond in the B-ring, and only the most stable phenoxyl radical is considered (lowest ΔH_f) to derive the correlation with the cytoprotective activity of flavonoids (Figure 18).

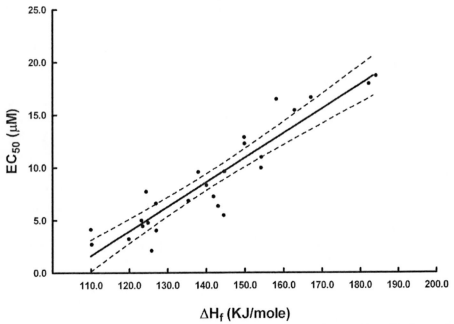

Figure 18. Correlation between EC_{50} (cytoprotective activity of flavonoids) and ΔH_f (the lowest heat of formation of the ArO-H bond of flavonoids from the A- or B-ring hydroxyl group) ($r^2 = 0.85$, n = 26).

As illustrated in Figure 18, a correlation was demonstrated between the calculated ΔH_f (the lowest differences in the enthalpy between each flavonoid's parent compound and its radical) values and the experimentally determined cytoprotective activity of flavonoids. There is a strong linear correlation between the lowest ΔH_f and the EC_{50} values and from the regression analysis a correlation with $r^2 = 0.85$ (n = 26) was obtained for the following equation 8:

$$EC_{50} = 0.23\,(\pm\,0.02)\,\Delta H_f - 23.97\,(\pm\,2.81)\,(n = 26) \qquad [8]$$

These findings suggest that a relatively low O-H bond dissociation enthalpy (BDE, approximation by the lowest ΔH_f), which facilitates the H-abstraction reaction between flavonoids and reactive oxygen species (ROS) and other hydroxyl groups may well have contributed to this reaction in the consequent steps. However, substitution of the hydroxyl group at the C_3 position of quercetin by the monosaccharide glucose in isoquercetin and disaccharide rutinose in rutin decreases the lowest ΔH_f values, but this does not result in an increase in the cytoprotective activity. This is probably due to the fact that glycosylation decreases the lipophilicity, and to the loss of the free hydroxyl group at the 3-position of the C-ring. An appropriate solubility, which improves the mobility of the antioxidant across cell membranes, is another important factor in explaining the cytoprotective effects of flavonoids.

Correlation between Partition Coefficient (Log P) and Cytoprotective Activity (EC50) of Flavonoids

As shown in Table 1, flavonoids with log P values that were high (log P > 3.0) or low (log P <1.0) had low cytoprotective activity, indicating that the cytoprotective activity of flavonoids is associated with their affinity and distribution in lipid membranes. This is presumably because a) at high values of log P, the flavonoid is dispersed in a lipid phase and not located at the lipid-water interface and, b) at low values of log P, the flavonoid is located in an aqueous phase and has insufficient solubility in the lipid phase. This can be important in terms of paracellular transport of flavonoids and the ability to enter the cell to participate in intracellular protection from oxidative damage. It has long been recognized that for a chemical to be biologically active, it must first be transported from its site of administration to its site of action and then it must bind to or react with its receptor or target, i.e. biological activity is a function of partitioning and reactivity (Barratt, 1998). It should be noted that the effect of membrane partitioning is not necessarily a direct relationship with lipophilicity. Beyeler and coworkers (Beyeler *et al.*, 1988), for example, reported that the effects of cianidanols on rat hepatic monooxygenase increased with lipophilicity, reached a plateau, decreased and then leveled off for the most lipophilic compounds.

As illustrated in Figure 19, for the 26 compounds tested, no correlation could be found between EC_{50} and log P (equation 9).

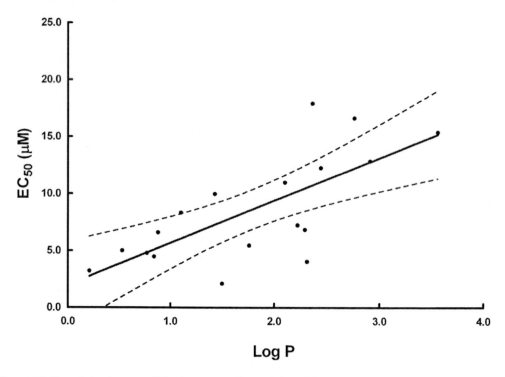

Figure 19. Correlation between EC_{50} (cytoprotective activity of flavonoids) and log P (calculated by CLogP program) of flavonoids ($r^2 = 0.15$, n = 26).

$$EC_{50} = 1.42 \ (\pm 0.68) \ \log P + 7.23 \ (\pm 1.20) \hspace{3cm} [9]$$

$$n = 26, \ r^2 = 0.15, \ p = 0.048$$

As mentioned above, glycosylation decreased the lipophilicity of flavonoid aglycones significantly and also decreased their cytoprotective activity depending on the nature of the sugar involved. Therefore, the balance of lipophilicity and lipophobicity allowing concentration at the interface is an important factor in the estimation of the antioxidant activity of flavonoids.

As demonstrated in Figure 20, there is a moderate linear correlation between the cytoprotective activities (EC_{50} values) and the partition coefficient (log P) values of flavonoid aglycones and from the regression analysis a correlation with $r^2 = 0.51$ (n = 18) was obtained for the following equation 10:

$$EC_{50} = 3.72 \ (\pm 0.92) \ \log P + 1.97 \ (\pm 1.82) \ (n = 18) \qquad\qquad [10]$$

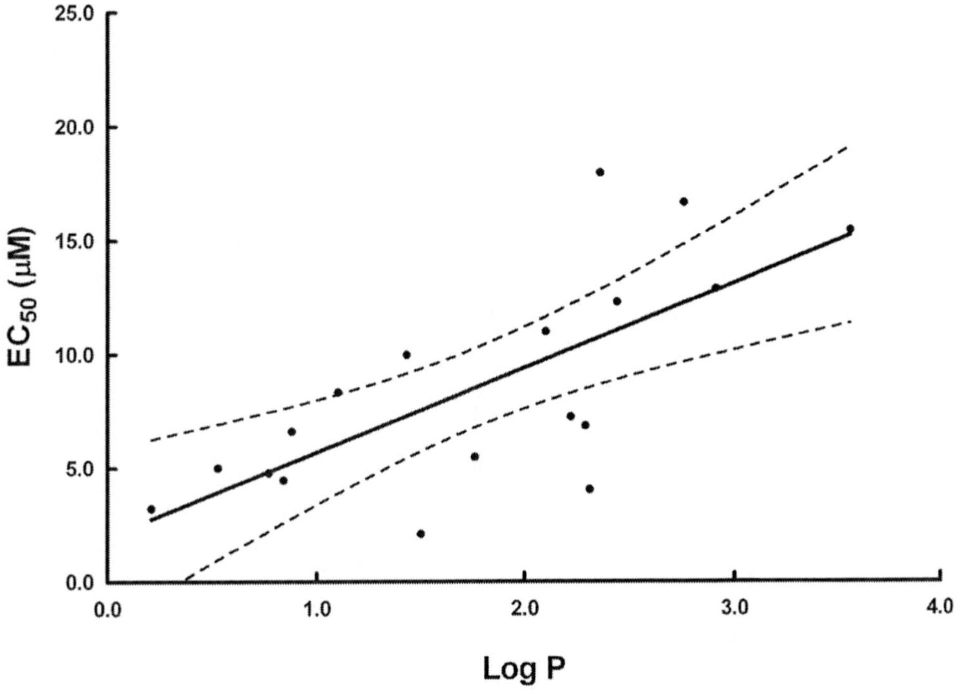

Figure 20. Correlation between EC_{50} (cytoprotective activity of flavonoids) and log P (calculated by CLogP program) of flavonoid aglycones (without sugar substitution) ($r^2 = 0.51$, n = 18).

Generally speaking, the cytoprotective activity of flavonoid aglycones decreases with increasing log P. However, this result also demonstrated that the cytoprotective activity of flavonoid aglycones is not solely dependant on their partition coefficient.

Quantitative Structure-Activity Relationship (QSAR) Model

The QSAR paradigm has been useful in elucidating the mechanisms of chemical-biological interactions in various biomolecules, particularly enzymes, membranes, organelles and cells (Hansch and Gao, 1997; Zhang et al., 2002a; Zhang et al., 2002b). The description of QSARs has been undertaken in order to find predictive models and/or mechanistic explanations for chemical as well as biological activities (Soffers et al., 2001). The underlying premise of SARs and QSARs is that the properties of a chemical are implicit in its molecular structure and the behavior of chemical compounds is dominated by their physicochemical properties (Hansch et al., 2000). If a QSAR model is deficient in modeling either partition or reactivity, only a partial correlation with the in vivo response is likely to be observed. The ΔH_f represents the stability of the free radical formed after H-abstraction and log P is an important parameter in chemical toxicology as it can indicate metabolic fate and biological transport properties.

The cytoprotection assay is a more biological measurement that accounts for some aspects of uptake, metabolism and location of flavonoids within cells. Here, a QSAR is modeled by starting from log P values and then incorporating ΔH_f.

With the introduction of ΔH_f (ease of H-abstraction) into equation 9, a two-parameter predictive model in the cytoprotection system could be derived based on the 26 compounds tested by step-wise regression as shown in equation 11.

$$EC_{50} = -0.45 \,(\pm 0.33)\, \log P + 0.25 \,(\pm 0.02)\, \Delta H_f - 25.75 \,(\pm 3.04) \qquad [11]$$

$$n = 26,\ r^2 = 0.86,\ p = 0.0000000001$$

The use of the new parameter (ΔH_f) increased the correlation coefficient r^2-value from 0.15 to 0.86. The significant increase in correlation coefficient upon the introduction of ΔH_f confirmed the importance of O-H bond strength (bond dissociation energy approximated by ΔH_f), which contributed most to the model. However, log P gave a negative contribution to the EC_{50} values in this model.

A QSAR model could also be derived by the introduction of ΔH_f to equation 9 for flavonoid aglycones through step-wise regression as shown in equation 12.

$$EC_{50} = 0.38 \,(\pm 0.65)\, \log P + 0.24 \,(\pm 0.03)\, \Delta H_f - 26.25 \,(\pm 4.04) \qquad [12]$$

$$n = 18,\ r^2 = 0.88,\ p = 0.000000072$$

Equation 12 indicated that log P gave a positive contribution to the EC_{50} values of flavonoid aglycones.

In conclusion, a QSAR model was derived from the cytoprotective activity and calculated theoretical parameters (enthalpy of hemolytic O-H bond cleavage ΔH_f and the partition coefficient). It demonstrated that the H-abstraction was not the sole mechanism responsible for the cytoprotective activity of flavonoids. It seems that the relative contribution of lipophilicity (log P) is much smaller than that of ΔH_f. These results demonstrated that it is feasible to estimate the cytoprotective activities of a flavonoid from the lipophilicity and the difference of heat of formations by using equation 11. The lipophilicity and heat of formation can be calculated purely by computer programs. Therefore, the QSAR model derived here could be useful in the selection of natural flavonoids with potential cytoprotective effects.

Conclusion

In summary, the cytoprotection assay provides information regarding cellular activity of antioxidants, which is important to our understanding of this area of antioxidant research. Traditionally, the antioxidant activity of phytochemicals has been measured using a range of chemically-defined laboratory-based assays. A cytoprotection assay that is a more biologically relevant method than the chemical antioxidant assays has been developed and can be adapted for use in other cell lines appropriate to tissues of interest. Using the cytoprotection assay, the effects of compounds on cells is determined, providing information regarding the cellular response to antioxidants, taking into account some aspects of uptake, metabolism, location of antioxidant compounds within cells and intracellular effects on signalling pathways and enzyme activity.

In the present study we showed that with a cell-based bioassay it is possible to identify natural-occurring flavonoids that are gastroprotective in a model of oxidant injury. By directly evaluating the effects of different classes of flavonoids using a lower dose of H_2O_2 and more chronic exposure, we showed that removal of excess ROS or suppression of their generation by flavonoids may be effective in preventing oxidative cell death.

In this study, we carried out a theoretical investigation into the possible mechanisms governing the cytoprotective activity of 24 different subclasses of flavonoids by computational chemistry, and explored the correlation between experimentally determined cytoprotective activities and physicochemical properties. It is reasonable to conclude that multiple mechanisms regulate the protective actions of flavonoid compounds although they contribute to the cytoprotective activity to different degrees. The cytoprotective activities of flavonoids were strongly correlated to their calculated enthalpy of hemolytic O-H bond cleavage (ΔH_f) but weakly correlated to their lipophilicity. It is concluded that the relative contribution of lipophilicity is much smaller than that of ΔH_f to their cytoprotective capacity. However, the balance of lipophilicity and lipophobicity is still critical in determining their abilities to protect human cells from oxidative damage.

Judging from the improvement in the correlation coefficient in the stepwise multiple-linear regression, we can conclude that the more precise the mechanistic information included in the QSAR model, the better the coefficient of relation that is obtained. It is reasonable to conclude that multiple mechanisms regulate the cytoprotection actions of flavonoids although they contribute to cytoprotective activity to different degrees. These results suggest the possibility of predicting the degree of contribution of different physicochemical factors among flavonoids by their *in vitro* actions against oxidative stress-induced cellular damage.

Acknowledgments

This work was funded by the Foundation for Research Science and Technology Wellness Food Programme Contract C06X0405. We thank Dr. Tony McGhie and Dr. Jeffery Greenwood for critically reviewing the manuscript.

References

Agullo G., Gamet-Payrastre L., Manenti S., Viala C., Rémésy C., Chap H., and Payrastre B. (1997). Relationship between flavonoid structure and inhibition of phosphatidylinositol 3-kinase: A comparison with tyrosine kinase and protein kinase C inhibition. *Biochemical Pharmacology* 53, 1649-1657.

Alonso-Salces R. M., Ndjoko K., Queiroz E. F., Ioset J. R., Hostettmann K., Berrueta L. A., Gallo B., and Vicente F. (2004). On-line characterisation of apple polyphenols by liquid chromatography coupled with mass spectrometry and ultraviolet absorbance detection. *Journal of Chromatography A* 1046, 89-100.

Andree H. A., Reutelingsperger C. P., Hauptmann R., Hemker H. C., Hermens W. T., and Willems G. M. (1990). Binding of vascular anticoagulant alpha (VAC alpha) to planar phospholipid bilayers. *Journal of Biological Chemistry* 265, 4923-4928.

Antunes F., and Cadenas E. (2001). Cellular titration of apoptosis with steady state concentrations of H_2O_2: submicromolar levels of H_2O_2 induce apoptosis through fenton chemistry independent of the cellular thiol state. *Free Radical Biology and Medicine* 30, 1008-1018.

Arora A., Nair M. G., and Strasburg G. M. (1998). Structure-activity relationships for antioxidant activities of a series of flavonoids in a liposomal system. *Free Radical Biology and Medicine* 24, 1355-1363.

Awad H. M., Boersma M. G., Boeren S., van Bladeren P. J., Vervoort J., and Rietjens I. M. (2001). Structure-activity study on the quinone/quinone methide chemistry of flavonoids. *Chemical Research in Toxicology* 14, 398-408.

Awad H. M., Boersma M. G., Boeren S., Van Bladeren P. J., Vervoort J., and Rietjens I. M. (2003). Quenching of quercetin quinone/quinone methides by different thiolate scavengers: Stability and reversibility of conjugate formation. *Chemical Research in Toxicology* 16, 822-831.

Bakalbassis E. G., Chatzopoulou A., Melissas V. S., Tsimidou M., Tsolaki M., and Vafiadis A. (2001). Ab initio and density functional theory studies for the explanation of the antioxidant activity of certain phenolic acids. *Lipids* 36, 181-190.

Barbouti A., Doulias P. T., Nousis L., Tenopoulou M., and Galaris D. (2002). DNA damage and apoptosis in hydrogen peroxide-exposed Jurkat cells: bolus addition versus continuous generation of H_2O_2. *Free Radical Biology and Medicine* 33, 691-702.

Barratt M. D. (1998). Integrating computer prediction systems with *in vitro* methods towards a better understanding of toxicology. *Toxicology Letters* 102-103, 617-621.

Behl C., Davis J. B., Lesley R., and Schubert D. (1994). Hydrogen peroxide mediates amyloid β−protein toxicity. *Cell* 77, 817-827.

Berkowitz J., Ellison G. B., and Gutman D. (1994). Three methods to measure RH bond energies. *Journal of Physical Chemistry* 98, 2744-2765.

Beyeler S., Testa B., and Perrissoud D. (1988). Flavonoids as inhibitors of rat liver monooxygenase activities. *Biochemical Pharmacology* 37, 1971-1979.

Bodor N., Gabanyi Z., and Wong C. K. (1989). A new method for the estimation of partition coefficient. *Journal of the American Chemical Society* 111, 3783-3786.

Boersma M. G., Vervoort J., Szymusiak H., Lemanska K., Tyrakowska B., Cenas N., Segura-Aguilar J., and Rietjens I. M. (2000). Regioselectivity and reversibility of the glutathione conjugation of quercetin quinone methide. *Chemical Research in Toxicology* 13, 185-191.

Bordwell F. G., and Zhang X.-M. (1993). From equilibrium acidities to radical stabilization energies. *Account in Chemical Research* 26, 510-517.

Borges dos Santos R. M., and Simoes J. A. M. (1998). Energetics of the O-H bond in phenol and substituted phenols: A critical evaluation of literature data. *Journal of Physical Chemistry Reference Data* 27, 707-739.

Borkowski T., Szymusiak H., Gliszczynska-Swiglo A., and Tyrakowska B. (2005). The effect of 3-O-[beta]-glucosylation on structural transformations of anthocyanidins. *Food Research International* 38, 1031-1037.

Bors W., Heller W., Michel C., and Saran M. (1990). Radical chemistry of flavonoid antioxidants. *Advances in Experimental Medicine and Biology* 264, 165-170.

Brigati G., Lucarini M., Mugnaini V., and Pedulli G. F. (2002). Determination of the substituent effect on the O-H bond dissociation enthalpies of phenolic antioxidants by the EPR radical equilibration technique. *Journal of Organic Chemistry* 67, 4828-4832.

Briviba K., Devasagayam T. P., Sies H., and Steenken S. (1993). Selective para hydroxylation of phenol and aniline by singlet molecular oxygen. *Chemical Research in Toxicology* 6, 548-553.

Brod S. A. (2000). Unregulated inflammation shortens human functional longevity. *Inflammation Research* 49, 561-570.

Brouillard R. (1983). The in vivo expression of anthocyanin colour in plants. *Phytochemistry* 22, 1311-1323.

Brouillard R., and Delaporte B. (1977a). Chemistry of anthocyanin pigments. 2. Kinetic and thermodynamic study of proton transfer, hydration, and tautomeric reactions of malvidin 3-glucoside. *Journal of the American Chemical Society* 99, 8461-8468.

Brouillard R., and Dubois J.-E. (1977b). Mechanism of the structural transformations of anthocyanins in acidic media. *Journal of the American Chemical Society* 99, 1359-1364.

Buchwald P., and Bodor N. (1998). Octanol-water partition of nonzwitterionic peptides: predictive power of a molecular size-based model. *Proteins* 30, 86-99.

Cantoni O., Cattabeni F., Stocchi V., Meyn R. E., Cerutti P., and Murray D. (1989). Hydrogen peroxide insult in cultured mammalian cells: Relationships between DNA single-strand breakage, poly(ADP-ribose) metabolism and cell killing. *Biochimica et Biophysica Acta* 1014, 1-7.

Car R. (2002). Introduction to density-functional theory and *ab-Initio* molecular mynamics. *Quantitative Structure-Activity Relationships* 21, 97-104.

Castle L., and Perkins M. J. (1986). Inhibition kinetics of chain-breaking phenolic antioxidants in SDS micelles. Evidence that intermicellar diffusion rates may be rate-limiting for hydrophobic inhibitors such as α-tocopherol. *Journal of the American Chemical Society* 108, 6382-6384.

Chen J. W., Zhu Z. Q., Hu T. X., and Zhu D. Y. (2002). Structure-activity relationship of natural flavonoids in hydroxyl radical-scavenging effects. *Acta Pharmacologica Sinica* 23, 667-672.

Chipman D. M., Liu R., Zhou X., and Pulay P. (1994). Structure and fundamental vibrations of phenoxyl radical. *Journal of Chemical Physics* 100, 5023-5035.

Choi J. S., Young C. H., Sik K. S., Jung J. M., Won K. J., Kyung N. J., and Ah J. H. (2002). The structure-activity relationship of flavonoids as scavengers of peroxynitrite. *Phytotherapy Research* 16, 232-235.

Colic M., and Pavelic K. (2000). Molecular mechanisms of anticancer activity of natural dietetic products. *Journal of Molecular Medicine* 78, 333-336.

Convard T., Dubost J. P., Le Solleu H., and Kummer E. (1994). SmilogP: A program for a fast evaluation of theoretical log P from smiles code of a molecule. *Quantitative Structure-Activity Relationships* 13, 34-37.

Cook N. C., and Samman S. (1996). Flavonoids--Chemistry, metabolism, cardioprotective effects, and dietary sources. *The Journal of Nutritional Biochemistry* 7, 66-76.

Cos P., Ying L., Calomme M., Hu J. P., Cimanga K., Van Poel B., Pieters L., Vlietinck A. J., and Berghe D. V. (1998). Structure-activity relationship and classification of flavonoids as inhibitors of xanthine oxidase and superoxide scavengers. *Journal of Natural Products* 61, 71-76.

Darzynkiewicz Z., Juan G., Li X., Gorczyca W., Murakami T., and Traganos F. (1997). Cytometry in cell necrobiology: analysis of apoptosis and accidental cell death (necrosis). *Cytometry* 27, 1-20.

Davies K. J. (1999). The broad spectrum of responses to oxidants in proliferating cells: a new paradigm for oxidative stress. *IUBMB Life* 48, 41-47.

Delgado-Vargas F., Jimenez A. R., Paredes-Lopez O., and Francis F. J. (2000). Natural pigments: Carotenoids, anthocyanins, and betalains - Characteristics, biosynthesis, processing, and stability. *Critical Reviews in Food Science and Nutrition* 40, 173-289.

Denisov E. T., and Khydyakov I. V. (1987). Mechanisms of action and reactivities of the free radicals of inhibitors. *Chemical Review* 87, 1313-1357.

Devaux P. F. (1991). Static and dynamic lipid asymmetry in cell membranes. *Biochemistry* 30, 1163-1173.

Dewar M. J. S., and Thiel W. (1977). Ground states of molecules. 38. The MNDO-method approximations and parameters. *Journal of the American Chemical Society* 99, 4899-4907.

Dewar M. J. S., Zoebisch E. G., Healy E. F., and Stewart J. J. P. (1985). AM1: A new general purpose quantum mechanical molecular model. *Journal of the American Chemical Society* 107, 3902-3909.

Diplock A. T., Charleux J. L., Crozier-Willi G., Kok F. J., Rice-Evans C., Roberfroid M., Stahl W., and Vina-Ribes J. (1998). Functional food science and defence against reactive oxidative species. *British Journal of Nutrition* 80 Suppl 1, S77-112.

Dziezak J. D. (1986). Preservatives: Antioxidants, the ultimate answer to oxidation. *Food Technology* 40 (9), 94-106.

Eadsforth C. V., and Moser P. (1983). Assessment of reverse-phase chromatographic methods for determining partition coefficients. *Chemosphere* 12, 1459-1475.

Eastwood M. A. (1999). Interaction of dietary antioxidants in vivo: how fruit and vegetables prevent disease? *Quarterly Journal of Medicine* 92, 527-530.

Fossen T., and Andersen Ø. M. (2006) Spectroscopic techniques applied to flavonoids, in *Flavonoids : Chemistry, biochemistry, and applications* (Andersen VM and Markham KR eds) pp 37-142, Taylor and Francis Group, Boca Raton, FL.

Fujita T., Iwasa J., and Hansch C. (1964). A new substituent constant, T, derived from partition coefficients. *Journal of the American Chemical Society* 86, 5175-5180.

Gardner A. M., Xu F. H., Fady C., Jacoby F. J., Duffey D. C., Tu Y., and Lichtenstein A. (1997). Apoptotic vs. nonapoptotic cytotoxicity induced by hydrogen peroxide. *Free Radical Biology and Medicine* 22, 73-83.

Ghose A. K., and Crippen G. M. (1987). Atomic physicochemical parameters for three-dimensional-structure-directed quantitative structure-activity relationships. 2. Modeling dispersive and hydrophobic interactions. *Journal of Chemical Information and Computer Sciences* 27, 21-35.

Gille J. J. P., and Joenje H. (1992). Cell culture models for oxidative stress: Superoxide and hydrogen peroxide versus normobaric hyperoxia. *Mutation Research/DNAging* 275, 405-414.

Giugliano D. (2000). Dietary antioxidants for cardiovascular prevention. *Nutrition, Metabolism and Cardiovascular Diseases* 10, 38-44.

Gotoh N., Noguchi N., Tsuchiya J., Morita K., Sakai H., Shimasaki H., and Niki E. (1996). Inhibition of oxidation of low density lipoprotein by vitamin E and related compounds. *Free Radical Research* 24, 123-134.

Gu L., kelm M. A., Hammerstone J. F., Beecher G., Holden J., Haytowitz D., and Prior R. L. (2003). Screening foods containing proanthocyanidins and their structural characterization using LC-MS/MS and thiolytic degradation. *Journal of Agriculture and Food Chemistry* 51, 7513-7521.

Guarnieri S., Riso P., and Porrini M. (2007). Orange juice vs vitamin C: effect on hydrogen peroxide-induced DNA damage in mononuclear blood cells. *British Journal of Nutrition* 97, 639-643.

Halliwell B. (1990). How to characterize a biological antioxidant. *Free Radical Research Communication* 9, 1-32.

Halliwell B. (1992). Reactive oxygen species and the central nervous system. *Journal of Neurochemistry* 59, 1609-1623.

Hansch C., and Gao H. (1997). Comparative QSAR: Radical reactions of benzene derivatives in chemistry and biology. *Chemical Review* 97, 2995-3060.

Hansch C., McKarns S. C., Smith C. J., and Doolittle D. J. (2000). Comparative QSAR evidence for a free-radical mechanism of phenol-induced toxicity. *Chemico-Biological Interactions* 127, 61-72.

Hansch C., Quinlan J. E., and Lawrence G. L. (1968). The linear free energy relationship between partition coefficients and the aqueous solubility of organic liquids. *Journal of Organic Chemistry* 33, 347-350.

Harborne J. B. (1962). Anthocyanins and their sugar components. *Fortschritte der Chemie Organischer Naturstoffe (Vienna)* 20, 165-199.

Harborne J. B., and Williams C. A. (2000). Advances in flavonoid research since 1992. *Phytochemistry* 55, 481-504.

Harborne J. B., and Williams C. A. (2001). Anthocyanins and other flavonoids. *Natural Product Reports* 18, 310-333.

Havsteen B. H. (2002). The biochemistry and medical significance of the flavonoids. *Pharmacology and Therapeutics* 96, 67-202.

Hedrickson H. P., Kaufman A. D., and Lunte C. E. (1994). Electrochemistry of catechol-containing flavonoids. *Journal of Pharmaceutical and Biomedical Analysis* 12, 325-334.

Herrmann K. M. (1976). Flavonoids and flavones in food plants: A review. *Journal of Food Technology* 11, 443-448.

Herrmann K. M. (1989). Occurrence and content of hydrocinnamic and hydrobenzoic acid compounds in foods. *Critical Review of Food Science and Nutrition* 28, 315-347.

Hollman P. C. H., and Arts I. C. W. (2000). Flavonols, flavones and flavanols - nature, occurrence and dietary burden. *Journal of the Science of Food and Agriculture* 80, 1081-1093.

Holt R. R., Lazarus S. A., Sullards M. C., Zhu Q. Y., Schramm D. D., Hammerstone J. F., Fraga C. G., Schmitz H. H., and Keen C. L. (2002). Procyanidin dimmer B2 [epicatechin-(4β-8)-epicatechin] in human plasma after the consumption of a flavanol-rich cococa. *Amercian Journal of Clinical Nutrition* 76, 798-804.

Hopia A., and Heinonen M. (1999). Antioxidant activity of flavonol aglycones and their glycosides in methyl linoleate. *Journal of the American Chemical Society* 76, 139-144.

Hoshino T. (1991). An approximate estimate of self-association constants and the self-stacking conformation of Malvin quinonoidal bases studied by 1H NMR. *Phytochemistry* 30, 2049-2055.

Hoshino T., and Goto T. (1990). Effects of pH and concentration on the self-association of malvin quinonoidal base -- electronic and circular dichroic studies. *Tetrahedron Letters* 31, 1593-1596.

Hoshino T., Matsumoto U., and Goto T. (1981). Self-association of some anthocyanins in neutral aqueous solution. *Phytochemistry* 20, 1971-1976.

Hyslop P. A., Zhang Z., Pearson D. V., and Phebus L. A. (1995). Measurement of striatal H_2O_2 by microdialysis following global forebrain ischemia and reperfusion in the rat: Correlation with the cytotoxic potential of H_2O_2 *in vitro. Brain Research* 671, 181-186.

Japertas P., Didziapetris R., and Petrauskas A. (2002). Fragmental methods in the design of new compounds. Applications of the advanced algorithm builder. *Quantitative Structure-Activity Relationships* 21, 23-37.

Kefford J. F., and Chandler B. V. (1970) *The chemical constituents of citrus fruits.* Academic Press, New York, NY.

Kim D. K., Cho E. S., and Um H. D. (2000). Caspase-dependent and -independent events in apoptosis induced by hydrogen peroxide. *Experimental Cell Research* 257, 82-88.

Klopman G., and Zhu H. (2001). Estimation of the aqueous solubility of organic molecules by the group contribution approach. *Journal of Chemical Information and Computer Sciences* 41, 439-445.

Kroon P. A., Clifford M. N., Crozier A., Day A. J., Donovan J. L., Manach C., and Williamson G. (2004). How should we assess the effects of exposure to dietary polyphenols *in vitro*? *American Journal of Clinical Nutrition* 80, 15-21.

Kumazawa Y., Kawaguchi K., and Takimoto H. (2006). Immunomodulating effects of flavonoids on acute and chronic inflammatory responses caused by tumor necrosis factor alpha. *Current Pharmaceutical Design* 12, 4271-4279.

Leo A., Hansch C., and Elkins D. (1971). Partition coefficients and their uses. *Chemical Review* 71, 525-616.

Leo A. J. (1991). Hydrophobic parameter: Measurement and calculation. *Methods in Enzymology* 202, 544-591.

Leo A. J. (1993). Calculating log P_{oct} from structures. *Chemical Review* 93, 1281-1306.

Lien E. J., Ren S., Bui H.-H., and Wang R. (1999). Quantitative structure-activity relationship analysis of phenolic antioxidants. *Free Radical Biology and Medicine* 26, 285-294.

Lipinski C. A., Lombardo F., Dominy B. W., and Feeney P. J. (1997). Experimental and computational approaches to estimate solubility and permeability in drug discovery and development settings. *Advanced Drug Delivery Reviews* 23, 3-25.

Lucarini M., Pedrielli P., and Pedulli G. F. (1996). Bond dissociation energies of O-H bonds in substituted from equilibration studies. *Journal of Organic Chemistry* 61, 9259-9263.

Lucarini M., and Pedulli F. (1994). Bond dissociation enthalpy of α–tocopherol and other phenolic antioxidants. *Journal of Organic Chemistry* 59, 5063-5070.

MacFarland J. W. (1970). On the parabolic relationship between drug potency and hydrophobicity. *Journal of Medicinal Chemistry* 13, 1192-1196.

Mahoney L. R., and DaRooge M. A. (1975). Kinetic behavior and thermochemical properties of phenoxy radicals. *Journal of the American Chemical Society* 97, 4722-4731.

Mannhold R., and Petrauskas A. (2003). Substructure versus whole-molecule approaches for calculating log P. *QSAR and Combinatorial Science* 22, 466-475.

Manthey J. A. (2000). Biological properties of flavonoids pertaining to inflammation. *Microcirculation* 7, S29-34.

Masuda J., Nakamura K., Kimura A., Takagi T., and Fujiwara H. (1997). Introduction of solvent-accessible surface area in the calculation of the hydrophobicity parameter log P from an atomistic approach. *Journal of Pharmaceutical Sciences* 86, 57-63.

McMurry J. (1992) Describing a reaction: Bond dissociation energies., in *McMurry Organic Chemistry.* (McMurry J eds) pp 156-159, Brooks/Cole Publishing Company, Belmont, California.

Metodiewa D., Jaiswal A. K., Cenas N., Dickancaite E., and Segura-Aguilar J. (1999). Quercetin may act as a cytotoxic prooxidant after its metabolic activation to semiquinone and quinoidal product. *Free Radical Biology and Medicine* 26, 107-116.

Meylan W. M., and Howard P. H. (1995). Atom/fragment contribution method for estimating octanol-water partition coefficients. *Journal of Pharmaceutical Sciences* 84, 83-92.

Middleton E., Jr., Kandaswami C., and Theoharides T. C. (2000). The effects of plant flavonoids on mammalian cells: Implications for inflammation, heart disease, and cancer. *Pharmacological Reviews* 52, 673-751.

Mora A., Paya M., Rios J. L., and Alcaraz M. J. (1990). Structure-activity relationships of polymethoxyflavones and other flavonoids as inhibitors of non-enzymic lipid peroxidation. *Biochemical Pharmacology* 40, 793-797.

Moridani M. Y., Galati G., and O'Brien P. J. (2002). Comparative quantitative structure toxicity relationships for flavonoids evaluated in isolated rat hepatocytes and HeLa tumor cells. *Chemico-Biological Interactions* 139, 251-264.

Mulder P., Saastad O. W., and Griller D. (1988). O-H bond dissociation energies in *para*-substituted phenols. *Journal of the American Chemical Society* 110, 4090-4092.

Murakami S., Muramatsu M., and Tomisawa K. (1999). Inhibition of gastric H+,K+-ATPase by flavonoids: A structure-activity study. *Journal of Enzyme Inhibition* 14, 151-166.

Noguchi N., Okimoto Y., Tsuchiya J., Cynshi O., Kodama T., and Niki E. (1997). Inhibition of oxidation of low-density lipoprotein by a novel antioxidant, BO-653, prepared by theoretical design. *Archives of Biochemistry and Biophysics* 347, 141-147.

O'Byrne K. J., and Dalgleish A. G. (2001). Chronic immune activation and inflammation as the cause of malignancy. *British Journal of Cancer* 85, 473-483.

Osterberg T., and Norinder U. (2001). Prediction of drug transport processes using simple parameters and PLS statistics: The use of ACD/logP and ACD/ChemSketch descriptors. *European Journal of Pharmaceutical Sciences* 12, 327-337.

Packer L., Rimbach G., and Virgili F. (1999). Antioxidant activity and biologic properties of a procyanidin-rich extract from pine (Pinus maritima) bark, pycnogenol. *Free Radical Biology and Medicine* 27, 704-724.

Passamonti S., Vrhovsek U., and Mattivi F. (2002). The interaction of anthocyanins with bilitranslocase. *Biochemical and Biophysical Research Communications* 296, 631-636.

Pople J. A., Beveridge D. L., and Doboshlc P. A. (1968). Molecular orbital theory of the electronic structure of organic compounds. 11. Spin densities in paramagnetic species. *Journal of the American Chemical Society* 90, 4201-4209.

Porter L. J. (1993). Flavans and proanthocyanidins. In: *The Flavonoids. Advances in Research since 1986* (Harborne JB eds), pp 23-55. Chapman & Hall, London, UK.

Porter W. L., Black E. D., and Drolet A. M. (1989). Use of polyamide oxidative fluorescence test on lipid emulsions: Contrast in relative effectiveness of antioxidants in bulk versus dispersed systems. *Journal of Agricultural and Food Chemistry* 37, 615-624.

Potapovich A. I., and Kostyuk V. A. (2003). Comparative study of antioxidant properties and cytoprotective activity of flavonoids. *Biochemistry (Mosc)* 68, 514-519.

Qin Y., and Wheeler R. A. (1995). Density-functional methods give accurate vibrational frequencies and spin densities for phenoxyl radical. *Journal of Chemical Physics* 102, 1689-1698.

Rastija V., and Medic-Saric M. (2009). QSAR study of antioxidant activity of wine polyphenols. *European Journal of Medicinal Chemistry* 44, 400-408.

Reddy A. M., Reddy V. S., Scheffler B. E., Wienand U., and Reddy A. R. (2007). Novel transgenic rice overexpressing anthocyanidin synthase accumulates a mixture of flavonoids leading to an increased antioxidant potential. *Metabolic Engineering* 9, 95-111.

Rice-Evans C. A., Miller N. J., Bolwell P. G., Bramley P. M., and Pridham J. B. (1995). The relative antioxidant activities of plant-derived polyphenolic flavonoids. *Free Radical Research* 22, 375-383.

Rice-Evans C. A., Miller N. J., and Paganga G. (1996). Structure-antioxidant activity relationships of flavonoids and phenolic acids. *Free Radical Biology and Medicine* 20, 933-956.

Riemersma R. A., Rice-Evans C. A., Tyrrell R. M., Clifford M. N., and Lean M. E. J. (2001). Tea flavonoids and cardiovascular health. *Quarterly Journal of Medicine* 94, 277-282.

Scalbert A., and Williamson G. (2000). Dietary Intake and Bioavailability of Polyphenols. *Journal of Nutrition* 130, 2073S-2085.

Schreck R., Rieber P., and Baeuerle P. A. (1991). Reactive oxygen intermediates as apparently widely used messengers in the activation of the NF-kappa B transcription factor and HIV-1. *Embo Journal* 10, 2247-2258.

Schwarz K., Frankel E. N., and German J. B. (1996). Partition behaviour of antioxidative phenolic compounds in heterophasic systems. *Lipid -Fett.* 98, 115-121.

Shahidi F., and Wanasundara P. K. (1992). Phenolic antioxidants. *Critical Review of Food Science and Nutrition* 32, 67-103.

Simonian N. A., and Coyle J. T. (1996). Oxidative stress in neurodegenerative diseases. *Annual Review of Pharmacology and Toxicology* 36, 83-106.

Soffers A. E. M. F., Boersma M. G., Vaes W. H. J., Vervoort J., Tyrakowska B., Hermens J. L. M., and Rietjens I. M. C. M. (2001). Computer-modeling-based QSARs for analyzing experimental data on biotransformation and toxicity. *Toxicology In Vitro* 15, 539-551.

Spencer J. P. E., Abd El Mohsen M. M., and Rice-Evans C. (2004). Cellular uptake and metabolism of flavonoids and their metabolites: implications for their bioactivity. *Archives of Biochemistry and Biophysics* 423, 148-161.

Spencer J. P. E., Kuhnle G. G., Williams R. J., and Rice-Evans C. (2003). Intracellular metabolism and bioactivity of quercetin and its in vivo metabolites. *Biochemical Journal* 372, 173-181.

Stack D. (1997) Phenolic metabolism., in *Plant Biochemistry* (Dey PM and Harborne JB eds) pp 387-417, Academic Press, London, UK.

Stewart J. P. J. (1989). Optimization of parameters for semiempirical methods. II. Applications. *Journal of Computational Chemistry* 10, 221-264.

Sugihara N., Kaneko A., and Furuno K. (2003). Oxidation of flavonoids which promote DNA degradation induced by bleomycin-Fe complex. *Biological and Pharmaceutical Bulletin* 26, 1108-1114.

Sun Y. M., Zhang H. Y., Chen D. Z., and Liu C. B. (2002). Theoretical elucidation on the antioxidant mechanism of curcumin: A DFT study. *Organic Letters* 4, 2909-2911.

Timberlake C. F., and Bridle P. (1967). Flavylium salts, anthocyanidins and anthocyanins. I. - Structural transformations in acid solutions. *Journal of the Science of Food and Agriculture* 18, 473-478.

Tournaire C., Croux S., Maurette M. T., Beck I., Hocquaux M., Braun A. M., and Oliveros E. (1993). Antioxidant activity of flavonoids: efficiency of singlet oxygen (1 delta g) quenching. *Journal of Photochemistry and Photobiology B* 19, 205-215.

van Acker S. A., de Groot M. J., van den Berg D. J., Tromp M. N., Donne-Op den Kelder G., van der Vijgh W. J., and Bast A. (1996). A quantum chemical explanation of the antioxidant activity of flavonoids. *Chemical Research in Toxicology* 9, 1305-1312.

van Acker S. A., Koymans L. M., and Bast A. (1993). Molecular pharmacology of vitamin E: Structural aspects of antioxidant activity. *Free Radical Biology and Medicine* 15, 311-328.

van Engeland M., Nieland L. J., Ramaekers F. C., Schutte B., and Reutelingsperger C. P. (1998). Annexin V-affinity assay: a review on an apoptosis detection system based on phosphatidylserine exposure. *Cytometry* 31, 1-9.

Vaya J., Mahmood S., Goldblum A., Aviram M., Volkova N., Shaalan A., Musa R., and Tamir S. (2003). Inhibition of LDL oxidation by flavonoids in relation to their structure and calculated enthalpy. *Phytochemistry* 62, 89-99.

Vedernikova I., Tollenaere J. P., and Haemers A. (1999). Quantum mechanical evaluation of the anodic oxidation of phenolic compounds. *Journal of Physical Organic Chemistry* 12, 144-150.

Vermes I., Haanen C., and Reutelingsperger C. (2000). Flow cytometry of apoptotic cell death. *Journal of Immunological Methods* 243, 167-190.

Ververidis F., Trantas E., Carl D., Guenter V., Georg K., and Panopoulos N. (2007). Biotechnology of flavonoids and other phenylpropanoid-derived natural products. Part I: Chemical diversity, impacts on plant biology and human health. *Biotechnology Journal* 2, 1214-1234.

Wang R., Fu Y., and Lai L. (1997). A new atom-additive method for calculating partition coefficients. *Journal of Chemical Information and Computer Sciences* 37, 615-621.

Wayner D. D., Lusztyk J. E., Page D., Ingold K. U., Mulder P., Laarhoven L. J. J., and Aldrichs H. S. (1995). Effects of solvation on the enthalpies of reaction of *tert*-butoxyl radicals with phenol and on the calculated O-H bond strength in phenol. *Journal of the American Chemical Society* 117, 8738-8744.

Wayner D. D. M., and Parker V. D. (1993). Bond energies in solution from electrode potentials and thermochemical cycles. A simplified and general approach. *Account in Chemical Research* 26, 287-294.

Wedworth S. M., and Lynch S. (1995). Dietary flavonoids in atherosclerosis prevention. *The Annals of Pharmacotherapy* 29, 627-628.

Williams R. J., Spencer J. P. E., and Rice-Evans C. (2004). Flavonoids: Antioxidants or signalling molecules? *Free Radical Biology and Medicine* 36, 838-849.

Winkel-Shirley B. (2001). Flavonoid Biosynthesis. A Colorful Model for Genetics, Biochemistry, Cell Biology, and Biotechnology. *Plant Physiology* 126, 485-493.

Wollenweber E., and Dietz V. H. (1981). Occurrence and distribution of free flavonoid aglycones in plants. *Phytochemistry* 20, 869-932.

Wright J. S., Carpenter D. J., McKay D. J., and Ingold K. U. (1997). Theoretical calculation of substituent effects on the O-H bond strength of phenolic antioxidants related to vitamin E. *Journal of the American Chemical Society* 119, 4245-4252.

Wright J. S., Johnson E. R., and DiLabio G. A. (2001). Predicting the activity of phenolic antioxidants: Theoretical method, analysis of substituent effects, and application to major families of antioxidants. *Journal of the American Chemical Society* 123, 1173-1183.

Yong D. C. (2001) *Computational chemistry: A practical guide for applying techniques to real-world problems.* Wiley Interscience, New York.

Zhang H.-Y., You-Min S., and Xiu-Li W. (2003a). Substituent Effects on O-H Bond Dissociation Enthalpies and Ionization Potentials of Catechols: A DFT Study and Its Implications in the Rational Design of Phenolic Antioxidants and Elucidation of Structure-Activity Relationships for Flavonoid Antioxidants. *Chemistry - A European Journal* 9, 502-508.

Zhang H. Y. (1998). Selection of theoretical parameter characterizing scavenging activity of antioxidants on free radicals. *Journal of the American Oil Chemists' Society* 75, 1705-1709.

Zhang H. Y., Ge N., and Zhang Z. Y. (1999). Theoretical elucidation of activity differences of five phenolic antioxidants. *Zhongguo Yao Li Xue Bao* 20, 363-366.

Zhang H. Y., Sun Y. M., and Wang X. L. (2002a). Electronic effects on O-H proton dissociation energies of phenolic cation radicals: A DFT study. *Journal of Organic Chemistry* 67, 2709-2712.

Zhang H. Y., and Wang L. F. (2002b). Theoretical elucidation on structure-antioxidant activity relationships for indolinonic hydroxylamines. *Bioorganic and Medicinal Chemistry Letters* 12, 225-227.

Zhang H. Y., Wang L. F., and Sun Y. M. (2003b). Why B-ring is the active center for genistein to scavenge peroxyl radical: A DFT study. *Bioorganic and Medicinal Chemistry Letters* 13, 909-911.

Zhang J., Melton L., Adaim A., and Skinner M. (2008). Cytoprotective effects of polyphenolics on H2O2-induced cell death in SH-SY5Y cells in relation to their antioxidant activities. *European Food Research and Technology* 228, 123-131.

Zhang J., Stanley R. A., Adaim A., Melton L. D., and Skinner M. A. (2006a). Free radical scavenging and cytoprotective activities of phenolic antioxidants. *Molecular Nutrition and Food Research* 50, 996-1005.

Zhang J., Stanley R. A., and Melton L. D. (2006b). Lipid peroxidation inhibition capacity assay for antioxidants based on liposomal membranes. *Molecular Nutrition and Food Research* 50, 714-724.

Ziegler T. (1991). Approximate density functional theory as a practical tool in molecular energetics and dynamics. *Chemical Review* 91, 651-667.

In: Encyclopedia of Vitamin Research
Editor: Joshua T. Mayer

ISBN: 978-1-61761-928-1
© 2010 Nova Science Publishers, Inc.

Chapter 40

Oligomeric Nature, Colloidal State, Rheology, Antioxidant Capacity and Antiviral Activity of Polyflavonoids[*]

A.Pizzi

ENSTIB-LERMAB, University Henry Poincare – Nancy 1,
Epinal, France

Abstract

The determination by Matrix-Assisted Laser Desorption/Ionization time–of-flight (MALDI-TOF) mass spectroscopy of the oligomeric nature of the two major industrial polyflvonoid tannins which exist, namely mimosa and quebracho tannins, and some of their modified derivatives indicates that: (i) mimosa tannin is predominantly composed of prorobinetinidins while quebracho is predominantly composed of profisetinidins, that (ii) mimosa tannin is heavily branched due to the presence of considerable proportions of "angular" units in its structure while quebracho tannin is almost completely linear. These structural differences also contribute to the considerable differences in viscoity of water solutions of the two tannins. (iii) the interflavonoid link is more easily hydrolysable, and does appear to sometime hydrolyse in quebracho tannin and profisetinidins, partly due to the linear structure of this tannin, and confirming NMR findings that this tannin is subject to polymerisation/depolymerisation equilibria. This tannin hydrolysis does not appear to occur in mimosa tannin in which the interflavonoid link is completely stable to hydrolysis. (iv) Sulphitation has been shown to influence the detachment of catechol B-rings much more than pyrogallol-type B-rings. (vi) The distribution of tannin oligomers, and the tannins number average degree of polymerisation obtained by MALDI-TOF, up to nonamers and decamers, appear to compare well with the results obtained by other techniques. As regards procyanidin tannins, it has been possible to determine for

---

[*] A version of this chapter was also published in *Flavonoids: Biosynthesis, Biological Effects and Dietary Sources, edited by Raymond B. Keller* published by Nova Science Publishers, Inc. It was submitted for appropriate modifications in an effort to encourage wider dissemination of research.

mangrove polyflavonoid tannins that: (i) procyanidins oligomers formed by catechin/epicatechin, epigallocatechin and epicatechin gallate monomers are present in great proportions. (ii) oligomers, up to nonamers, in which the repeating unit at 528-529 Da is a catechin gallate dimer that has lost both the gallic acid residues and an hydroxy group are the predominant species. (iii) oligomers of the two types covalently linked to each other also occur.

Water solution of non-purified polyflavonoid extracts appear to be incolloidal state, this being due mainly to the hydrocolloid gums extracted with the tannin as well as to the tannin itself.

Commercial, industrially produced mimosa, quebracho, pine and pecan polyflavonoid tannin extracts water solutions of different concentrations behave mainly as viscous liquids at the concentrations which are generally used for their main industrial applications. Clear indications of viscoelastic response are also noticeable, among these the cross-over of the elastic and viscous moduli curves at the lower concentrations of the range investigated, with some differences being noticeable between each tannin and the others, pine and quebracho tannin extracts showing the more marked viscoelastic behaviour. Other than pH dependence (and related structural considerations), the parameters which were found to be of interest as regards the noticeable viscoelastic behaviour of the tannin extracts were the existence in the solutions of labile microstructures which can be broken by applied shear. This is supported by the well known thixotropic behaviour of concentrated, commercial polyflavonoid tannin extracts water solutions.

Such microstructures appear to be due or (i) to the known colloidal interactions of these materials, or (ii) to other types of secondary interactions between tannin oligomers and particularly between tannin and carbohydrate oligomers. The latter is supported by the dependence of this effect from both the average molecular masses of the tannin and of the carbohydrate oligomers.

The behaviour of polyflavonoid tannins as regards their antioxydant capacity and radical scavenging ability has been examined. Radical formation and radical decay reactions of some polyflavonoid and hydrolysable tannins has been followed, and comparative kinetics determined, for both light induced radicals and by radical transfer from a less stable chemical species to the tannin as part of an investigation of the role of tannin as antioxidants.

The five parameters which appear to have a bearing on the very complex pattern of the rates of tannin radical formation and radical decay were found to be (i) the extent of the colloidal state of the tannin in solution (ii) the stereochemical structure at the interflavonoid units linkage (iii) the ease of heterocyclic pyran ring opening, (iv) the relative numbers of A- and B-rings hydroxy groups and (v) solvation effects when the tannin is in solution. It is the combination of these five factors which appears to determine the behaviour as an antioxidant of a particular tannin under a set of application conditions.

The chapter ends with some recent results on the antiviral activity of polyflavonoid tannins for a great variety of viruses.

Introduction

Polyflavonoids also called condensed tannins are natural polyphenolic materials. Industrial polyflavonoid tannin extracts are mostly composed of flavan-3-ols repeating units, and smaller fractions of polysaccharides and simple sugars. Two types of phenolic rings having different reactivities are present on each flavan-3-ol repeating unit, namely A-rings and B-rings, with each repeating unit being linked 4,6 or 4,8 with the units which precede and follow it.

Recently, the radical and ionic mechanisms of the reaction of autocondensation and networking of polyflavonoid tannins induced by bases and by weak Lewis acids has been described [2-8]. Different polyflavonoid tannins however present different structures and different average molecular masses, and as a consequence often present peculiarly different behaviour in their application [10]. The most common method of examination of the relative structures of polyflavonoid tannins, and of their differences, is by ^{13}C NMR [10].

The Oligomeric Nature of Polyflavonoids

Since its introduction by Karas and Hillenkamp in 1987 [11], Matrix-Assisted Laser Desorption/Ionization (MALDI) mass spectrometry has greatly expanded the use of mass spectrometry towards large molecules and has revealed itself to be a powerful method for the characterization of both synthetic and natural polymers [12-17]. Fragmentation of analyte molecules upon laser irradiation can be substantially reduced by embedding them in a light absorbing matrix. As a result intact analyte molecules are desorbed and ionized along with the matrix and can be analysed in a mass spectrometer. This soft ionization technique is mostly combined with time-of-flight (TOF) mass analysers. This is so as TOF-MS present the advantage of being capable to provide a complete mass spectrum per event, for its virtually unlimited mass range, for the small amount of analyte necessary and the relatively low cost of the equipment.

Matrix-Assisted Laser Desorption/Ionization Time-of-Flight (MALDI-TOF) mass spectrometry (MS) is a technique that has revealed itself to be a very useful tool in defining the oligomeric structure of polyflavonoids, much more pointed than other techniques used before. As an example even oligomers up to and even of more than 10 flavonoid repeating units have been clearly detected in commercial polyflavonoid extracts by using such a technique. The technique was used to compare the structures of the most common industrial polyflavonoid condensed tannins.

Profisetinindin and Prorobinetinidin Type Polyflavonoids

The profisetinidin/prorobinetinidin type of polyflavonoid tannins are the most common extracted industrially [1]. The great majority of the flavonoid units are linked C4 to C6 to form the oligomers, but certain units, in the minority are also linked C4 to C8. Quebracho tannin and Mimosa tannin are the two main exponents of this class. Quebracho gave clear spectra showing the degree of polymerization of the building units and oligomer series with masses of the repeat units of 272 Da and 288 Da (Figure 1a; Table 1). For each oligomer, substructures with mass increments of 16 Da appear, indicating different combinations of various substructures. As quebracho is mainly based on combinations of resorcinol, catechol and pyrogallol building blocks the following monoflavonoids and their oligomers can be expected to be present:

A   **B**

The masses of units A and B are 274 Da and 290 Da respectively. Combinations of these masses can be used to calculate the masses of the oligomer peaks in the spectra according to the expression $M+Na^+ = 23(Na) + 2$ (endgroups, 2xH) $+ 272A + 288B$ (Table 1). As can be seen in the spectra, there are more peak series which are due to different endgroups. They have the same repeat units, for example 683-956 Da and 1555-1827 Da in Figure 1. The peak at 683 is very near to a result of 688 Da which would be obtained by the loss of both a B-ring plus the three-carbons chain from the heterocycle of the lower terminal repeat unit, be this of type B or of type A, to yield two flavonoid units linked to a resorcinol phenoxy anion.

687

The peak at 585 Da is also explained by the presence of a dimer according to the same equation above composed of a A-unit plus a B-unit plus 2 H endgroups plus Na^+. The peak at 375 Da is obtained from the 585 Da dimer by elimination of a catecholic B-ring (585-110 = 375).

Table 1. MALDI fragmentation peaks for industrial quebracho tannin extract. Note that the predominant repeat units in this tannin is 272 Da, indicating that this tannin is predominantly a profisetinidin

M+Na+	M+Na+	Unit type	
(exp) (calc.) A			B
Dimers			
585	586	1	1
601	601	--	2
Trimers			
842	841	3	--
*857	857	2	1
874	873	1	2
Tetramers			
1114	1113	4	--
*1130	1129	3	1
1146	1145	2	2
Pentamers			
1387	1385	5	--
*1402	1401	4	1
1420	1417	3	2
1435	1433	2	3
Hexamers			
1658	1659	6	--
1675	1673	5	1
*1692	1689	4	2
1708	1705	3	3
Heptamers			
1948	1945	6	1
*1965	1961	5	2
1982	1977	4	3
Octamers			
*2237	2233	6	2
Nonamers			
*2510	2505	7	2
Decamers			
*2782	2777	8	2
2798	2793	7	3

*Dominant fragment.

There is however an alternate, and more correct explanation for the 683 Da peak. Industrial quebracho tannin extract is sulphited/bisulphited, which introduces a sulphite or sodium sulphite group on the C1 of the flavonoid structure and causes the opening of the heterocycle ring. Thus, if one of the flavonoid units of a 857 Da trimer loses its catechol B-ring (-110) from a type A repeat unit as well as the $-SO_2^-$ group (-64), the 683 Da signal is obtained.

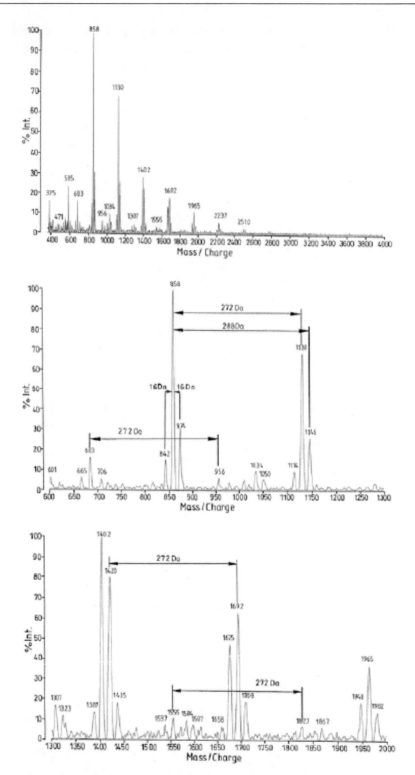

Figure 1. MALDI mass spectrum of (A) natural sulphited quebracho tannin extract. (B) details of the 600-1300 Da range with indication of the relevant 272 Da repeat unit. (C) details of the 1300-2000 Da range with indication of the relevant 272 Da repeat unit.

This is more likely as the introduction of the $-SO_2^-$ group should favour under certain conditions the elimination of the B-ring of the unit. The origin of the much smaller 665 Da peak is the same but by elimination of the $-SO_2H$ group (-65) and of a pyrogallol B-ring (-126) from a type B repeat unit. The fact that the intensity of the 665 Da peak is considerably lower than that of the 683 Da peak indicates the novel finding that as a consequence of sulphitation catechol rings appear to be much more easily detached than pyrogallol ones from a flavonoid unit. That the 683 peak is caused by the presence of the sulphonic group on C1 and the relative ease of decomposition indicated above is shown by the fact that in mimosa tannin which in general is not sulphited the 683 Da peak does not exist while presenting a very small peak at 687 Da which come from the first explanation (Figure 2a).

Also of interest are the existence of peaks at 1965, 2237, 2510 and 2800 Da for commercial quebracho tannin, these representing respectively heptamers, octamers, nonamers and decamers (Figure 1). Tannins are not easily water soluble at this higher molecular weight and thus it is of interest to find definite proof of the existence of such higher molecular weight oligomers in a commercial tannin extract. The sample in question had been found by ^{13}C NMR to have a number average degree of polymerization of 6.74 [19,20] which appears to confirm the existence of such higher molar mass oligomers in this commercial tannin extract. The same type of pattern is obtained for solvent purified commercial quebracho extract (MALDI spectrum not reported here), in which all the carbohydrates have been eliminated, confirming that the patterns observed are really due to the polyflavonoid components of the tannin extract. It is, however, of interest to note that the tannin extract which has undergone an acid/base treatment [18] to obtain an adhesive intermediate gives at best a pentamer at 1967 Da, see Figure 2. This is accompanied by a considerable increase in the proportion of the 858 Da trimers, of the 727 degraded trimers (2 flavonoid units + 1 A-ring + its C4), of degradation product composed of a single flavonoid unit linked to a single A-ring of another flavonoid unit (375 da) and also an increase in the 1130 Da tetramers confirming that the treatment to yield a tannin adhesive intermediate clearly induces some level of hydrolysis of the interflavonoid bond and hence some level of depolymerization in quebracho tannin.

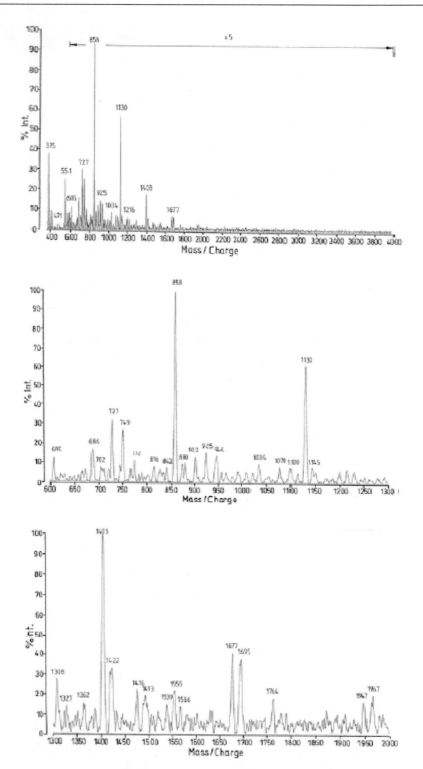

Figure 2. MALDI mass spectrum of (a) acid/base treated modified quebracho tannin extract. (b) details of the 600-1300 Da range, (c) details of the 1300-2000 Da range.

This confirms previous findings [6-8,18] obtained by ^{13}C NMR that contrary to what widely thought the interflavonoid bond in the profisetinidins/prorobinetinidins of quebracho tannin are fairly labile and that this particular type of tannin can be subject to some depolymerization. It also confirms what has been up to now only a suspicion, namely that the decrease in viscosity [18] of tannin solutions as a consequence of acid/base treatments is not only due to hydrolysis of the hydrocolloid polymeric carbohydrates present in the extract, but also to the decrease in degree of polymerization of the tannin itself, this at least in the case of quebracho tannin. It is also interesting to observe a definite, clear peak at 605 Da (see Figure 2) which can only belong to a pure robinetinidin dimer (289+289+25 = 605), MALDI-TOF analysis appearing to indicate here that it is the interflavonoid inter-fisetinidin link, or at least links in which fisetinidin units are involved which appear to be more sensitive to cleavage. The acid/base treatment to produce a tannin adhesive intermediate involves the use of acetic anhydride or maleic anhydride for the acid hydrolysis phase. As the treatment is done in water solution but being the tannin extract strongly colloidal in nature a question of interest is to know if some of the tannin –OH groups have been acetylated within the micelles present in the solution and before the induced hydrolysis has drastically decreased the level of colloidality of the system. Past investigations by ^{13}C NMR and by other techniques [18] indicate that a certain amount (small) of acetylation appears also to occur, this being of importance in accelerating subsequently, on application, the polycondensation of tannins with aldehydes. MALDI-TOF appears to confirm this by the presence of small but detected peaks at 772 Da (in theory 769) and 902 Da (see Figure 2), respectively a flavonoid dimer and a flavonoid trimer both monoacetylated.

The MALDI-TOF analysis of mimosa tannin extract (Figure 3) indicates the presence in the tannin of oligomers to the maximum of octamers (2333 Da) in line with the lower number average degree of polymerzation of 4.90 obtained by other means for this tannin [19,20], and the distribution obtained is shown in Table 2. The flavonoid repeating units present in this tannin extract are of type A and B as for quebracho but with a relatively important proportion of units of type C.

C

The correct equation to calculate the different possibilities does then become $M+Na^+ = 23(Na) + 2$ (endgroups, 2xH) + 272A + 288B + 304C (Table 2). Table 2 indicates that many valid combinations of different repeating units are possible. There are however some cases in which unequivocal assignement of the structure can indeed be done.

Table 2. MALDI fragmentation peaks for industrial mimosa tannin extract. Note that the predominant repeat units in this tannin is 288 Da, indicating that this tannin is predominantly a prorobinetinidin

M+Na+ (exp.)	M+Na+ (calc.)		Unit type			
			A	B	C	
Dimers						
602	601		--	2	--	
Trimers						
858	857		2	1	--	
874	873		1	2	--	
		or	2	--	1	angular tannin
*890	889		1	1	1	
		or	--	3	--	
*906	905		--	2	1	angular tannin
		or	1	--	2	angular tannin
922	921		--	1	2	a "diangular" structure
Tetramers						
1147	1145		2	2	--	
		or	3	--	1	
1163	1161		1	3	--	
		or	2	1	1	
*1179	1177		--	4	--	
		or	1	2	1	
		or	2	--	2	
1195	1193		--	3	1	angular tannin
		or	1	1	2	
1211	1209		--	2	2	angular tannin
		or	1	--	3	a "diangular" structure
Pentamers						
1467	1465					
Hexamers						
1756	1753					
Heptamers						
2045	2041					
Octamers						
2333	2329					

*Dominant fragment.

This is the case of angular tannins, namely oligomers in which a repeating unit of type C is bound through both its 6 and its 8 A-ring sites to A and B type units, with its C4 sites equally bound and unbound.

These structures were discovered by high temperature ^{1}H NMR on rotational isomers [1,21,22]. The MALDI-TOF analysis also shows clearly the existence of fragments of angular tannins by the presence of definite peaks at 906, 1195 and 1211 Da. Their presence in mimosa tannin extract, where it is known that angular tannins exist, underlines their total absence in the otherwise similar quebracho tannin extract. It is not possible to say with the data available if angular tannins are naturally absent in quebracho tannin extract or if their absence is the result of the fairly heavy sulphitation this tannin has always to undergo for solubility reasons. The high relative intensity of the very marked peaks of the angular trimer at 906 Da and of the angular tetramer at 1195 Da in Figure 3 indicate that the frequence of angular structures in mimosa tannin extract is rather high. The lower viscosity of solutions of mimosa extract, much lower than solutions of quebracho tannin extract at equal concentration and under the same conditions, is not only due then to mimosa tannin lower number average degree of polymerization [19,20] but also to its more "branched" structure as opposed to the fundamentally "linear" structure of quebracho tannin. The susceptibility to hydrolysis of the interflavonoid bond of quebracho tannin remarked about above, in relation to the well-known total lack of it in mimosa tannin [2,18] , could then be ascribed also to this conformational difference between the two otherwise similar profisetinidin/prorobinetinidin tannins. This observation is of importance indicating for the first time that the difference in spacial structure is one of the main contributing reasons why two tannins of fundamentally very similar chemical composition (they are both profisetinidins/prorobinetinidins) do behave rather differently under several aspects. In the case of mimosa tannin of even greater interest is the the existence of a well definite and clear peak at 1211 Da: this is formed by 4 flavonoid repeating units two of which are of type C. If the sample was just a dimer one could claim that this was a procyanidin fragment, namely two C-type units linked 4,8 and conclude that a certain number of separate procyanidin units exists in mimosa tannin. That the fragment is instead a tetramer first of all negates that the phloroglucinol A-ring units can exist in mimosa tannin as separate procyanidins, but confirms that in this tannin such units are exclusively present reacted as an "angular" within the profisetinidin/prorobinetinidin predominant structures. Second, this fragment is clearly then a di-"angular" unit never observed or isolated before, again confirming the high frequence of angular structures in mimosa tannin.

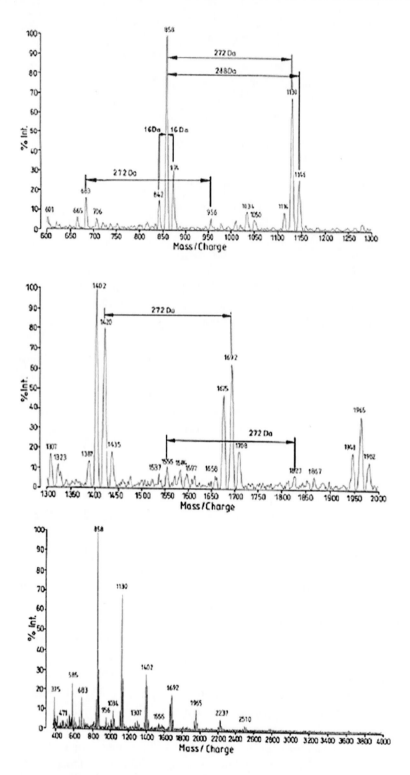

Figure 3. MALDI mass spectrum of (a) natural mimosa tannin extract. (b) details of the 600-1300 Da range with indication of the relevant 288 Da repeat unit. (c) details of the 1300-2000 Da range.

A further interesting difference between mimosa and quebracho tannins can be observed by comparing the results in Figures 1 and 3 and Tables 1 and 2. In quebracho the predominant repeat unit has 272 Da (a type A unit), while in mimosa the predominant repeating unit is of 288 Da (a type B unit). This is particularly evident in the higher oligomers for the two tannins. Based on this, on the dominant fragments for different oligomers and on the relative intensities for the different peaks in Figures 1 and 3 it is possible to conclude that quebracho tannin is composed of between 20% and 30% of B units and of between 70% and 80% of A-type units. Quebracho is then predominantly a profisetinidin. Mimosa tannin instead is composed predominantly of between 50% and 70% of type B units and only of between 15% and 25% of type A units. Mimosa tannin is then predominantly a prorobinetinidin. It is also interesting to note that the number average degree of polymerization obtained from the MALDI-derived oligomer distributions yield values of 6.25 and 5.4 for quebracho and mimosa tannins respectively. Considering the variability of such natural materials, these values compare well with the DP_n values of 6.74 and 4.9 for the same tannins obtained by ^{13}C NMR and other techniques [19,20].

It must be born in mind that in some mainly prorobinetinidin/profisetinidin tannins the structure of the oligomers present is not fixed and immutable. There are almost pure procyanidin oligomers present mixed with pure prorobitenidin oligomers, mixed with hybrid prorobinetinidin/profisetinidin oligomers and with hybrid prorobinetinidin/ profisetinidin/ procyanidin oligomers. An example of this is the case of the flavonoids from the bark of *Acacia mangium*, a species now extensively cultivated in Brazil and in South East Asia (Figure 4). This tannin presents two main "mixed" patterns of oligomers overimposed one on the other. As an example (Figure 4):

(1) Starting from the 1210 peak if one adds 289 Da the series 1210-1499-1788-2076.7-2365.4 etc up to the 3535 peak (that is very small) is observed in Figure 4, thus a pure prorobinetinidin pattern of trimers, tetramers, pentamers etc., up to oligomers comprised of 13 repeating units (although their proportion is quite low). This indicates that pure prorobinetidin oligomers , thus pure B type units linked together with perhaps one or two C units but without any A units linked to them do indeed exist.

(2) Starting again from the 1210 Da peak also a pattern adding 272-273 Da is present, namely 1210 - 1483 - 1756 Da but this stops there and the intensity of the peaks is lower, thus they are less abundant. This is hence a mixed prorobinetinidin/ profisetinidin series of oligomers. The fisetinidin repeating unit is less abundant, as also indicated by the intensity of these peaks. Adding a 289 Da B unit then one passes to the 2044.9 mass oligomer. Another 289 unit will bring to the 2334 oligomer. Equally, starting from the 1499 peak adding 272-273 Da one also gets the sequence 1499 - 1772 - 2044.9 and again it stops there. Adding a 289 Da unit to the 2044.9 peak and oligomer one gets the peak at 2334 Da, indicating clearly that fisetinidins and robinetinidins mixed oligomers, where both units of type A and B are linked together exist (still with a majority of B units). It also indicates that some peaks such as the 2044.9 Da, for example ,are the superposition of two different types of oligomers.

(3) In Figure 4 there is also a very interesting, clearly identifiable, very low intensity pattern 752 - 1041 - 1330 - 1635 - 1924 - 2217 - 2506 where all the peaks are

separated by a 288-290 repeating motive except for the 1330 - 1635 one that is separated by a 304 Da C unit. This is a definite series of angular oligomers up to at least a 7 repeating units one. Thus, a series of angular tannins of 3+1, 3+2 and 3+3 robinetinidin units linked to a branching C unit. (an angular tannin means there is a C branching unit). It is angular if there are two flavonoid units linked both to the A ring of the C unit, it is branched if on top of this there is another flavonoid series attached to the C4 of the C unit. The pattern indicated is almost certainly a series of angular or branched oligomers of a length never determined before. By the way, whenever there is a C unit linked to A and B units one could have an angular tannin. However in cases where several C-units linked to each other are present, then one has definetely a prodelphinidin or procyanidin oligomer. Furthermore the 289 Da unit can equally be a prorobinetinidin but also a catechin unit, hence one could also have angular tannins with the 289 B unit if one of the -OHs is situated on the A ring rather than the B-ring.

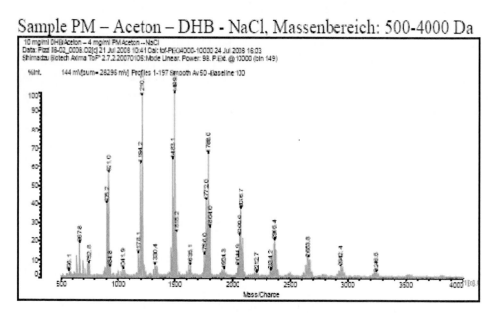

Figure 4. MALDI mass spectrum of *Acacia mangium* tannin extract.

Procyanidin and Prodelphinidin Type Polyflavonoids

An example of procyanidin type tannins, in which the great majority, almost the totality of the flavonoid units are linked C4 to C8 are pine tannin and mangrove polyflavonoid tannins. The greater majority of all polyflavonoids fall into this category. They are a class very diffuse, present in many foodstuffs, apple skins, fruit juices etc. Mangrove polyflavonoids are the one that have been examined most in depth as regards their oligomeric structure.

Mangrove tannins can come from a variety of different *Rhizophora* species. In the case of *Rhizophora apiculata* the tannins found are of the procyanidin type [23,24]. These are the most common tannins existing in nature. *Rhizophora apiculata* mangrove tannin most common monomer constituents are catechin, epicatechin, epigallocatechin and epicatechin gallate with molecular weights (MW) respectively of 290.3 Da, 290.3 Da, 306.3 Da and 442.4 Da.

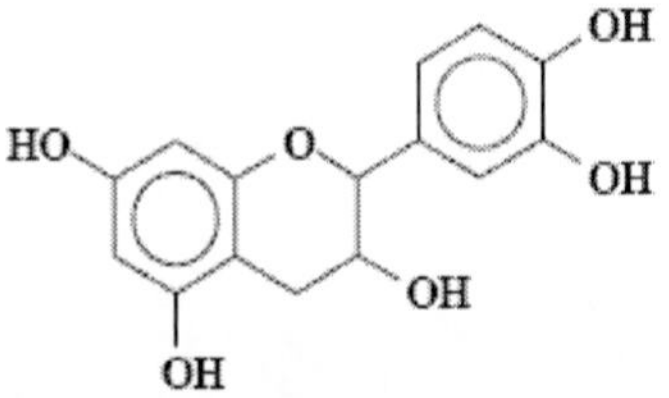

CATECHIN / EPICATECHIN
MW = 290
A

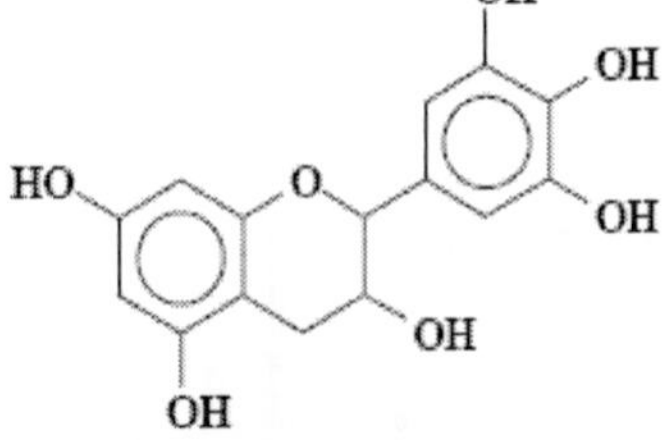

EPIGALOCATECHIN
MW = 306
B

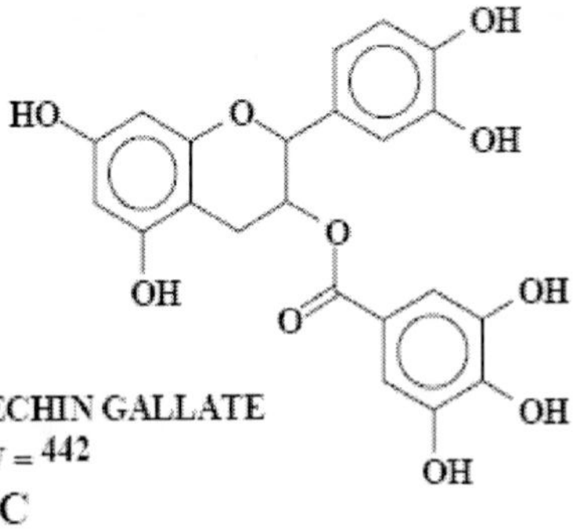

EPICATECHIN GALLATE
MW = 442
C

For *Rhizophora apiculata* mangrove tannins, the MALDI –TOF spectra in Figure 5a,b,c indicates clearly that alternate repeating units with mass increments of 264-264.9 Da occur. These have not been identified by previous analysis by other methods [23-26] in mangrove tannins indicating possibly the presence also of other monomers than those shown in Figure 1 and/or different combinations of various structures. Combination of the masses of the catechinin monomers shown in Figure 5 can be used to calculate the masses of the oligomer peaks in the spectra according to the expression $M+Na+ = 23(Na) + 2$ (endgroups, 2xH) + 290.3 (-2H)A + 306.3 (-2H)B + 442.4 (-2H)C (Table 3). The only problem about this is the presence of a repeating structure the MW of which is regular at 264.0 – 264.9 Da.

This unit has not been identified before, and we will call it here structure D. Calculation of the MALDI masses indicate that certain peaks can only be explained by the presence of epicatechin gallate units in which the gallic acid residue has being removed of 274.3 Da (structure E), these being related to the unknown structure. The equation than becomes $M+Na+ = 23(Na) + 2$ (endgroups, 2xH) + 290.3 (-2H)A + 306.3 (-2H)B + 442.4 (-2H)C + 274.3 (-2H)E. In Table 3 are shown the results of the combination of monomer units forming the different oligomers observed by MALDI-TOF. It must be noticed that only very few of the dominant peaks (Figure 5a) can be explained only on the basis of the catechinic structures A, B and C. Some mass peaks however are not easily explained without the use of structure D. The majority of the dominant peaks are shown in Tables 4 and 5.

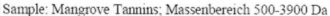

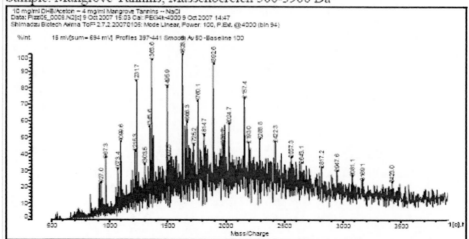

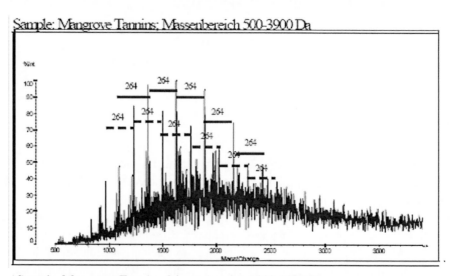

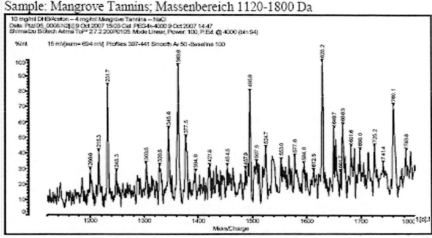

Figure 5. MALDI mass spectrum of (a) mixed *Rhizophora apiculata* mangrove tannin extract, 500-3900 Da range. (b) indication of the relevant 264 Da repeat unit.. (c) details of the 1120-1800 Da range.

Table 3. MALDI fragmentation peaks for mixed *Rhizophora spp* mangrove tannin extract. Note that the predominant repeat unit in this tannin indicate that it is predominantly a procyanidin

M+Na+ (exp.)	M+Na+ (calc.)	A	B	C	Unit type D	E (C-gallic)
Da		290.3	306.3	442.4	264/265	274.3
835	841.9	--	--	--	--	3
927	921.9	1	2	--	--	--
967*	see Table 3					
1073.4	1074	--	2	1	--	--
1099.6*	1094.1	1	--	2	--	--
or	1098.6	--	--	--	2	2
1200	1200		3		1	
1215.3	1210.2	--	3	--	--	1
or	1210.1	--	1	--2		
or	1210.2	2	2			
1231.7*	1226.2	1	3	--	--	--
or						
1248.3	1242.2	--	4			
1328.5	1330.3	1	1	1	--	1
1345.6	1346.2	--	--	3		
or	1346.3	2	1	1		
or	1346.3	--	2	1	--	1
1363*	1362.3	1	2	1		
1377.5	1378.3	--	3	1		
1454.5	1450.5	4	--	--	--	1
1487.9	1482.5	--	3	--	--	2
1507.5	1507.2	--	4	--	1	
1649.7	1650.5	--	1	3		
or	1650.6	2	2	1		
1666.3	1666.3	1	3	1		
1681.6	1682.6	--	4	1		
1725.2	1722.8	4	--	--	--	2
1741.4	1738.8	5	--	--	--	1
or	1738.7	1	--	2	--	2
	1738.8	3	1	--	--	2
1892.6*	1890.9	4	--	1	--	1
2193	2195.2	6	--	1		
2557.3	2556.2	--	6	1	1	
2817.2	2819.7	3	2	3		
or	2819.6	1	1	5		
2947.6	2940.0	--	6	--	--	4
or	2940.0	2	5	--	--	3
	2939.9	--	4	2	--	3
3081	3076.1	4	3	1	--	2
or	3076.0	2	2	3	--	2
	3076.0	--	3	3	--	3
3169.1	3164.2	5	--	2	--	3
or	3164.3	7	1	--	--	3

*Dominant fragment.

Table 4. MALDI fragmentation peaks for mixed *Rhizophora spp* mangrove tannin extract. Note that the predominant repeat units in this tannin is 528-530 Da, indicating that in its main series of peaks this tannin may present pure profisetinidin oligomers as predominant components

M+Na$^+$ (exp.) Da	M+Na$^+$ (calc.)	Unit type				
		A 290.3	B 306.3	C 442.4	E 274.3	D 264-264.9
835	841.9	--	--	--	3	--
1099.6*	1105.6	--	--	--	3	1
1363.6*	1362.3	1	2	1		
1628.2*	1628.2	1	2	1	--	1
1892.6*	1892.6	1	2	1	--	2
2157.4*	2157.4	1	2	1	--	3
2422.3*	2422.3	1	2	1	--	4

*Dominant fragment.

Table 5. MALDI fragmentation peaks for mixed *Rhizophora spp* mangrove tannin extract. Note that the predominant repeat units in this tannin is still 528-530 Da, indicating that in this MALDI series of peaks this tannin may present predominantly a profisetinidin component but linked to procyanidins units too

M+Na$^+$ (exp.) Da	M+Na$^+$ (calc.)	Unit type					DPn Tot	DPn E unit
		A 290.3	B 306.3	C 442.4	E (C-gallic) 274.3	D 264-264.9		
967.3	967.7			1	1	1 (-2xO)	3	1
1231.7*	1226.2	1	3				4	-
1495.9*	1497.7			1	1	3 (-2xO)	5	3
1760.1*	1756	1	3			2	6	2
2024.7*	2025.7			1	1	5 (-2xO)	7	5
2288.8*	2285.8	1	3			4	8	4
2557.3	2553.7			1	1	7 (-2xO)	9	7

*Dominant fragment.

E

274·3

Structure D cannot be inserted in the equation simply because no known flavonoid structure could be found with such a molecular weight. However, this structure partecipates markedly, from peak intensities in Figure 5a its partecipation being predominant to the formation of the mangrove tannin oligomers. Two series of the most intense MALDI mass peaks rely on the repetition of this 264 Da structure. Thus, the oligomers of the series of peaks at 835 Da, 1099 Da, 1363 Da, 1628 Da, 1892 Da, 2157 Da, 2422 Da are separated by the 264 Da motive recurring six times. Equally, the oligomers of the series of peaks at 967 Da, 1231 Da, 1495 Da, 1760 Da, 2024 Da, 2288 Da, 2557 Da are separated by the 264 Da motive again recurring six times. Which means that attached to the starting oligomer to an hexamer of the 264 Da unit is progressively linked to the starting oligomer, whatever this may be. Tables 4 and 5 show the interpretation of the two predominant series present.

It is of interest to find out what structure corresponds to 264 Da. No known monoflavonoid corresponds to such a structure. If one takes structure E however, for a E repeating unit at 272.3 Da, the difference with 264 Da is always of 8 Da, that does not correspond to the mass of any leaving functional group. However, if one considers that there is an –OH group less in a dimer formed by two joined E structures this will give the loss of 16 Da, hence of an oxygen. It means that the repeating unit of the system is not 264 Da but appears to be 264x2 = 528 Da. Thus, the repeating unit is a dimer of structure E whith a –OH group missing. The unit has a single phenolic –OH group which has been lost, as shown below, the alcoholic –OH groups in C3 having already been lost at the separation of the gallic acid.

Thus, in Table 4 is shown the main series of dominant MALDI masses indicating that oligomers of this unit appear to occur in *apiculata* mangrove tannins. This is the most likely case seeing the regular progression from trimer to octamer in Table 4.Thus, mixed oligomers where a procyanidin oligomer formed by structures of type A, B and C (1363.6 Da) is linked to progressively increasing number of D structure oligomers are possible. The results in Table 3 of the second more important series of recurrent MALDI peaks clearly confirms that mixed procyanidin and D oligomers covalently linked do exist in such mangrove tannins because none of the masses of the series 835 Da, 1099 Da, 1363 Da, 1628 Da, 1892 Da, 2157 Da, 2422 Da can be explain without having units of structures A, B and C linked to the D oligomers. It appears most likely then that both pure oligomers of the two types as well as linked mixed oligomers do coexist in this tannin.

A mainly prodelphinidin tannin, namely pecan nut tannin extract was also examined (Figure 6) [33]. The main prodelphinidin repeat unit has a molar mass of 306 Da and the main fragments found arrived only up to trimers (304+304+288+2+23 = 921 Da). This unusual result leads to two consequences. In pecan nut tannin extract robinetinidin units are linked within the prodelphinidin main oligomers, and that the interflavonoid bond of prodelphinidins is particularly prone to cleavage (this is known to be so). It means that the finding of trimers only , when the number average degree of polymeryzation of this tannin is known to be of 5.50 [19,20] , indicates that the cleavage of the interflavonoid bond here is mainly a fabrication of the method of analysis used and if MALDI-TOF has to be used in this case much milder conditions needed to be used.

In conclusion MALDI-TOF is a suitable method for examining polyflavonoid tannin oligomers and one that is able to determine through this technique facts on polyflavonoid tannins which are already known by using other approaches. It also appears capable however to determine aspects of the structure and characteristics of the tannins which are too difficult to determine by other techniques.

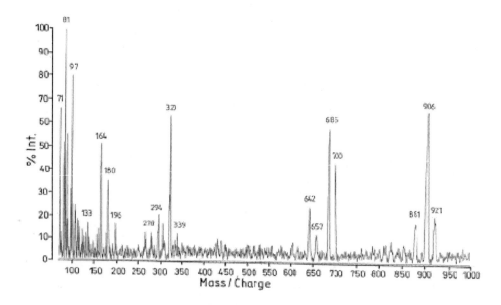

Figure 6. MALDI mass spectrum of natural pecan nut tannin extract.

In the present investigation of the two major commercial polyflavonoid tannins it has been possible to determine by MALDI-TOF that: (i) mimosa tannin is predominantly composed of prorobinetinidins while quebracho is predominantly composed of profisetinidins, that (ii) mimosa tannin is heavily branched due to the presence of considerable proportions of "angular" units in its structure while quebracho tannin is almost completely linear. These structural differences also contribute to the considerable differences in viscoity of water solutions of the two tannins. (iii) the interflavonoid link is more easily hydrolysable, and does appear to sometime hydrolyse in quebracho tannin and profisetinidins, partly due to the linear structure of this tannin, and confirming NMR findings that this tannin is subject to polymerisation / depolymerisation equilibrium. This is not the case for mimosa tannin in which the interflavonoid link is completely stable to hydrolysis. (iv) Sulphitation has been shown to influence the detachment of catechol B-rings much more than pyrogallol-type B-rings. (v) The distribution of tannin oligomers, and the tannins number average degree of polymerisation obtained by MALDI-TOF appear to compare well with the results obtained by other techniques.

Colloidal State of Polyflavonoid Extracts

Raw polyflavonoid extracts present colloidal behaviour. Of importance is the presence in the polyflavonoid extracts of consistent amounts of polymeric carbohydrates (in general hemicellulose fragments, sometime called hydrocolloid gums) extracted together with the tannins. These are always present unless the tannin has undergone special purification, such as the case of their use for medical and pharmaceutical use. These polymeric carbohydrates contribute to maintain the water solutions of polyflavonoid tannin extracts in colloidal state, rendering sometime possible reactions on the tannin that otherwise are not or are less likely to occur in just a water solution. The reactions that can occur under these conditions appear to rely on the surfactant-like action of the hydrocolloid gums and also on the tannin oligomers themselves, hence on their capability to form micelles in water. The ζ-potential of a solution is correlated to the extent of its colloidal state. In Table 6 are reported the The ζ-potentials of water solutions of four industrial polyflavonoid tannin extracts, of a monomer model compound, catechin, and of catechin in gum arabic to imitate the solution of a tannin extract. These show that the colloidal state of a water solution of polyflavonoid tannin is quite definite, but very variable according to the tannin type. Thus, pecan nut pith tannin extract which is known to contain a very small proportion of hydrocolloid gums, around 4%, is clearly much less colloidal than mimosa or quebracho tannin extracts where the amount of hydrocolloid gums is much higher between 10 and 20%. Thus, it must be pointed out that both reactions and structural modifications of the tannins that occur independently of the colloidal state of the solution, as well as reactions that are dependent on their colloidal state , may greatly contribute to the performance of the polyflavonoid extracts. This area has been explored only for application to wood adhesives [27], but no work on this appears to have been carried out in the neutraceutical or pharmaceutical fields where it may be also of importance.

Table 6. Comparative ζ-potentials measurements in mV of natural tannin extracts

Mimosa tannin extract 40% water solution	11.3
Quebracho tannin extract 40% water solution	14.5
Pine tannin extract 40% water solution	2.4
Pecan nut tannin extract 40% water solution	4.9
Catechin water solution	0
Gum arabic 23% water solution	5.2
Catechin/gum arabic mix 23% warter solution	5.2

Rheology of Industrial Polyflavonoids

Polyflavonoid tannin extracts have been produced and used industrially for many applications since the end of the 19th century [1,28]. Among these uses are the early one as dyes for silk, and their predominat use to-day as tanning agents for the manufacture of leather [28] as well as their use as wood adhesives [1] plus the growing proportion of food, medical, pharmaceutical and nutracetical applications. Considering the relevance of their rheological characteristics on their main fields of industrial application the literature is almost completely devoid of rheological studies on these materials. It is for this reason that what is known of their rheology is worthwhile to know. Some early rheology work has concentrated on tannins extracted in non-traditional manner, different from industrial practice [29-31] while more recent work investigated the rheology of the major commercially avalaible polyflavonoid tannin extracts [32] extracted by standard industrial practice.

Figures 7-10 show plots of elastic modulus G' and viscous modulus G'' over various concentrations (20% -50%) of water solutions of four natural polyflavonoid extracts, namely mimosa, quebracho, pine and pecan nut tannin extracts [32]. Dynamic oscillatory measurements were carried out in order to examine the shear sensitive associations of molecules and clusters at low deformations. Dynamic moduli (storage modulus G' and loss modulus G'') of the different extracts were measured as a function of strain amplitude at a fixed frequency to obtain the linear viscoelastic region. The strain sweep for the four natural extracts at various concentrations (20%, 30%, 40%, 50%) measured at 1 rad s^{-1} frequency are shown in Figures 7-10. These figures show that in general G'' > G' for the solutions of all the tannin and hence that the solutions of industrial polyflavonoid tannin extracts behave as viscous liquids even at the higher (50%) concentration. This indicates that commercial tannin extracts are primarily composed of relatively short oligomers which do not appear to show the entanglement and elasticity of higher molecular weight polymers. This is supported by measures of number and weight average molecular masses for the four tannins obtained by different techniques [19,20] which show that typical number average degree of polymerization (DP$_n$) of mimosa, quebracho, pine and pecan industrial tannin extracts [19,20] are respectively of 4.9, 6.7, 5.9 and 5.5. A level of entanglement is however possible for the higher molecular mass fractions of the tannins if one considers that typical values of the weight average degree of polymerization (DP$_w$) are of respectively 8.8, 12.3, 10.9, 9.5 for mimosa, quebracho, pine and pecan tannins, and the great number of polar hydroxy groups present on these molecules [19,20,33].

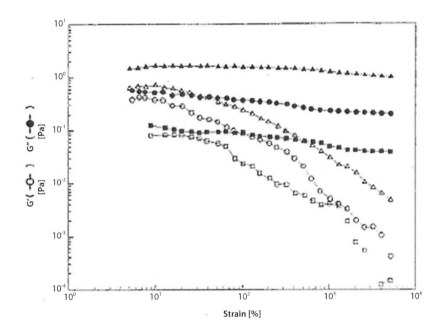

Figure 7. Strain sweeps at ω = 1 rad s⁻¹ for mimosa tannin extract solutions at different concentrations: (□) 30%, (o) 40%, (Δ) 50% concentration. (o) G′ curves; (•) G″ curves.

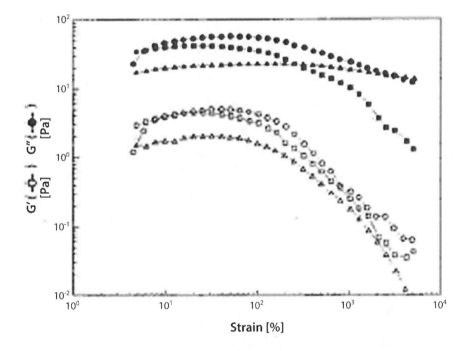

Figure 8. Strain sweeps at ω = 1 rad s⁻¹ for quebracho tannin extract solutions at different concentrations: (□) 30%, (o) 40%, (Δ) 50% concentration. (o) G′ curves; (•) G″ curves.

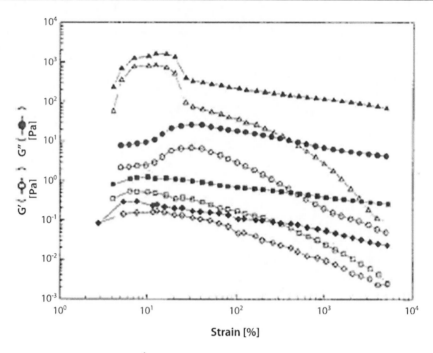

Figure 9. Strain sweeps at $\omega = 1$ rad s^{-1} for pine tannin extract solutions at different concentrations: (♣) 20% ; (□) 30%, (o) 40%, (Δ) 50% concentration. (o) G' curves; (•) G'' curves.

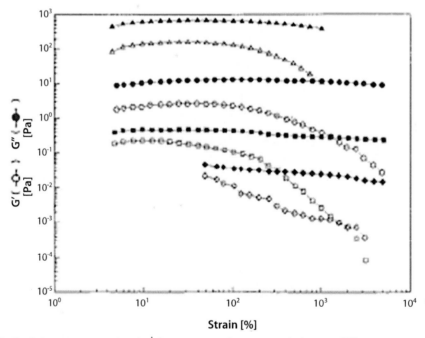

Figure 10. Strain sweeps at $\omega = 1$ rad s^{-1} for pecan tannin extract solutions at different concentrations: (♣) 20% ; (□) 30%, (o) 40%, (Δ) 50% concentration. (o) G' curves; (•) G'' curves.

These figures also indicate that in the low percentage strain region both moduli appear to be fairly independent of the applied strain amplitude as shown from the almost parallel trend

of the two moduli curves. However, when the percentage strain increases the value of G'
starts to decrease significantly in relation to the value of G", a trend which becomes slightly
more evident the lower is the concentration studied. Furthermore, the G### linearity limit
appears to decrease somewhat with increasing concentration. This indicates that,
notwithstanding the purely viscous liquid behaviour of these tannin extract solutions, (i)
microstructures exists for these extracts in solution , a fact supported by the known colloidal
interactions for these materials already reported [27,29-32,34-39], and (ii) that such
microstructures are labile as they are significantly broken with applied shear, leading to a
critical strain after which a significant decline in the elastic modulus results, a fact supported
by the well known thixotropic behaviour of concentrated, commercial polyflavonoid tannin
extracts water solutions [1,27,30,34,36]. For the two higher concentrations used, and also for
the 30% concentration, with only one exception, as the extracts where used at their natural pH
which is in the 4.2-5.1 range there was no case where G' > G" and no concentration occurred
at which G' = G", as this behaviour has been associated with much higher alkalinity ranges
[30].

While these are general trends for all the four polyflavonoid tannins, some important
difference between the tannins also exists, mainly based on their differences in viscosity.
Firstly, G' starts decreasing according to the different typical molecular masses of each
tannin: to a higher molecular mass corresponds a later start in the decrease of G'. The main
difference occurs for pine tannin extract solutions where two plateau for G' and G" occurs
with this becoming more evident the higher is the tannin solution concentration. The
existence of another transition at lower percentage strain also indicates the presence of
another type of labile microstructure. Secondary forces associations between tannin oligomers
and oligomeric sugars, derived from degraded hemicelluloses which are always present in
consistant proportions in these extracts, are well known [1,19,20,30]. They have often caused
in the past the incorrect determination of absurdly high molecular masses for tannin
oligomers due to the formation of ionic polymers between tannins and carbohydrate
oligomers. This transition is particularly evident in Figure 9 for the pine tannin extract. It is
not possible to conclude from the available data if this is the cause of the additional transition
in pine tannin, or rather if the affinity of carbohydrates for tannins is the transition that occurs
for all the four tannins. The decrease of these secondary forces associations at higher
percentage strains will cause the system to appear to behave as composed of species of lower
average molecular mass with the consequent trend observed for G' in Figures 7-10.

Figures 11-14 show the variation of G' and G" with frequency for the four tannins each at
four different concentrations. The lower the slope of the curves the closer to a newtonian
behaviour is the behaviour of the tannin extract solution. For all the tannins and for all the
concentrations examined G' values are smaller than G" and all G" values are relatively low
and increase progressively with increasing frequency: the tannin extracts are behaving
essentially as a viscous liquid as discussed earlier, the only exceptions being the tannin
extract solutions at 20% concentration where G' and G" cross-over points do indeed occur.
For concentrations higher than 20% this appears to suggest that the tannin oligomers are well
separated and that, once the interactions with the carbohydrate are eliminated or minimized,
there is little possibility of molecular interaction and entanglement, even at the higher
concentration.

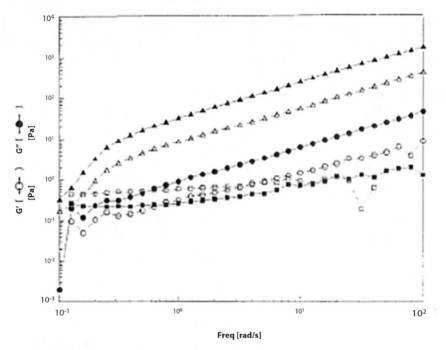

Figure 11. Elastic modulus (G′) and viscous modulus (G″) as a function of frequency (ω) for mimosa tannin extract solutions at different concentrations: (□) 30%, (o) 40%, (Δ) 50% concentration. (o) G′ curves; (•) G″ curves.

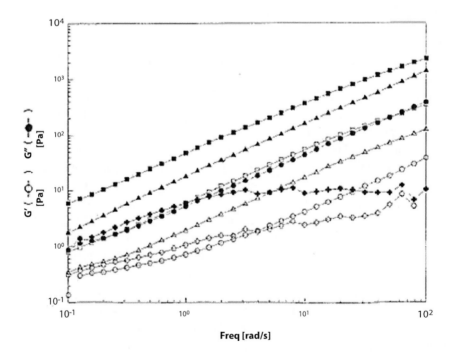

Figure 12. Elastic modulus (G′) and viscous modulus (G″) as a function of frequency (ω) for quebracho tannin extract solutions at different concentrations: (♣) 20% ; (□) 30%,(o) 40%, (Δ) 50% concentration. (o) G′ curves; (•) G″ curves.

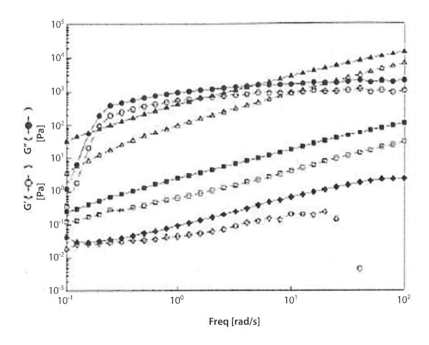

Figure 13. Elastic modulus (G') and viscous modulus (G″) as a function of frequency (ω) for pine tannin extract solutions at different concentrations: (♣) 20% ; (□) 30%, (o) 40%, (Δ) 50% concentration. (o) G' curves; (•) G″ curves.

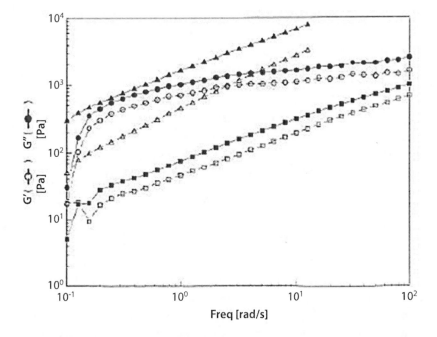

Figure 14. Elastic modulus (G') and viscous modulus (G″) as a function of frequency (ω) for pecan tannin extract solutions at different concentrations: (♣) 20% ; (□) 30%, (o) 40%, (Δ) 50% concentration. (o) G' curves; (•) G″ curves.

Thus, is there little interaction in the tannin extracts, resulting in smaller elastic contributions, or must one consider also other parameters? In this respect there are some differences in the curves of the four natural extracts. Considering the differences in percentage strain which had to be used for the different tannin solutions it can be noticed that the value of the two moduli are quite different passing from one tannin to the other (mimosa and quebracho appear for example to have have similar G' and G" values; in reality this is not the case as the two figures are respectively at 100% and 10% strain respectively (Figures 11, 12). This partly reflects the level of molecular association occurring in each different extract. However, (Figure 13) in the pine tannin extract solutions the differences in value between G' and G", at the same imposed frequency, are smaller than for the other three tannins, and the value of both moduli is higher (Figure 13). This means that at parity of conditions the elastic component of a pine tannin extract solutions is both in absolute and proportionally greater than in the solutions of the other tannin extracts. This indicates that the determining parameters as regards the elastic response of a tannin extract solution are both (i) the greater average molecular mass of the tannin as well as (ii) the intensity of the tannin interaction with the carbohydrate oligomers present in the extract, which is related to both the amount of carbohydrate oligomers present and to their average molecular mass as well as to (i) above, however feeble such interactions might be. The first of these two parameters would lead to pine and quebracho tannin solutions having the higher moduli values, followed by pecan tannin extract and mimosa tannin extract (which is indeed the case if one considers the differences in percentage strain which had to be used, and the average molecular masses reported above [19,20]). The second of these two parameters would place the elastic response of the tannin as highest for pine and quebracho (the first mainly but not only for the higher proportion of carbohydrates, and the second for their and their carbohydrates higher molecular mass), followed by pecan (the carbohydrates content of which is very low) and last mimosa. In Figures 11-14 pine tannins and quebracho are the ones with higher numerical values of elastic response (if one considers the differences in percentage strain which had to be used) and pine also presenting the higher proportional value, followed by pecan and by mimosa.

Figures 11-14 also indicate that G' and G" present a pronounced frequency dependence for mimosa and quebracho tannin extracts, as indicated by the sharper slope of the moduli curves. The same figures indicate that G' and G" present instead little or no frequency dependence for pine and pecan tannin extracts.

A case apart appears to be the 20% concentration case for the three tannins for which such a concentration was also used (mimosa was not used at 20% concentration). A G' and G" cross-over point (G' = G", and then at increasing frequency G' > G") occurs for all the three tannin extracts, as it also occurs for mimosa tannin solutions at 30% concentration, in all four cases at the extreme range of the frequency used (Figures 11-14). This again confirms that on top of the effect of the pH [30] , the viscoelastic response of the tannin extracts obtained in these cases is due to intermolecular associations. It is a very clear indication that molecular associations between tannin molecules, and particularly between tannin molecules and carbohydrates to form labile structures of greater apparent molecular mass by either colloidal or other interactions, do indeed occur. An example of the behaviour of a solution of a polymeric carbohydrate, such as gum arabic, at the same four concentrations used for the tannins (Figure 15) indicates both a clear rubbery plateau at the two higher concentrations, but also that G' = G" cross-over points occur. At the two lower concentrations (20%-30%), at the extreme of the frequency range used, it is is indeed the value of G' which becomes higher than the value of G", imitating what seen for the tannin extracts at the same concentration, again confirming the partecipation of carbohydrate oligomers in imparting under certain conditions viscoelastic behaviour to tannin extract solutions, a purified tannin without any carbohydrates rather behaving as a viscous liquid only [37-39].

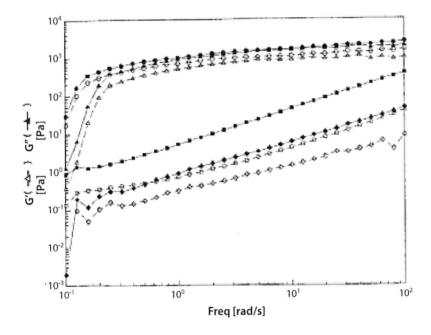

Figure 15. Elastic modulus (G') and viscous modulus (G") as a function of frequency (ω) for gum arabic solutions at different concentrations: (♣) 20% ; (□) 30%, (o) 40%, (Δ) 50% concentration. (o) G' curves; (•) G" curves.

In conclusion commercial, industrially produced mimosa, quebracho, pine and pecan nut polyflavonoid tannin extracts water solutions of different concentrations were examined by rheometry by measuring dynamic moduli both as a function of strain amplitude and at varying frequency. The water solutions of these materials have been found to behave in general mainly as viscous liquids at the concentrations which are generally used for their main industrial applications [1,27,40]. Clear indications of viscoelastic response are also noticeable, among these the cross-over of the elastic and viscous moduli curves at the lower concentrations of the range investigated, with some differences being noticeable between each tannin and the others, pine and quebracho tannin extracts showing the more marked viscoelastic behaviour. Other than pH dependence (and related structural considerations), the parameters which were found to be of interest as regards the noticeable viscoelastic behaviour of the tannin extracts were the existence in the solutions of labile microstructures which can be broken by applied shear. This is supported by the well known thixotropic behaviour of concentrated, commercial polyflavonoid tannin extracts water solution [1,30,34,36]. Such microstructures appear to be due or (i) to the known colloidal interactions of these materials already reported [1,30,34,35,37-39,41], or (ii) to other types of secondary interactions [35,37-39] between tannin oligomers and particularly between tannin and carbohydrate oligomers present in the extracts. The latter is supported by the dependence of this effect from both the average molecular masses of the tannin and of the carbohydrate oligomers.

Anti-Oxydant Capability of Polyflavonoids

The capability of phenols to produce rather stable phenoxyl radicals, capable by their presence of retarding or even inhibiting the progress of radical addition polymerisation is well known [42,43]. In the ambit of research on the improvement of antioxidant capabilities, natural phenolic and polyphenolic materials such as hydrolysable and polyflavonoid tannins, and their model compounds, have been shown by the use of stopped-flow techniques to be capable of similar, but rather more intense effects [44,45]. However, both a simpler to handle and more rapid technique to measure tannins antioxidant capabilities, as well as a screening of the antioxidant capabilities of a variety of different hydrolysable and polyflavonoid tannins has been developed.

Polyflavonoids contain an elevated number of phenolic hydroxyls and their characteristic structure lends itself to the stabilisation of radicals not only by mechanisms characteristic of all phenols but also by the existance of side reactions such as heterocycle pyran ring opening and others.

Electron spin resonance (ESR), among other techniques has been used with good results to study the reactions of radical formation and decay induced by bases and weak Lewis acids in polyflavonoid tannins [37-39,46] and their model compounds [38,45-47]. It is for this reason that ESR has been used as rapid technique for the determination of the antioxidant properties of polyflavonoids [45].

What has been studied is how (i) the structure of different tannins influences the rate of radical transfer from the stable 2,2-diphenyl-1-picrylhydrazyl (DPPH) radical to a tannin and the subsequent rate of radical decay of the phenoxyl radical formed; (ii) the effect of the presence or absence of solvent, and of the type of solvent; but it was mainly aimed at (iii) studying the rate of increase in phenoxyl radical concentration by light irradiation in different tannins, and the subsequent radical decay rate once the inducing light is removed. All these aspect refer to their antioxydanrt capacity.

The tannins used were commercial mimosa (*Acacia mearnsii* formerly *mollissima,* de Wildt) bark tannin extract, a mainly prorobinetinidin tannin; commercial quebracho (*Schinopsis balansae*, variety chaqueno) wood tannin extract, also a mainly prorobinetinidin tannin but with greater percentages od fisetinedin units in it; commercial pecan (*Carya illinoensis*) nut pith tannin extract, a almost totally prodelphinidin tannin; commercial gambier (*Uncaria gambir*) shoots tannin extract, commercial pine (*Pinus radiata*) bark tannin extract, both being mainly procyanidin type tannins. All these are polyflavonoid tannins, plus for comparison commercial oak (*Quercus spp.*) tannin extract, an hydrolysable tannin. Also the tannin extract of chestnut (*Castanea sativa*) wood, an hydrolysable tannin, was tested but far too variable results were obtained and thus the results for this tannin were not reported in the study [45].

One of the more necessary steps to take at the start of such a type of study is to define what is intended for antioxidant capabilities of a tannin. In relation to light-induced degradation of a material, to measure the antioxidant capabilities of any surface finish could be defined as the measurement of two different parameters. These are:

(i) The rate at which the tannin is able to form a radical; this is determined either by the rate of radical transfer from a pre-existing radical species to the tannin to form a more stable phenoxyl radical, or by the rate of radical formation on light irradiation of the tannin, and

(ii) The rate of radical decay of tannin phenoxyl radicals formed.

The first parameter defines the ease and readiness of the tannin in subtracting a radical from, for instance, the substrate; the easier and the more rapid this transfer is, the greater are the antioxidant capabilities of the tannin. The second parameter defines how stable is the tannin phenoxyl radical. Here two interpretations are possible: (i) in general the more stable is the radical, hence the slower is the rate of radical decay, the more marked is the inhibition of radical degradation of the substrate and hence the better are the antioxidant properties of the tannin, but (ii) in the case of tannin radicals considerably more reactive than the substrate, hence where radical termination reactions between two tannin radicals are favourite, the faster the rate of radical decay, hence the faster the quenching between themselves of the tannin radicals formed, the better are the antioxidant properties of the tannin. Cases (i) and (ii) define two different effects: while case (i) has general applicability in all cases, case (ii) might assume disproportionate importance in the case of experiments, like those reported here, in which the substrate is not present. This discussion is then limited at evaluating the importance of the radical decay reaction only from the point of view of case (ii): the slower the radical decay rate, the greater is the antioxidant power of the tannin. An example of the type of cumulative curve obtained is shown in Figures 16 and 17.

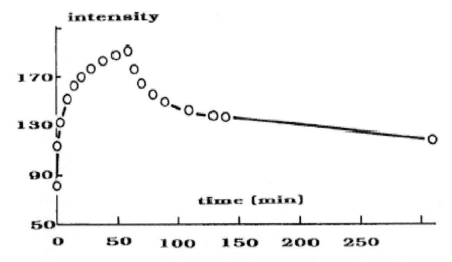

Figure 16. Intensity increase and decrease of the average of the two opposite symmetrical peaks representing the ESR signal during UV irradiation experiments of Quebracho flavonoid tannin extract powder without vacuum, in air, and in a quartz sample-holder. The initial part of the curve up to the maximum of intensity describes the increase in radical concentration as a function of time during irradiation while the decreasing intensity section describes the radical decay reaction from the moment the UV lamp has been switched off.

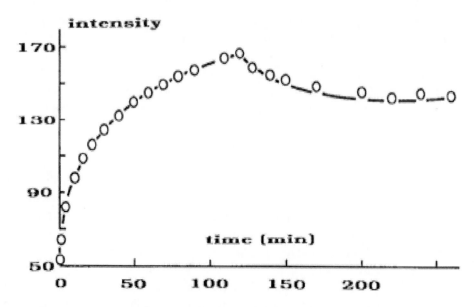

Figure 17. Intensity increase and decrease of the average of the two symmetrical, opposite peaks representing the ESR signal during UV irradiation experiments of Mimosa flavonoid tannin extract powder under vacuum and in a glass sample-holder. The initial part of the curve up to the maximum of intensity describes the increase in radical concentration as a function of time during irradiation while the decreasing intensity section describes the radical decay reaction from the moment the UV lamp has been switched off.

The increase in intensity of the ESR signal, which corresponds to the reaction of radical formation due to the irradiation of the three flavonoid and one hydrolysable tannins examined, can be modelled by a first order kinetic law of the type $I/I_o=ae^{kt}$ (Table 7).

Comparison of the rate constants or of the semitransformation times $t_{1/2}$ allows a few deductions, namely

1. In absence of vacuum, thus in presence of singlet oxygen, mimosa and quebracho tannins present the faster radical formation reaction, while pecan and oak tannins are somewhat slower.
2. In vacuum, thus in absence of singlet oxygen, mimosa tannin shows the more rapid rate of formation, followed by quebracho and pecan tannins which are almost comparable, finally followed by oak tannin which is the slowest of them all.
3. With a few exceptions, the results in quartz and glass cells are comparable.

Thus, in air, the above results (Table 7) indicate that mimosa and quebracho should present the best antioxidant characteristics, with the results of mimosa under vacuum indicating a greater consistency, while pecan and oak tannin appears to have poorer antioxidant characteristics.

Equally, the decrease in intensity as a function of time of the ESR signal after stopping the irradiation of the specimen, hence the radical decay reaction itself, is correctly described by first order kinetics of the form $I/I_0=a'e^{-k't}$ and shown in Table 8 and indicates that

1. In general without vacuum, oak and pecan mantain the radical for much longer than quebracho and even longer than mimosa tannin.
2. In general with vacuum, quebracho presents the slowest radical decay reaction, followed by oak, then pecan and last by mimosa tannin.
3. Differences in the behaviour between quartz and glass cells are noticeable. With vacuum for instance, pecan in a glass cell appears to have the slowest radical decay rate, an unexpected occurrence considering all the other results.

Table 7. Radical formation (= First reaction step) kinetics according to a first order kinetic law derived from electron spin resonance experiments. ($I/I_0 = a\ e^{kt}$)

Tannin	Vacuum Conditions	Cell Material	Parameters			
			a	$k(s^{-1})$	r	$t_{1/2}(s)$
Mimosa	Without	quartz	1.4974	1.549×10^{-4}	0.809	4474
	Vacuum	glass	1.5069	1.510×10^{-4}	0.786	4604
	With	quartz	1.7192	1.120×10^{-4}	0.838	6187
	Vacuum	glass	1.6806	1.148×10^{-4}	0.839	6038
Quebracho	Without	quartz	1.5546	1.513×10^{-4}	0.785	4580
	Vacuum	glass	1.6545	1.605×10^{-4}	0.770	4316
	With	quartz	1.4770	0.580×10^{-4}	0.832	11939
	Vacuum	glass	1.8611	0.744×10^{-4}	0.806	9319
Pecan	Without	quartz	1.1835	0.442×10^{-4}	0.668	15671
	Vacuum	glass	1.2018	0.463×10^{-4}	0.672	14968
	With	quartz	1.6345	0.652×10^{-4}	0.827	10634
	Vacuum	glass	1.6595	0.558×10^{-4}	0.823	12424
Oak	Without	quartz	1.1748	0.610×10^{-4}	0.792	11360
	Vacuum	glass	1.2057	0.581×10^{-4}	0.742	11927
	With	quartz	1.1050	0.383×10^{-4}	0.898	18079
	Vacuum	glass	1.2253	0.496×10^{-4}	0.902	13962

Thus, in radical formation the order of faster to slower rate remains the same with just differences in relative rates determined by the conditions used (vacuum or not, quartz or glass), and is

mimosa=quebracho>>pecan>/=oak

In the radical decay reaction instead the slower to faster rate changes quite considerably according to the conditions, particularly but not only according to the presence or absence of vacuum. Thus, without vacuum and the air singlet oxygen present the rate of radical decay is

mimosa>quebracho>>pecan=oak (> faster than)

while under vacuum

mimosa>pecan>/=oak>>quebracho

In air then, the balance of the two reactions indicate that the differences between the various tannins should not be major. As, however, radicals have to form before they can decay, the rapidity of radical assumption or formation is the most likely important factor, and thus mimosa and quebracho should be considerably better as antioxidants than the other two tannins. If it is considered that quebracho is as rapid as mimosa to form radicals but that its radicals definitely present a slower radical decay rate, the first conclusion which could be drawn is that quebracho appears to have a slightly better overall antioxidant behaviour than mimosa, but that such a difference is not likely to be very marked. All three flavonoid tannins appear to have considerably better behaviour as antioxidants than the hydrolysable tannin.

The general behaviour of tannins described above can also be seen however from a point of view of relative intensity of the ESR signals, thus total radicals formed, rather than just from a purely kinetic rate point of view (table 8). Table 9 puts in perspective the relative quantities of radicals formed, directly related to the surge in intensity during a fixed period of time of 60 minutes (which in all the cases without vacuum corresponds to the peak of maximum radical concentration obtained at which the inducing light was switched off).

From Table 9 it is easy to see that differences in ESR intensity units, hence in radical concentration, is much higher for quebracho (111, 101, Table 9) than for all the other three tannins. The results for the other three tannins are comparable to each other, presenting only minor differences.

Table 8. Radical decay (=second reaction step) kinetics according to a first order kinetic law derived from electron spin resonance experiments. $(I/I_o = a'e^{-k't})$.

Tannin	Vacuum Conditions	Cell Material	Parameters			
			a	$k(s^{-1})$	r	$t_{1/2}(s)$
Mimosa	Without	quartz	0.909	0.874×10^{-4}	0.92	7931
	Vacuum	glass	0.928	0.639×10^{-4}	0.90	10839
	With	quartz	0.927	0.227×10^{-4}	0.89	30586
	Vacuum	glass	0.951	0.148×10^{-4}	0.87	46896
Quebracho	Without	quartz	0.901	0.559×10^{-4}	0.91	11571
	Vacuum	glass	0.846	0.379×10^{-4}	0.81	18294
	With	quartz	0.950	0.024×10^{-4}	0.92	289665
	Vacuum	glass	0.920	0.028×10^{-4}	0.92	249264
Pecan	Without	quartz	0.886	0.163×10^{-4}	0.71	42402
	Vacuum	glass	0.886	0.076×10^{-4}	0.61	91184
	With	quartz	0.951	0.147×10^{-4}	0.86	47185
	Vacuum	glass	0.936	0.020×10^{-4}	0.75	344069
Oak	Without	quartz	0.931	0.102×10^{-4}	0.74	68177
	Vacuum	glass	0.934	0.197×10^{-4}	0.71	35102
	With	quartz	0.987	0.043×10^{-4}	0.80	160107
	Vacuum	glass	0.997	0.055×10^{-4}	0.93	127249

Expressing the same results (Table 9) in percentages show mimosa to give comparable results to those of quebracho: this gives a faulse idea of the situation because it is the difference in units which is directly related to the increase in radical concentration on the tannin, and thus the percentage should not be considered. The percentages are shown in Table 9 to warn about this error in interpretation. These results confirm again that quebracho has the best antioxidant characteristics, but also show that there is not much difference between the other tannins.

Table 9. Radical formation reaction. Maximum intensity (10^{-5}) and starting intensity (10^{-5}) in intensity units of ESR signal and of relative radical concentration

Tannin	Vacuum Conditions	Cell Material	Peak intensity (relative radical concentration)			
			Maximum (at 60 min.)	Starting (at 0 min.)	difference	
					units	%
Mimosa	Without	quartz	95	41	54	132
	Vacuum	glass	67	29	38	131
	With	quartz	179	65	114	177
	Vacuum	glass	145	53	92	174
Quebracho	Without	quartz	191	80	111	139
	Vacuum	glass	164	63	101	160
	With	quartz	450	230	220	96
	Vacuum	glass	311	115	196	170
Pecan	Without	quartz	182	137	45	33
	Vacuum	glass	147	109	38	35
	With	quartz	471	207	264	128
	Vacuum	glass	343	153	190	124
Oak	Without	quartz	222	160	62	39
	Vacuum	glass	182	128	54	42
	With	quartz	651	511	140	27
	Vacuum	glass	349	229	120	52

In the cases with vacuum in which the role of the singlet oxygen is minimized (radical formation in flavonoids is generally considerably easier in presence rather than absence of air, hence of singlet oxygen as shown by both more rapid radical formation and decay without rather than with vacuum in Tables 7, 8 and 9) the real dependence of radical formation from just the characteristic structure of the tannin can be deduced. Here the difference in units follows the order

pecan>/=quebracho>>oak>mimosa

It is interesting to relate such a scale to the structural and chemical characteristics of the three flavonoid tannins in question. Formation of radicals on the flavonoid B-rings generally leads to heterocycle ring opening, and pyran ring opening is much favourite in prodelphinidins (pecan) because of their pyrogallol B-ring/phloroglucinol A-ring structure which ensures better stabilization by delocalisation of the radical on a greater number of possible sites. For this reason mimosa (a 70% prorobinetinidin) should then be better than quebracho (mainly a profistinidin) which is not the case. There must then be at least another major structural reaction influencing the above scale. The other frequent bond cleavage reaction characteristic of flavonoid polymers is the cleavage of the interflavonoid linkage. Radical formation is also likely to be stabilised through this reaction. Interflavonoid bond cleavage is relatively easy in pecan and quebracho tannins and notoriously difficult in mimosa tannin [18,48]. It appears that it is the ease of this reaction superimposed onto the ease of pyran ring opening which is likely to lead to the scale shown above.

ease of pyran ring opening =   pecan=mimosa>quebracho
                                                     +
ease of interflavonoid bond cleavage=   pecan=quebracho>>mimosa

This appears to indicate that in general the higher is the number of -OHs on the flavonoid B-rings, but particularly the higher is the number of -OHs on the flavonoids A-rings the greater appears to be the antioxidant behaviour of the flavonoid tannin, although this characteristic is again overcome by the ease of interflavonoid bond cleavage. The fact that interflavonoid bond cleavage appear to be strongly related to antioxidant behaviour under vacuum might not mean that this reaction determines radical formation or stability. It might only mean that the stereochemistry of tannins which present easier bond cleavage is such, for instance the structure is more open, that radical formation and uptake are facilitated.

The structural parameters which influence the antioxidant properties of the tannins change of importance in presence of air, hence in presence of singlet oxygen. The total scale is mimosa=quebracho>>pecan>/=oak. Here it appears that there is a clear inverse relationship between the number of A-rings -OHs and of ease of interflavonoid bond cleavage with the rates of radical formation and decay, namely: in presence of air the greater the number of A-rings -OHs and the easier the interflavonoid links cleavage the lesser is the antioxidant activity of the tannin. Thus, the parameters of importance are the same in presence or absence of air, but the effect is exactly opposite in the two cases. This indicates that another tannin property might also have a bearing on the antioxidant capability of the tannin, namely its colloidal state. Flavonoid tannins present decreasing colloidal state according to the scale mimosa=quebracho>pecan [27]. In presence of singlet oxygen the effect of migration of such a radical species within the colloidal micelles will afford much more rapid radical formation or uptake by the tannin, thus improve its radical uptake characteristics (and at the same time possibly also accelerate radical decay within the micelles). This is indeed the case from the results in Tables 1 and 2. If the singlet oxygen is not present, hence in absence of air, the effect of the colloidal state is non-existent for the radical formation reaction and radical formation is much slower. The effect might have very little bearing on the radical decay reaction, although with the data available it is impossible to say.

In conclusion the four parameters the combination of which appears to have a bearing on the antioxidant capabilities of a tannin are (i) the extent of its colloidal state, (ii) the ease of interflavonoid bond cleavage (or better its stereochemical structure), (iii) the ease of pyran ring opening and (iv) the relative numbers of A- and B-rings -OH groups. It is the combination of these four factors which will determine the behaviour as an antioxidant of a particular tannin under each set of particular application conditions. With the data presently available it is impossible to quantify the relative extent of the four effects as a function of application conditions.

Table 10. First order kinetics of radical decay reaction after radical transfer to tannin from DPPH, in methanol

Tannin	Radical decay reaction					Radical formation
	a'	$k'(s^{-1})$	r	$t_{1/2}(s^{-1})$	Max peak Intensity $(x10^5)$	
Quebracho	1.092	$-8.3x10^{-5}$	0.978	8349	38	15 int. units in 1200 s
Mimosa	0.972	$-1.7x10^{-5}$	0.952	40765	5	too fast to measure
Pecan	0.932	$-5.5x10^{-5}$	0.988	12600	19	too fast to measure
Pine	0.977	$-1.03x10^{-5}$	0.848	67282	55	44 int. units in 1200 s
Gambier	0.999	$-0.14x10^{-5}$	0.945	498561	117	105 int.units/13000 s
Oak	0.934	$-1.96x10^{-5}$	0.708	35357	21	too fast to measure

* In dioxane only two radical decay rates could be reliably measured:
Quebracho ($a'=0.900$, $k'=4.24x10^{-5}$ s^{-1}, $r=0.960$) and Gambier ($a'=1.053$, $k'=6.7x10^{-5}$ s^{-1}, $r=0.953$).

The experiments of radical transfer from DPPH to a tannin in solution also gave some interesting results. Three solvents were tried: tetrahydrofurane was discarded because did not dissolve the tannins. Dioxane dissolved the tannin but presented problems of radical transfer between DPPH and tannin: some of the few reliable results in dioxane are reported in Table 10. Solutions of tannin and DPPH in methanol instead gave reliable results: these are also shown in Table 10. These show that as regards the radical decay reaction mimosa is slower, thus has better antioxidant power than quebracho, this result closely matching and supporting what already obtained by radical transfer in solvent with the stopped-flow apparatus experiments [44]. This result supports again the use of ESR techniques for this type of determination. As regards the other tannins the increasing order of the rate of the radical decay reaction (thus passing from the slowest to the fastest radical decay rate) (Table 10) is as follows

gambier<pine=/<mimosa=/<oak<pecan<quebracho

which presents quite a different order from the experiments done without solvent and simply by light irradiation. The order of quebracho, pecan and oak in the above scale reproduces what obtained without vacuum in the experiments without solvent, except for the relative position of mimosa tannin in the scale which is now completely different. It is clear then, that solvation parameters also appear to play an important role under certain conditions. This goes to shaw the complexity of the interrelation of parameters in tannins radical reactions. As regards the radical formation reaction the results obtained can be calculated only in a very few cases, the reaction in the other cases being either too fast or too unreliable (Table 10).

Antiviral Activity of Polyflavonoids

Tannins are well known to have antimicrobial activity. This is logical as their capability to tan proteins means that they will complex irreversibly also with the protein in bacterial membranes, inhibiting any activity they might have. Thus, pharmaceutical containing tannins and aimed at curing bacterial intestinal infections have been around already for some time. Some studies on their anticaries effectiveness have also been conducted [49]. Independently from these, almost obvious, pharmaceutical applications of tannins several experimental studies on their use for other pharmaceutical/medical applications have been reported. Particularly well reported are the studies on their antitumor and anticancer activity [50-53]. More recently, work on their antiviral effectiveness has been investigated [54,55]. The data which follow in Tables 11-18 are the preliminary results obtained on the the antiviral activity of 12 different flavonoid and hydrolysable tannins which were carried out by the medical dept. of Leuven university [54,55].

Table 11. Tannins concentration required to protect CEM cells against the cytopathogenicity of HIV by 50 %

Anti-HIV-1 and -HIV-2 activity of the compounds		
in human T-lymphocyte (CEM) cells		
	EC_{50} (µg/ml)	EC_{50} (µg/ml)
Compound	HIV-1	HIV-2
1. Mimosa tannin	6.0 ± 0.0	>20
2. Mimosa tanin intermediate[33,56]	5.0 ± 1.4	>20
3. Chestnut tannin	1.4 ± 0.5	>20
4. Tara+Chestnut mix	5.0 ± 1.4	>20
5. Quebracho standard	6.5 ± 0.7	>20
6. Quebracho highly purified	7.5 ± 0.7	>20
7. Quebracho highly sulphited	7.0 ± 1.4	>20
8. Pecan nut tannin	5.0 ± 1.4	>20
9. Cube Gambier	9.0 ± 1.4	>20
10. Radiata Pine Tannin	7.0 ± 1.4	>20
11. Maritime Pine Tannin	7.5 ± 0.7	>20
12. Sumach Tannin	11.0 ± 1.4	>20
13. Spruce Tannin	>100	>100
EC_{50} = effective concentration or concentration required to protect CEM cells against the cytopathogenicity of HIV by 50 %		

Table 12. Cytotoxicity and antiviral activity of compounds in HEL cell cultures, Herpes and vesicular stomatitis viruses. Tannins added before virus administration

Cytotoxicity and antiviral activity of compounds in E_6SM cell cultures						
Compound	Minimum cytotoxic concentration[a] (µg/ml)	Minimum inhibitory concentration[b] (µg/ml)				
		Herpes simplex virus-1 (KOS)	Herpes simplex virus-2 (G)	Vaccinia virus	Vesicular stomatitis virus	Herpes simplex virus-1 TK⁻ KOS ACV[r]
1	200	40	16	16	>80	40
2	≥40	40	16	16	>80	40
3	≥40	40	16	16	>80	47
4	≥40	40	48	16	>80	47
5	40	47	36	16	>80	47
6	40	80	36	16	>80	47
7	≥40	40	40	16	>80	36
8	40	16	16	16	>80	36
9	8	>80	>80	>80	>80	>80
10	40	40	>80	16	>80	40
11	40	>80	>80	80	>80	47
12	40	36	36	16	>80	36
13	40	>16	>16	>16	>16	>16
Brivudin	>400	0.128	400	16	>400	>400
Ribavirin	>400	>400	>400	400	>400	>400
Acyclovir	>400	0.384	0.128	>400	>400	48
Ganciclovir	>100	0.0064	0.0064	100	>100	2.4

[a]Required to cause a microscopically detectable alteration of normal cell morphology.
[b]Required to reduce virus-induced cytopathogenicity by 50 %.

The results in Tables 11-18 evaluate both the effectiveness of 12 different tannins as measured by the Minimum Inhibitory Concentration (MIC) of the tannin required to reduce virus-induced cytopathogenicity by 50 %. The lower is the MIC value the better is the compound as an antiviral substance.

Equally important, the results in the tables measure the Minimum Cytotoxic Concentration (MCC) required to cause a microscopically detectable alteration of normal cell morphology. The higher the MCC the less toxic to the patient's cells is the compound and the better is the compound as an antiviral substance.

Thus, what is looked for is the lowest possible MIC and the highest possible MCC. These results are in vitro screening tests. A good results must be still translated into being effective by the carrier used to deliver it and the way the substance is delivered to the relevant site where it is needed. Nonetheless as these are very advanced results and they should be recorded , they are reported in full here. It is evident that different tannins can be very effective against different viruses, polyphenolic grouping being the cause of this behaviour. Most likely, they tan the proteins and they associate with the carbohydrates of the virus membrane. In all an effect similar to their well known association with hide proteins to give leather and with carbohydrates.

Table13. Cytotoxicity and antiviral activity of compounds in HEL cell cultures, vesicular stomatitis, Coxsackie and respiratory syncytial viruses

Cytotoxicity and antiviral activity of compounds in HeLa cell cultures				
Compound	Minimum cytotoxic concentration[a] (µg/ml)	Minimum inhibitory concentration[b] (µg/ml)		
		Vesicular Stomatitis virus	Coxsackie virus B4	Respiratory syncytial virus
1	400	>80	>80	12 +/-5
2	400	>80	>80	12 +/-5
3	400	>80	>80	43 +/-4
4	400	43.4 +/-4	>80	35 +/-7
5	400	>80	>80	40 +/-0.2
6	400	>80	>80	40 +/-0.2
7	400	>80	>80	43 +/-5
8	400	>80	>80	9 +/-1
9	400	>80	>80	>80
10	400	>80	>80	40 +/-0.2
11	400	>80	>80	40 +/-0.2
12	80	>16	>16	>16
13	≥80	>80	>80	>80
Brivudin	>400	>400	>400	>400
(S)-DHPA	>400	400	>400	>400
Ribavirin	>400	48	240	9.4

[a]Required to cause a microscopically detectable alteration of normal cell morphology.
[b]Required to reduce virus-induced cytopathogenicity by 50 %.

Table 14. Inhibitory effects of tannins on the proliferation of murine leukemia cells (L1210/0), murine mammary carcinoma cells (FM3A) and human T-lymphocyte cells (Molt4/C8, CEM/0)

Compound	IC50 (µg/ml)			
	L1210/0	FM3A/0	Molt4/C8	CEM/0
1	18 ± 0	153 ± 66	74 ± 18	58 ± 0
2	16 ± 1	148 ± 74	66 ± 27	61 ± 1
3	17 ± 0	141 ± 7	98 ± 22	65 ± 2
4	17 ± 0	114 ± 1	75 ± 57	56 ± 0
5	12 ± 4	76 ± 16	20 ± 1	51 ± 30
6	15 ± 2	79 ± 27	33 ± 21	45 ± 27
7	14 ± 2	82 ± 26	40 ± 27	55 ± 25
8	21 ± 6	≥ 200	81 ± 7	66 ± 11
9	13 ± 4	80 ± 22	17 ± 2	18 ± 1
10	65 ± 4	≥ 200	65 ± 28	71 ± 9
11	53 ± 23	≥ 200	94 ± 1	111 ± 40
12	17 ± 0	18 ± 1	17 ± 0	18 ± 2
13	49 ± 16	> 200	145 ± 78	83 ± 20

[a]50% inhibitory concentration.

Table 15. Cytotoxicity and antiviral activity of compounds in HEL cell cultures, influenza viruses

Cytotoxicity and antiviral activity of compounds in MDCK cell cultures							
Compound	Minimum cytotoxic concentration[a] (µg/ml)	EC_{50}					
		Influenza A H1N1		Influenza A H3N2		Influenza B	
		MTS		MTS		MTS	
1	100	3.3 +/-1.2		1.7 +/-1.3		2.3 +/-1.9	
2	100	2.2 +/-0.1		1.7 +/-0.6		2.3 +/-1.5	
3	100	4.0 +/-2.8		2.0 +/-0		1.4 +/-0.8	
4	33.3	4.1 +/-2.8		2.2 +/-0.8		1.4 +/-0.9	
5	100	1.7 +/-0.1		2.1 +/-0.4		3.5 +/-3.2	
6	100	5.4 +/-3.8		3.7 +/-1.6		3.6 +/-3.0	
7	100	4.4 +/-2.8		1.9 +/-0.4		3.4 +/-3.0	
8	33.3	2.1 +/-0.1		3.0 +/-1.5		1.8 +/-1.1	
9	100	5.5 +/-4.6		4.4 +/-3.6		2.7 +/-2.6	
10	100	4.2 +/-3.1		2.7 +/-1.0		2.7 +/-2.7	
11	100	2.9 +/-1.2		2.2 +/-0.3		1.5 +/-1.1	
12	20	2.0 +/-1.6		0.9 +/-0.2		2.6 +/-1.9	
13	100	9.9 +/-5.7		9.5 +/-4.8		1.9 +/-1.9	
Oseltamivir carboxylate (µM)	>100	0.05		0.65		10.65	
Ribavirin (µM)	60	4.55		6.32		9.07	
Amantadin (µM)	>100	21.39		0.78		>100	
Rimantadin (µM)	>100	18.45		0.05		>100	

[a]Required to cause a microscopically detectable alteration of normal cell morphology.
Compounds added prior to virus administration.

Table 16. Cytotoxicity and antiviral activity of compounds in HEL cell cultures, Corona viruses

	Feline CORONA	virus (FIPV)	Human Corona (SARS)	virus
	EC50 (µg/ml)	CC50 (µg/ml)	EC50 (µg/ml)	CC50 (µg/ml)
1	52 ± 19	> 100	> 100	> 100
2	67 ± 47	> 100	> 100	> 100
3	49 ± 17	> 100	> 100	> 100
4	43 ± 2	> 100	> 100	> 100
5	49 ± 10	☐ 100	44 ± 10	> 100
6	55 ± 19	> 100	49 ± 21	> 100
7	32 ± 1	> 100	40 ± 1	> 100
8	72 ± 40	> 100	> 100	> 100
9	☐100	> 100	> 100	> 100
10	20 ± 21	> 100	> 100	> 100
11	44 ± 5	> 100	56 ± 13	> 100
12	7.8 ± 8.0	81 ± 13	> 100	> 100
13	63 ± 32	> 100	> 100	> 100

Table 17. Cytotoxicity and antiviral activity of compounds in HEL cell cultures, Herpes and Vaccinia viruses. Tannins added after virus administration

Cytotoxicity and antiviral activity of compounds in HEL cell cultures						
Compound	Minimum cytotoxic concentration[a] (µg/ml)	Minimum inhibitory concentration[b] (µg/ml)				
		Herpes simplex virus-1 (KOS)	Herpes simplex virus-2 (G)	Vaccinia virus	Vesicular stomatitis virus	Herpes simplex virus-1 TK⁻ KOS ACV[r]
1	200	6 +/-2	1.8 +/-0.2	>40	>40	6 +/-2
2	200	4 +/-0	2 +/-1	8 +/-0	>40	4 +/-0
3	200	15 +/-1	3 +/-1	24 +/-1	>40	17 +/-3
4	200	15 +/-1	8 +/-0	24 +/-1	>40	20 +/-2
5	≥40	>40	>40	20 +/-2	>40	>40
6	≥40	>40	8 +/-0	>40	>40	>40
7	≥40	8 +/-0	>40	20 +/-2	>40	>40
8	40	4 +/-0	4 +/-0	8 +/-0	>8	4 +/-0
9	≥40	>40	>40	>40	>40	>40
10	40	8 +/-0	4 +/-0	8 +/-0	>8	>8
11	40	>8	8 +/-0	>8	>8	>8
12	40	>8	8 +/-0	>8	>8	>8
13	200	>40	>40	>40	>40	>40
Brivudin (µM)*	>250	0.016	10	6	>250	50
Ribavirin (µM)*	>250	250	50	30	50	250
Acyclovir (µM)*	>250	0.08	0.08	>250	>250	50
Ganciclovir (µM)*	>100	0.0064	0.032	>100	>100	12

Compounds added prior to virus administration.
[a]Required to cause a microscopically detectable alteration of normal cell morphology.
[b]Required to reduce virus-induced c ytopathogenicity by 50 %.
* Controls.

References

[1]   Pizzi A. Wood Adhesives Chemistry and Technology, Vol. 1. New York: Dekker, 1983.

[2]   Meikleham N, Pizzi A, Stephanou A. *J. Appl. Polymer Sci.* 1994; 54: 1827.

[3]   Pizzi A, Meikleham N, Stephanou A. *J. Appl. Polymer Sci.* 1995; 55: 929.

[4]   Pizzi A., Meikleham N. *J. Appl. Polymer Sci.* 1995; 55: 1265.

[5]   Merlin A, Pizzi A. J. Appl. Polymer Sci.. 1996; 59: 945.

[6]   Masson E, Merlin A, Pizzi A. *J. Appl. Polymer Sci..* 1996; 60: 263.

[7]   Masson E, Pizzi A, Merlin A. *J. Appl. Polymer Sci..* 1996; 60: 1655.

[8]   Masson E, Pizzi A, Merlin A. *J. Appl. Polymer Sci..* 1997; 64: 243.

[9]   Pizzi A, Meikleham N, Dombo B, Roll W. Holz Roh Werkstoff 1995; 53: 201.

[10]   Pizzi A. Advanced Wood Adhesives Technology. New York: Dekker, 1994.

[11]   Karas M, Bachmann D, Bahr U, Hillenkamp F. *Int. J. Mass Spectrom Ion. Proc.* 1987; 78: 53.

[12]   Bahr U, Deppe A, Karas M, Hillenkamp F, Giessmann U. *Anal. Chem.* 1992; 64: 2866.

[13]   Ehring H, Karas M, Hillenkamp F, *Org. Mass Spectrom.* 1992; 27: 472.

[14]   Danis PO, Karr DE, Mayer F, Holle A, Watson CH. *Org. Mass Spectrom.* 1992; 27: 843.

[15]   Danis PO, Karr DE. *Org. Mass Spectrom.* 1993; 28: 923.

[16]   Pasch H, Resch M. *GIT Fachz Lab.* 1996; 40: 90.

[17]   Pasch H, Gores F. *Polymer* 1995; 36: 1999.

[18]   Pizzi A, Stephanou A. *J. Appl. Polymer Sci..* 1994; 51: 2109.

[19]   Thompson D, Pizzi A. *J. Appl. Polymer Sci..* 1995; 55: 107.

[20]   Fechtal M, Riedl B. *Holzforschung* 1993; 47: 349.

[21]   Botha JJ, Ferreira D, Roux DG. J Chem Soc, *Chem. Commun.* 1978: 700.

[22]   Pizzi A, Cameron FA, Eaton NJ. *J. Macromol Sci. Chem. Ed.* 1986; A23(4): 515.

[23]   Rahim, AA. PhD thesis, University Sains Malaysia, Penang, Malaysia 2005.

[24]   Oo CW, Pizzi A, Pasch H, Kassim MJ, *J.Appl.Polymer Sci.,* 2008, 109(2): 963-967.

[25]   Oo, CW PhD thesis, University of sains Malaysia, Penang, Malaysia 2008.

[26]   Rahim, AA, Rocca E, Steinmetz J, Kassim M J, Adnan R, Sani Ibrahim M. *Corrosion Science* 2007, 49, 402.

[27]   Pizzi A and Stephanou A, *J.Appl.Polymer Sci.,* 1994, 51: 2125-2130.

[28]   Colleri L. Le Fabbriche Italiane di Estratto di Castagno; Milanostampa S.p.A.: Farigliano (CN), Italy, 1989.

[29]   Kim, S.R.; Saratchandra, D.; Mainwaring, D.E. *J. Appl. Polym Sci.* 1995, 56, 905.

[30]   Kim, S.R.; Saratchandra, D.; Mainwaring, D.E. *J. Appl. Polym Sci.* 1995, 56, 915.

[31]   Kim, S.R.; Mainwaring, D.E. *Holzforschung* 1996, 50, 42.

[32]   Garnier, S.; Pizzi, A.; Vorster, O.C.; Halasz, L. J.Appl.Polymer Sci., 2001, 81(7): 1634-1642.

[33]   Pasch, H.; Pizzi, A.; Rode, K. Polymer, 2001, 42, 7531.

[34]   Pizzi, A. *Forest Prod. J.* 1978, 28(12), 42.

[35]   Pizzi, A.; Meikleham, N.; Stephanou, A. *J. Appl. Polym Sci.* 1995, 55, 929.

[36]   Pizzi, A.; Vogel, M.C. *J. Macromol. Sci. Chem. Ed* 1983, A19(2), 369.

[37]   Masson, E.; Merlin, A.; Pizzi, A. *J. Appl. Polym Sci.* 1996, 60, 263.

[38] Masson, E.; Pizzi, A.; Merlin, A. *J. Appl. Polym Sci.* 1996, 60, 1655.

[39] Masson, E.; Pizzi, A.; Merlin, A. *J. Appl. Polym Sci.* 1997, 64, 243.

[40] Roux, D.G. in Mimosa Extract, LIRI Leather Industries Research Inst.: Grahamstown, South Africa, 1965, pages 33-51.

[41] Pizzi, A. Advanced Wood Adhesives Technology, Marcel Dekker: New York, 1994.

[42] Allcock, H.R. and Lampe, F.W., 1990, Contemporary Polymer Chemistry, Prentice Hall,New Jersey.

[43] Seymour; R.B. and Carraher, C.E., 1992, Polymer Chemistry, an introduction, Dekker, New York.

[44] Martin, F., 1995, Ph.D. thesis, University of Nancy 1, Vandoeuvre, France.

[45] Noferi, M.; Masson, E.; Merlin, A.; Pizzi, A. and Deglise, X. *J. Appl. Polymer Sci.*, 1997, 63, 475-482.

[46] Merlin, A. and Pizzi, A., *J. Appl. Polymer Sci.*, 1996, 59: 945-952.

[47] Jensen, O.H. and Pedersen, J.A., *Tetrahedron,* 1983, 39, 1609.

[48] Pizzi, A. and Stephanou, A., *J. Appl. Polymer Sci.*, 1993, 50, 2105.

[49] Mitsunaga, T. in Plant Polyphenols 2 – (G.G.Gross, R.W.Hemingway, T.Yoshida Eds.), Kluwer Academic/Plenum Publishers, New York, pp. 555-574, 1999.

[50] L.-L.Yang, L.-L., Wang, C.-C., Yen, K.-Y., Yoshida, T., Hatano, T., Okuda, T., in Plant Polyphenols 2 – (G.G.Gross, R.W.Hemingway, T.Yoshida Eds.), Kluwer Academic/Plenum Publishers, New York, pp. 615-628, 1999.

[51] Nakamura, Y., Matsuda, M., Honma, T., Tomita, I., Shibata, N., Warashina, T., Noro, T., Hara, Y. in Plant Polyphenols 2 – (G.G.Gross, R.W.Hemingway, T.Yoshida Eds.), Kluwer Academic/Plenum Publishers, New York, pp. 629-642, 1999.

[52] Miyamoto, K., Murayama, T., Hatano, T., Yoshida, T., Okuda, T. in Plant Polyphenols 2 – (G.G.Gross, R.W.Hemingway, T.Yoshida Eds.), Kluwer Academic/Plenum Publishers, New York, pp. 643-664, 1999.

[53] Noro, T., Ohki, T., Noda, Y., Warashina, T., Noro, K., Tomita, I., Nakamura, Y. in Plant Polyphenols 2 – (G.G.Gross, R.W.Hemingway, T.Yoshida Eds.), Kluwer Academic/Plenum Publishers, New York, pp. 665-674, 1999.

[54] Balzarini, J., Persoons, L., Absillis, A., Van Berckelaer, L., Pizzi, A. Rijk Universiteit Leuven, Belgium and University of Nancy 1, France, unpublished results (2006).

[55] Pizzi, A., Tannins: major sources, properties and applications, Chapter 8 in Monomers, Polymers and Composites from Renewable Resources (M.N.Belgacem and A.Gandini Eds.), Elsevier, Amsterdam (2008), pp179 – 199.

[56] Pizzi, A., Stephanou, A. *Holzforschung Holzverwertung*, 1992, 44(4): 62-68

In: Encyclopedia of Vitamin Research
Editor: Joshua T. Mayer

ISBN: 978-1-61761-928-1
© 2011 Nova Science Publishers, Inc.

Chapter 41

Grapefruit Flavonoids: Naringin and Naringinin[*]

Ricky W. K. Wong[†] and A. Bakr M. Rabie

Biomedical and Tissue Engineering, the University of Hong Kong

Abstract

Naringin is the flavonoid compound found in grapefruit that gives grapefruit its characteristic bitter flavor. Grapefruit processors attempt to select fruits with a low naringin content, and often blend juices obtained from different grapefruit varieties to obtain the desired degree of bitterness. Naringin is believed to enhance our perception of taste by stimulating the taste buds; some people consume a small amount of grapefruit juice before a meal for this reason.

Naringin and its aglycone naringinin are commonly used health supplements; they exert a variety of biological actions. This article attempts to review their pharmacokinetics and pharmacological actions from scientific publications up to November 2008 including effects on the cardiovascular system, on the skeletal system, on smooth muscle, on the gastric intestinal system, on the endocrine system, also effects against tumours, protection against toxins in chemotherapy drugs and the environment, antioxidant effects, drug interactions, anti-inflammatory effects, and the newly discovered osteogenic and antibacterial actions.

Keywords: Naringin, Narginenin, antioxidant effect, drug interactions, osteogenic effect, antibacterial effect, anti-inflammatory effect.

---

[*] A version of this chapter was also published in *Flavonoids: Biosynthesis, Biological Effects and Dietary Sources, edited by Raymond B. Keller* published by Nova Science Publishers, Inc. It was submitted for appropriate modifications in an effort to encourage wider dissemination of research.

[†] Tel: 852-28590554; Fax: 852-25593803; E-mail: fyoung@hkucc.hku.hk

Introduction

Naringin is the flavonoid compound found in grapefruit that gives grapefruit its characteristic bitter flavor. Grapefruit processors attempt to select fruits with a low naringin content, and often blend juices obtained from different grapefruit varieties to obtain the desired degree of bitterness. Naringin is believed to enhance our perception of taste by stimulating the taste buds (some people consume a small amount of grapefruit juice before a meal for this reason). Naringin may be instrumental in inhibiting cancer-causing compounds and thus may have potential chemotherapeutic value. Studies have also shown that naringin interferes with enzymatic activity in the intestines and, thus, with the breakdown of certain drugs, resulting in higher blood levels of the drug. A number of drugs that are known to be affected by the naringin in grapefruit include calcium channel blockers, estrogen, sedatives, medications for high blood pressure, allergies, AIDS, and cholesterol-lowering drugs. Caffeine levels and effects of caffeine may also be extended by consuming grapefruit or grapefruit juice. While the effect of naringin on the metabolism of a drug can increase the drug's effectiveness, it can also result in dosages that are inadvertently too high. Therefore, it's best not to take any drugs with grapefruit juice unless the interaction with the drug is known. In addition, the effects of drinking grapefruit juice is cumulative, which means that if you drank a glass of grapefruit juice daily with your medication for a week, the drug interaction would be stronger at the end of the week than at the beginning.

Research on naringin and naringinin shows the following effects:

(A) Effects on cardiovascular system

Reference	Robbins et al., 1988
Study	The effect on hematocrits of adding grapefruit to the daily diet was determined using 36 human subjects (12 F, 24 M) over a 42-day study.
Results	The effect on hematocrits of adding grapefruit to the daily diet was determined using 36 human subjects (12 F, 24 M) over a 42-day study.
Conclusion	Ingestion of grapefruit lowers elevated hematocrits in human subjects.

Reference	Bok et al., 1999
Study	The cholesterol-lowering effects of tangerine peel extract and a mixture of two citrus flavonoids were tested.
Results	The inhibition of HMG-CoA reductase and ACAT activities resulting from either tangerine-peel extract or its bioflavonoids could account for the decrease in fecal neutral sterol.
Conclusion	Plasma and hepatic cholesterol and hepatic activities of 3-hydroxy-3-methyl-glutaryl-CoA (HMG-CoA) reductase and acyl CoA: cholesterol transferase (ACAT) are lower in rats fed citrus peel extract or a mixture of citrus bioflavonoids.

Reference	Shin et al., 1999
Study	The effects of the citrus bioflavonoid naringin were tested by using it as a supplement in a high-cholesterol diet.
Results	The combination of the inhibited HMG-CoA reductase (-24.4%) and ACAT (-20.2%) activities as a result of naringin supplementation could account for the decrease of fecal neutral sterols.
Conclusion	Hypocholesterolemic effect of naringin associated with hepatic cholesterol regulating enzyme changes in rats.

Reference	Lee et al., 2001
Study	The anti-atherogenic effects of the citrus flavonoids, naringin and naringenin, were evaluated in high cholesterol-fed rabbits.
Results	The anti-atherogenic effect of the citrus flavonoids, naringin and naringenin, is involved with a decreased hepatic ACAT activity and with the downregulation of VCAM-1 and MCP-1 gene expression.
Conclusion	Anti-atherogenic effect of citrus flavonoids, naringin and naringenin.

Reference	Choi et al., 2001
Study	The interactive effect of naringin and vitamin E was studied with respect to cholesterol metabolism and antioxidant status in high-cholesterol-fed rats.
Results	Naringin lowers the plasma lipid concentrations when the dietary vitamin E level is low. The HMG-CoA reductase-inhibitory effect of naringin was more potent when dietary vitamin E was at a normal level.
Conclusion	Interactive effect of naringin and vitamin E on cholesterol biosynthesis.

Reference	Choe et al., 2001
Study	This study evaluated the effect of naringin on blood lipid levels and aortic fatty streaks, and its action mechanism in hypercholesterolemic rabbits.
Results	Naringin treatment inhibited hypercholesterolemia-induced intercellular adhesion molecule-1 (ICAM-1) expression on endothelial cells. Hypercholesterolemia caused fatty liver and elevation of liver enzymes, which was prevented by naringin but not by lovastatin.
Conclusion	Naringin has an antiatherogenic effect with the inhibition of intercellular adhesion molecule-1 in hypercholesterolemic rabbits.

Reference	da Silva et al., 2001
Study	The effect of naringin and rutin on the metabolism lipidic of chicks hypercholesterolemic was evaluated.
Results	Naringin and rutin reduced the levels of total cholesterol significantly, cholesterol-LDL, cholesterol-VLDL and triglycerols, not presenting, however, reductions in the levels of cholesterol-HDL.
Conclusion	Hypocholesterolemic effect of naringin and rutin flavonoids

Reference	Naderi et al., 2003
Study	The susceptibility of LDL to in vitro oxidation was assessed. LDL oxidation were monitored by change in 234-absorbance in the presence and absence of pure flavonoids.
Results	Genistein, morin and naringin have stronger inhibitory activity against LDL oxidation than biochanin A or apigenin.
Conclusion	Flavonoids prevent in vitro LDL oxidation and probably would be important to prevent atherosclerosis.

Reference	Jung et al., 2003
Study	The effect of naringin on hypercholesterolemic subjects was studied. A hypercholesterolemic group (n=30) and healthy control group (n=30) were established.
Results	Naringin supplementation was found to lower the plasma total cholesterol by 14% and low-density lipoprotein cholesterol concentrations by 17%, apolipoprotein B levels were significantly lowered, erythrocyte superoxide dismutase and catalase activities were significantly increased.
Conclusion	Naringin may play an important role in lowering plasma cholesterol and regulating the antioxidant capacity in hypercholesterolemic subjects.

Reference	Kim et al., 2004
Study	The lipid lowering and antioxidant capacity of naringin was evaluated in LDL receptor knockout (LDLR-KO) mice fed a cholesterol (0.1 g/100 g) diet.
Results	The hepatic HMG-CoA reductase activity was significantly lower in the naringin and lovastatin supplemented groups than in the control group, the superoxide dismutase, catalase, and glutathione reductase activities were all significantly higher in the naringin-supplemented group than in the control group.

| Conclusion | Naringin lowers the plasma cholesterol level via the inhibition of hepatic HMG-CoA reductase activity and improve the activities of hepatic antioxidant enzymes against oxidative stress. |

Reference	Chiou and Xu, 2004
Study	Effects of flavonoids to improve retinal function recovery after ischemic insult were studied. Electroretinography was used to measure the b-wave recovery as an indication of retinal function recovery.
Results	Naringenin, hesperetin, and rutin were found to produce marked positive effects on b-wave recovery, whereas naringin, hesperidin, and quercetin showed poor recovery of b-wave after ischemic insult of the retina.
Conclusion	Flavonoids that showed strong increase of ocular blood flow also showed marked increase of retinal function recovery.

Reference	Singh and Chopra, 2004
Study	The protective effect of naringin against the damage inflicted by ROS during renal I/R was investigated in Sprague-Dawley rats using histopathological and biochemical parameters.
Results	Pretreatment of animals with naringin markedly attenuated renal dysfunction, morphological alterations, reduced elevated TBARS levels and restored the depleted renal antioxidant enzymes.
Conclusion	Reactive oxygen species (ROS) play a causal role in renal ischemia/reperfusion (I/R) induced renal injury and naringin exert renoprotective effects probably by the radical scavenging and antioxidant activities.

Reference	Jeon et al., 2004
Study	To confirm the hypocholesterolemic role of naringin, male rabbits were fed 0.5% high-cholesterol diet or high-cholesterol diet supplemented with either 0.05% naringin or 0.03% lovastatin for 8 weeks.
Results	The naringin and lovastatin supplements significantly lowered plasma total- and LDL-cholesterol and hepatic lipids levels, while significantly increasing HDL-C/total-C ratio compared to the control group.
Conclusion	Both naringin and lovastatin contributed to hypocholesterolemic action. Naringin seemed to preserve tissue morphology from damages induced by high cholesterol diet.

Reference	Orallo et al., 2005
Study	The potential vasorelaxant, antioxidant and cyclic nucleotide PDE inhibitory effects of the citrus-fruit flavonoids naringin and (+/-)-naringenin were comparatively studied.
Results	(+/-)-naringenin relaxed, in a concentration-dependent manner, the contractions elicited by phenylephrine (PHE, 1 microM) or by a high extracellular KCl concentration (60 mM) in intact rat aortic rings.
Conclusion	The vasorelaxant effects of (+/-)-naringenin seem to be basically related to the inhibition of phosphodiesterase (PDE)1, PDE4 and PDE5 activities.

Reference	Reshef et al., 2005
Study	Patients with stage I hypertension, the antihypertensive effect of juice of the so-called sweetie fruit (a hybrid between grapefruit and pummelo) with and without high flavonoid content were studied.
Results	The high-flavonoid (HF) sweetie juice was more effective than LF sweetie juice in reducing diastolic blood pressure.
Conclusion	The active ingredients associated with the antihypertensive effect of sweetie juice are the flavonoids naringin and narirutin.

Reference	Jung et al., 2006
Study	The effect of the flavonoids hesperidin and naringin on glucose and lipid regulation in C57BL/KsJ-db/db mice was studied.
Results	Hesperidin and naringin effectively lowered the plasma free fatty acid and plasma and hepatic triglyceride levels, and simultaneously reduced the hepatic fatty acid oxidation and carnitine palmitoyl transferase activity.
Conclusion	Hesperidin and naringin are beneficial for improving hyperlipidemia and hyperglycemia in type-2 diabetic animals.

Reference	Rajadurai and Prince, 2006
Study	The preventive effect of naringin in isoproterenol (ISO)-induced myocardial infarction (MI) in rats was studied.
Results	Pretreatment with naringin significantly decreased the levels of total, ester, and free cholesterol, triglycerides, and free fatty acids in serum and heart and increased phospholipids in heart.
Conclusion	Naringin has a lipid-lowering effect in ISO-induced MI rats.

Reference	Rajadurai and Prince, 2006
Study	The cardioprotective potential of naringin on lipid peroxides, enzymatic and nonenzymatic antioxidants and histopathological findings in isoproterenol (ISO)-induced myocardial infarction (MI) in rats were evaluated.
Results	Oral administration of naringin to ISO-induced rats showed a significant decrease in the levels of lipid peroxidative products and improved the antioxidant status. Histopathological findings of the myocardial tissue showed the protective role of naringin in ISO-induced rats.
Conclusion	Naringin possess anti-lipoperoxidative and antioxidant activity in experimentally induced cardiac toxicity.

Reference	Rajadurai and Prince, 2007
Study	The preventive role of naringin on cardiac troponin T (cTnT), lactate dehydrogenase (LDH)-isoenzyme, cardiac marker enzymes, electrocardiographic (ECG)-patterns and lysosomal enzymes in isoproterenol (ISO)-induced myocardial infarction (MI) in male Wistar rats were investigated.
Results	Pretreatment with naringin positively altered the levels of cTnT, intensity of the bands of the LDH1 and LDH2-isoenzyme and the activities of cardiac marker enzymes, ECG-patterns and lysosomal hydrolases in ISO-induced rats.
Conclusion	Naringin possess cardioprotective effect in ISO-induced MI in rats.

Reference	Kim et al., 2006
Study	Naringin was investigated for its differential effects on hepatic cholesterol regulation when supplemented for 3 weeks and 6 weeks in Sprague-Dawley rats.
Results	Supplementation with naringin did not exhibit a hypolipidemic effect when given with a HFHC diet. Naringin can, however, be beneficial for lowering hepatic cholesterol biosynthesis and levels of plasma lipids in this animal model.
Conclusion	Naringin time-dependently lowers hepatic cholesterol biosynthesis and plasma cholesterol in rats fed high-fat and high-cholesterol diet.

Reference	Rajadurai and Prince, 2007
Study	The preventive role of naringin on heart weight, blood glucose, total proteins, albumin/globulin (A/G) ratio, serum uric acid, serum iron, plasma iron binding capacity and membrane bound enzymes and glycoproteins such as hexose, hexosamine, fucose and sialic acid in isoproterenol (ISO)-induced myocardial infarction (MI) in rats and in vitro free radical scavenging assay were studied. The preventive role of naringin on mitochondrial enzymes in isoproterenol (ISO)-induced myocardial infarction in male albino Wistar rats was studied.
Results	Pretreatment with naringin exhibited a significant effect and altered these biochemical parameters positively in ISO-induced rats. Naringin also scavenges. 1,1-diphenyl-2-picrylhydrazyl,2,2'-azinobis-(3-ethyl-benzothiazoline-6-sulfonic acid) and nitric oxide radicals in vitro. Oral pretreatment with naringin to ISO-induced rats daily for a period of 56 days significantly minimized the alterations in all the biochemical parameters and restored the normal mitochondrial function. Transmission electron microscopic observations also correlated with these biochemical findings.
Conclusion	Naringin has cardioprotective role in ISO-induced MI in rats

Reference	Morikawa et al., 2008
Study	The effect of some flavanones on the adipocytic conversion of the human preadipocyte cell line, AML-I.
Results	Among four structure-related flavanones including naringenin, naringenin-7-rhamnoglucoside (naringin), hesperetin, and hesperetin-7-rhamnoglucoside (hesperidin), the aglycones such as naringenin and hesperetin exhibited the growth arrest of AML-I cells.
Conclusion	Apoptosis by flavanones does not inhibit the adipocytic conversion of AML-I preadipocytes.

Reference	Lee et al., 2008
Study	The exact molecular mechanisms underlying the roles of integrated cell cycle regulation and MAPK signaling pathways in the regulation of naringin-induced inhibition of cell proliferation in vascular smooth muscle cells (VSMCs)
Results	Naringin treatment resulted in significant growth inhibition and G(1)-phase cell cycle arrest mediated by induction of p53-independent p21WAF1 expression; expression of cyclins and CDKs in VSMCs was also down-regulated.
Conclusion	The Ras/Raf/ERK pathway participates in p21WAF1 induction, leading to a decrease in cyclin D1/CDK4 and cyclin E/CDK2 complexes and in naringin-dependent inhibition of cell growth. These novel and unexpected findings provide a theoretical basis for preventive use of flavonoids to the atherosclerosis disease.

Reference	Rajadurai and Prince, 2008
Study	To evaluate the preventive role of naringin on mitochondrial lipid peroxides, antioxidants and lipids in isoproterenol (ISO)-induced myocardial infarction (MI) in male Wistar rats.
Results	Oral pretreatment with naringin (10, 20 and 40 mg/kg) to ISO-induced rats daily for a period of 56 days significantly decreased the levels of mitochondrial lipid peroxides with a significant increase in the activities/levels of mitochondrial antioxidants and significantly minimized the alterations in the mitochondrial lipid levels in ISO-induced rats.
Conclusion	Naringin prevents alterations in mitochondrial lipid peroxides, antioxidants and lipids in ISO-induced MI in rats.

(B) Effects on skeletal system

Reference	Wood, 2004
Study	The influence of dietary bioflavonoid (rutin [R], quercetin [Q], and naringin [N]) supplementation on physiological molar crestal alveolar bone(CAB)-cemento-enamel junction (CEJ) distances in young male albino rats was studied.
Results	The N group demonstrated the lowest CAB-CEJ distance, followed by the R and Q groups (P <.001-.05), except in the mandibular lingual region, where the Q group had a lower CAB-CEJ distance than the N and R groups (P <.05). The control group showed the largest CAB-CEJ distances.
Conclusion	Rutin, quercetin, and naringin supplementation reduce molar crestal alveolar bone-cemento-enamel junction distance in young rats.

Reference	Wong and Rabie, 2006
Study	The amount of new bone produced by naringin in collagen matrix to that produced by bone grafts and collagen matrix in rabbits was compared.
Results	A total of 284% and 490% more new bone was present in defects grafted with naringin in collagen matrix than those grafted with bone and collagen, respectively.
Conclusion	Naringin in collagen matrix have the effect of increasing new bone formation locally and can be used as a bone graft material.

Reference	Wong and Rabie, 2006
Study	The effect of naringin, which was also a HMG-CoA reductase inhibitor, was studied in UMR 106 osteoblastic cell line in vitro.
Results	Naringin significantly increased bone cell activities in vitro.
Conclusion	Besides statin, this provided another example of HMG-CoA reductase inhibition that increases the bone cell activities

Reference	Li et al., 2006
Study	The osteoblastic activity of extracts of Drynaria fortunei (Kunze) J. Sm. rhizome was assayed in the UMR106 cell line cultured in vitro.
Results	The ethanol extract, and its ethyl acetate and n-butanol fractions exhibited stimulating activity.
Conclusion	Two active constituents were isolated and identified as naringin and neoeriocitrin.

Reference	Wei et al., 2007
Study	A retinoic acid-induced osteoporosis model of rats was used to assess whether naringin has similar bioactivity against osteoporosis in vitro.
Results	A blood test showed that naringin-treated rats experienced significantly lower activity of serum alkaline phosphatase and had higher femur bone mineral density, compared to untreated rats.
Conclusion	These outcomes suggest that naringin offer a potential in the management of osteoporosis in vitro.

Reference	Mandadi et al., 2008
Study	Effects of feeding citrus bioactive compounds and crude extract on bone quality in orchidectomized rats were evaluated.
Results	The citrus crude extract or the purified bioactive compounds increased ($p<0.05$) the plasma antioxidant status, plasma IGF-I, and bone density, preserved ($p<0.05$) the concentration of calcium in the femur and in the 5th lumbar, and numerically improved bone strength.
Conclusion	Potential benefit of the citrus crude extract and its bioactive compounds on bone quality appears to preserve bone calcium concentration and increase antioxidant status.

Reference	Wu et al., 2008
Study	Naringin was shown to enhance alkaline phosphatase activity, osteocalcin level, osteopontin synthesis and cell proliferation in primary cultured osteoblasts.
Results	Naringin increased mRNA and protein levels of BMP-2 using Western blot, ELISA and RT-PCR assay, also prevented the decreasing of BMP-2 and bone loss inducing by ovariectomy in vivo.
Conclusion	Naringin increase BMP-2 expression and enhance osteogenic response via the phosphoinositide 3-kinase (PI3K), Akt, c-Fos/c-Jun and AP-1-dependent signaling pathway.

(C) Effects on smooth muscle

Reference	Herrera and Marhuenda, 1993
Study	Effect of naringin and naringenin on contractions induced by noradrenaline in rat vas deferens was studied.
Results	Naringin significantly increased contractions induced by noradrenaline in rat vas deferens. Naringenin increased the contractile effect of noradrenaline and was dose dependent.
Conclusion	Naringin and naringinin increased contractions induced by noradrenaline in rat vas deferens.

Reference	
Study	The potency, structure-activity relationship, and mechanism of vasorelaxation of flavonols: fisetin, rutin, quercetin; flavones: chrysin, flavone, baicalein; flavanones: naringenin, naringin; isoflavones: diadzein and flavanes: epigallo catechin gallate, were examined in the isolated rat aorta.
Results	Most of the flavonoids tested showed concentration dependent relaxant effects against K+ (80 mM) and phenylephrine (PE, 0.1 microM)-induced contractions with a greater inhibition of the responses to the alpha1-adrenoceptor agonist.
Conclusion	Relaxant effects of flavonoids on vascular smooth muscle of the isolated rat thoracic aorta.

Reference	Saponara et al., 2006
Study	The mechanical and electrophysiological effects of (+/-)-naringenin were investigated In vascular smooth muscle cells.
Results	(+/-)-Naringenin induced concentration-dependent relaxation in endothelium-denuded rat aortic rings.
Conclusion	The vasorelaxant effect of the naturally-occurring flavonoid (+/-)-naringenin on endothelium-denuded vessels was due to the activation of BK (Ca) channels in myocytes.

(D) Effects on gastric intestinal system

Reference	Parmar, 1983
Study	The gastric anti-ulcer activity of a specific histidine decarboxylase inhibitor naringenin, has been studied on the various types of ulcers experimentally induced in rats, viz., pylorus-ligated (Shay method) and restraint ulcers, and on the gastric mucosal damage induced by aspirin, phenylbutazone or reserpine.
Results	Naringenin possessed significant anti-ulcer activity in all these models, manifesting a dose-dependent anti-ulcer effect.
Conclusion	Naringenin, a specific histidine decarboxylase inhibitor, has gastric anti-ulcer activity.

Reference	Martín et al., 1994
Study	To determine the gastroprotective properties of naringin on and the involvement of endogenous prostaglandins in mucosal injury produced by absolute ethanol.
Results	Oral pretreatment with the highest dose of naringin (400 mg/kg), 60 min before absolute ethanol was the most effective antiulcer treatment.
Conclusion	Naringin has a 'cytoprotective' effect against ethanol injury in the rat, but this property appears to be mediated by non-prostaglandin-dependent mechanisms.

Reference	Fenton and Hord, 2004
Study	Whether specific flavonoids induce cell migration in colon epithelial cells either wild type or heterozygous for Apc genotype was studied.
Results	Naringin and hesperidin induced the greatest migratory response in IMCE cells at 1 microM and induced migration greater than untreated control cells.
Conclusion	Flavonoids promote cell migration in nontumorigenic colon epithelial cells differing in Apc genotype.

(E) Effects on endocrine system

Reference	Divi and Doerge, 1996
Study	A structure-activity study of 13 commonly consumed flavonoids was conducted to evaluate inhibition of thyroid peroxidase (TPO), the enzyme that catalyzes thyroid hormone biosynthesis.
Results	Inhibition by the more potent fisetin, kaempferol, naringenin, and quercetin, was consistent with mechanism-based inactivation of TPO as previously observed for resorcinol and derivatives. Myricetin and naringin inhibited TPO by different mechanisms.
Conclusion	Dietary flavonoids inhibit thyroid peroxidase.

Reference	Déchaud et al., 1999
Study	This study reports on some environmental chemicals with estrogenic activity (xenoestrogens) and their binding interaction for human plasma sex-hormone binding globulin (hSHBG).
Results	The flavonoid phytoestrogens genistein and naringenin were also identified as hSHBG ligands, whereas their glucoside derivatives, genistin and naringin, had no binding activity for hSHBG.
Conclusion	Naringinin interacts with human sex hormone-binding globulin.

Reference	Asgary et al., 2002
Study	Several flavonoids, such as rutin, kaempferol, quercetin, apigenin, naringin, morin and biochanin A were selected to determine their antioxidant effects on in vitro insulin, hemoglobin and albumin glycosylation.
Results	Biochanin A, the best inhibitor of insulin and hemoglobin glycosylation, inhibits their glycosylation 100% and 60%, respectively. Glycosylation of albumin was inhibited 100% by both biochanin A and apigenin.
Conclusion	Plants containing flavonoids may have preventive effects in diabetic complications.

Reference	Jung et al., 2004
Study	The effect of citrus bioflavonoids on blood glucose level, hepatic glucose-regulating enzymes activities, hepatic glycogen concentration, and plasma insulin levels was studied, and assessed the relations between plasma leptin and body weight, blood glucose, and plasma insulin.
Results	Hesperidin and naringin supplementation significantly reduced blood glucose compared with the control group. Naringin also markedly lowered the activity of hepatic glucose-6-phosphatase and phosphoenolpyruvate carboxykinase compared with the control group.
Conclusion	Hesperidin and naringin prevent the progression of hyperglycemia, by increasing hepatic glycolysis and glycogen concentration and/or by lowering hepatic gluconeogenesis.

Reference	Ali and El Kader, 2004
Study	The effect of various doses of naringin was studied on streptozotocin (STZ)-induced hyperglycaemic rats to evaluate the possible hypoglycaemic and antioxidant activity of naringin in diabetes.
Results	Exogenous administration of naringin to hyperglycaemic rats causes a dose-dependent decrease of the glucose level, an increase of the insulin concentration, a decrease of the H_2O_2 and TBARS levels, as well as the increase of the total antioxidant status.
Conclusion	Naringin provided a significant amelioration of hypoglycaemic and antioxidant activity in STZ-induced diabetic rats.

Reference	Li et al., 2006
Study	Using purified intestinal brush border membrane vesicles and everted intestinal sleeves, glucose uptake in intestine was studied with naringinin and naringin.
Results	Naringenin, but not naringin, significantly inhibited glucose uptake in the intestine.
Conclusion	Inhibition of intestinal glucose uptake and renal glucose reabsorption explains, the antihyperglycemic action of naringenin and its derivatives.

Reference	Punithavathi et al., 2008
Study	The combined protective role of low dose of naringin (15 mg kg(-1)) and vitamin C (25 mg kg(-1)) and high dose of naringin (30 mg kg(-1)) and vitamin C (50 mg kg(-1)) on streptozotocin (STZ)-induced toxicity was studied in male Wistar rats.
Results	Oral administration of high doses of naringin (30 mg kg(-1)) and vitamin C (50 mg kg(-1)) to diabetic rats for a period of 21 days normalized all the above-mentioned biochemical parameters.
Conclusion	The antihyperglycemic and antioxidant effects of naringin and vitamin C in STZ-induced type II diabetes mellitus in rats.

(F) Effects against tumour

Reference	So et al., 1996
Study	Two citrus flavonoids, hesperetin and naringenin, and four noncitrus flavonoids, baicalein, galangin, genistein, and quercetin, were tested singly and in one-to-one combinations for their effects on proliferation and growth of a human breast carcinoma cell line, MDA-MB-435. These compounds, were tested for their ability to inhibit development of mammary tumors in female Sprague-Dawley rats.
Results	IC50 values for the one-to-one combinations ranged from 4.7 micrograms/ml (quercetin + hesperetin, quercetin + naringenin) to 22.5 micrograms/ml (naringenin + hesperetin). Rats given orange juice had a smaller tumor burden than controls, although they grew better than any of the other groups.
Conclusion	Citrus flavonoids are effective inhibitors of human breast cancer cell proliferation in vitro, especially when paired with quercetin.

Reference	Calomme et al., 1996
Study	The antimutagenicity of the Citrus flavonoids naringin, hesperidin, nobiletin, and tangeretin against the mutagens benzo[a]pyrene, 2-aminofluorene, quercetin, and nitroquinoline N-oxide was investigated in the Salmonella/microsome assay.
Results	Naringin and hesperidin showed a weak antimutagenic activity against benzo[a]pyrene.
Conclusion	The antimutagenic properties the Citrus flavonoids, especially tangeretin and nobiletin, might prevent cancer.

Reference	Le Marchand et al., 2000
Study	To investigate the possible relationship between intake of flavonoids-powerful dietary antioxidants that may also inhibit P450 enzymes-and lung cancer risk, we conducted a population-based, case-control study in Hawaii.
Results	Authors found statistically significant inverse associations between lung cancer risk and the main food sources of the flavonoids quercetin (onions and apples) and naringin (white grapefruit).
Conclusion	Foods rich in certain flavonoids may protect against certain forms of lung cancer. Decreased bioactivation of carcinogens by inhibition of CYP1A1 should be explored.

Reference	Russo et al., 2000
Study	Authors investigated the free-radical scavenging capacity of bioflavonoids (rutin, catechin, and naringin) and the effects of these polyphenols on xanthine oxidase activity, spontaneous lipid peroxidation, and DNA cleavage.
Results	The bioflavonoids under examination showed a dose-dependent free-radical scavenging effect, a significant inhibition of xanthine oxidase activity, and an antilipoperoxidative capacity. In addition, they showed a protective effect on DNA cleavage.
Conclusion	Bioflavonoids as antiradicals, antioxidants and DNA cleavage protectors.

Reference	Kanno et al., 2005
Study	The effect of naringenin on tumor growth in various human cancer cell lines and sarcoma S-180-implanted mice was studied.
Results	Naringenin inhibited tumor growth in sarcoma S-180-implanted mice, following intraperitoneal or peroral injection once a day for 5 d. Naringin also inhibited tumor growth by peroral injection but not intraperitoneal injection.
Conclusion	Inhibitory effects of naringenin on tumor growth in human cancer cell lines and sarcoma S-180-implanted mice.

Reference	Ugocsai et al., 2005
Study	The effects of various flavonoids and carotenoids on Rhodamine 123 accumulation in MDR Colo 320 human colon cancer cells expressing MDR1/LRP were studied. The Colo 205 cell line was used as a drug-sensitive control.
Results	Catechin, Neohesperidin, Naringin, Robinin, Phloridzin, Dihydrobinetin and Sakuranetin, had only marginal effects on Rhodamine 123 accumulation.
Conclusion	The tested flavonoids were weak apoptosis inducers on multidrug-resistant (MDR) and parent cells.

Reference	Vanamala et al., 2006
Study	The hypothesis that untreated and irradiated grapefruit as well as the isolated citrus compounds naringin and limonin would protect against azoxymethane (AOM)-induced aberrant crypt foci (ACF) by suppressing proliferation and elevating apoptosis through anti-inflammatory activities was examined.
Results	Lower levels of iNOS and COX-2 are associated with suppression of proliferation and upregulation of apoptosis, which may have contributed to a decrease in the number of high multiplicity ACF in rats provided with untreated grapefruit and limonin.
Conclusion	Consumption of grapefruit or limonin may help to suppress colon cancer development.

Reference	Schindler and Mentlein, 2006
Study	Whether secondary plant constituents, i.e., flavonoids, tocopherols, curcumin, and other substances regulate VEGF in human tumor cells in vitro was studied by measuring VEGF release by ELISA from MDA human breast cancer cells and, for comparison, U-343 and U-118 glioma cells.
Results	The rank order of VEGF inhibitory potency was naringin > rutin > alpha-tocopheryl succinate > lovastatin > apigenin > genistein > alpha-tocopherol >or= kaempferol > gamma-tocopherol; chrysin and curcumin were inactive except at a concentration of 100 micromol/L. Glioma cells were similarly sensitive, with U343 more than U118, especially for alpha-TOS and tocopherols.
Conclusion	Glycosylated flavonoids (i.e., naringin, a constituent of citrus fruits, and rutin, a constituent of cranberries) induced the greatest response to treatment at the lowest concentration in MDA human breast cancer cells.

Reference	Luo et al., 2008
Study	the effects of 12 different flavonoids and other substances on cell proliferation and VEGF expression in human ovarian cancer cells, OVCAR-3 were studied.
Results	The rank order of VEGF protein secretion inhibitory potency was genistein > kaempferol > apigenin > quercetin > tocopherol > luteolin > cisplatin > rutin > naringin > taxifolin.
Conclusion	Genistein, quercetin, and luteolin have shown strong inhibition to cell proliferation and VEGF expression of human ovarian cancer cells, and they show promising in the prevention of ovarian cancers.

Reference	Miller et al., 2008
Study	Six citrus flavonoids were tested for antineoplastic activity. The hamster cheek pouch model was utilized, and the solutions of the flavonoids (2.0-2.5%) and the solution of the carcinogen, 7,12-dimethylbenz[a]anthracene (0.5%), were applied topically to the pouches.
Results	The results with naringin and naringenin show that both of these flavonoids significantly lowered tumor number [5.00 (control group), 2.53 (naringin group), and 3.25 (naringenin group)]. Naringin also significantly reduced tumor burden [269 mm(3)(control group) and 77.1 mm(3)(naringin group)].
Conclusion	Naringin and naringenin, 2 flavonoids found in high concentrations in grapefruit, may be able to inhibit the development of cancer.

Reference	Kim et al., 2008
Study	Identified a novel mechanism of the anticancer effects of naringin in urinary bladder cancer cells.
Results	Naringin treatment resulted in significant dose-dependent growth inhibition together with G(1)-phase cell-cycle arrest at a dose of 100 microM (the half maximal inhibitory concentration) in 5637 cells. Naringin treatment strongly induced p21WAF1 expression, independent of the p53 pathway, and downregulated expression of cyclins and cyclin dependent kinases (CDKs).
Conclusion	The Ras/Raf/ERK pathway participates in p21WAF1 induction, subsequently leading to a decrease in the levels of cyclin D1/CDK4 and cyclin E-CDK2 complexes and naringin-dependent inhibition of cell growth. These provide a theoretical basis for the therapeutic use of flavonoids to treat malignancies.

(G) Protections against toxins in chemotherapy drugs and the environment

Reference	Gordon et al., 1995
Study	55 different flavonoids were tested for their effect on okadaic acid-inhibited autophagy, measured as the sequestration of electroinjected [3H] raffinose.
Results	Naringin (naringenin 7-hesperidoside) and several other flavanone and flavone glycosides (prunin, neoeriocitrin, neohesperidin, apiin, rhoifolin, kaempferol 3-rutinoside) offered virtually complete protection against the autophagy-inhibitory effect of okadaic acid.
Conclusion	Naringin and other okadaic acid-antagonistic flavonoids could have potential therapeutic value as protectants against pathological hyperphosphorylations, environmental toxins, or side effects of chemotherapeutic drugs.

Reference	Kawaguchi et al., 1999
Study	Suppressive effects of naringin on lipopolysaccharide-induced tumor necrosis factor (TNF) release followed by liver injury were investigated.
Results	Treatment with naringin 3 h prior to lipopolysaccharide challenge resulted in complete protection from lipopolysaccharide lethality in D-galactosamine-sensitized mice.
Conclusion	Action of naringin is mediated through suppression of lipopolysaccharide-induced TNF production.

Reference	Blankson et al., 2000
Study	The protein phosphatase-inhibitory algal toxins, okadaic acid and microcystin-LR, induced overphosphorylation of keratin and disruption of the keratin cytoskeleton in freshly isolated rat hepatocytes. In hepatocyte cultures, the toxins elicited DNA fragmentation and apoptotic cell death within 24 h.
Results	All these toxin effects could be prevented by the grapefruit flavonoid, naringin. The cytoprotective effect of naringin was apparently limited to normal hepatocytes, since the toxin-induced apoptosis of hepatoma cells, rat or human, was not prevented by the flavonoid.
Conclusion	Prevention of toxin-induced cytoskeletal disruption and apoptotic liver cell death by the grapefruit flavonoid, naringin.

Reference	Bear and Teel, 2000a
Study	Authors investigated the effects of five citrus phytochemicals on the in vitro metabolism of the tobacco-specific nitrosamine NNK and on the dealkylation of methoxyresorufin (MROD) and pentoxyresorufin (PROD) in liver and lung microsomes of the Syrian golden hamster.
Results	Results suggest that naringenin and quercetin from citrus fruits inhibit the activity of cytochrome P450 (CYP) isoforms that activate NNK and may afford protection against NNK-induced carcinogenesis.
Conclusion	Naringenin inhibits the activity of cytochrome P450 (CYP) isoforms that activate NNK

Reference	Bear and Teel, 2000b
Study	Using Aroclor 1254 induced rat liver S9, four citrus flavonoids: diosmin, naringenin, naringin and rutin were tested for their effects on the mutagenicity of HCA's MeIQx, Glu-P-1*, IQ and PhIP in Salmonella typhimurium TA98.
Results	MeIQx induced mutagenesis and PhIP induced mutagenesis in S. typhimurium were significantly inhibited by all four flavonoids. Glu-P-1 induced mutagenesis was inhibited by rutin and naringenin. IQ induced mutagenesis was significantly inhibited by each flavonoid except diosmin.
Conclusion	Diosmin, naringin, naringenin and rutin are chemoprotective towards CYP1A2 mediated mutagenesis of heterocyclic amines (HCA's)

Reference	Jagetia and Reddy, 2002
Study	The effect of various doses of naringin was studied on the alteration in the radiation-induced micronucleated polychromatic (MPCE) and normochromatic (MNCE) erythrocytes in mouse bone marrow exposed to 2 Gy of 60Co gamma-radiation.
Results	naringin is able to protect mouse bone marrow cells against the radiation-induced DNA damage and decline in the cell proliferation as observed by a reduction in the micronucleus frequency and an increase in PCE/NCE ratio, respectively, in the naringin-pretreated irradiated group.
Conclusion	Naringin protects against the radiation-induced genomic instability in the mice bone marrow.

Reference	Seo et al., 2003
Study	The effect of naringin supplements on the alcohol, lipid, and antioxidant metabolism in ethanol-treated rats was investigated.
Results	Naringin would appear to contribute to alleviating the adverse effect of ethanol ingestion by enhancing the ethanol and lipid metabolism as well as the hepatic antioxidant defense system.
Conclusion	Naringin supplement regulate lipid and ethanol metabolism

Reference	Kanno et al., 2003
Study	The effects of naringin on H_2O_2-induced cytotoxicity and apoptosis in mouse leukemia P388 cells were investigated.
Results	H_2O_2-induced cytotoxicity was significantly attenuated by naringin or the reduced form of glutathione, a typical intracellular antioxidant. Naringin suppressed chromatin condensation and DNA damage induced by H_2O_2.
Conclusion	Naringin from natural products is a useful drug having antioxidant and anti-apoptopic properties.

Reference	Jagetia et al., 2003
Study	The radioprotective action of 2 mg/kg naringin in the bone marrow of mice exposed to different doses of (60)Co gamma-radiation was studied by scoring the frequency of asymmetrical chromosomal aberrations.
Results	Naringin at 5 μM scavenged the 2,2-azino-bis-3-ethyl benzothiazoline-6-sulphonic acid cation radical very efficiently, where a 90% scavenging was observed.
Conclusion	Naringin can protect mouse bone marrow cells against radiation-induced chromosomal damage.

Reference	Kumar et al., 2003
Study	The effect of naringin and naringenin protect hemoglobin from nitrite-induced oxidation to methemoglobin was studied.
Results	Naringenin was more effective than naringin, probably because of the extra phenolic group in the aglycone.
Conclusion	Naringin and naringenin inhibit nitrite-induced methemoglobin formation.

Reference	Kawaguchi et al., 2004
Study	The protective effect of the naringin was studied in an endotoxin shock model based on Salmonella infection. Intraperitoneal (i. p.) infection with 10 (8) CFU Salmonella typhimurium aroA caused lethal shock in lipopolysaccharide (LPS) -responder but not LPS-non-responder mice.
Results	Administration of 1 mg naringin 3 h before infection resulted in protection from lethal shock, similar to LPS-non-responder mice. Also resulted not only in a significant decrease in bacterial numbers in spleens and livers, but also in a decrease in plasma LPS levels.
Conclusion	Suppression of infection-induced endotoxin shock in mice by naringin.

Reference	Kanno et al., 2004
Study	The effect of naringin on the cytotoxicity and apoptosis in mouse leukemia P388 cells treated with Ara-C. Ara-C caused cytotoxicity in a concentration and time-dependent manner in the cells was examined.
Results	Naringin remarkably attenuated the Ara-C-induced apoptosis and completely blocked the DNA damage caused by Ara-C treatment at 6 h using the Comet assay.
Conclusion	Naringin blocked apoptosis caused by Ara-C-induced oxidative stress, resulting in the inhibition of the cytotoxicity of Ara-C.

Reference	Singh et al., 2004a
Study	The effect of naringin, a bioflavonoid with anti-oxidant potential, was studied on Fe-NTA-induced nephrotoxicity in rats.
Results	Pre-treatment of animals with naringin, 60 min before Fe-NTA administration, markedly attenuated renal dysfunction, morphological alterations, reduced elevated TBARS, and restored the depleted renal anti-oxidant enzymes.
Conclusion	There is a protective effect of naringin on Fe-NTA-induced nephrotoxicity in rats.

Reference	Singh et al., 2004b
Study	The effect of naringin, a bioflavonoid with anti-oxidant potential, was studied in glycerol-induced ARF in rats.
Results	Pretreatment of animals with naringin 60 min prior to glycerol injection markedly attenuated renal dysfunction, morphological alterations, reduced elevated thiobarbituric acid reacting substances (TBARS), and restored the depleted renal antioxidant enzymes.
Conclusion	There is a protective effect of naringin in glycerol-induced renal failure in rats.

Reference	Jagetia et al., 2004
Study	Whether naringin treatment may help to overcome the iron-induced toxic effects in vitro was studied.
Results	Pretreatment of HepG2 cells with naringin resulted in an elevation in all the antioxidant enzymes.
Conclusion	Enhanced antioxidant status by naringin could compensate the oxidative stress and may facilitate an early recovery from iron-induced genomic insult in vitro.

Reference	Jagetia and Reddy, 2005
Study	The alteration in the antioxidant status and lipid peroxidation was investigated in Swiss albino mice treated with 2 mg/kg b.wt. naringin, a citrus flavoglycoside, before exposure to 0.5, 1, 2, 3, and 4 Gy gamma radiation.
Results	The alteration in the antioxidant status and lipid peroxidation was investigated in Swiss albino mice treated with 2 mg/kg b.wt. naringin, a citrus flavoglycoside, before exposure to 0.5, 1, 2, 3, and 4 Gy gamma radiation.
Conclusion	Naringin protects mouse liver and intestine against the radiation-induced damage by elevating the antioxidant status and reducing the lipid peroxidation

Reference	Yeh et al., 2005
Study	The interaction of beta-carotene with three flavonoids-naringin, rutin and quercetin-on DNA damage induced by ultraviolet A (UVA) in C3H10T1/2 cells was studied.
Results	All three flavonoids had some absorption at the UVA range, but the effects were opposite to those on DNA damage and beta-carotene oxidation.
Conclusion	A combination of beta-carotene with naringin, rutin or quercetin may increase the safety of beta-carotene.

Reference	Shiratori et al., 2005
Study	The efficacy of naringin and naringenin on endotoxin- induced uveitis (EIU) in rats was studied. EIU was induced in male Lewis rats by a footpad injection of lipopolysaccharide (LPS).
Results	40 microM/kg of naringin and naringenin suppressed increases in cell count owing to LPS treatment by 31% and 38%, respectively.
Conclusion	Possible mechanism for the antiocular inflammatory effect may be the suppression of PGE_2 and NO by naringin and naringenin.

Reference	Kanno et al., 2006)
Study	The effect of naringin, on LPS-induced endotoxin shock in mice and NO production in RAW 264.7 macrophages was studied.
Results	Naringin suppressed LPS -induced production of NO and the expression of inflammatory gene products such as iNOS, TNF-alpha, COX-2 and IL-6 as determined by RT-PCR assay.
Conclusion	Suppression of the LPS-induced mortality and production of NO by NG is due to inhibition of the activation of NF-kappaβ

Reference	Jagetia et al., 2005
Study	The effect of naringin, a grapefruit flavonone was studied on bleomycin-induced genomic damage and alteration in the survival of cultured V79 cells.
Results	Treatment of cells with naringin before exposure to different concentrations of bleomycin arrested the bleomycin-induced decline in the cell survival accompanied by a significant reduction in the frequency of micronuclei when compared with bleomycin treatment alone.
Conclusion	Naringin reduced the genotoxic effects of bleomycin and consequently increased the cell survival and therefore may act as a chemoprotective agent in clinical situations.

Reference	Hori et al., 2007
Study	A diversity of antioxidants and plant ingredients were examined for their protective effect in cultured Balb/c 3T3 cells against ultraviolet A (UVA)-induced cytotoxicities of extracted air pollutants and benz[a]pyrene (B[a]P).
Results	The B[a]P phototoxicity was not eliminated by well-known antioxidants but was markedly diminished by diversity of plant ingredients.
Conclusion	Among the plant ingredients tested in the current study, morin, naringin, and quercetin were found to be desirable protectors against B[a]P phototoxicity.

Reference	Attia, 2008
Study	Anti-mutagenic effects of naringin, against lomefloxacin-induced genomic instability in vivo were evaluated in mouse bone marrow cells by chromosomal aberration and micronucleus (MN) assays.
Results	Naringin was neither genotoxic nor cytotoxic in mice at doses equivalent to 5 or 50 mg/kg. Pre-treatment of mice with naringin significantly reduced lomefloxacin-induced chromosomal aberrations and the MN formation in bone marrow.
Conclusion	Naringin has a protective role in the abatement of lomefloxacin-induced genomic instability that resides, at least in part, in its anti-radical effects.

Reference	Benković et a., 2008
Study	The radioprotective effects of water-soluble derivate of propolis (WSDP) collected in Croatia, and single flavonoids, caffeic acid, chrysin and naringin in the whole-body irradiated CBA mice were investigated.
Results	Possible genotoxic effects of all test components were assessed on non-irradiated animals. The higher efficiency of test components was observed when given preventively.
Conclusion	Propolis and related flavonoids given to mice before irradiation protected mice from lethal effects of whole-body irradiation and diminish primary DNA damage in their white blood cells as detected by the alkaline comet assay.

(H) Antioxidant effects

Reference	Younes and Siegers, 1981
Study	Depletion of hepatic glutathione in phenobarbital-induced rats by phorone (diisopropylidene acetone) led to an enhancement of spontaneous lipid peroxidation in vitro. Addition of exogenous glutathione, dithiocarb or one of the flavonoids (+)-catechin, (-)-epicatechin, 3-O-methylcatechin, quercetin, taxifolin, rutin, naringin or naringenin led in every case to a dose-dependent inhibition of this peroxidative activity.
Results	The concentration values yielding 50% inhibition (I (50)) varied from 1.0×10^{-6} M for glutathione to 1.9×10^{-5} M for naringenin.
Conclusion	Some flavonoids have inhibitory action on enhanced spontaneous lipid peroxidation following glutathione depletion.

Reference	Kroyer, 1986
Study	The antioxidant properties of freeze-dried citrus fruit peels (orange, lemon, grapefruit) and methanolic extracts from the peel were studied.
Results	Freeze-dried orange peel showed the highest, lemon peel somewhat less and grapefruit peel the lowest but still remarkable antioxidant activity.
Conclusion	Citrus fruit peels have antioxidant activity.

Reference	Affany et al., 1987
Study	Cumene hydroperoxide induces in vitro the peroxidation of erythrocyte membrane. The protective effect of various flavonoids was compared to that of butylated hydroxytoluene (BHT). Protective effect was evaluated by the inhibition of peroxidation product formation.
Results	Quercetin and catechin showed a protective effect against lipid peroxidation as high as that of BHT. Morin, rutin, trihydroxyethylrutin, and naringin were active but to a lesser degree.
Conclusion	Flavonoids have protective effect against lipid peroxidation of erythrocyte membranes.

Reference	Ratty and Das, 1988
Study	The in vitro effects of several flavonoids on nonenzymatic lipid peroxidation in the rat brain mitochondria was studied. The lipid peroxidation was indexed by using the 2-thiobarbituric acid test.
Results	The flavonoids, apigenin, flavone, flavanone, hesperidin, naringin, and tangeretin promoted the ascorbic acid-induced lipid peroxidation.
Conclusion	Polyhydroxylated substitutions on rings A and B, a 2,3-double bond, a free 3-hydroxyl substitution and a 4-keto moiety confer antiperoxidative properties.

Reference	Chen et al., 1990
Study	The superoxide anions scavenging activity and antioxidation of seven flavonoids were studied. The superoxide anions were generated in a phenazin methosulphate-NADH system and were assayed by reduction of nitroblue tetrazolium.
Results	The scavenging activity ranked: rutin was the strongest, and quercetin and naringin the second, while morin and hispidulin were very weak.
Conclusion	Flavonoids are superoxide scavengers and antioxidants.

Reference	Ng et al., 2000
Study	A variety of flavonoids, lignans, an alkaloid, a bisbenzyl, coumarins and terpenes isolated from Chinese herbs was tested for antioxidant activity as reflected in the ability to inhibit lipid peroxidation in rat brain and kidney homogenates and rat erythrocyte hemolysis. The pro-oxidant activities of the aforementioned compounds were assessed by their effects on bleomycin-induced DNA damage.
Results	The flavonoid rutin and the terpene tanshinone I manifested potent antioxidative activity in the lipid peroxidation assay but no inhibitory activity in the hemolysis assay. The lignan deoxypodophyllotoxin, the flavonoid naringin and the coumarins columbianetin, bergapten and angelicin slightly inhibited lipid peroxidation in brain and kidney homogenates.
Conclusion	Aromatic hydroxyl group is very important for antioxidative effects of the compounds. None of the compounds tested exerted an obvious pro-oxidant effect.

Reference	Jeon et al., 2001
Study	To determine the antioxidative effects of the citrus bioflavonoid, naringin, a potent cholesterol-lowering agent, compared to the cholesterol-lowering drug, lovastatin, in rabbits fed a high cholesterol diet.
Results	Naringin regulate antioxidative capacities by increasing the SOD and catalase activities, up-regulating the gene expressions of SOD, catalase, and GSH-Px, and protecting the plasma vitamin E. Lovastatin exhibited an inhibitory effect on the plasma and hepatic lipid peroxidation and increased the hepatic catalase activity.
Conclusion	Antioxidative activity of naringin and lovastatin in high cholesterol-fed rabbits.

Reference	Jeon et al., 2002
Study	Twenty male rabbits were served a high-cholesterol diet or high-cholesterol diet supplemented with naringin or probucol for 8 weeks to compare the antioxidative effects of the naringin and antioxidative cholesterol-lowering drug (probucol).
Results	The probucol supplement was very potent in the antioxidative defense system, whereas naringin exhibited a comparable antioxidant capacity based on increasing the gene expressions in the antioxidant enzymes, increasing the hepatic SOD and CAT activities, sparing plasma vitamin E, and decreasing the hepatic mitochondrial H_2O_2 content.
Conclusion	Antioxidant effects of naringin and probucol in cholesterol-fed rabbits

Reference	Yu et al., 2005
Study	A variety of in vitro models such as beta-carotene-linoleic acid, 1,1-diphenyl-2-picryl hydrazyl (DPPH), superoxide, and hamster low-density lipoprotein (LDL) were used to measure the antioxidant activity of 11 citrus bioactive compounds.
Results	Flavonoids, which contain a chromanol ring system, had stronger antioxidant activity as compared to limonoids and bergapten, which lack the hydroxy groups.
Conclusion	Several structural features were linked to the strong antioxidant activity of flavonoids.

Reference	Gorinstein et al., 2005
Study	The influence of naringin versus red grapefruit juice on plasma lipid levels and plasma antioxidant activity in rats fed cholesterol-containing and cholesterol-free diets was compared.
Results	After 30 days of different feeding, it was found that diets supplemented with red grapefruit juice and to a lesser degree with naringin improved the plasma lipid levels mainly in rats fed cholesterol and increased the plasma antioxidant activity.
Conclusion	Naringin is a powerful plasma lipid lowering and plasma antioxidant activity increasing flavonone. However, fresh red grapefruit is preferable than naringin.

Reference	Hsu and Yen 2006
Study	The relationship between the influence of flavonoids on cell population growth and their antioxidant activity was studied.
Results	The inhibition of flavonoids (naringenin, rutin, hesperidin, resveratrol, naringin and quercetin) on 3T3-L1 pre-adipocytes was 28.3, 8.1, 11.1, 33.2, 5.6 and 71.5%, respectively.
Conclusion	Induction of cell apoptosis in 3T3-L1 pre-adipocytes by flavonoids is associated with their antioxidant activity.

Reference	Pereira et al., 2007
Study	In order to understand the contribution of the metal coordination and the type of interaction between a flavonoid and the metal ion, in this study a new metal complex of Cu (II) with naringin was synthesized and characterized by FT-IR, UV-VIS, mass spectrometry (ESI-MS/MS), elemental analysis and 1H-NMR.
Results	The results of these analyses indicate that the complex has a Cu (II) ion coordinated via positions 4 and 5 of the flavonoid.
Conclusion	The Naringin-Cu (II) complex 1 showed higher antioxidant, anti-inflammatory and tumor cell cytotoxicity activities than free naringin without reducing cell viability. Naringin and naringinin have been identified as prooxidants independent of transition metal catalysed autoxidation reactions.

Reference	Nafisi et al., 2008
Study	To examine the interactions of three flavonoids; morin (Mor), apigenin (Api) and naringin (Nar) with yeast RNA in aqueous solution at physiological conditions
Results	Spectroscopic evidence showed major binding of flavonoids to RNA with overall binding constants of K(morin)=9.150x10(3)M(-1), K(apigenin)=4.967x10(4)M(-1), and K(naringin)=1.144x10(4)M(-1).
Conclusion	The affinity of flavonoid-RNA binding is in the order of apigenin>naringin>morin.

Reference	Zielińska-Przyjemska and Ignatowicz., 2008
Study	Three citrus flavonoids - naringin, naringenin and hesperidin - have been examined for their ability to activate caspase-3, a marker of apoptosis execution, in human polymorphonuclear neutrophils in vitro, stimulated and non-stimulated with phorbol 12-myristate 13-acetate.
Results	Flavonoids inhibited the neutrophil ability to generate superoxide radical and 10-100 microm hesperidin appeared the most active phytochemical.
Conclusion	Reactive oxygen species may inhibit apoptosis via caspase-3 inhibition and the antioxidant action of citrus flavonoids may reverse this process.

Reference	Nafisi et al., 2008
Study	To examine the interactions of morin (Mor), naringin (Nar), and apigenin (Api) with calf thymus DNA in aqueous solution at physiological conditions,
Results	Spectroscopic evidence shows both intercalation and external binding of flavonoids to DNA duplex with overall binding constants of K(morin) = 5.99 x 10(3) M(-1), K(apigenin) = 7.10 x 10(4) M(-1), and K(naringin) = 3.10 x 10(3) M(-1).
Conclusion	The affinity of ligand-DNA binding is in the order of apigenin > morin > naringin. DNA aggregation and a partial B- to A-DNA transition occurs upon morin, apigenin, and naringin complexion.

(I) Antimicrobial effects

Reference	Ng et al., 1996
Study	Coumarins, flavonoids and polysaccharopeptide were tested for antibacterial activity. The bacteria used for this study included clinical isolates of Staphylococcus aureus, Shigella flexneri, Salmonella typhi, Escherichia coli and Pseudomonas aeruginosa.
Results	When tested at the dose of 128 mg/l, the flavonoids (rutin, naringin and baicalin) inhibited 25% or less of P. aeruginosa and only baicalin was active against S. aureus.
Conclusion	Naringin inhibited P. aeruginosa.

Reference	Paredes et al., 2003
Study	The effect of hesperetin, naringenin and its glycoside form on the Sindbis neurovirulent strain (NSV) replication in vitro was studied. All flavanones tested were not cytotoxic on Baby Hamster cells 21 clone 15 (BHK-21).
Results	Hesperetin and naringenin had inhibitory activity on NSV infection. However their glycosides, hesperidin and naringin did not have inhibitory activity. Implying that the presence of rutinose moiety of flavanones blocks the antiviral effect.
Conclusion	Anti-Sindbis activity of flavanones hesperetin and naringenin.

Reference	Cvetnić and Vladimir-Knezević, 2004
Study	Antibacterial and antifungal activity of ethanolic extract of grapefruit (Citrus paradisi Macf., Rutaceae) seed and pulp was examined against 20 bacterial and 10 yeast strains
Results	Ethanolic extract exibited the strongest antimicrobial effect against Salmonella enteritidis (MIC 2.06%, m/V). Other tested bacteria and yeasts were sensitive to extract concentrations ranging from 4.13% to 16.50% (m/V).
Conclusion	There exist antimicrobial activity of grapefruit seed and pulp ethanolic extract.

Reference	Wood, 2007
Study	The present study evaluates two separate, but related, dietary trials-trial 1, dietary naringenin (NAR) supplementation; and trial 2, dietary rutin (R), quercetin (Q), and naringin (N) supplementation-on dental caries formation in 40 different male albino rats, at the expense of dextrose, for periods of 42 days.
Results	An inverse dose-dependent relationship was established among the NAR experimental groups and control group. In dietary trial 2, statistically significant reductions in occlusal caries were observed for R, Q, and N in the maxillary molars and for Q and N in the mandibular molars compared with the control group.
Conclusion	Selected bioflavonoids may show promise as an alternative means of reducing dental caries.

Reference	Tsui et al., 2007
Study	The effects of naringin on the growth of periodontal pathogens such as A. actinomycetemcomitans and P. gingivalis were studied in vitro. For comparison, the effects of naringin on several oral microbes were also studied.
Results	Naringin also had an inhibitory effect against all bacteria and yeasts tested.
Conclusion	Naringin possesses significant antimicrobial properties on periodontal pathogens in vitro. It also has an inhibitory effect on some common oral microorganisms in low concentrations.

(J) Drug interactions

Reference	Fuhr et al., 1993
Study	The effects of grapefruit juice and naringenin on the activity of the human cytochrome P450 isoform CYP1A2 were evaluated using caffeine as a probe substrate.
Results	In vitro naringin was a potent competitive inhibitor of caffeine 3-demethylation by human liver microsomes ($K_i = 7$-29 microM). In vivo grapefruit juice decreased the oral clearance of caffeine and prolonged its half-life.
Conclusion	Grapefruit juice and naringenin inhibit CYP1A2 activity in man.

Reference	Bailey et al., 1993a
Study	The pharmacokinetics of felodipine and its single primary oxidative metabolite, dehydrofelodipine, were studied after drug administration with 200 ml water, grapefruit juice, or naringin in water at the same concentration as the juice in a randomized crossover trial of nine healthy men.
Results	Grapefruit juice produces a marked and variable increase in felodipine bioavailability. Naringin solution produced much less of an interaction, showing that other factors were important.
Conclusion	Grapefruit juice produces a marked and variable increase in felodipine bioavailability.

Reference	Bailey et al., 1993b
Study	The pharmacokinetics of nisoldipine coat-core tablet were studied in a Latin square-designed trial in which 12 healthy men were administered the drug with water, grapefruit juice, or encapsulated naringin powder at the same amount as that assayed in the juice.
Results	The bioavailability of some dihydropyridine calcium antagonists can be markedly augmented by grapefruit juice. The naringin capsule did not change nisoldipine pharmacokinetics.
Conclusion	The bioavailability of some dihydropyridine calcium antagonists can be augmented by grapefruit juice but does not involve naringin.

Reference	Runkel et al., 1997
Study	To investigate whether the presence of naringin is demanded for the inhibition of the coumarin 7-hydroxylase in man or other compounds are responsible for it.
Results	While increasing amounts of grapefruit juice delay the excretion of 7-hydroxycoumarin by 2 h, increasing doses of naringin in water up to twofold do not cause any alteration in the time course of excretion.
Conclusion	As naringin alone is ineffective, the inhibitory effect of grapefruit juice on the metabolism of coumarin is caused by at least one compound other than naringin.

Reference	Fuhr et al., 1998
Study	A randomized crossover interaction study on the effects of grapefruit juice on the pharmacokinetics of nimodipine and its metabolites.
Results	Grapefruit juice increases oral nimodipine bioavailability.
Conclusion	To avoid the interaction, nimodipine should not be taken with grapefruit juice.

Reference	Bailey et al., 1998
Study	To test whether naringin or 6',7'-dihydroxybergamottin is a major active substance in grapefruit juice-felodipine interaction in humans.
Results	The findings show the importance of in vivo testing to determine the ingredients in grapefruit juice responsible for inhibition of cytochrome P450 3A4 in humans.
Conclusion	Naringin and 6',7'-dihydroxybergamottin are not the major active ingredients, although they may contribute to the grapefruit juice-felodipine interaction.

Reference	Ubeaud et al., 1999
Study	NRG's inhibition of the metabolism of SV in rat hepatocytes (the intrinsic clearance of SV) was studied.
Results	Naringenin present in grapefruit juice inhibits in vitro the metabolism of simvastatin, a HMG-CoA reductase inhibitor.
Conclusion	In vitro inhibition of simvastatin (SV) metabolism in rat and human liver by naringenin (NRG).

Reference	Ueng et al., 1999
Study	In vitro and in vivo effects of naringin on microsomal monooxygenase were studied to evaluate the drug interaction of this flavonoid.
Results	Naringenin is a potent inhibitor of benzo(a)pyrene hydroxylase activity in vitro and naringin reduces the P450 1A2 protein level in vivo.
Conclusion	These effects may indicate a chemopreventive role of naringin against protoxicants activated by P450 1A2.

Reference	Mitsunaga et al., 2000
Study	To see whether grapefruit juice bioflavonoids alter the permeation of vincristine across the blood-brain barrier, we conducted experiments with cultured mouse brain capillary endothelial cells (MBEC4 cells) in vitro and ddY mice in vivo.
Results	The in vivo brain-to-plasma concentration ratio of [3H]vincristine in ddY mice was decreased by coadministration of 0.1 mg/kg quercetin, but increased by 1.0 mg/kg quercetin. Kaempferol had a similar biphasic effect. Cchrysin, flavon, hesperetin, naringenin increased [3H]vincristine uptake in the 10-50 microM range, and glycosides (hesperidin, naringin, rutin) were without effect.
Conclusion	Patients taking drugs which are P-glycoprotein substrates may need to restrict their intake of bioflavonoid-containing foods and beverages, such as grapefruit juice.

Reference	Ho et al., 2001
Study	33 flavonoids, occurring ubiquitously in foods of plant origin, were tested for their ability to alter the transport of the beta-lactam antibiotic cefixime via the H+-coupled intestinal peptide transporter PEPT1 in the human intestinal epithelial cell line Caco-2. To evaluate the inhibition of CYP3A4 activity in human liver microsomes by flavonoids, furanocoumarins and related compounds and investigate possibly more important and potential inhibitors of CYP3A4 in grapefruit juice.
Results	Quercetin, genistein, naringin, diosmin, acacetin, and chrysin increased uptake of [14C] cefixime dose dependently by up to 60%. Bergapten (5-methoxypsoralen) with the lowest IC50 value (19-36 microM) was the most potent CYP3A4 inhibitor.
Conclusion	Flavonoids with EGF-receptor tyrosine kinase inhibitory activities enhance the intestinal absorption of the beta-lactam antibiotic cefixime in Caco-2 cells. Bergapten appears to be a potent inhibitor of CYP3A4, and may therefore be primarily responsible for the effect of grapefruit juice on CYP3A4 activity.

Reference	Choi and Shin, 2005
Study	The effect of naringin on the bioavailability and pharmacokinetics of paclitaxel after oral administration of paclitaxel or its prodrug coadministered with naringin to rats was studied.
Results	The bioavailability of paclitaxel coadministered as a prodrug with or without naringin was remarkably higher than the control.
Conclusion	Enhanced paclitaxel bioavailability after oral coadministration of paclitaxel prodrug with naringin to rats.

Reference	Kim and Choi, 2005
Study	The pharmacokinetics of verapamil and one of its metabolites, norverapamil, were investigated after oral administration of verapamil at a dose of 9 mg/kg without or with oral naringin at a dose of 7.5 mg/kg in rabbits. With naringin, the total area under the plasma concentration-time curve (AUC) of verapamil was significantly greater, the AUC(verapamil)/AUC(norverapamil) ratio was considerably greater.
Results	With naringin, the total area under the plasma concentration-time curve (AUC) of verapamil was significantly greater, the AUC(verapamil)/AUC(norverapamil) ratio was considerably greater.
Conclusion	The metabolism of verapamil and the formation of norverapamil were inhibited by naringin possibly by inhibition of CYP3A in rabbits.

Reference	Choi and Han, 2005
Study	Pharmacokinetic parameters of diltiazem and desacetyldiltiazem were determined in rats following an oral administration of diltiazem to rats in the presence and absence of naringin.
Results	Absolute and relative bioavailability values of diltiazem in the presence of naringin were significantly higher than those from the control group.
Conclusion	The concomitant use of naringin significantly enhanced the oral exposure of diltiazem in rats.

Reference	Yeum and Choi, 2006
Study	The effect of naringin on the pharmacokinetics of verapamil and its major metabolite, norverapamil in rabbits were studied.
Results	Pretreatment of naringin enhanced the oral bioavailability of verapamil.
Conclusion	Verapamil dosage should be adjusted when given with naringin or a naringin-containing dietary supplement.

Reference	Lim and Choi, 2006
Study	The effects of oral naringin on the pharmacokinetics of intravenous paclitaxel in rats were studied.
Results	After intravenous administration of paclitaxel, the AUC was significantly greater, and Cl was significantly slower than controls.
Conclusion	The inhibition of hepatic P-gp by oral naringin could also contribute to the significantly greater AUC of intravenous paclitaxel by oral naringin.

Reference	Bailey et al., 2007
Study	Inhibition of OATP1A2 transport by flavonoids in grapefruit (naringin) and orange (hesperidin) was conducted in vitro. Two randomized, crossover, pharmacokinetic studies were performed clinically.
Results	Naringin most probably directly inhibited enteric OATP1A2 to decrease oral fexofenadine bioavailability. Inactivation of enteric CYP3A4 was probably not involved.
Conclusion	Naringin is a major and selective clinical inhibitor of organic anion-transporting polypeptide 1A2 (OATP1A2) in grapefruit juice.

Reference	Li et al., 2007
Study	The esterase-inhibitory potential of 10 constitutive flavonoids and furanocoumarins toward p-nitrophenylacetate (PNPA) hydrolysis was investigated.
Results	In Caco-2 cells, demonstrated to contain minimal CYP3A activity, the permeability coefficient of the prodrugs lovastatin and enalapril was increased in the presence of the active flavonoids kaempferol and naringenin, consistent with inhibition of esterase activity.
Conclusion	Kaempferol and naringenin are shown to mediate pharmacokinetic drug interaction with the prodrugs lovastatin and enalapril due to their capability of esterase inhibition.

Reference	de Castro et al., 2007
Study	The potential interaction between selected ingredients of grapefruit juice and, the transport of talinolol, a P-gp substrate, across Caco-2 cells monolayers was determined in the absence and presence of distinct concentrations of grapefruit juice, bergamottin, 6',7'-dihydroxybergamottin, 6',7'-epoxybergamottin, naringin, and naringenin.
Results	The flavonoid aglycone naringenin was around 10-fold more potent than its glycoside naringin with IC(50) values of 236 and 2409 microM, respectively.
Conclusion	The in vitro data suggest that compounds present in grapefruit juice are able to inhibit the P-gp activity modifying the disposition of drugs that are P-gp substrates such as talinolol.

Reference	Shim et al., 2007
Study	The cellular uptake of benzoic acid was examined in the presence and the absence of naringin, naringenin, morin, silybin and quercetin in Caco-2 cells.
Results	All the tested flavonoids except naringin significantly inhibited the cellular uptake of [(14)C]-benzoic acid. Particularly, naringenin and silybin exhibited strong inhibition effects.
Conclusion	Some flavonoids appeared to be competitive inhibitors of monocarboxylate transporter 1 (MCT1)

Reference	Shirasaka et al., 2008
Study	The impact of P-gp and Oatp on intestinal absorption of the beta(1)-adrenoceptor antagonist talinolol.
Results	Naringin inhibited talinolol uptake by Oatp1a5 (IC (50) = 12.7 muM).
Conclusion	The absorption behavior of talinolol can be explained by the involvement of both P-gp and Oatp, based on characterization of talinolol transport by Oatp1a5 and P-gp, and the effects of naringin.

Reference	Taur and Rodriguez-Proteau, 2008
Study	To study cimetidine as a substrate of P-glycoprotein (P-gp) and organic cation transport systems and the modulatory effects of eight flavonoid aglycones and glycosides on these transport systems using Caco-2 and LLC-PK1 cells.
Results	Intracellular uptake rate of (14)C-tetraethylammonium (TEA) was reduced in the presence of quercetin, naringenin and genistein in LLC-PK1 cells.
Conclusion	Quercetin, naringenin, genistein, and xanthohumol reduced P-gp-mediated transport and increased the basolateral uptake rate of cimetidine. Quercetin, naringenin, genistein, but not xanthohumol, reduced intracellular uptake rate of TEA in LLC-PK1 cells. These results suggest that flavonoids may have potential to alter the disposition profile of cimetidine and possibly other therapeutics that are mediated by P-gp and/or cation transport systems.

Reference	de Castro et al., 2008
Study	grapefruit juice (white and ruby red) and its selected components (naringin, naringenin, and bergamottin) was investigated on the activity of the P-glycoprotein (P-gp) in male Sprague-Dawley rats.
Results	The flavonoids naringenin (0.7 mg/kg) and naringin (2.4 and 9.4 mg/kg) had a similar effect increasing the talinolol C max and AUC (0-infinity) by 1.5- to 1.8-fold, respectively.
Conclusion	the effect of GFJ on P-gp activity seems to depend on the variety, the concentration of compounds in the juice, and the composition of different ingredients.

(K) Anti-inflammatory effects

Reference	Lambev et al., 1980a
Study	Experiments are carried out on 35 male albino rats. The effect of the flavonoids naringin and rutin on the level of mastocytic and nonmastocytic histamine is studied, as well as on its release induced by compound 48/80 (2 mg/kg i. p.). The histamine content is determined fluorimetrically.
Results	Naringin and rutin have no effect on the levels of mastocytic and nonmastocytic histamine. They prevent the release of mastocytic histamine, induced by compound 48/80.
Conclusion	Flavonoids with antioxidant action (naringin and rutin) prevent the release of mastocytic and nonmastocytic histamine.

Reference	Lambev et al., 1980b
Study	The authors examined antiexudative activity of bioflavonoids naringin and rutin in comparative aspect in two models of acute inflammation. The experiments were carried out on 180 male white rats and 24 guinea pigs.
Results	The two flavonoids manifested marked antiexudative effect in rats with experiments peritonitis.
Conclusion	Naringin has antiexudative effect of in experimental pulmonary edema and peritonitis.

Reference	Middleton and Drzewiecki, 1984
Study	Eleven flavonoids included flavone, quercetin, taxifolin, chalcone, apigenin, fisetin, rutin, phloretin, tangeretin, hesperetin, and naringin were studied for their effects on human basophil histamine release triggered by six different stimuli.
Results	The flavonols, quercetin and fisetin, and the flavone, apigenin, exhibited a predilection to inhibit histamine release stimulated by IgE-dependent ligands (antigen, anti-IgE, and con A). The flavanone derivatives, taxifolin and hesperetin, were inactive, as were the glycosides, rutin and naringin. The open chain congeners, chalcone and phloretin, also possessed inhibitory activity.
Conclusion	Flavonoid inhibited human basophil histamine release stimulated by various agents.

Reference	Park et al., 2005
Study	The passive cutaneous anaphylaxis-inhibitory activity of the flavanones isolated from the pericarp of Citrus unshiu (Family Rutaceae) and the fruit of Poncirus trifoliata (Family Rutaceae) was studied.
Results	Naringenin, hesperetin and ponciretin potently inhibited IgE-induced beta-hexosaminidase release from RBL-2H3 cells and the PCA reaction.
Conclusion	Flavanone glycosides can be activated by intestinal bacteria, and may be effective toward IgE-induced atopic allergies.

Reference	Fujita et al., 2008
Study	The competitive inhibitory effects of extracts from immature citrus fruit on CYP activity.
Results	Extracts having relatively strong inhibitory effects for CYP3A4 tended to contain higher amounts of naringin, bergamottin and 6',7'-dihydroxybergamottin.
Conclusion	Citrus extracts containing high levels of narirutin and hesperidin and lower levels of furanocoumarins such as C. unshiu are favorable as antiallergic functional ingredients.

(L) Other effects

Reference	Chan et al., 1999
Study	Flavonoids containing phenol B rings, e.g. naringenin, naringin, hesperetin and apigenin, were studied if they formed prooxidant metabolites that oxidised NADH upon oxidation by peroxidase/H_2O_2.
Results	Prooxidant phenoxyl radicals formed by these flavonoids cooxidise NADH to form NAD radicals which then activated oxygen.
Conclusion	Naringin and naringinin have been identified as prooxidants independent of transition metal catalysed autoxidation reactions.

References

Affany, A., Salvayre, R. and Douste-Blazy, L. (1987). Comparison of the protective effect of various flavonoids against lipid peroxidation of erythrocyte membranes (induced by cumene hydroperoxide). *Fundam. Clin. Pharmacol.,* 1(6): 451-7.

Ajay, M., Gilani, A.U. and Mustafa, M.R. (2003). Effects of flavonoids on vascular smooth muscle of the isolated rat thoracic aorta. *Life Sci.,* 74(5): 603-12.

Ali, M.M. and El Kader, M.A. (2004). The influence of naringin on the oxidative state of rats with streptozotocin-induced acute hyperglycaemia. *Z. Naturforsch. [C],* 59(9-10): 726-33.

Ameer, B., Weintraub, R.A., Johnson, J.V., Yost, R.A. and Rouseff, R.L. (1996). Flavanone absorption after naringin, hesperidin, and citrus administration. *Clin. Pharmacol. Ther.,* 60(1): 34-40.

Asgary, S., Naderi, G.A., Zadegan, N.S. and Vakili, R. (2002). The inhibitory effects of pure flavonoids on in vitro protein glycosylation. *J. Herb. Pharmacother.,* 2(2): 47-55.

Attia, S.M. (2008) Nov. Abatement by naringin of lomefloxacin-induced genomic instability in mice. *Mutagenesis,* 23(6): 515-2. Epub 2008 Aug 28.

Bailey, D.G., Arnold, J.M., Munoz, C. and Spence, J.D. (1993a). Grapefruit juice--felodipine interaction: mechanism, predictability, and effect of naringin. *Clin. Pharmacol. Ther.,* 53(6): 637-42.

Bailey, D.G., Arnold, J.M., Strong, H.A., Munoz, C. and Spence, J.D. (1993b). Effect of grapefruit juice and naringin on nisoldipine pharmacokinetics. *Clin. Pharmacol. Ther.,* 54(6): 589-94.

Bailey, D.G., Dresser, G.K., Leake, B.F. and Kim, R.B. (2007). Naringin is a major and selective clinical inhibitor of organic anion-transporting polypeptide 1A2 (OATP1A2) in grapefruit juice. *Clin. Pharmacol. Ther.,* 81(4): 495-502.

Bailey, D.G., Kreeft, J.H., Munoz, C., Freeman, D.J. and Bend, J.R. (1998). Grapefruit juice-felodipine interaction: effect of naringin and 6', 7' -dihydroxybergamottin in humans. *Clin. Pharmacol. Ther.,* 64(3): 248-56.

Bear, W.L. and Teel, R.W. (2000a.) Effects of citrus phytochemicals on liver and lung cytochrome P450 activity and on the in vitro metabolism of the tobacco-specific nitrosamine NNK. *Anticancer Res.,* 20(5A): 3323-9.

Bear, W.L. and Teel, R.W. (2000b). Effects of citrus flavonoids on the mutagenicity of heterocyclic amines and on cytochrome P450 1A2 activity. *Anticancer Res.,* 20(5B): 3609-14.

Benković, V., Orsolić, N., Knezević, A.H., Ramić, S., Dikić, D., Basić, I. and Kopjar, N. (2008) Jan. Evaluation of the radioprotective effects of propolis and flavonoids in gamma-irradiated mice: the alkaline comet assay study. *Biol. Pharm. Bull,* 31(1): 167-72.

Blankson, H., Grotterød, E.M. and Seglen, P.O. (2000). Prevention of toxin-induced cytoskeletal disruption and apoptotic liver cell death by the grapefruit flavonoid, naringin. *Cell Death Differ.,* 7: 739-746.

Bok, S.H., Lee, S.H., Park, Y.B., Bae, K.H., Son, K.H., Jeong, T.S. and Choi, M.S. (1999). Plasma and hepatic cholesterol and hepatic activities of 3-hydroxy-3-methyl-glutaryl-CoA reductase and acyl CoA: cholesterol transferase are lower in rats fed citrus peel extract or a mixture of citrus bioflavonoids. *J. Nutr.,* 129(6): 1182-5.

Calomme, M., Pieters, L., Vlietinck, A. and Vanden Berghe, D. (1996). Inhibition of bacterial mutagenesis by Citrus flavonoids. *Planta Med.,* 62(3): 222-6.

Chan, T., Galati, G. and O'Brien, P.J. (1999). Oxygen activation during peroxidase catalysed metabolism of flavones or flavanones. *Chem. Biol. Interact.,* 122(1): 15-25.

Chen, Y.T., Zheng, R.L., Jia, Z.J. and Ju, Y. (1990). Flavonoids as superoxide scavengers and antioxidants. *Free Radic. Biol. Med.,* 9(1): 19-21.

Chiou, G.C. and Xu, X.R. (2004). Effects of some natural flavonoids on retinal function recovery after ischemic insult in the rat. *J. Ocul. Pharmacol. Ther.,* 20(2): 107-13.

Choe, S.C., Kim, H.S., Jeong, T.S., Bok, S.H. and Park, Y.B. (2001). Naringin has an antiatherogenic effect with the inhibition of intercellular adhesion molecule-1 in hypercholesterolemic rabbits. *J. Cardiovasc. Pharmacol,* 38(6): 947-55.

Choi, M.S., Do, K.M., Park, Y.S., Jeon, S.M., Jeong, T.S., Lee, Y.K., Lee, M.K. and Bok, S.H. (2001) Effect of naringin supplementation on cholesterol metabolism and antioxidant status in rats fed high cholesterol with different levels of vitamin E. *Ann. Nutr. Metab.,* 45(5): 193-201.

Choi, J.S. and Han, H.K. (2005). Enhanced oral exposure of diltiazem by the concomitant use of naringin in rats. *Int. J. Pharm.,* 305(1-2): 122-8.

Choi, J.S. and Shin, S.C. (2005). Enhanced paclitaxel bioavailability after oral coadministration of paclitaxel prodrug with naringin to rats. *Int. J. Pharm.,* 292(1-2):149-56.

Cvetnić, Z. and Vladimir-Knezević, S. (2004). Antimicrobial activity of grapefruit seed and pulp ethanolic extract. *Acta. Pharm.,* 54(3): 243-50.

da Silva, R.R., de Oliveira, T.T., Nagem, T.J., Pinto, A.S., Albino, L.F., de Almeida, M.R., de Moraes, G.H. and Pinto, J.G. (2001). Hypocholesterolemic effect of naringin and rutin flavonoids. *Arch. Latinoam Nutr.,* 51(3): 258-64.

de Castro, W.V., Mertens-Talcott, S., Derendorf, H. and Butterweck, V. (2007). Grapefruit juice-drug interactions: Grapefruit juice and its components inhibit P-glycoprotein (ABCB1) mediated transport of talinolol in Caco-2 cells. *J. Pharm. Sci.,* 96(10): 2808-17.

Déchaud, H., Ravard, C., Claustrat, F., de la Perrière, A.B. and Pugeat, M. (1999). Xenoestrogen interaction with human sex hormone-binding globulin (hSHBG). *Steroids,* 64(5): 328-34.

Divi, R.L. and Doerge, D.R. (1996). Inhibition of thyroid peroxidase by dietary flavonoids. *Chem. Res. Toxicol.,* 9(1): 16-23.

Fenton, J.I. and Hord, N.G. (2004). Flavonoids promote cell migration in nontumorigenic colon epithelial cells differing in Apc genotype: implications of matrix metalloproteinase activity. *Nutr. Cancer,* 48(2): 182-8.

Fuhr, U., Klittich, K. and Staib, A.H. (1993). Inhibitory effect of grapefruit juice and its bitter principal, naringenin, on CYP1A2 dependent metabolism of caffeine in man. *Br J Clin Pharmacol,* 35(4): 431-6.

Fuhr, U., Maier-Brüggemann, A., Blume, H., Mück, W., Unger, S., Kuhlmann, J., Huschka, C., Zaigler, M., Rietbrock, S. and Staib, A.H. (1998). Grapefruit juice increases oral nimodipine bioavailability. *Int. J. Clin. Pharmacol. Ther.,* 36(3): 126-32.

Fujita, T. Kawase, A. Niwa, T. Tomohiro, N. Masuda, M. Matsuda, H. and Iwaki, M. (2008) May. Biol. Pharm. Bull. *Comparative evaluation of 12 immature citrus fruit extracts for the inhibition of cytochrome P450 isoform activitie, 31(5): 925-30.*

Gordon, P.B., Holen, I. and Seglen, P.O. (1995). Protection by naringin and some other flavonoids of hepatocytic autophagy and endocytosis against inhibition by okadaic acid. *J. Biol. Chem.,* 270(11): 5830-8.

Herrera, M.D. and Marhuenda, E. (1993). Effect of naringin and naringenin on contractions induced by noradrenaline in rat vas deferens--I. Evidence for postsynaptic alpha-2 adrenergic receptor. *Gen. Pharmacol.,* 24(3): 739-42.

Ho, P.C., Saville, D.J. and Wanwimolruk, S. (2001). Inhibition of human CYP3A4 activity by grapefruit flavonoids, furanocoumarins and related compounds. *J. Pharm. Pharm. Sci.,* 4(3): 217-27.

Hori, M., Kojima, H., Nakata, S., Konishi, H., Kitagawa, A. and Kawai, K. (2007). A search for the plant ingredients that protect cells from air pollutants and benz[a]pyrene phototoxicity. *Drug Chem. Toxicol.,* 30(2): 105-16.

Hsiu, S.L., Huang, T.Y., Hou, Y.C., Chin, D.H. and Chao, P.D. (2002). Comparison of metabolic pharmacokinetics of naringin and naringenin in rabbits. *Life Sci.,* 70(13): 1481-9.

Hsu, C.L. and Yen, G.C. (2006). Induction of cell apoptosis in 3T3-L1 pre-adipocytes by flavonoids is associated with their antioxidant activity. *Mol. Nutr. Food Res.,* 50(11): 1072-9.

Jagetia, A., Jagetia, G.C. and Jha, S. (2007). Naringin, a grapefruit flavanone, protects V79 cells against the bleomycin-induced genotoxicity and decline in survival. *J. Appl. Toxicol.,* 27(2): 122-32.

Jagetia, G.C. and Reddy, T.K. (2002). The grapefruit flavanone naringin protects against the radiation-induced genomic instability in the mice bone marrow: a micronucleus study. *Mutat Res,* 519(1-2): 37-48.

Jagetia, G.C. and Reddy, T.K. (2005). Modulation of radiation-induced alteration in the antioxidant status of mice by naringin. *Life Sci.,* 77(7): 780-94.

Jagetia, G.C., Reddy, T.K., Venkatesha, V.A. and Kedlaya, R. (2004). Influence of naringin on ferric iron induced oxidative damage in vitro. *Clin. Chim. Acta,* 347(1-2): 189-97.

Jagetia, G.C., Venkatesha, V.A. and Reddy, T.K. (2003). Naringin, a citrus flavonone, protects against radiation-induced chromosome damage in mouse bone marrow. *Mutagenesis,* 18(4): 337-43.

Jeon, S.M., Bok, S.H., Jang, M.K., Kim, Y.H., Nam, K.T., Jeong, T.S., Park, Y.B. and Choi, M.S. (2002). Comparison of antioxidant effects of naringin and probucol in cholesterol-fed rabbits. *Clin. Chim. Acta,* 317(1-2): 181-90.

Jeon, S.M., Bok, S.H., Jang, M.K., Lee, M.K., Nam, K.T., Park, Y.B., Rhee, S.J. and Choi, M.S. (2001). Antioxidative activity of naringin and lovastatin in high cholesterol-fed rabbits. *Life Sci.,* 69(24): 2855-66.

Jeon, S.M., Park, Y.B. and Choi, M.S. (2004). Antihypercholesterolemic property of naringin alters plasma and tissue lipids, cholesterol-regulating enzymes, fecal sterol and tissue morphology in rabbits. *Clin. Nutr.,* 23(5): 1025-34.

Jung, U.J., Kim, H.J., Lee, J.S., Lee, M.K., Kim, H.O., Park, E.J., Kim, H.K., Jeong, T.S. and Choi, M.S. (2003). Naringin supplementation lowers plasma lipids and enhances erythrocyte antioxidant enzyme activities in hypercholesterolemic subjects. *Clin. Nutr.,* 22(6): 561-8.

Jung, U.J., Lee, M.K., Park, Y.B., Kang, M.A. and Choi, M.S. (2006). Effect of citrus flavonoids on lipid metabolism and glucose-regulating enzyme mRNA levels in type-2 diabetic mice. *Int. J. Biochem. Cell Biol.,* 38(7): 1134-45.

Jung, U.J., Lee, M.K., Jeong, K.S. and Choi, M.S. (2004). The hypoglycemic effects of hesperidin and naringin are partly mediated by hepatic glucose-regulating enzymes in C57BL/KsJ-db/db mice. *J. Nutr.,* 134(10): 2499-503.

Kanaze, F.I., Bounartzi, M.I., Georgarakis, M. and Niopas, I. (2007). Pharmacokinetics of the citrus flavanone aglycones hesperetin and naringenin after single oral administration in human subjects. *Eur. J. Clin. Nutr.,* 61(4): 472-7.

Kanno, S., Shouji, A., Asou, K. and Ishikawa, M. (2003). Effects of naringin on hydrogen peroxide-induced cytotoxicity and apoptosis in P388 cells. *J. Pharmacol. Sci.,* 92(2): 166-70.

Kanno, S., Shouji, A., Hirata, R., Asou, K. and Ishikawa, M. (2004). Effects of naringin on cytosine arabinoside (Ara-C)-induced cytotoxicity and apoptosis in P388 cells. *Life Sci.,* 75(3): 353-65.

Kanno, S., Shouji, A., Tomizawa, A., Hiura, T., Osanai, Y., Ujibe, M., Obara, Y., Nakahata, N. and Ishikawa, M. (2006). Inhibitory effect of naringin on lipopolysaccharide (LPS)-induced endotoxin shock in mice and nitric oxide production in RAW 264.7 macrophages. *Life Sci.,* 78(7): 673-81.

Kanno, S., Tomizawa, A., Hiura, T., Osanai, Y., Shouji, A., Ujibe, M., Ohtake, T., Kimura, K. and Ishikawa, M. (2005). Inhibitory effects of naringenin on tumor growth in human cancer cell lines and sarcoma S-180-implanted mice. *Biol. Pharm. Bull,* 28(3): 527-30.

Kawaguchi, K., Kikuchi, S., Hasegawa, H., Maruyama, H., Morita, H. and Kumazawa, Y. (1999). Suppression of lipopolysaccharide-induced tumor necrosis factor-release and liver injury in mice by naringin. *Eur. J. Pharmacol.,* 368(2-3): 245-50.

Kawaguchi, K., Kikuchi, S., Hasunuma, R., Maruyama, H., Ryll, R. and Kumazawa, Y. (2004). Suppression of infection-induced endotoxin shock in mice by a citrus flavanone naringin. *Planta Med.,* 70(1): 17-22.

Kim, D.I., Lee, S.J., Lee, S.B., Park, K., Kim, W.J. and Moon, S.K. (2008) Sep. Requirement for Ras/Raf/ERK pathway in naringin-induced G1-cell-cycle arrest via p21WAF1 expression. *Carcinogenesis, 29(9): 1701-9.* Epub 2008 Feb 22.

Kim, H.J. and Choi, J.S. (2005). Effects of naringin on the pharmacokinetics of verapamil and one of its metabolites, norverapamil, in rabbits. *Biopharm Drug Dispos,* 26(7): 295-300.

Kim, S.Y., Kim, H.J., Lee, M.K., Jeon, S.M., Do, G.M., Kwon, E.Y., Cho, Y.Y., Kim, D.J., Jeong, K.S., Park, Y.B., Ha, T.Y. and Choi, M.S. (2006). Naringin time-dependently lowers hepatic cholesterol biosynthesis and plasma cholesterol in rats fed high-fat and high-cholesterol diet. *J. Med. Food,* 9(4): 582-6.

Kim, H.J., Oh, G.T., Park, Y.B., Lee, M.K., Seo, H.J. and Choi, M,S. (2004). Naringin alters the cholesterol biosynthesis and antioxidant enzyme activities in LDL receptor-knockout mice under cholesterol fed condition. *Life Sci.,* 74(13): 1621-34.

Kroyer, G. (1986). The antioxidant activity of citrus fruit peels. *Z. Ernahrungswiss.,* 25(1): 63-9.

Kumar, M.S., Unnikrishnan, M.K., Patra, S., Murthy, K. and Srinivasan, K.K. (2003). Naringin and naringenin inhibit nitrite-induced methemoglobin formation. *Pharmazie,* 58(8): 564-6.

Lambev, I., Belcheva, A. and Zhelyazkov, D. (1980a). Flavonoids with antioxidant action (naringin and rutin) and the release of mastocytic and nonmastocytic histamine. *Acta. Physiol. Pharmacol. Bulg.,* 6(2): 70-5.

Lambev, I., Krushkov, I., Zheliazkov, D. and Nikolov, N. (1980b). Antiexudative effect of naringin in experimental pulmonary edema and peritonitis. *Eksp. Med. Morfol.,* 19(4): 207-12.

Le Marchand, L., Murphy, S.P., Hankin, J.H., Wilkens, L.R. and Kolonel, L.N. (2000). Intake of flavonoids and lung cancer. *J. Natl. Cancer Inst.,* 92(2): 154-60.

Lee, C.H., Jeong, T.S., Choi, Y.K., Hyun, B.H., Oh, G.T., Kim, E.H., Kim, J.R., Han, J.I. and Bok, S.H. (2001). Anti-atherogenic effect of citrus flavonoids, naringin and naringenin, associated with hepatic ACAT and aortic VCAM-1 and MCP-1 in high cholesterol-fed rabbits. *Biochem. Biophys. Res. Commun.,* 284(3): 681-8.

Lee, E.J., Moon, G.S., Choi, W.S., Kim, W.J. and Moon, S.K. (2008) Oct 8. Naringin-induced p21WAF1-mediated G(1)-phase cell cycle arrest via activation of the Ras/Raf/ERK signaling pathway in vascular smooth muscle cell. *Food Chem. Toxicol.,* [Epub ahead of print].

Li, P., Callery, P.S., Gan, L.S. and Balani, S.K. (2007). Esterase inhibition by grapefruit juice flavonoids leading to a new drug interaction. *Drug Metab Dispos,* 35(7): 1203-8.

Li, J.M., Che, C.T., Lau, C.B., Leung, P.S. and Cheng, C.H. (2006). Inhibition of intestinal and renal Na+-glucose cotransporter by naringenin. *Int. J. Biochem. Cell Biol.,* 38(5-6): 985-95.

Li, F., Meng, F., Xiong, Z., Li, Y., Liu, R. and Liu, H. (2006). Stimulative activity of Drynaria fortunei (Kunze) J. Sm. extracts and two of its flavonoids on the proliferation of osteoblastic like cells. *Pharmazie,* 61(11): 962-5.

Lim, S.C. and Choi, J.S. (2006). Effects of naringin on the pharmacokinetics of intravenous paclitaxel in rats. *Biopharm Drug Dispos,* 27(9): 443-7.

Luo, H., Jiang, B.H., King, S.M. and Chen, Y.C. (2008). Inhibition of cell growth and VEGF expression in ovarian cancer cells by flavonoids. *Nutr. Cance,* 60(6): 800-9.

Mandadi, K., Ramirez, M., Jayaprakasha, G.K., Faraji, B., Lihono, M., Deyhim, F. and Patil, B.S. (2008) Oct 18. Itrus bioactive compounds improve bone quality and plasma antioxidant activity in orchidectomized rats. *Phytomedicine,* [Epub ahead of print].

Martín, M.J., Marhuenda, E., Pérez-Guerrero, C. and Franco, J.M. (1994). Antiulcer effect of naringin on gastric lesions induced by ethanol in rats. *Pharmacology,* 49(3): 144-50.

Mata-Bilbao Mde, L., Andrés-Lacueva, C., Roura, E., Jáuregui, O., Escribano, E., Torre, C., and Lamuela-Raventós, R.M. (2007). Absorption and pharmacokinetics of grapefruit flavanones in beagles. *Br. J. Nutr.,* 98(1): 86-92.

Middleton, E. Jr. and Drzewiecki, G. (1984). Flavonoid inhibition of human basophil histamine release stimulated by various agents. *Biochem Pharmacol,* 33(21): 3333-8.

Miller, E.G., Peacock, J.J., Bourland, T.C., Taylor, S.E., Wright, J.M. and Patil, B.S. (2008) Jan-Feb. Inhibition of oral carcinogenesis by citrus flavonoids, *Nutr. Cancer,* 60(1): 69-74.

Mitsunaga. Y., Takanaga, H., Matsuo, H,, Naito, M., Tsuruo, T., Ohtani, H. and Sawada, Y. (2000). Effect of bioflavonoids on vincristine transport across blood-brain barrier. *Eur. J. Pharmacol.,* 395(3): 193-201.

Morikawa, K., Nonaka, M., Mochizuki, H., Handa, K., Hanada, H. anf Hirota, K. (2008) Nov 4. Naringenin and Hesperetin Induce Growth Arrest, Apoptosis, and Cytoplasmic Fat Deposit in Human Preadipocytes. *J. Agric. Food Chem.,* [Epub ahead of print].

Naderi, G.A., Asgary, S., Sarraf-Zadegan, N. and Shirvany, H. (2003). Anti-oxidant effect of flavonoids on the susceptibility of LDL oxidation. *Mol. Cell Biochem.,* 246(1-2): 193-6.

Nafisi, S., Shadaloi, A., Feizbakhsh, A. and Tajmir-Riahi, H.A. (2008) Aug 30. RNA binding to antioxidant flavonoids. *J. Photochem. Photobiol. B,* [Epub ahead of print].

Nafisi, S., Hashemi, M., Rajabi, M. and Tajmir-Riahi, H.A. (2008) Aug. DNA Cell Biol. *DNA adducts with antioxidant flavonoids: morin, apigenin, and naringin, 27(8): 433-42.*

Ng, T.B., Ling, J.M., Wang, Z.T., Cai, J.N. and Xu, G.J. (1996). Examination of coumarins, flavonoids and polysaccharopeptide for antibacterial activity. *Gen. Pharmacol.,* 27(7): 1237-40.

Ng, T.B., Liu, F. and Wang, Z.T. (2000). Antioxidative activity of natural products from plants. *Life Sci.,* 66(8): 709-23.

Orallo, F., Camiña, M., Alvarez, E., Basaran, H. and Lugnier, C. (2005). Implication of cyclic nucleotide phosphodiesterase inhibition in the vasorelaxant activity of the citrus-fruits flavonoid (+/-)-naringenin. *Planta Med.,* 71(2): 99-107.

Paredes, A., Alzuru, M., Mendez, J. and Rodríguez-Ortega, M. (2003). Anti-Sindbis activity of flavanones hesperetin and naringenin. *Biol. Pharm. Bull.* 26(1):108-9.

Park, S.H., Park, E.K. and Kim, D.H. (2005). Passive cutaneous anaphylaxis-inhibitory activity of flavanones from Citrus unshiu and Poncirus trifoliata. *Planta Med.,* 71(1): 24-7.

Parmar, N.S. (1983). The gastric anti-ulcer activity of naringenin, a specific histidine decarboxylase inhibitor. *Int. J. Tissue React,* 5(4): 415-20.

Pereira, R.M., Andrades, N.E., Paulino, N., Sawaya, A.C., Eberlin, M.N., Marcucci, M.C., Favero G.M., Novak, E.M. and Bydlowski, S.P. (2007). Synthesis and characterization of a metal complex containing naringin and Cu, and its antioxidant, antimicrobial, antiinflammatory and tumor cell cytotoxicity. *Molecules,* 12(7): 1352-66.

Punithavathi, V.R., Anuthama, R. and Prince, P.S. (2008) Aug. Combined treatment with naringin and vitamin C ameliorates streptozotocin-induced diabetes in male Wistar rats. *J. Appl. Toxicol.*, 28(6): 806-13.

Rajadurai, M. and Stanely Mainzen Prince, P. (2006). Preventive effect of naringin on lipids, lipoproteins and lipid metabolic enzymes in isoproterenol-induced myocardial infarction in Wistar rats. *J. Biochem. Mol. Toxicol.,* 20(4): 191-7.

Rajadurai M., and Stanely Mainzen Prince, P. (2006). Preventive effect of naringin on lipid peroxides and antioxidants in isoproterenol-induced cardiotoxicity in Wistar rats: biochemical and histopathological evidences. *Toxicology,* 228(2-3): 259-68.

Rajadurai, M. and Stanely Mainzen Prince, P. (2007). Preventive effect of naringin on cardiac markers, electrocardiographic patterns and lysosomal hydrolases in normal and isoproterenol-induced myocardial infarction in Wistar rats. *Toxicology,* 230(2-3): 178-88.

Rajadurai, M. and Prince, P.S. (2007). Preventive effect of naringin on isoproterenol-induced cardiotoxicity in Wistar rats: an in vivo and in vitro study. *Toxicology,* 232(3): 216-25.

Rajadurai, M. and Prince, P.S. (2007). Preventive effect of naringin on cardiac mitochondrial enzymes during isoproterenol-induced myocardial infarction in rats: a transmission electron microscopic study. *J. Biochem. Mol. Toxicol.,* 21(6): 354-61.

Rajadurai, M. and Prince, P.S. (2008) Oct 10. Naringin ameliorates mitochondrial lipid peroxides, antioxidants and lipids in isoproterenol-induced myocardial infarction in Wistar rat. *Phytother Res*, [Epub ahead of print].

Ratty, A.K. and Das, N.P. (1988). Effects of flavonoids on nonenzymatic lipid peroxidation: structure-activity relationship. *Biochem Med. Metab. Biol.* 39(1): 69-79.

Reshef. N., Hayari, Y., Goren, C., Boaz, M., Madar, Z. and Knobler, H. (2005). Antihypertensive effect of sweetie fruit in patients with stage I hypertension. *Am. J. Hypertens,* 18(10): 1360-3.

Robbins, R.C., Martin, F.G. and Roe, J.M. (1988). Ingestion of grapefruit lowers elevated hematocrits in human subjects. *Int. J. Vitam Nutr. Res,* 58(4): 414-7.

Runkel, M., Bourian, M., Tegtmeier, M. and Legrum, W. (1997). The character of inhibition of the metabolism of 1,2-benzopyrone (coumarin) by grapefruit juice in human. *Eur. J. Clin. Pharmacol.,* 53(3-4): 265-9.

Russo, A., Acquaviva, R., Campisi, A., Sorrenti, V., Di Giacomo, C., Virgata, G., Barcellona, M.L. and Vanella, A. (2000). Bioflavonoids as antiradicals, antioxidants and DNA cleavage protectors. *Cell Biol. Toxicol.,* 16(2): 91-8.

Sansone, F., Aquino, R.P., Gaudio, P.D., Colombo, P. and Russo, P. (2008) Nov 1. Physical characteristics and aerosol performance of naringin dry powders for pulmonary delivery prepared by spray-drying. *Eur. J. Pharm. Biopharm.,* [Epub ahead of print].

Saponara, S., Testai, L., Iozzi, D., Martinotti, E., Martelli, A., Chericoni, S., Sgaragli, G., Fusi, F. and Calderone, V. (2006). (+/-)-Naringenin as large conductance Ca(2+)-activated K+ (BKCa) channel opener in vascular smooth muscle cells. *Br. J. Pharmacol.,* 149(8): 1013-21.

Schindler, R. and Mentlein, R. (2006). Flavonoids and vitamin E reduce the release of the angiogenic peptide vascular endothelial growth factor from human tumor cells. *J. Nutr.,* 136(6): 1477-82.

Seo, H.J., Jeong, K.S., Lee, M.K., Park, Y.B., Jung, U.J., Kim, H.J. and Choi, M.S. (2003). Role of naringin supplement in regulation of lipid and ethanol metabolism in rats. *Life Sci.,* 73(7): 933-46.

Shim, C.K., Cheon, E.P., Kang, K.W., Seo, K.S. and Han, H.K. (2007). Inhibition effect of flavonoids on monocarboxylate transporter 1 (MCT1) in Caco-2 cells. *J. Pharm. Pharmacol.,* 59(11): 1515-9.

Shin, Y.W., Bok, S.H., Jeong, T.S., Bae, K.H., Jeoung, N.H., Choi, M.S., Lee, S.H. and Park, Y.B. (1999). Hypocholesterolemic effect of naringin associated with hepatic cholesterol regulating enzyme changes in rats. *Int. J. Vitam Nutr. Res.,* 69(5): 341-7.

Shirasaka, Y., Li, Y., Shibue, Y., Kuraoka, E., Spahn-Langguth, H., Kato, Y. Langguth, P. and Tamai, I. (2008). Nov 12. Concentration-Dependent Effect of Naringin on Intestinal Absorption of beta(1)-Adrenoceptor Antagonist Talinolol Mediated by P-Glycoprotein and Organic Anion Transporting Polypeptide (Oatp). *Pharm Res,* [Epub ahead of print].

Shiratori, K., Ohgami, K., Ilieva, I., Jin, X.H., Yoshida, K., Kase, S. and Ohno, S. (2005). The effects of naringin and naringenin on endotoxin-induced uveitis in rats. *J. Ocul. Pharmacol. Ther.,* 21(4): 298-304.

Singh, D., Chander, V. and Chopra, K. (2004a). Protective effect of naringin, a bioflavonoid on ferric nitrilotriacetate-induced oxidative renal damage in rat kidney. *Toxicology,* 201(1-3): 1-8.

Singh, D., Chander, V. and Chopra, K. (2004b). Protective effect of naringin, a bioflavonoid on glycerol-induced acute renal failure in rat kidney. *Toxicology,* 201(1-3): 143-51.

Singh, D. and Chopra, K. (2004). The effect of naringin, a bioflavonoid on ischemia-reperfusion induced renal injury in rats. *Pharmacol Res.,* 50(2): 187-93.

So, F.V., Guthrie, N., Chambers, A.F., Moussa, M. and Carroll, K.K. (1996). Inhibition of human breast cancer cell proliferation and delay of mammary tumorigenesis by flavonoids and citrus juices. *Nutr. Cancer,* 26(2): 167-81.

Taur, J.S. and Rodriguez-Proteau, R. (2008) Oct 24. Effects of dietary flavonoids on the transport of cimetidine via P-glycoprotein and cationic transporters in Caco-2 and LLC-PK1 cell models. *Xenobiotica,* [Epub ahead of print].

Tsui, V.W., Wong, R.W. and Rabie, A.B. (2007). The inhibitory effects of naringin on the growth of periodontal pathogens in vitro. Phytother Res. [Epub ahead of print]

Ubeaud, G., Hagenbach, J., Vandenschrieck, S., Jung, L. and Koffel, J.C. (1999). In vitro inhibition of simvastatin metabolism in rat and human liver by naringenin. *Life Sci.,* 65(13): 1403-12.

Ueng, Y.F., Chang, Y.L., Oda, Y., Park, S.S., Liao, J.F., Lin, M.F. and Chen, C.F. (1999). In vitro and in vivo effects of naringin on cytochrome P450-dependent monooxygenase in mouse liver. *Life Sci.,* 65(24): 2591-602.

Ugocsai, K., Varga, A., Molnár, P., Antus, S. and Molnár, J. (2005). Effects of selected flavonoids and carotenoids on drug accumulation and apoptosis induction in multidrug-resistant colon cancer cells expressing MDR1/LRP. *In:* Vivo. 19(2): 433-8.

Vanamala, J., Leonardi, T., Patil, B.S., Taddeo, S.S., Murphy, M.E., Pike, L.M., Chapkin, R.S., Lupton, J.R. and Turner, N.D. (2006). Suppression of colon carcinogenesis by bioactive compounds in grapefruit. *Carcinogenesis,* 27(6): 1257-65.

Wei, M., Yang, Z., Li,P., Zhang, Y. and Sse, W.C. (2007). Anti-osteoporosis activity of naringin in the retinoic acid-induced osteoporosis model. *Am. J. Chin. Med.,* 35(4): 663-7.

Wenzel, U., Kuntz, S. and Daniel, H. (2001). Flavonoids with epidermal growth factor-receptor tyrosine kinase inhibitory activity stimulate PEPT1-mediated cefixime uptake into human intestinal epithelial cells. *J. Pharmacol. Exp. Ther.,* 299(1): 351-7.

Wong, R.W. and Rabie, A.B. (2006). Effect of naringin collagen graft on bone formation. *Biomaterials,* 27(9): 1824-31.

Wong, R.W. and Rabie, A.B. (2006). Effect of naringin on bone cells. *J. Orthop. Res.,* 24(11): 2045-50.

Wood, N. (2004). The effects of dietary bioflavonoid (rutin, quercetin, and naringin) supplementation on physiological changes in molar crestal alveolar bone-cemento-enamel junction distance in young rats. *J. Med. Food,* 7(2): 192-6.

Wood, N. (2007). The effects of selected dietary bioflavonoid supplementation on dental caries in young rats fed a high-sucrose diet. *J. Med. Food,* 10(4): 694-701.

Wu, J.B., Fong, Y.C., Tsai, H.Y., Chen, Y.F., Tsuzuki, M. and Tang, C.H. (2008) Jul 7. Naringin-induced bone morphogenetic protein-2 expression via PI3K, Akt, c-Fos/c-Jun and AP-1 pathway in osteoblasts. *Eur. J. Pharmacol,* 588(2-3): 333-41. Epub 2008 May 19.

Yeh, S.L., Wang, W.Y., Huang, C.H. and Hu, M.L. (2005). Pro-oxidative effect of beta-carotene and the interaction with flavonoids on UVA-induced DNA strand breaks in mouse fibroblast C3H10T1/2 cells. *J. Nutr. Biochem.,* 16(12): 729-35.

Yeum, C.H. and Choi, J.S. (2006). Effect of naringin pretreatment on bioavailability of verapamil in rabbits. *Arch. Pharm. Res.,* 29(1): 102-7.

Younes, M. and Siegers, C.P. (1981). Inhibitory Action of some Flavonoids on Enhanced Spontaneous Lipid Peroxidation Following Glutathione Depletion. *Planta,* 43(11): 240-4.

Yu, J., Wang, L., Walzem, R.L., Miller, E.G., Pike, L.M. and Patil, B.S. (2005). Antioxidant activity of citrus limonoids, flavonoids, and coumarins. *J. Agric Food Chem.,* 53(6): 2009-14.

Zielińska-Przyjemska, M. and Ignatowicz, E. (2008) Sep 19. Citrus fruit flavonoids influence on neutrophil apoptosis and oxidative metabolism. *Phytother Res.,* [Epub ahead of print].

In: Encyclopedia of Vitamin Research
Editor: Joshua T. Mayer

ISBN: 978-1-61761-928-1
© 2011 Nova Science Publishers, Inc.

Chapter 42

Development of Promising Naturally Derived Molecules to Improve Therapeutic Strategies[*]

***Dominique Delmas[†1,2], Frédéric Mazué[1,2], Didier Colin[1,2],
Patrick Dutartre[1,2] and Norbert Latruffe[1,2]***
[1]Inserm U866, Dijon, F-21000, France
[2]Université de Bourgogne, Faculté des Sciences Gabriel,
Centre de Recherche-Biochimie Métabolique et Nutritionnelle (LBMN),
Dijon, F-21000, France

Abstract

Numerous epidemiological studies show that some nutrients may protect against vascular diseases, cancers and associated inflammatory effects. Consequently, the use of phytoconstituents, namely those from the human diet, as therapeutic drugs is relevant. Various studies report the efficiency of phyto-molecules which have cellular targets similar to those of the new drugs developed by pharmaceutical companies. Indeed, more than 1600 patents are currently reported concerning flavonoids and 3000 patents concerning polyphenols. Pleiotropic pharmaceutical activities are claimed in fields such as cancer, inflammation arthritis, eye diseases and many other domains. The increase of activities after combination with other natural compounds or therapeutic drugs is also patented. In addition, the aforementioned molecules, from natural origin, generally exhibit low toxicities and often a multipotency which allow them to be able to simultaneously interfere with several signalling pathways. However, several in vivo studies revealed that polyphenols / flavonoids are efficiently absorbed by the organism,

---

[*] A version of this chapter was also published in *Flavonoids: Biosynthesis, Biological Effects and Dietary Sources, edited by Raymond B. Keller* published by Nova Science Publishers, Inc. It was submitted for appropriate modifications in an effort to encourage wider dissemination of research.
[†] Phone : 33 3 80 39 62 37, Fax : 33 3 80 39 62 50, Email : ddelmas@u-bourgogne.fr

but unfortunately have a low level of bioavailability, glucuronidation and sulphation being limiting factors. Therefore, many laboratories are developing elements to increase bioavailability and consequently the biological effects of these natural molecules. For example, the modifications in the lipophilicity of molecules increase the cellular uptake and consequently involve a best absorption without loss of their activities. Moreover isomerisation and methylation of hydroxyl groups of polyphenols (e.g. resveratrol) change the cell molecular targets and are crucial to improve the molecule efficiency in blocking cell proliferation. In this review, we focus on the relevance of using flavonoid and polyphenol combinations or chemical modifications to enhance their biological effects. We discuss the innovative directions to develop a new type of drugs which may especially be used in combination with other natural components or pharmacological conventional drugs in order to obtain synergistic effects.

A) Introduction

A wide variety of plant-derived compounds, including polyphenols and flavonoids, is present in the human diet and may protect against vascular diseases, cancers and associated inflammatory effects (Figure 1).

The impetus sparking of this scientific inquiry was the result of many epidemiologic studies. For example, in France, as compared with other western countries with a fat-containing diet, the strikingly low incidences of coronary heart diseases is partly attributed to the consumption of red wine, which contains high levels of polyphenols [1]. Similarly, benefit effects may be attributed to the flavonoids of green tea.

Indeed, several cohort studies demonstrate a significant inverse association between flavonoid consumption and cardiovascular risk [2]. Interestingly, other epidemiological studies reveal that phytoconstituents or micronutrients can protect against cancers [3]. Especially, Levi et al. show an inverse relation between resveratrol (a non-flavonoid polyphenol) and breast cancer risk [4]. Another cohort study in Finland [5] shows a link between flavonol consumption and reduced risk of lung cancer. These findings lead to the suggestion that polyphenols and flavonoids have beneficial health effects. Various reports from in vitro and in vivo show the pleiotropic activities of theses compounds, and interestingly, these phytoconstituents. These compounds seem to exert similar actions against general processes such as oxidation, kinases activation pathways or pro-inflammatory substances production found as well in coronary as in cancerous pathologies. In this review, we briefly summarize the pathway by which dietary microcomponents may inhibit carcinogenesis by affecting the molecular events in the initiation, promotion and progression stages. Nevertheless, there appears to be a large discrepancy between the potential effects of these compounds, as observed in vitro, and observed effects in in vivo. We show and discuss the relationship between polyphenols / flavonoids metabolism and their biological effects, and how the modifications in the lipophilicity of these molecules and the phytonaturals combinations could enhance their activities. For these practical reasons, many pharmaceutical groups develop new types of drugs that may especially be used in combination with other natural components or pharmacological conventional drugs in order to obtain synergistic effects.

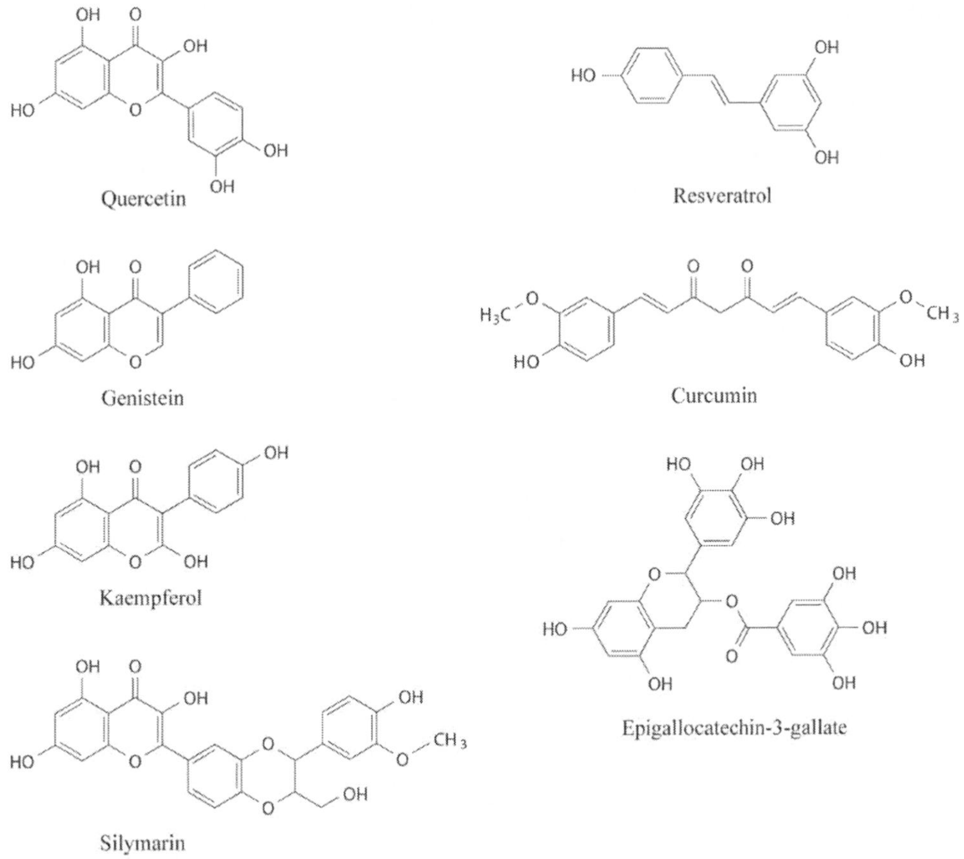

Figure 1. Examples of stilbenes / flavonoids chemical structures.

B) Phytochemicals Prevent Carcinogenesis Pathways

Carcinogenesis is commonly described by three stages—initiation, promotion and progression. The initiating event can consist of a single exposure to a carcinogenic agent or, in some cases, it may be an inherited genetic defect. The initiated cell may remain dormant for months or years and unless a promoting event occurs, it may never develop into a clinical cancer case. The promotion phase is the second major step in the carcinogenesis process in which specific agents *(referred to as promoters)* trigger the further development of the initiated cells. Promoters often, but not always, interact with the cellular DNA and influence the further expression of the mutated DNA so that the initiated cell proliferates and progresses further through the carcinogenesis process. Finally, the ultimate carcinogenesis phase is the progression which is associated with the evolution of the initiated cells into a biologically malignant cell population. In this stage, a portion of the benign tumor cells may be converted into malignant forms leading to a true cancer.

1. Anti-Initiation Activities of Phytonatural Compounds

The anti-initiation activity of polyphenols and flavonoids is linked to the suppression of the metabolic activation of carcinogens and / or the detoxifying increases via a modulation of the drug-metabolizing enzymes involved either in phase I or in phase II (Figure 2).

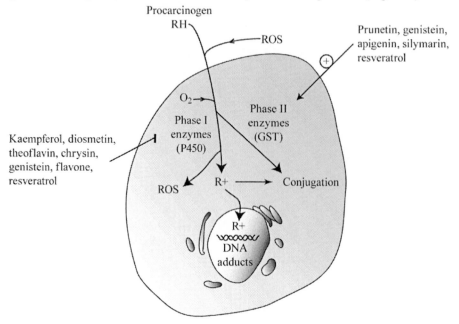

Figure 2. Polyphenols effects on tumor initiation. Polyphenols are able to prevent initiation phase by inhibition of carcinogen activation (R+) induction of carcinogen deactivation and subsequently blocking interaction between DNA and carcinogen (R+).

For example, resveratrol and genistein are able to antagonize the transactivation of genes regulated by the aryl hydrocarbon receptor (AhR) ligand, such as the 7,12-dimethylbenz[a]anthracen (DMBA) [6]. Consequently, compounds are able to reduce the number of DNA adducts induced by various chemical agents.

Moreover, polyphenolic compounds and flavonoids could induce phase II enzyme which generally protects tissues and cells from endogen and/or exogen intermediate carcinogens. Activation of phase II detoxifying enzymes by flavonoids / non flavonoids, such as UDP-glucuronyl transferase [7-9], glutathione S-transferase (GST) [10], quinone reductase [11, 12], and sulfotransferase [13] result in the detoxification of carcinogens and represent one mechanism of their anticarcinogenic effects (Figure 2).

For example, Kong et al. propose a model where an antioxidant such as butylated hydroxyanisol (BHA) and isothiocyanate sulforafane (SUL) may modulate the mitogen-activated protein kinases (MAPKs) pathway leading to transcriptional activation of the nuclear factor erythroid 2p45 related factor, Nrf2 (a basic leucine zipper transcription factor) and of the antioxidant electrophile response element (ARE), with subsequent induction of phase II detoxifying enzymes such as hemeoxygenase (HO-1), GST, NAD(P)H:quinine reductase (NQO-1) [14].

Recently, quercetin was reported to protect human hepatocytes from ethanol-induced cellular damage and this beneficial effect was mediated by a pathway involving extracellular signal-regulated protein kinase (ERK), p38, and Nrf2, with the induction of HO-1 expression [15].

In addition, the activation of Nrf2 up-regulated the induction of a phase II enzyme, NQO-1, in HepG2 cells [16]. In the same manner, resveratrol is able to up-regulate NQO-1 gene expression in human ovarian cancer PA-1 cells [17] by its activation of kinase pathways. Furthermore, a study using a resveratrol affinity column shows that the dihydronicotinamide riboside quinone reductase 2 (NQO-2) binds resveratrol and could constitute a potential target in cancer cells [18].

2. Anti-Promotion Activities of Phytonatural Compounds

The promotion phase is the second major step in the carcinogenesis process in which specific agents *(referred to as promoters)* trigger the further development of the initiated cells. Promoters often, but not always, interact with the cellular DNA and influence the further expression of the mutated DNA so that the initiated cell proliferates and progresses further through the carcinogenesis process (Figure 3).

An intricate network of signalling pathways is involved in these control mechanisms, especially the cell cycle and the induction of apoptosis. This induction of cell death in precancerous or malignant cells is considered to be a promising strategy for chemopreventive or chemotherapeutic purpose. Natural compounds, like many cytotoxic agents, affect cell proliferation by disturbing the normal progress of the cell cycle. In fact, both stilbenes and flavonoids are able to block cell progression through the cell cycle, this blockage depends on the cell type, the natural compound concentration, and the treatment duration. Various studies report that checkpoint at both G1/S and G2/M of the cell cycle is found to be perturbed by the phyto chemicals [19-21]. Checkpoints are controlled by a family of protein kinase complexes, and each complex is composed minimally of a catalytic subunit, cyclin-dependent kinases (cdks), and its essential activating partner, cyclin.

Cyclins play a key regulatory role in this process by activating their partner cdks and targeting them to the respective protein substrates [22]. Complexes-formed in this way are activated at specific intervals during the cell cycle and their inhibition blocks the cell cycle at the corresponding control point. These key regulators can be affected by these flavonoids and stilbenes leading to an arrest of the cell cycle. For example, epigallocatechin-3-gallate (EGCG), a green tea polyphenol, mediates a G1 phase arrest in various cancer cell lines such as ovarian, pancreatic through a modulation of cyclin D1 and $p21^{WAF1}$ [23, 24]. The balance between pro- and anti-apoptotic Bcl-2 family proteins favors apoptosis in prostate cancer cells also arrested in G0/G1 phase [25]. In the same manner, treatment by curcumin, resveratrol or silymarin involve an increase of $p21^{WAF1}$ and $p27^{KIP1}$ expressions and inhibit the expression of cyclin E and cyclin D1, and hyperphosphorylation of retinoblastoma (Rb) protein [26-31].

Concerning the G2/M phase, some phytochemicals can arrest the cell cycle at the transition from G2 stage to M stage such as genistein [32-35], resveratrol [36-38], curcumin and quercetin [39] in various cancer cell types (Figure 3). Biochemical analysis demonstrates that the disruption of G2 phase progression by polyphenolic compounds is accompanied by an upregulation of $p21^{WAF1}$ and an inactivation of cyclin-dependent kinase, Cdk1 [31, 35, 36, 38, 40].

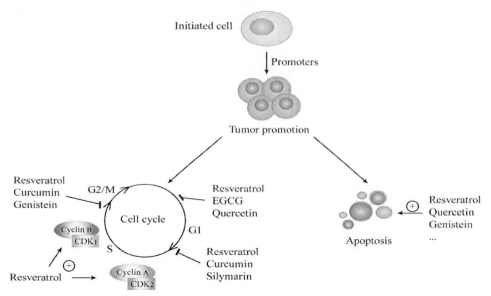

Figure 3. Polyphenols effects on tumor progression. Polyphenols are able to prevent promotion phase by inhibition of cell cycle progression and are able to induce apoptosis.

In addition to cell cycle arrest, another specialized event of polyphenol compounds action involves the induction of apoptosis (Figure 3). Induction of apoptosis in precancerous or malignant cells is considered to be a promising strategy for chemopreventive or chemotherapeutic purposes. The induction of apoptosis triggered by polyphenolic compounds has been observed in various cell types with different pathways. Indeed it has been demonstrated that polyphenols are able to activate cell death by the mitochondrial pathway or by the death receptor pathway.

The mitochondrial pathway is activated in response to extracellular signals and internal disturbances such as DNA damages. We and others have shown that polyphenols such as resveratrol [41], quercetin [42, 43], genistein [44-47] induce apoptosis in various tumor cell lines by modulating pro-apoptotic Bcl-2 family proteins which are known as "BH3-only proteins" behaving as sensors of cellular damage and initiating the agents of death process. We and others have shown that polyphenols and flavonoids down-regulate Bcl-2 protein expression [41, 48-53] and gene expression [54-56], which normally stabilizes the mitochondrial potential of the membrane ($\Delta\varphi_m$), and inhibits ROS production. Cytochrome c, in the cytosol, induces oligomerization of the adapter molecule Apaf-1 to generate a complex, the apoptosome, in which caspase-9 is activated. Active caspase-9 then triggers the catalytic maturation of caspase-3 and other resultant caspases, thus leading to cell death.

Major external signals triggering apoptosis are mediated by receptor/ligand interactions (such as CD95 and tumor necrosis factor receptor). The binding of ligand to receptor induces receptor clustering and the formation of death inducing signalling complex (DISC). This complex recruits via the adaptator FADD (Fas-associated death domain protein), multiple procaspase-8 molecules resulting in caspase-8 activation. It can activate the proteolytic cascade or / and converge on the mitochondrial pathway through the activation of pro-apoptotic members of the Bcl-2 family. We and others have shown that polyphenols/ flavonoids can involve this pathway in various cells lines.

The action of different polyphenols/flavonoids on the cell cycle at different stages, on the apoptosis cascade, or on the metabolizing enzymes, depends on their cellular targets, the concentrations used and the cellular type. These findings suggest a very specific mechanism of action of these phytochemical compounds. An association of these compounds or chemical modifications can modify their primary targets and amplify their biological effects.

3. Anti-Progression Activities of Phytonatural Compounds

Finally, stilbenes and flavonoids can act on the third step of carcinogenesis, the progression which is associated with the evolution of the initiated cells into a biologically malignant cell population. In this stage, a portion of the benign tumor cells may be converted into malignant forms leading to a true cancer. At this stage, tumor progression is certainly too advanced for chemopreventive intervention but not for a chemotherapeutic intervention. During tumor progression, polyphenols (resveratrol, curcumin, EGCG, silymarin, ...), as previously described, can act as antiproliferative agents by blocking cell cycle progression and inducing apoptosis of cancer cells. The phytochemical compounds can also act on events more specific of the progression / invasion step. In this final stage, invasion, can break away and start new clones of growth distant from the original site of development of the tumor. It is reported that resveratrol, quercetin, genistein show an anti-proliferative effect on highly invasive breast carcinoma cells (MDA-MB-435) [45, 49, 57]. In fact, these polyphenols can modify the key regulators of angiogenesis such as vascular endothelial growth factor (VEGF) and could inhibit matrix metalloproteinase. Indeed, resveratrol, genistein, quercetin and silymarin inhibit VEGF expression in various cancer cell lines [58-67]. One hypothesis is that polyphenols inhibition of VEGF-induced angiogenesis is mediated by disruption of ROS-dependent Src kinase activation and the subsequent VE-cadherin tyrosine phosphorylation. Efficient tumor invasion also requires partial degradation of the extracellular matrix (ECM) at the invasion front. The matrix metalloproteinases (MMPs) are the main proteases involved in remodeling the ECM contributing to invasion and metastasis, as well as tumor angiogenesis [68]. Concerning the human MMPs, the expression levels of gelatinase-A (MMP-2) and gelatinase-B (MMP-9) are associated with tumor metastasis for various human cancers [69, 70]. Resveratrol [71-73], silibin [74] and genistein [75, 76] are able to decrease the MMP-9 expression via diminished MAP kinases activation.

C) Polyphenols as Chemosensitizer Agents

An important cause of failure in cancer therapies is due to a defect of drug accumulation in cancer cells. Indeed, the action of chemopreventive or chemotherapeutic agents can be nullified by a failure of their absorption, distribution, metabolism or an increase in their excretion. Moreover, there appears to be a large discrepancy between the potential effect, as observed in vitro, and observed in vivo or in human subjects. This difference could be due to the poor bioavailability of flavonoids and polyphenols to target tissue in vivo. Metabolism of polyphenols occurs via a common pathway [77]. The chemical structure of polyphenols determines their rate and extent of intestinal absorption and the nature of the metabolites circulating in the plasma. The few bioavailability studies in humans show that the quantities of polyphenols found intact in urine vary from one phenolic compound to another [78-80]. They are particularly low for quercetin and rutin, a glycoside of quercetin (0.3–1.4%), but reach higher values for catechins from green tea, isoflavones from soy, flavanones from citrus fruits or anthocyanidins from red wine (3–26%). Interindividual variations have also been observed: 5–57% of the naringin consumed with grapefruit juice is found in urine according to the individual [81]. A major part of the polyphenols ingested (75–99%) is not found in urine. This implies they are not absorbed through the gut barrier, but excreted in the bile or metabolized by the colonic microflora or other tissues. In the same manner to chemical drugs, animal cells react to plant polyphenols exposure by recognizing these molecules as xenobiotics. As consequence, the cells transform these compounds in order to eliminate them as quick and as extended as possible. The pharmacokinetic is an essential parameter to select natural compounds based on their biological activity, especially their possible anticancer properties. For example, resveratrol is a well known promising anticancer natural molecule [82], but this molecule exhibits a low bioavailability [9, 83]. To overcome this problem, it is interesting to used: 1) phytochemicals combinations, 2) phytochemicals / therapeutics drugs association, 3) chemically modified natural polyphenols.

1. Phytochemical Combinations

The synergistic activity of phytochemical combinations can be easily tested in vitro and the combination treatment might represent a new strategy that can play a major role in the future of cancer chemoprevention [84]. Various reports show that the combination of several natural molecules or one phytochemical compound with an anticancer drug might be more effective in cancer prevention or in cancer therapy than a single molecule (Table I). By their pleiotropic actions, the use of several polyphenols can operate many cellular targets and/or decrease the phenomena of metabolisation, glucuronidation and sulfation, being limiting factors, and consequently increase the bioavailability and the biological effects of these natural molecules. It is the case for the EGCG glucuronidation [85] which is inhibited by the association with an alkaloid derived from black pepper, the piperine in the small intestine [86]. So, the bioavailability of EGCG is enhanced in mice. In a same manner, it is reported that coadministration of piperine and curcumin to humans and rats enhanced the bioavailability of curcumin by 2000% and 154%, respectively [87]. The use of flavonoids can also enhance the bioavailability of other polyphenols such as resveratrol. Indeed, many flavonoids can inhibit the hepatic glucuronidation and the hepatic/ duodenal sulphation of resveratrol and such inhibition may improve the bioavailability of this compound [88-90].

The modifications of bioavailability can enhance the toxicity of phytochemicals on cancer cells through synergistic or additive actions. For example, an antiproliferative synergy between resveratrol, quercetin and catechin is observed on human breast cancer cells [91]. No modifications is observed when compounds are used alone, but at only 0.5 μM, they significantly reduce cell proliferation and block cell cycle progression in vitro and at 5 mg/kg reduce breast tumor growth in a nude mouse model. The essential steps in tumor progression are the cell cycle and apoptosis alteration (see previously). Ellagic acid and quercetin interact synergistically with resveratrol in the induction of apoptosis and cause transient cell cycle arrest in human leukemia cells [92]. This apoptosis effect may be due to p21 overexpression and a greater p53 phosphorylation [93]. The MAP kinases, JNK1,2, and p38 are also activated in a "more than additive" manner.

Table I. Phytochemicals combination effects on cancer cell lines

Cell system	Compounds	Concentration	Action	Biological Effect	References
human platelets	quercetin	5 µM	synergy	Antagonizing the intracellular production of hydrogen peroxide	[95]
	catechin	25 µM			
B16M-F10	quercetin	20 µM	synergy	Inhibits metastatic activity	[96]
	pterostilbene	40 µM			
MOLT-4 (human leukemia cells)	quercetin	5 µM / 10 µM each	synergy	Antiproliferation, Cytotoxicity, Apoptosis	[97]
	ellagic acid				
	quercetin	20 µM each	synergy	p21, p53 and MAPK activation	[92]
	ellagic acid				
	quercetin	10 µM each	synergy	Apoptosis, cell cycle arrest	
	resveratrol				
	ellagic acid	10 µM each	synergy	Apoptosis, cell cycle arrest	[93]
	resveratrol				
	quercetin	10 µM each	synergy	Apoptosis, cell cycle arrest	
	ellagic acid				
	resveratrol				
3T3-L1 (adipocytes)	quercetin	25 µM each	synergy	Inhibition of adipogenesis, apoptosis	[98]
	resveratrol				
MDA-MB-231 (human breast cancer cells)	resveratrol	0,5 µM each	synergy	Antiproliferation, Apoptosis	[91]
	quercetin				
	catechin				

The caspase-3 activity can be synergistically induced by combinations of ellagic acid and reveratrol (combination index 0,64) or quercetin and resveratrol (combination index 0,68) [92]. A combination of EGCG and curcumin synergistically suppresses MDA-MB-231 estrogen receptor-alpha-breast cancer cells by cytotoxic effects and cell cycle arrest [94].

All those studies lead to think that polyphenols are mostly efficient against cancer when used in combinations or with other natural compounds in a plant-rich diet [95-98].

2. Polyphenols as Adjuvant for Chemosensitization

The increase in chemosensitivity is clinically relevant as it is often a limiting factor for the use of these compounds. Therefore, an increase in sensitivity should lead to a decrease of therapeutic thresholds. Taking into account the chemosensitizing agents in conventional therapy would potentially offer the possibility to improve the survival rate and decrease the toxicity of these substances for patients.

For example, the green tea polyphenol epigallocatechin-3-gallate shows synergy with 5-fluorouracil on human carcinoma cell lines [99]. Besides EGCG, various flavonoids or stilbenes can present a synergy or an additive action with anticancer drugs through a modification of anticancer drug metabolism or multiple actions on various targets. For example, various phenolic antioxidants (catechin, epicatechin, fisetin, gallic acid, morin, myricetin, naringenin, quercetin and resveratrol) can modify the paclitaxel metabolism. Indeed, Paclitaxel metabolites are virtually inactive in comparison with the parent drug. Some reports show that phenolic substances might increase paclitaxel blood concentrations during chemotherapy by inhibiting. cytochrome p450-catalyzed metabolism of paclitaxel [100]. Moreover the enhancement of paclitaxel action can be due to a complementary effect on targets [101, 102]. In resistant non-Hodgkin's lymphoma (NHL) and multiple myeloma (MM), resveratrol and paclitaxel selectively modify the expression of regulatory proteins in the apoptotic signalling pathway. Indeed, combination treatment results in apoptosis through the formation of tBid, mitochondrial membrane depolarization, cytosolic release of cytochrome c and Smac/DIABLO, activation of the caspase cascade, and cleavage of poly(adenosine diphosphate-ribose) polymerase. Combination of resveratrol with paclitaxel have minimal cytotoxicity against quiescent and mitogenically stimulated human peripheral blood mononuclear cells. Inhibition of Bcl-x(L) expression by resveratrol is critical for chemosensitization and its functional impairment mimics resveratrol-mediated sensitization to paclitaxel-induced apoptosis. Interestingly, a simultaneous exposure does not amplify the antiproliferative or pro-apoptotic effects of paclitaxel [103]. In fact, a pretreatment with resveratrol induces $p21^{WAF1}$ expression suggesting a possible arrest of cell cycle favoring the effect of paclitaxel action. This could be the case of the combination with 5-fluorouracil (5-Fu) which is a classic drug used in colorectal and hepatoma chemotherapy. Indeed, it was reported that resveratrol can exert synergic effect with this drug to inhibit hepatocarcinoma cell proliferation by the induction of apoptosis [104, 105].

Concerning cytokines, we and others have shown that polyphenols (resveratrol, quercetin, kaempferol, silibinin, genistein, apigenin) are able to sensitive to TRAIL (tumor necrosis factor-related apoptosis-inducing ligand)-induced apoptosis in cancer cells [106-114]. For example, in human colon cancer cell lines, some phytochemicals, resveratrol, quercetin, kaempferol can sensitize these cells to TRAIL-induced apoptosis [106, 108, 109, 112]. This sensitization by quercetin and resveratrol involves an increase of formation of a functional DISC at plasma membrane level [108, 112] and activates a caspase-dependent pathway that escapes Bcl-2-mediated expression [112]. The cholesterol sequestering agent nystatin prevents resveratrol or quercetin-induced death receptor redistribution and cell sensitization to death receptor stimulation, suggesting that polyphenols-induced redistribution of death receptors in lipid rafts is an essential step in their sensitizing effects expression [108, 112]. The sensitization by resveratrol involves also a cell cycle arrest-mediated survivin depletion and an upregulation of p21 [106].

3. Chemical Modifications of Natural Polyphenols to Improve Their Efficacy

Previous studies have documented that stilbenes and flavonoids, despite an efficient absorption by the organism, have unfortunately a low level bioavailability, glucuronidation and sulfation being limiting factors [78-80].

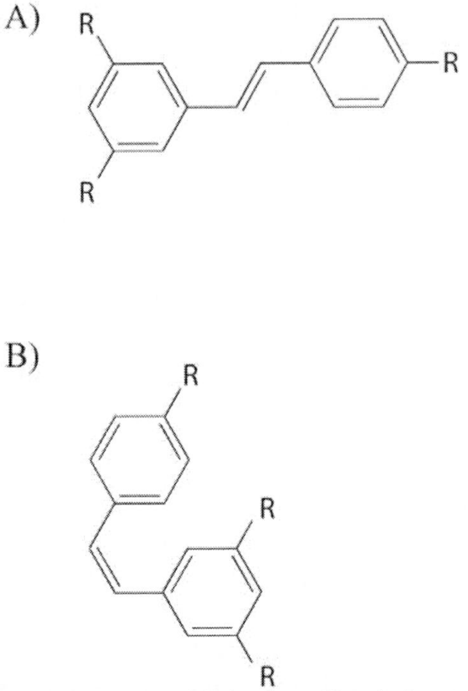

Figure 4. Chemical structures of resveratrol and derivatives. Chemical structures of *Trans* (A) or *Cis* (B) resveratrol (R=OH); resveratrol triacetate (R=CH₃COO); trimethoxyresveratrol (R=CH₃O).

Nevertheless, some elements may increase phytochemicals bioavailability such as the acetylation of polyphenol molecules (Figure 4). Indeed, recent studies show that acetylation can enhance biological activities and increase bioavailability of natural compounds such as epigallocatechin-3-gallate [115, 116]. Besides these compounds, we have recently developed acetylated forms of resveratrol and oligomers, showing that acetylation of *trans*-resveratrol inhibits colon cancer cell proliferation in the same manner as resveratrol [117]. It seems that the acetylation of the molecules does not change the targets compared to the parent molecule such as the cyclin in the cell cycle progression or the caspase activation in the apoptosis induction. These results attract major interest since an esterification of the three phenol groups leads to important modifications in the lipophilicity of the molecule and could therefore improve their intestinal absorption and cell permeability [118]. Consequently, the enhancement of cellular uptake of these molecules without loss of their activities is of great interest such as is observed with the anticancer drug, declopramide [119].

On the contrary, the isomerization of molecules and the methylation of hydroxyl groups change the cell molecular targets and are crucial to strengthened efficiency of the molecule such as resveratrol for blocking the cell cycle. Indeed, Cardile *et al.* prepared a series of acylated, methylated and hydrogenated resveratrol analogs and subjected them to bioassay towards human prostate tumor cell cultures DU-145 [120]. The results shows that the most active compound is the *cis* (Z)-3,5,4'-trimethoxystilbene, which is considerably more efficient than *trans* (E) resveratrol. Other literature data [121] reports that polymethoxystilbenes and related compounds as resveratrol analogs show interesting antitumor properties such as potent antiproliferative, pro-apoptotic activity or strong inhibition of TNFα-induced activation of NF-*k*B [122]. Further studies indicate that polymethoxystilbenes undergo different metabolic conversion and have a higher bioavailability with respect to resveratrol. Recently, Saiko et al., reported the influence of several *trans*-resveratrol analogs on HT 29 human colon cancer cell proliferation inhibition and apoptosis [123]. Indeed, a poor effect with 3,5, 4',5' tetramethoxy-*trans*-resveratrol is observed while a strong effect of 3,5 4' trimethoxy-*trans*-resveratrol and of 3,3',4,5'-tetramethoxy-*trans*-stilbene lead to remarkable changes of the cell cycle distribution on HT29 cells. Interestingly, after treatment with 3,5 4' trimethoxy-*trans*-resveratrol, growth arrest occurrs mainly in the G2-M phase, whereas incubation with 3,3',4,5'-tetramethoxy-*trans*-stilbene resulted in arrest in the G0-G1 phase of the cell cycle. The presence of hydroxylated group does not significantly change the antiproliferative effect. This is in agreement with results of Ovesna *et al.*, reporting that hydroxylation mainly protect against DNA damage [124]. However experiments are done on established cell lines which are already initiated. The only visible effect can be seen on promotion step.

Moreover, the isomerisation could modulate the activity of these compounds. Indeed, methoxylated Z-stilbenoids have a structural analogy with combretastatin A4, a potent antimitotic which interacts with tubulin like colchicines [125]. In the majority of cases where pairs of *E*- and *Z*-isomers were evaluated for antitumor activity, the *cis* (Z)-isomers proved significantly more active effects than their *trans* (E) analogs; nevertheless, the antiproliferative / apoptotic activity ratio between the *E/Z* isomers reported show wide variations and in some cases both either have comparable activities or the *E*-isomer may be even more active, as for *E* and *Z*-resveratrol. The strong effect of *cis* (Z) 3,5,4'-trimethylresveratrol is due to its inhibition of the microtubule polymerisation [126, 127], leading to a blockade of the cell division. This blockade provokes an increase of cell death, probably by mitotic catastrophe [128]. Other compounds exhibit a similar antiproliferative activity to *trans* (E) resveratrol, but their action mechanism is very different: resveratrol accumulates cells in S phase, while most of the other synthetic derivatives stop mitosis (M phase). The stronger effect of *cis* (Z) methoxy derivatives than the *trans* (E) counterparts is not linked to the lack of anti-oxidative effect (diseappearence of hydroxyl groups) but would be due to a steric mechanism leading to interference with different pathways as compared to the *trans* derivatives.

When the analogs of phenolics compounds is used, it is important to choose the methods to estimate the biological effects such as antiproliferative activity. Indeed, we and others have shown that methods commonly used to measure cytotoxic and/or antiproliferative effects could lead to a pitfall resulting from a differential sensitivity to natural compounds [117, 129]. For example, in the human colorectal cancer cell, SW480, we observed that resveratrol triacetate and a preparation containing resveratrol (16 %) and ε-viniferin (20 %) can induce an increase in the MTT-reducing activity [117]. These observations are very important since the MTT test can mask antiproliferative activities and could be a possible pitfall in cell sensitization determination. In genistein-treated cells, it was suggest that this increase of MTT-reducing activity could be due to an increase of the cell volume and of the number of mitochondria [130]. Similarly, resveratrol and its acetylated form induce an increase in cell volume and also induce an accumulation of SW480 cells in S phase [117]. Bernhard et al. [129] suggest that this phenomenon is associated with the differentiation process. This hypothesis is supported by the ability of resveratrol to induce differentiation of colon carcinoma cells via nuclear receptor [131]. However, it was not the case with ε-viniferin and its acetylated form which have no effect on the cell volume and differentiation, probably because these polyphenols may interact with the redox activities of mitochondria and consequently contribute to the reduction of MTT.

Consequently, it is necessary to evaluate methods used for cytotoxic determinations and to evaluate the absence of toxicities in normal cells. Several studies have shown that polyphenols compounds such as resveratrol and viniferin have no cytotoxic effect on normal hematopoietic progenitor cells, in contrast to leukemic cells. In addition, resveratrol shows specific cytotoxic effects toward tumor cells when compared with normal lung [132] and blood cells [133]. Furthermore, at the concentrations inducing growth inhibition and cell cycle arrest in colon carcinoma cells, polyphenols compounds and vineatrol did not impair the viability of human normal peripheral blood mononuclear cells (PBMC) and much higher concentrations were required to induce a cytotoxic effect in these cells [52], but what are the effects of derivatives compounds on the normal cells ? This point is very critical for a potential use of these compounds in therapeutics and more studies should be carried out to determine the absence of toxicity on normal cell and in animal models.

E) Pattern of Various Combinations of Chemical Modifications

Increase of activities after combination with natural compounds or therapeutic drugs or chemical modifications is also protected. In addition, these molecules, from natural origin, generally exhibit a lower toxicity and often a multipotency which allow them to be able to simultaneously interfere with several signalling pathways.

Although a large number of patents are available in data bases (more than 3000 results using the text word "polyphenol" on November 6th, 2008 in Esp@cenet.com worldwide) patent filing remains at a very high level.

Diversity of technical and scientific approaches as well as patent arguments is still a subject of surprise for people not familiar with the words polyphenol and flavonoid. Pharmacology activity profile of flavonoid is focused on cancer, control of inflammation, hair loss skin disorders and color.

Apart the "classical" anticancer and cardiovascular activity profile of polyphenol such as resveratrol new applications are claimed especially in cosmetic field, central nervous system, food complements and preparations etc... As described in figure 5, four approaches can be identified to develop innovation in polyphenol and flavonoid use:

1) modification of the production methods leads to increase of production or identification of new compounds;
2) in a second way new chemical structures are obtained by total synthesis or hemi synthesis from raw materials;

3) the third approach is related to formulation leading to increase of compliance and
    activity;

4) and finally combination therapy with various other components leads to increase or
    even synergy of activity. Due to the large of amount patents and projects this review
    will focus only on the more recent information.

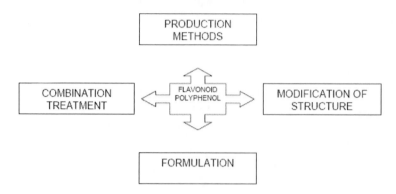

Figure 5. The four approaches for innovation in polyphenol use.

1. Production Methods

New plants are reported to be powerful producers of polyphenols with strong activity in
traditional pharmaceutical domains (inflammation, cancer, cardiovascular...) including algae
(EP1977756) and a new plant species from *Fallopia* named *igniscum* (DE102007011676)
(Table II).

Table II. Optimization of production methods for polyphenols

Patent Number and date of filling	Inventor, company	Claims and commentaries
EP1977756, 2008-10-08	M Besnard, Diana Naturals	High quantity of polyphenols in the phylum of brown algae (Phaeophyceae) is reported with activity in inflammation domain
DE102007011676 2008-09-18	J H Wilhelm	Active substances from the leafage and/or the rhizome of the new plant species from Fallopia named igniscum is claimed
JP2008037839 2008-02-21	K Masao Cosmo Oil Ltd	The agent for increasing the polyphenol content in a plant contains 5-aminolevulinic acid derivatives
CA2621922 2007-03-15	J Page Nat. Res. Council	DNA Sequences involved in prenylflavonoid synthesis in hops are use for modification of prenylflavonoid plants production
CN101199355 2008-06-18	W Liu High Tech Res Cter of Shangai	Improvement of the resveratrol production by a genetically modified peanut kernel with a full-long resveratrol synthase gene and a specific promoter Arah1P.
JP2007089430 2007-04-12	Y Tsurunaga Matsushita Ltd	Irradiation of leaves by a white lamp 2 emitting visible light, and a fluorescent light 3 emitting UV-B light. To increase polyphenol production.
CN101160393 2008-04-09	M Katz Fluxome Sciences	Metabolically engineered cells for the production of resveratrol or an oligomeric or glycosidically-bound

Table III. Optimization of production methods for flavonoids

Patent Number and date of filling	Inventor, company	Claims and commentaries
CN101229328 2008-07-30	Central South Univ of FO	*Method of extracting eucalyptus and bamboo wood flavonoid*
WO2008125433 2008-10-23	Poole Mervin C UNILEVER	The invention relates to a method for producing a plant tissue, preferably a fruit with an increased content of a flavonoid component and to a plant tissue obtained by transfection of transcripts of TDR4.
WO2008096354 2008-08-14	Levin I Israel State	*Means and methods for providing an AFT gene encoding a protein characterized by at least 80% identity with the amino acid sequence from LA1996 Seq is reported. The AFT gene confers higher concentrations of flavonoids to the plants compared with prior art cultivated plants. Transgenic plants expressing metabolites of the flavonoid pathway, especially anthocyanin or flavonols, in plants, plant parts or seeds thereof, carrying particular DNA sequences recombinable into a plurality of one or more transformation and/or expression vectors, useful for transformation and/or expression in plants are disclosed. Methods of obtaining same are disclosed.*
US2008200537 2008-08-21	Cleveland T	Increased biosynthesis of the isoflavonoid phytoalexin compounds, Glyceollins I, II and III, in soy plants is obtained after grown under stressed conditions (elicited soy). Compounds exhibit marked anti-estrogenic effects on ER function with inhibition of proliferation of ER-positive estrogen dependent breast cancer cells and inhibiting ER-dependent gene expression of progesterone receptor (PgR) and stromal derived factor-1 (SDF1/CXCL12).
JP2008161184 2008-07-17	Chin-Wen H Tatung Univ	The in vitro flavonoid-rich rhizome tissue of N. gracilis, which is obtained from a tissue culture-prepared product variable in the flavonoid content of Neomarica gracilis, contains tectorigenin which is not the case from the original plant
US2008134356 2008-06-05	Rommens C	The present invention relates to increasing at least one antioxidant level in a plant or plant product by expressing a polynucleotide that encodes a transcription factor, which is active in a flavonoid pathway. Overexpression of, for instance, a novel and newly-identified gene, the mCai gene, in a plant, results in increased accumulation of chlorogenic acid and other related phenolics, which, in turn, increases the levels of beneficial antioxidant in the plant
NZ543387 (A) 2008-04-30	Spangenberg G Agres Ltd	The present invention relates to nucleic acids and nucleic acid fragments encoding amino acid sequences for flavonoid biosynthetic enzymes in plants, and the use thereof for the modification of flavonoid biosynthesis in plants. (chalcone isomerase (CHI), chalcone synthase (CHS), chalcone reductase (CHR), dihydroflavonol 4-reductase (DFR), leucoanthocyanidin reductase (LCR), flavonoid 3', 5' hydrolase (F3'5'H), flavanone 3-hydroxylase (F3H), flavonoid 3'-hydroxylase (F3'H), phenylalanine ammonia-olyase (PAL) and vestitone reductase (VR)) (originating from WO03031622 2003-04-17)

Optimization of polyphenol production is obtained by stimulation of production by compounds (JP2008037839), genetic manipulations (CA2621922 and CN101199355) as well as treatment of plants before final extraction (JP2007089430 using lamp illumination of plants). Modification of bacteria for production of polyphenols is also feasible (CN101160393). Concerning more specifically flavonoids, new plants are reported to be powerful producer of flavonoids with strong activity in traditional pharmaceutical domains (inflammation, cancer cardiovascular…). Development of new extraction method to obtain significant quantity of compounds is claimed especially from China unfortunately without direct translation of patents (See bamboo origin in CN101229328) (Table III). Genetic transformation of plants is also used to increase flavonoid production by the use of genes involved in the synthesis pathway or transcription factors (WO2008125433, WO2008096354 US2008134356).

In a more simple approach, stress induction of production is also described in soybeans for example (US2008200537). In vitro culture is also reported to induce original production of flavonoid (JP2008161184).

2. Modification of Structures

Syntheses of new analogs of polyphenol remain a good approach for innovation (Table IV). In CA2617213 inhibition of inflammation, recruitment and cell proliferation is claimed according to chemical modifications. Rather complex compounds are also reported (example in EP1901735 or CN101115763) with questionable possibility for final pharmaceutical production (Figure 6A). Chemical modification of resveratrol remains hardly explored especially in anticancer and cardiovascular fields (see US2005240062 as an example). Association of polyphenols with fatty acids is again reported for increased activity (US2008176956 and WO2007099162).

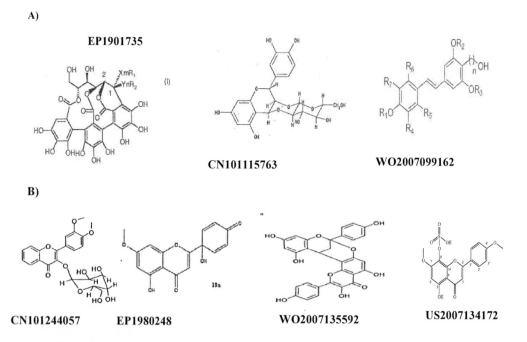

Figure 6. Some examples of structures with a patent.

Table IV. Chemical modifications by synthesis or hemi synthesis of polyphenol drugs

Patent Number and date of filling	1st Inventor, company	Claims and commentaries
CA2617213 2007-02-08	F Chiacchia Resverlogix Corp	Polyphenol-like compounds that are useful f or inhibiting VCAM-1 expression, MCP-1 expression and/or SMC proliferation for inflammation and cardiovascular problems
EP1901735 2008-03-26	G Depierre Bordeaux Univ	Polyphenols active on cell proliferation especially on cancer cells
CN101115763 2008-01-30	K Nagamine Nichirei Biosciences Inc	Polyphenol glycoside from acerola associated with an antioxidant, a glucosidase inhibitor, a food, a cosmetic, and a skin preparation for external use, each of which comprises such compound
US2005240062 2005-10-27	G Pettit	Structural modifications of resveratrol and combretastatin A-4 for the production of novel compounds having antineoplastic and antimicrobial activity
US2008176956 2008-07-24	S Hsu Georgia Res Inst	Production of green tea polyphenols with one on more ester-linked fatty acids.
WO2007099162 2007-09-07	L Bang CNRS	Hydroxylated long chain resveratrol derivatives useful as neurotrophic agents.
CN101072815 2007-11-14	T Numata Univ Tsukuba	Therapeutic agent for mitochondrial disease for preventive/therapeutic agent for diabetes mellitus with polymeric polphenol extracted for fermented tea

Table V. Chemical modifications by synthesis or hemi synthesis of flavonoid drugs

Patent Number and date of filling	1st Inventor, company	Claims and commentaries
US2008287374 2008-11-20	Yamazaki R	Flavonoid and glycosides, esters, or salts mixed with an anticancer agent are claimed to be anticancer agent (no structure available) with inhibition of BCRP (an ABC transporter)
CN101244057 2008-08-20	Yongsheng J Second Military Med Univ	"3-substituted oxygen group-3',4'-dimethoxy flavonoid compound with blood fat reducing function" (Patent in Chinese language)
EP1980248 2008-10-15	A-Shen Lin Kaohsiung Med Univ.	Flavonoid compound with modification of rings with increased anticancer activity.
US2007134172 2007-06-14	Buchholz H	Novel flavonoid derivative, to an extract comprising the flavonoid derivative, to the cosmetic and pharmaceutical use thereof, to preparations comprising the flavonoid derivative or extract, and to a process for the preparation of the flavonoid derivative or extract.
WO2008076767 2008-06-26	Cushman M Purdue Res Found.	Substituted flavonoid compounds, and pharmaceutical formulations of flavonoid compounds are described. Optimization of structure on cell proliferation and apoptosis induction is reported
CN101205233 2008-06-25	Yonghong L South Chiba Sea Inst Ocean.	Novel dimeric flavonoid compound for the treatment of cancers, especially the cervical cancer, gastric cancer and liver cancer, from the roots of the Ephedra sinica. Activity is reported on HeLa cervical carcinoma cells, SGC-7901 gastric cancer cells and HepG2 hepatocellular carcinoma cells.
WO2007135592 2007-11-29	Chan T Univ Hong Kong Polytech.	A series of flavonoid dimers are found to be efficient P-gp modulators that increase cytotoxicity of anticancer drugs in vitro and dramatically enhance their intracellular drug accumulation.

Surprisingly, polymerization of natural polyphenols is claimed to increase pharmacologic activity in metabolic disease (CN101072815) (Table IV). Concerning syntheses of new analogs of flavonoids remain as well as polyphenols a good approach for innovation (Table V). In US2008287374 and EP1980248 flavonoids and esters are demonstated as anticancer agents. WO2008076767 reports substituted flavonoid compounds, and more specifically, racemic abyssinone II, zapotin, and analogs useful for treating cancer. Substituted flavonoids in CN101244057 are described to be hypolipidemic agents (Figure 6B).

3. Formulation

Polyphenol administration is complex due to high level of astringency and bitterness and low absorption associated with questionable gut stability. Therefore new ways for increasing compliance and oral availability are under study in many companies. Microencapsulation (US2008213441) or association with new vehicle (WO2008072155) as well as nanoencapsulation (CN101214225) and nanocrystallization (CN101195559) are good ways to increase stability and facilitate absorption (Table VI).

Table VI. New formulation approaches for polyphenols use

Patent Number and date of filling	1[rst] Inventor , company	Claims and commentaries
US2008213441 2008-09-04	C J Ludwig	Reduction of astringency in polyphenol and protection from oxidation, enzymatic degradation, while maintaining gastrointestinal bioavailability within the digestive system by microencapsulation
WO2008072155 2008-06-19	E Amal Firmenich and Cie	The ingredient delivery system comprises polyphenol in combination with porous apatite grains and an amorphous metal salt in order to increase stability and availability
CN101214225 2008-07-09	Ouyangwuqing Northwest univ	Production of a resveratrol nano-emulsion anticancer drug which is characterized in that the particle size of the nano-emulsion anticancer drug is between 1nm and 100nm
CN101195559 2008-06-11	Y Wang	Resveratrol nano-crystallization relates to skin-care cosmetic technical field, relates to a method for preparing white chenopodium album alcohol nanometer crystal and application
S2008095866 2008-04-24	L Declercq Ajinomoto Monichem	Phosphorylated polyphenols combination with a carrier provide a means for delayed delivery to keratinous tissues, such as skin, hair and nails, with enzymes of the keratinous tissue dephosphorylating the polyphenol, and returning it to its native active form.
EP1893555 2008-03-05	S Delaire Rhone Poulenc Chimie	Bioprecursor of formula [A]n -PP - [B]m wherein: PP represents a polyphenol radical where each hydroxyl function is protected by a group a saturated or unsaturated alkyl chain, comprising 1 to 20 carbon atoms able to form the initial polyphenol after enzymatic digestion.
US2008213456 2008-09-04	M Chimel Mars Inc	Bars and Confectioneries with a high cocoa polyphenol content and sterol/stanol esters are produced with processes able to maintain high level of active compounds.

If required optimization of topical use of polyphenol is also hardly worked for the treatment of skin disorders. S2008095866 claims increase of topical availability of polyphenols with phosphorylated polyphenols. An original approach with the synthesis of bioprecursors of polyphenol is also reported in EP1893555 especially for topic targets. In that case bioprocessing of these molecules will lead to in situ production of active polyphenols. Food industry is also concerned by polyphenol use as demonstrated by US2008213456 showing incorporation of extracts into bars (Table VI).

Flavonoid usage is also complex due to instability of the compounds. Topical use is limited due to interaction with UV light, therefore stabilization of the drug with antioxidant compounds is necessary (WO2008140440) (Table VII).

Table VII. New formulation approaches for flavonoid use

Patent Number and date of filling	1st Inventor, company	Claims and commentaries
WO2008140440 2008-11-20	Mercier M F	Stable flavonoid solutions including antioxidant drugs in combination with other compounds and the use of these solutions in treating dermatologic conditions are reported.
JP2008174553 2008-07-31	Glico Daily Products Co	Promoting the absorption of flavonoid with pectin derived from an apple or a citrus as an effective ingredient.
JP2008174507 2008-07-31	Suntory Ltd	Production of a flavonoid (catechin or its methylated form) glycoside (from maltotriose residue-containing carbohydrate (preferably, maltotriose, maltotetraose, maltopentaose, maltohexaose, maltoheptaose, a dextrin, [gamma]-cyclodextrin, a soluble starch) highly soluble in water, better in taste and increased in stability.
DE102007005507 2008-08-07	Wellness and Health Care GMBH	Mixture of Piperin (black pepper), flavonoids (grapefruit), and a third component containing amino acids (lysine) and niacin.
CN101180319 (A) 2008-05-14	Lang Zhuo Agency Sciencde Techn and Res.	Polymer carrier with C6 or C8 position of the flavonoid A ring is used to form delivery vehicles to deliver high doses of flavonoids, and may also be used as delivery vehicles to deliver an additional bioactive agent.
GB2443576 2008-05-07	Managoli N B Sahajanand Biotech Ltd.	Implantable medical devices, such as stents, that comprise a composition for controlled delivery of flavonoids or a derivative thereof.
JP2007223914 2007-09-06	Takayanagi K Unitika Ltd	Oral administration formulation with, a carotenoid such as cryptoxanthin or its fatty acid ester, a flavonoid such as hesperidin, its derivative or hesperitin and/or its derivative and has anti-diabetes action and/or an ameliorative action for impaired glucose tolerance.

In order to increase oral availability mixture with pectin from citrus and other origin is also reported (JP2008174553). Modification of taste and increase of water solubility is obtained after glycosylation of compounds (JP2008174507). Complex mixtures are also claimed to increase oral absorption (DE102007005507). In CN101180319 chemical linkage with polymer is shown to increase local availability of flavonoid even after in vivo injection. Local effect of flavonoid is also found after inclusion of compound into medical devices for example in implantable stents for the prevention of restenosis (GB2443576) (Table VII).

4. Combination Treatment

A mixture of natural compounds is an old pharmaceutical approach in polyphenol use. However a clear synergy of activity is rarely demonstrated. Some recent patents describe this type of result (combination of fatty acids and polyphenol in US2008234361 and US2008004342 and combination of natural extracts in CN101156839, WO2008120220, EP1782802, US2007219146 and US2007054868) (Table VIII). Example of synergy of activity on cancer cell proliferation in vitro is shown in figure 7. Sophisticated in vitro demonstration of activity is under development (see SNARE target in WO2008111796 for the demonstration of compound activity on central nervous system diseases or inhibition of proteasome in US2008015248 for inhibition of cancer cell proliferation). AMPK target is also reported for control of cancer cells (US2007244202) and sirtuins for the control of aging (US2008255382).

Use of polyphenols as a nutrient is claimed in UA80692 or US2008262081 leading to improvements of cancer and inflammation. In rather the same domain WO2007009187 reports a combination with probiotics in order to increase cardiovascular health. In another approach (N101138569) polyphenols are claimed to increase antineoplastic activity of drugs such as indol-3-methanol. It is also remarkable to notice that biological activity is not necessary while ORAC value appears to be acceptable for patent filling. (US2008254135) (*ORAC Value* Is the *Value* Given to a Fruit's Oxygen Radical Absorbance Capacity). Activity on metabolic disease such as diabetes and obesity is increasing especially in patent from Asia (example in CN101199647).

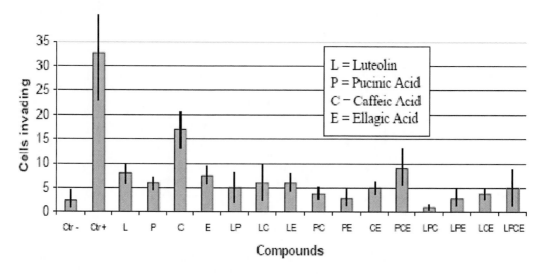

Figure 7. Synergy of activity after mixing polyphenol and conjugated fatty acids on prostate cancer cells. (US2008234361) (according to patent number US2008234361).

The patent approach remains especially active in the polyphenol field. New formulations and mixtures seem to be especially appreciated. New mechanisms of action in relation with published scientific results can be observed (sirtuin phenomenon). The number of patents is relatively stable according to a year of filing, indicating that the situation will remain relatively stable for the future.

Table VIII. Combination treatment

Patent Number and date of filling	1st Inventor, company	Claims and commentaries
US2008234361 2008-09-25 US2008004342 2008-01-03	E Lansky Rimonest Ltd G P Zaloga	Mixture of conjugated fatty acid(s) and polyphenol(s) for the treatment of obesity, diabetes, cancer and heart disease. The biologically active formulation of a fatty acid and a complex phenol is used to inhibit mammalian cell growth and/or metastasis of malignant cells.
CN101156839 2008-04-09	S Zhang Beijing Xinghao Med St	Resveratrol in combination with other drugs demonstrates synergism and enhancement function on prevention and treatment of ischemia-refilling cardiac muscle cell.
WO2008120220 2008-10-09	G Ganra Raju	Enriched 3- O-acetyl-11-keto-ss-boswellic acid and enriched demethylated curcuminoids, demonstrate synergistic effect on specific inhibition of- COX-2 and 5-LOX with anti-inflammatory, antiulcerogenic and antioxidant activities.
EP17828022007-05-09	J M Estrela Ariquel Univ Valencia	Combined use of pterostilbene and quercetin for the production of cancer treatment medicaments with decrease of cell proliferation inv tro and in in vivo experiments.
US200721914620 07-09-20	B Sunil	Diabetes Mellitus is treated by synergistic mixture of polyphenol of concentration ranging between 85 to 95% (w/w) GAE, theobromine of concentration ranging between 1 to 5% (w/w), and moisture content ranging between 0.5 to 10% (v/w).
US2007054868 2007-03-08	I B Weinstein	Treating or preventing cancer in a subject with a Synergistic Polyphenol Compound or composition thereof (no results available)
WO2008111796 2008-09-18	W Dae-Hyuk Sungkyunkwan Univ	Naturally extracted polyphenols suppresses the formation of a SNARE complex with claimed about the control of central nervous system dysfunction.
US2008015248 2008-01-17	Q P Dou	Synthetic green tea derived polyphenolic compounds are produced and used for inhibition of proteasomal activity for treating cancers
US2007244202 2007-10-18	M Takatoshi Kao Corp	AMPK activator containing resveratrol as an active ingredient was described
US2008255382 2008-10-16	A Merritt Univ Brigham	Novel sirtuin activating compounds and methods for making the same with methods for preparing resveratrol, resveratrol esters and substituted and unsubstituted stilbenes
UA80692 2007-10-25	M Rat	Nutrient pharmaceutical formulation with ascorbic acid, L-lysine, L-proline and polyphenol compound are used for the treatment if cancer
US2008262081 2008-10-23	D Raerdersorff	Nutraceutical compositions with Resveratrol for delaying aging and/or for the treatment or prevention of age-related diseases in animals, in particular in mammals including humans
WO2007009187 2007-01-25	S Keith Tarac Tech	Polyphenol from grape seed, apple, pear, green tea or cocoa extracts, in combination with lactobacilli and bifidobacteria species improves cardiovascular health
N101138569 2008-03-12	J Zhou Beijing Weimingbao Bio	Increase of the curative effect of anti-cancer Indole-3-methanol (I3C) and derivatives with resveratrol
US2008254135 2008-10-16	M Heuer	Components having high ORAC values and supplying polyphenols and antioxidants in amounts equal to or greater than the recommended daily requirements found in fruits and vegetables are able to enhance cardioprotective and immune system functions.
CN101199647 2008-06-18	B Zhao Chinese Acad Sci	Mixture of epigallocatechin-3-gallate, any kind of tea polyphenol and cyclocarya paliurus (Batal.) iljinsk water extracts are active on type II diabetes mellitus and reverse insulin resistance

Conclusion

We have established that one of the goals is to increase bioavailability and consequently the biological effects of natural molecules. Increase in the lipophilicity of molecules should improve the cellular uptake and consequently lead to better absorption without loss of their activities. We presented the idea that isomerisation and methylation of hydroxyl groups of some polyphenols especially resveratrol are crucial to improve the molecule efficiency in blocking cell proliferation by changing the cell molecular targets. We focused on the relevance of using flavonoid and polyphenol combinations or chemical modifications to enhance their biological effects. We suggested innovative directions to develop new types of drugs which may especially be used in combination with other natural components or pharmacological conventional drugs in order to obtain a synergistic effect.

Acknowledgments

This project was supported by the "Conseil Régional de Bourgogne", BIVB and Ligue contre le Cancer, comités Côte d'Or et Jura.

References

[1]	Frankel, E.N., Waterhouse, A.L. and Kinsella, J.E., Inhibition of human LDL oxidation by resveratrol, *Lancet*. 1993, *341*, 1103-1104.

[2]	Maron, D.J., Flavonoids for reduction of atherosclerotic risk, *Curr Atheroscler Rep*. 2004, *6*, 73-78.

[3]	Renaud, S.C., Gueguen, R., Schenker, J. and d'Houtaud, A., Alcohol and mortality in middle-aged men from eastern France, *Epidemiology*. 1998, *9*, 184-188.

[4]	Levi, F., Pasche, C., Lucchini, F., Ghidoni, R., Ferraroni, M. and La Vecchia, C., Resveratrol and breast cancer risk, *Eur J Cancer Prev*. 2005, *14*, 139-142.

[5]	Knekt, P., Jarvinen, R., Seppanen, R., Hellovaara, M., Teppo, L., Pukkala, E. and Aromaa, A., Dietary flavonoids and the risk of lung cancer and other malignant neoplasms, *Am J Epidemiol*. 1997, *146*, 223-230.

[6]	Chan, H.Y. and Leung, L.K., A potential protective mechanism of soya isoflavones against 7,12-dimethylbenz[a]anthracene tumour initiation, *Br J Nutr*. 2003, *90*, 457-465.

[7]	Walle, T., Otake, Y., Galijatovic, A., Ritter, J.K. and Walle, U.K., Induction of UDP-glucuronosyltransferase UGT1A1 by the flavonoid chrysin in the human hepatoma cell line hep G2, *Drug Metab Dispos*. 2000, *28*, 1077-1082.

[8]	Galijatovic, A., Walle, U.K. and Walle, T., Induction of UDP-glucuronosyltransferase by the flavonoids chrysin and quercetin in Caco-2 cells, *Pharm Res*. 2000, *17*, 21-26.

[9]	Lancon, A., Hanet, N., Jannin, B., Delmas, D., Heydel, J.M., Lizard, G., Chagnon, M.C., Artur, Y. and Latruffe, N., Resveratrol in human hepatoma HepG2 cells:

metabolism and inducibility of detoxifying enzymes, *Drug Metab Dispos*. 2007, *35*, 699-703.

[10] Nijhoff, W.A., Bosboom, M.A., Smidt, M.H. and Peters, W.H., Enhancement of rat hepatic and gastrointestinal glutathione and glutathione S-transferases by alpha-angelicalactone and flavone, *Carcinogenesis*. 1995, *16*, 607-612.

[11] Miranda, C.L., Aponso, G.L., Stevens, J.F., Deinzer, M.L. and Buhler, D.R., Prenylated chalcones and flavanones as inducers of quinone reductase in mouse Hepa 1c1c7 cells, *Cancer Lett*. 2000, *149*, 21-29.

[12] Yannai, S., Day, A.J., Williamson, G. and Rhodes, M.J., Characterization of flavonoids as monofunctional or bifunctional inducers of quinone reductase in murine hepatoma cell lines, *Food Chem Toxicol*. 1998, *36*, 623-630.

[13] Eaton, E.A., Walle, U.K., Lewis, A.J., Hudson, T., Wilson, A.A. and Walle, T., Flavonoids, potent inhibitors of the human P-form phenolsulfotransferase. Potential role in drug metabolism and chemoprevention, *Drug Metab Dispos*. 1996, *24*, 232-237.

[14] Kong, A.N., Yu, R., Hebbar, V., Chen, C., Owuor, E., Hu, R., Ee, R. and Mandlekar, S., Signal transduction events elicited by cancer prevention compounds, *Mutat Res*. 2001, *480-481*, 231-241.

[15] Murakami, A., Ashida, H. and Terao, J., Multitargeted cancer prevention by quercetin, *Cancer Lett*. 2008, *269*, 315-325.

[16] Tanigawa, S., Fujii, M. and Hou, D.X., Action of Nrf2 and Keap1 in ARE-mediated NQO1 expression by quercetin, *Free Radic Biol Med*. 2007, *42*, 1690-1703.

[17] Yang, S.H., Kim, J.S., Oh, T.J., Kim, M.S., Lee, S.W., Woo, S.K., Cho, H.S., Choi, Y.H., Kim, Y.H., Rha, S.Y., Chung, H.C. and An, S.W., Genome-scale analysis of resveratrol-induced gene expression profile in human ovarian cancer cells using a cDNA microarray, *Int J Oncol*. 2003, *22*, 741-750.

[18] Wang, Z., Hsieh, T.C., Zhang, Z., Ma, Y. and Wu, J.M., Identification and purification of resveratrol targeting proteins using immobilized resveratrol affinity chromatography, *Biochem Biophys Res Commun*. 2004, *323*, 743-749.

[19] Traganos, F., Ardelt, B., Halko, N., Bruno, S. and Darzynkiewicz, Z., Effects of genistein on the growth and cell cycle progression of normal human lymphocytes and human leukemic MOLT-4 and HL-60 cells, *Cancer Res*. 1992, *52*, 6200-6208.

[20] Hosokawa, N., Hosokawa, Y., Sakai, T., Yoshida, M., Marui, N., Nishino, H., Kawai, K. and Aoike, A., Inhibitory effect of quercetin on the synthesis of a possibly cell-cycle-related 17-kDa protein, in human colon cancer cells, *Int J Cancer*. 1990, *45*, 1119-1124.

[21] Zi, X., Grasso, A.W., Kung, H.J. and Agarwal, R., A flavonoid antioxidant, silymarin, inhibits activation of erbB1 signaling and induces cyclin-dependent kinase inhibitors, G1 arrest, and anticarcinogenic effects in human prostate carcinoma DU145 cells, *Cancer Res*. 1998, *58*, 1920-1929.

[22] Morgan, D.O., Principles of CDK regulation, *Nature*. 1995, *374*, 131-134.

[23] Huh, S.W., Bae, S.M., Kim, Y.W., Lee, J.M., Namkoong, S.E., Lee, I.P., Kim, S.H., Kim, C.K. and Ahn, W.S., Anticancer effects of (-)-epigallocatechin-3-gallate on ovarian carcinoma cell lines, *Gynecol Oncol*. 2004, *94*, 760-768.

[24] Hsieh, T.C. and Wu, J.M., Suppression of cell proliferation and gene expression by combinatorial synergy of EGCG, resveratrol and gamma-tocotrienol in estrogen receptor-positive MCF-7 breast cancer cells, *Int J Oncol*. 2008, *33*, 851-859.

[25] Hastak, K., Gupta, S., Ahmad, N., Agarwal, M.K., Agarwal, M.L. and Mukhtar, H., Role of p53 and NF-kappaB in epigallocatechin-3-gallate-induced apoptosis of LNCaP cells, *Oncogene*. 2003, *22*, 4851-4859.

[26] Lah, J.J., Cui, W. and Hu, K.Q., Effects and mechanisms of silibinin on human hepatoma cell lines, *World J Gastroenterol*. 2007, *13*, 5299-5305.

[27] Srivastava, R.K., Chen, Q., Siddiqui, I., Sarva, K. and Shankar, S., Linkage of curcumin-induced cell cycle arrest and apoptosis by cyclin-dependent kinase inhibitor p21(/WAF1/CIP1), *Cell Cycle*. 2007, *6*, 2953-2961.

[28] Ahmad, N., Adhami, V.M., Afaq, F., Feyes, D.K. and Mukhtar, H., Resveratrol causes WAF-1/p21-mediated G(1)-phase arrest of cell cycle and induction of apoptosis in human epidermoid carcinoma A431 cells, *Clin Cancer Res*. 2001, *7*, 1466-1473.

[29] Adhami, V.M., Afaq, F. and Ahmad, N., Involvement of the retinoblastoma (pRb)-E2F/DP pathway during antiproliferative effects of resveratrol in human epidermoid carcinoma (A431) cells, *Biochem Biophys Res Commun*. 2001, *288*, 579-585.

[30] Kim, Y.A., Lee, W.H., Choi, T.H., Rhee, S.H., Park, K.Y. and Choi, Y.H., Involvement of p21WAF1/CIP1, pRB, Bax and NF-kappaB in induction of growth arrest and apoptosis by resveratrol in human lung carcinoma A549 cells, *Int J Oncol*. 2003, *23*, 1143-1149.

[31] Deep, G. and Agarwal, R., Chemopreventive efficacy of silymarin in skin and prostate cancer, *Integr Cancer Ther*. 2007, *6*, 130-145.

[32] Lian, F., Bhuiyan, M., Li, Y.W., Wall, N., Kraut, M. and Sarkar, F.H., Genistein-induced G2-M arrest, p21WAF1 upregulation, and apoptosis in a non-small-cell lung cancer cell line, *Nutr Cancer*. 1998, *31*, 184-191.

[33] Pagliacci, M.C., Smacchia, M., Migliorati, G., Grignani, F., Riccardi, C. and Nicoletti, I., Growth-inhibitory effects of the natural phyto-oestrogen genistein in MCF-7 human breast cancer cells, *Eur J Cancer*. 1994, *30A*, 1675-1682.

[34] Casagrande, F. and Darbon, J.M., p21CIP1 is dispensable for the G2 arrest caused by genistein in human melanoma cells, *Exp Cell Res*. 2000, *258*, 101-108.

[35] Davis, J.N., Singh, B., Bhuiyan, M. and Sarkar, F.H., Genistein-induced upregulation of p21WAF1, downregulation of cyclin B, and induction of apoptosis in prostate cancer cells, *Nutr Cancer*. 1998, *32*, 123-131.

[36] Wolter, F., Akoglu, B., Clausnitzer, A. and Stein, J., Downregulation of the cyclin D1/Cdk4 complex occurs during resveratrol-induced cell cycle arrest in colon cancer cell lines, *J Nutr*. 2001, *131*, 2197-2203.

[37] Schneider, Y., Vincent, F., Duranton, B., Badolo, L., Gosse, F., Bergmann, C., Seiler, N. and Raul, F., Anti-proliferative effect of resveratrol, a natural component of grapes and wine, on human colonic cancer cells, *Cancer Lett*. 2000, *158*, 85-91.

[38] Delmas, D., Passilly-Degrace, P., Jannin, B., Malki, M.C. and Latruffe, N., Resveratrol, a chemopreventive agent, disrupts the cell cycle control of human SW480 colorectal tumor cells, *Int J Mol Med*. 2002, *10*, 193-199.

[39] Choi, J.A., Kim, J.Y., Lee, J.Y., Kang, C.M., Kwon, H.J., Yoo, Y.D., Kim, T.W., Lee, Y.S. and Lee, S.J., Induction of cell cycle arrest and apoptosis in human breast cancer cells by quercetin, *Int J Oncol*. 2001, *19*, 837-844.

[40] Liang, Y.C., Tsai, S.H., Chen, L., Lin-Shiau, S.Y. and Lin, J.K., Resveratrol-induced G2 arrest through the inhibition of CDK7 and p34CDC2 kinases in colon carcinoma HT29 cells, *Biochem Pharmacol*. 2003, *65*, 1053-1060.

[41] Delmas, D., Rebe, C., Lacour, S., Filomenko, R., Athias, A., Gambert, P., Cherkaoui-Malki, M., Jannin, B., Dubrez-Daloz, L., Latruffe, N. and Solary, E., Resveratrol-induced apoptosis is associated with Fas redistribution in the rafts and the formation of a death-inducing signaling complex in colon cancer cells, *J Biol Chem*. 2003, *278*, 41482-41490.

[42] Mouria, M., Gukovskaya, A.S., Jung, Y., Buechler, P., Hines, O.J., Reber, H.A. and Pandol, S.J., Food-derived polyphenols inhibit pancreatic cancer growth through mitochondrial cytochrome C release and apoptosis, *Int J Cancer*. 2002, *98*, 761-769.

[43] Granado-Serrano, A.B., Martin, M.A., Bravo, L., Goya, L. and Ramos, S., Quercetin induces apoptosis via caspase activation, regulation of Bcl-2, and inhibition of PI-3-kinase/Akt and ERK pathways in a human hepatoma cell line (HepG2), *J Nutr*. 2006, *136*, 2715-2721.

[44] Li, Y., Upadhyay, S., Bhuiyan, M. and Sarkar, F.H., Induction of apoptosis in breast cancer cells MDA-MB-231 by genistein, *Oncogene*. 1999, *18*, 3166-3172.

[45] Li, Y., Bhuiyan, M. and Sarkar, F.H., Induction of apoptosis and inhibition of c-erbB-2 in MDA-MB-435 cells by genistein, *Int J Oncol*. 1999, *15*, 525-533.

[46] Alhasan, S.A., Pietrasczkiwicz, H., Alonso, M.D., Ensley, J. and Sarkar, F.H., Genistein-induced cell cycle arrest and apoptosis in a head and neck squamous cell carcinoma cell line, *Nutr Cancer*. 1999, *34*, 12-19.

[47] Katdare, M., Osborne, M. and Telang, N.T., Soy isoflavone genistein modulates cell cycle progression and induces apoptosis in HER-2/neu oncogene expressing human breast epithelial cells, *Int J Oncol*. 2002, *21*, 809-815.

[48] Kim, Y.A., Choi, B.T., Lee, Y.T., Park, D.I., Rhee, S.H., Park, K.Y. and Choi, Y.H., Resveratrol inhibits cell proliferation and induces apoptosis of human breast carcinoma MCF-7 cells, *Oncol Rep*. 2004, *11*, 441-446.

[49] Hsieh, T.C., Burfeind, P., Laud, K., Backer, J.M., Traganos, F., Darzynkiewicz, Z. and Wu, J.M., Cell cycle effects and control of gene expression by resveratrol in human breast carcinoma cell lines with different metastatic potentials, *Int J Oncol*. 1999, *15*, 245-252.

[50] Surh, Y.J., Hurh, Y.J., Kang, J.Y., Lee, E., Kong, G. and Lee, S.J., Resveratrol, an antioxidant present in red wine, induces apoptosis in human promyelocytic leukemia (HL-60) cells, *Cancer Lett*. 1999, *140*, 1-10.

[51] Roman, V., Billard, C., Kern, C., Ferry-Dumazet, H., Izard, J.C., Mohammad, R., Mossalayi, D.M. and Kolb, J.P., Analysis of resveratrol-induced apoptosis in human B-cell chronic leukaemia, *Br J Haematol*. 2002, *117*, 842-851.

[52] Billard, C., Izard, J.C., Roman, V., Kern, C., Mathiot, C., Mentz, F. and Kolb, J.P., Comparative antiproliferative and apoptotic effects of resveratrol, epsilon-viniferin and vine-shots derived polyphenols (vineatrols) on chronic B lymphocytic leukemia cells and normal human lymphocytes, *Leuk Lymphoma*. 2002, *43*, 1991-2002.

[53] Lee, D.H., Szczepanski, M. and Lee, Y.J., Role of Bax in quercetin-induced apoptosis in human prostate cancer cells, *Biochem Pharmacol*. 2008, *75*, 2345-2355.

[54] Zhou, H.B., Yan, Y., Sun, Y.N. and Zhu, J.R., Resveratrol induces apoptosis in human esophageal carcinoma cells, *World J Gastroenterol*. 2003, *9*, 408-411.

[55] Kaneuchi, M., Sasaki, M., Tanaka, Y., Yamamoto, R., Sakuragi, N. and Dahiya, R., Resveratrol suppresses growth of Ishikawa cells through down-regulation of EGF, *Int J Oncol*. 2003, *23*, 1167-1172.

[56] Zhou, H.B., Chen, J.J., Wang, W.X., Cai, J.T. and Du, Q., Anticancer activity of resveratrol on implanted human primary gastric carcinoma cells in nude mice, *World J Gastroenterol*. 2005, *11*, 280-284.

[57] Dechsupa, S., Kothan, S., Vergote, J., Leger, G., Martineau, A., Berangeo, S., Kosanlavit, R., Moretti, J.L. and Mankhetkorn, S., Quercetin, Siamois 1 and Siamois 2 induce apoptosis in human breast cancer MDA-mB-435 cells xenograft in vivo, *Cancer Biol Ther*. 2007, *6*, 56-61.

[58] Aggarwal, B.B., Bhardwaj, A., Aggarwal, R.S., Seeram, N.P., Shishodia, S. and Takada, Y., Role of resveratrol in prevention and therapy of cancer: preclinical and clinical studies, *Anticancer Res*. 2004, *24*, 2783-2840.

[59] Brakenhielm, E., Cao, R. and Cao, Y., Suppression of angiogenesis, tumor growth, and wound healing by resveratrol, a natural compound in red wine and grapes, *Faseb J*. 2001, *15*, 1798-1800.

[60] Kim, J.D., Liu, L., Guo, W. and Meydani, M., Chemical structure of flavonols in relation to modulation of angiogenesis and immune-endothelial cell adhesion, *J Nutr Biochem*. 2006, *17*, 165-176.

[61] Luo, H., Jiang, B.H., King, S.M. and Chen, Y.C., Inhibition of cell growth and VEGF expression in ovarian cancer cells by flavonoids, *Nutr Cancer*. 2008, *60*, 800-809.

[62] Guo, Y., Wang, S., Hoot, D.R. and Clinton, S.K., Suppression of VEGF-mediated autocrine and paracrine interactions between prostate cancer cells and vascular endothelial cells by soy isoflavones, *J Nutr Biochem*. 2007, *18*, 408-417.

[63] Kim, M.H., Flavonoids inhibit VEGF/bFGF-induced angiogenesis in vitro by inhibiting the matrix-degrading proteases, *J Cell Biochem*. 2003, *89*, 529-538.

[64] Jiang, C., Agarwal, R. and Lu, J., Anti-angiogenic potential of a cancer chemopreventive flavonoid antioxidant, silymarin: inhibition of key attributes of vascular endothelial cells and angiogenic cytokine secretion by cancer epithelial cells, *Biochem Biophys Res Commun*. 2000, *276*, 371-378.

[65] Yang, S.H., Lin, J.K., Chen, W.S. and Chiu, J.H., Anti-angiogenic effect of silymarin on colon cancer LoVo cell line, *J Surg Res*. 2003, *113*, 133-138.

[66] Garvin, S., Ollinger, K. and Dabrosin, C., Resveratrol induces apoptosis and inhibits angiogenesis in human breast cancer xenografts in vivo, *Cancer Lett*. 2006, *231*, 113-122.

[67] Cao, Z., Fang, J., Xia, C., Shi, X. and Jiang, B.H., trans-3,4,5'-Trihydroxystibene inhibits hypoxia-inducible factor 1alpha and vascular endothelial growth factor expression in human ovarian cancer cells, *Clin Cancer Res*. 2004, *10*, 5253-5263.

[68] Sternlicht, M.D. and Werb, Z., How matrix metalloproteinases regulate cell behavior, *Annu Rev Cell Dev Biol*. 2001, *17*, 463-516.

[69] Sato, H., Takino, T., Okada, Y., Cao, J., Shinagawa, A., Yamamoto, E. and Seiki, M., A matrix metalloproteinase expressed on the surface of invasive tumour cells, *Nature*. 1994, *370*, 61-65.

[70] Sato, H. and Seiki, M., Regulatory mechanism of 92 kDa type IV collagenase gene expression which is associated with invasiveness of tumor cells, *Oncogene*. 1993, *8*, 395-405.

[71] Li, Y.T., Shen, F., Liu, B.H. and Cheng, G.F., Resveratrol inhibits matrix metalloproteinase-9 transcription in U937 cells, *Acta Pharmacol Sin*. 2003, *24*, 1167-1171.

[72]   Woo, J.H., Lim, J.H., Kim, Y.H., Suh, S.I., Min do, S., Chang, J.S., Lee, Y.H., Park, J.W. and Kwon, T.K., Resveratrol inhibits phorbol myristate acetate-induced matrix metalloproteinase-9 expression by inhibiting JNK and PKC delta signal transduction, *Oncogene*. 2004, *23*, 1845-1853.

[73]   Gunther, S., Ruhe, C., Derikito, M.G., Bose, G., Sauer, H. and Wartenberg, M., Polyphenols prevent cell shedding from mouse mammary cancer spheroids and inhibit cancer cell invasion in confrontation cultures derived from embryonic stem cells, *Cancer Lett.* 2006.

[74]   Lee, S.O., Jeong, Y.J., Im, H.G., Kim, C.H., Chang, Y.C. and Lee, I.S., Silibinin suppresses PMA-induced MMP-9 expression by blocking the AP-1 activation via MAPK signaling pathways in MCF-7 human breast carcinoma cells, *Biochem Biophys Res Commun*. 2007, *354*, 165-171.

[75]   Owen, J.L., Torroella-Kouri, M. and Iragavarapu-Charyulu, V., Molecular events involved in the increased expression of matrix metalloproteinase-9 by T lymphocytes of mammary tumor-bearing mice, *Int J Mol Med*. 2008, *21*, 125-134.

[76]   Li, Y. and Sarkar, F.H., Down-regulation of invasion and angiogenesis-related genes identified by cDNA microarray analysis of PC3 prostate cancer cells treated with genistein, *Cancer Lett.* 2002, *186*, 157-164.

[77]   Scalbert, A. and Williamson, G., Dietary intake and bioavailability of polyphenols, *J Nutr*. 2000, *130*, 2073S-2085S.

[78]   Xu, X., Wang, H.J., Murphy, P.A., Cook, L. and Hendrich, S., Daidzein is a more bioavailable soymilk isoflavone than is genistein in adult women, *J Nutr*. 1994, *124*, 825-832.

[79]   Hollman, P.C., van Trijp, J.M., Buysman, M.N., van der Gaag, M.S., Mengelers, M.J., de Vries, J.H. and Katan, M.B., Relative bioavailability of the antioxidant flavonoid quercetin from various foods in man, *FEBS Lett*. 1997, *418*, 152-156.

[80]   Lee, M.J., Wang, Z.Y., Li, H., Chen, L., Sun, Y., Gobbo, S., Balentine, D.A. and Yang, C.S., Analysis of plasma and urinary tea polyphenols in human subjects, *Cancer Epidemiol Biomarkers Prev*. 1995, *4*, 393-399.

[81]   Fuhr, U. and Kummert, A.L., The fate of naringin in humans: a key to grapefruit juice-drug interactions? *Clin Pharmacol Ther*. 1995, *58*, 365-373.

[82]   Delmas, D., Lancon, A., Colin, D., Jannin, B. and Latruffe, N., Resveratrol as a chemopreventive agent: a promising molecule for fighting cancer, *Curr Drug Targets*. 2006, *7*, 423-442.

[83]   [83] Niles, R.M., Cook, C.P., Meadows, G.G., Fu, Y.M., McLaughlin, J.L. and Rankin, G.O., Resveratrol is rapidly metabolized in athymic (nu/nu) mice and does not inhibit human melanoma xenograft tumor growth, *J Nutr*. 2006, *136*, 2542-2546.

[84]   Sporn, M.B. and Suh, N., Chemoprevention: an essential approach to controlling cancer, *Nat Rev Cancer*. 2002, *2*, 537-543.

[85]   Lambert, J.D., Lee, M.J., Lu, H., Meng, X., Hong, J.J., Seril, D.N., Sturgill, M.G. and Yang, C.S., Epigallocatechin-3-gallate is absorbed but extensively glucuronidated following oral administration to mice, *J Nutr*. 2003, *133*, 4172-4177.

[86]   Lambert, J.D., Hong, J., Kim, D.H., Mishin, V.M. and Yang, C.S., Piperine enhances the bioavailability of the tea polyphenol (-)-epigallocatechin-3-gallate in mice, *J Nutr*. 2004, *134*, 1948-1952.

[87] Shoba, G., Joy, D., Joseph, T., Majeed, M., Rajendran, R. and Srinivas, P.S., Influence of piperine on the pharmacokinetics of curcumin in animals and human volunteers, *Planta Med.* 1998, *64*, 353-356.

[88] de Santi, C., Pietrabissa, A., Mosca, F. and Pacifici, G.M., Glucuronidation of resveratrol, a natural product present in grape and wine, in the human liver, *Xenobiotica.* 2000, *30*, 1047-1054.

[89] De Santi, C., Pietrabissa, A., Spisni, R., Mosca, F. and Pacifici, G.M., Sulphation of resveratrol, a natural compound present in wine, and its inhibition by natural flavonoids, *Xenobiotica.* 2000, *30*, 857-866.

[90] De Santi, C., Pietrabissa, A., Spisni, R., Mosca, F. and Pacifici, G.M., Sulphation of resveratrol, a natural product present in grapes and wine, in the human liver and duodenum, *Xenobiotica.* 2000, *30*, 609-617.

[91] Schlachterman, A., Valle, F., Wall, K.M., Azios, N.G., Castillo, L., Morell, L., Washington, A.V., Cubano, L.A. and Dharmawardhane, S.F., Combined resveratrol, quercetin, and catechin treatment reduces breast tumor growth in a nude mouse model, *Transl Oncol.* 2008, *1*, 19-27.

[92] Mertens-Talcott, S.U. and Percival, S.S., Ellagic acid and quercetin interact synergistically with resveratrol in the induction of apoptosis and cause transient cell cycle arrest in human leukemia cells, *Cancer Lett.* 2005, *218*, 141-151.

[93] Mertens-Talcott, S.U., Bomser, J.A., Romero, C., Talcott, S.T. and Percival, S.S., Ellagic acid potentiates the effect of quercetin on p21waf1/cip1, p53, and MAP-kinases without affecting intracellular generation of reactive oxygen species in vitro, *J Nutr.* 2005, *135*, 609-614.

[94] Somers-Edgar, T.J., Scandlyn, M.J., Stuart, E.C., Le Nedelec, M.J., Valentine, S.P. and Rosengren, R.J., The combination of epigallocatechin gallate and curcumin suppresses ER alpha-breast cancer cell growth in vitro and in vivo, *Int J Cancer.* 2008, *122*, 1966-1971.

[95] Pignatelli, P., Pulcinelli, F.M., Celestini, A., Lenti, L., Ghiselli, A., Gazzaniga, P.P. and Violi, F., The flavonoids quercetin and catechin synergistically inhibit platelet function by antagonizing the intracellular production of hydrogen peroxide, *Am J Clin Nutr.* 2000, *72*, 1150-1155.

[96] Ferrer, P., Asensi, M., Segarra, R., Ortega, A., Benlloch, M., Obrador, E., Varea, M.T., Asensio, G., Jorda, L. and Estrela, J.M., Association between pterostilbene and quercetin inhibits metastatic activity of B16 melanoma, *Neoplasia.* 2005, *7*, 37-47.

[97] Mertens-Talcott, S.U., Talcott, S.T. and Percival, S.S., Low concentrations of quercetin and ellagic acid synergistically influence proliferation, cytotoxicity and apoptosis in MOLT-4 human leukemia cells, *J Nutr.* 2003, *133*, 2669-2674.

[98] Yang, J.Y., Della-Fera, M.A., Rayalam, S., Ambati, S., Hartzell, D.L., Park, H.J. and Baile, C.A., Enhanced inhibition of adipogenesis and induction of apoptosis in 3T3-L1 adipocytes with combinations of resveratrol and quercetin, *Life Sci.* 2008, *82*, 1032-1039.

[99] Navarro-Peran, E., Cabezas-Herrera, J., Campo, L.S. and Rodriguez-Lopez, J.N., Effects of folate cycle disruption by the green tea polyphenol epigallocatechin-3-gallate, *Int J Biochem Cell Biol.* 2007, *39*, 2215-2225.

[100] Vaclavikova, R., Horsky, S., Simek, P. and Gut, I., Paclitaxel metabolism in rat and human liver microsomes is inhibited by phenolic antioxidants, *Naunyn Schmiedebergs Arch Pharmacol.* 2003, *368*, 200-209.

[101] Jazirehi, A.R. and Bonavida, B., Resveratrol modifies the expression of apoptotic regulatory proteins and sensitizes non-Hodgkin's lymphoma and multiple myeloma cell lines to paclitaxel-induced apoptosis, *Mol Cancer Ther.* 2004, *3*, 71-84.

[102] Duraj, J., Bodo, J., Sulikova, M., Rauko, P. and Sedlak, J., Diverse resveratrol sensitization to apoptosis induced by anticancer drugs in sensitive and resistant leukemia cells, *Neoplasma.* 2006, *53*, 384-392.

[103] Kubota, T., Uemura, Y., Kobayashi, M. and Taguchi, H., Combined effects of resveratrol and paclitaxel on lung cancer cells, *Anticancer Res.* 2003, *23*, 4039-4046.

[104] Sun, Z.J., Pan, C.E., Liu, H.S. and Wang, G.J., Anti-hepatoma activity of resveratrol in vitro, *World J Gastroenterol.* 2002, *8*, 79-81.

[105] Fuggetta, M.P., D'Atri, S., Lanzilli, G., Tricarico, M., Cannavo, E., Zambruno, G., Falchetti, R. and Ravagnan, G., In vitro antitumour activity of resveratrol in human melanoma cells sensitive or resistant to temozolomide, *Melanoma Res.* 2004, *14*, 189-196.

[106] Fulda, S. and Debatin, K.M., Sensitization for tumor necrosis factor-related apoptosis-inducing ligand-induced apoptosis by the chemopreventive agent resveratrol, *Cancer Res.* 2004, *64*, 337-346.

[107] Russo, M., Nigro, P., Rosiello, R., D'Arienzo, R. and Russo, G.L., Quercetin enhances CD95- and TRAIL-induced apoptosis in leukemia cell lines, *Leukemia.* 2007, *21*, 1130-1133.

[108] Psahoulia, F.H., Drosopoulos, K.G., Doubravska, L., Andera, L. and Pintzas, A., Quercetin enhances TRAIL-mediated apoptosis in colon cancer cells by inducing the accumulation of death receptors in lipid rafts, *Mol Cancer Ther.* 2007, *6*, 2591-2599.

[109] Yoshida, T., Konishi, M., Horinaka, M., Yasuda, T., Goda, A.E., Taniguchi, H., Yano, K., Wakada, M. and Sakai, T., Kaempferol sensitizes colon cancer cells to TRAIL-induced apoptosis, *Biochem Biophys Res Commun.* 2008, *375*, 129-133.

[110] Son, Y.G., Kim, E.H., Kim, J.Y., Kim, S.U., Kwon, T.K., Yoon, A.R., Yun, C.O. and Choi, K.S., Silibinin sensitizes human glioma cells to TRAIL-mediated apoptosis via DR5 up-regulation and down-regulation of c-FLIP and survivin, *Cancer Res.* 2007, *67*, 8274-8284.

[111] Jin, C.Y., Park, C., Cheong, J., Choi, B.T., Lee, T.H., Lee, J.D., Lee, W.H., Kim, G.Y., Ryu, C.H. and Choi, Y.H., Genistein sensitizes TRAIL-resistant human gastric adenocarcinoma AGS cells through activation of caspase-3, *Cancer Lett.* 2007, *257*, 56-64.

[112] Delmas, D., Rebe, C., Micheau, O., Athias, A., Gambert, P., Grazide, S., Laurent, G., Latruffe, N. and Solary, E., Redistribution of CD95, DR4 and DR5 in rafts accounts for the synergistic toxicity of resveratrol and death receptor ligands in colon carcinoma cells, *Oncogene.* 2004, *23*, 8979-8986.

[113] Gill, C., Walsh, S.E., Morrissey, C., Fitzpatrick, J.M. and Watson, R.W., Resveratrol sensitizes androgen independent prostate cancer cells to death-receptor mediated apoptosis through multiple mechanisms, *Prostate.* 2007, *67*, 1641-1653.

[114] Horinaka, M., Yoshida, T., Shiraishi, T., Nakata, S., Wakada, M. and Sakai, T., The dietary flavonoid apigenin sensitizes malignant tumor cells to tumor necrosis factor-related apoptosis-inducing ligand, *Mol Cancer Ther*. 2006, *5*, 945-951.

[115] Lambert, J.D., Sang, S., Hong, J., Kwon, S.J., Lee, M.J., Ho, C.T. and Yang, C.S., Peracetylation as a means of enhancing in vitro bioactivity and bioavailability of epigallocatechin-3-gallate, *Drug Metab Dispos*. 2006, *34*, 2111-2116.

[116] Fragopoulou, E., Nomikos, T., Karantonis, H.C., Apostolakis, C., Pliakis, E., Samiotaki, M., Panayotou, G. and Antonopoulou, S., Biological activity of acetylated phenolic compounds, *J Agric Food Chem*. 2007, *55*, 80-89.

[117] Marel, A.K., Lizard, G., Izard, J.C., Latruffe, N. and Delmas, D., Inhibitory effects of trans-resveratrol analogs molecules on the proliferation and the cell cycle progression of human colon tumoral cells, *Mol Nutr Food Res*. 2008, *52*, 538-548.

[118] Riva, S., Monti, D., Luisetti, M. and Danieli, B., Enzymatic modification of natural compounds with pharmacological properties, *Ann N Y Acad Sci*. 1998, *864*, 70-80.

[119] Hua, J., Sheng, Y., Bryngelsson, C., Kane, R. and Pero, R.W., Comparison of antitumor activity of declopramide (3-chloroprocainamide) and N-acetyl-declopramide, *Anticancer Res*. 1999, *19*, 285-290.

[120] Cardile, V., Lombardo, L., Spatafora, C. and Tringali, C., Chemo-enzymatic synthesis and cell-growth inhibition activity of resveratrol analogues, *Bioorg Chem*. 2005, *33*, 22-33.

[121] Pettit, G.R., Grealish, M.P., Jung, M.K., Hamel, E., Pettit, R.K., Chapuis, J.C. and Schmidt, J.M., Antineoplastic agents. 465. Structural modification of resveratrol: sodium resverastatin phosphate, *J Med Chem*. 2002, *45*, 2534-2542.

[122] Heynekamp, J.J., Weber, W.M., Hunsaker, L.A., Gonzales, A.M., Orlando, R.A., Deck, L.M. and Jagt, D.L., Substituted trans-stilbenes, including analogues of the natural product resveratrol, inhibit the human tumor necrosis factor alpha-induced activation of transcription factor nuclear factor KappaB, *J Med Chem*. 2006, *49*, 7182-7189.

[123] Saiko, P., Pemberger, M., Horvath, Z., Savinc, I., Grusch, M., Handler, N., Erker, T., Jaeger, W., Fritzer-Szekeres, M. and Szekeres, T., Novel resveratrol analogs induce apoptosis and cause cell cycle arrest in HT29 human colon cancer cells: inhibition of ribonucleotide reductase activity, *Oncol Rep*. 2008, *19*, 1621-1626.

[124] Ovesna, Z., Kozics, K., Bader, Y., Saiko, P., Handler, N., Erker, T. and Szekeres, T., Antioxidant activity of resveratrol, piceatannol and 3,3',4,4',5,5'-hexahydroxy-trans-stilbene in three leukemia cell lines, *Oncol Rep*. 2006, *16*, 617-624.

[125] de Lima, D.P., Rotta, R., Beatriz, A., Marques, M.R., Montenegro, R.C., Vasconcellos, M.C., Pessoa, C., de Moraes, M.O., Costa-Lotufo, L.V., Frankland Sawaya, A.C. and Eberlin, M.N., Synthesis and biological evaluation of cytotoxic properties of stilbene-based resveratrol analogs, *Eur J Med Chem*. 2008.

[126] Schneider, Y., Fischer, B., Coelho, D., Roussi, S., Gosse, F., Bischoff, P. and Raul, F., (Z)-3,5,4'-Tri-O-methyl-resveratrol, induces apoptosis in human lymphoblastoid cells independently of their p53 status, *Cancer Lett*. 2004, *211*, 155-161.

[127] Seiler, N., Schneider, Y., Gosse, F., Schleiffer, R. and Raul, F., Polyploidisation of metastatic colon carcinoma cells by microtubule and tubulin interacting drugs: effect on proteolytic activity and invasiveness, *Int J Oncol*. 2004, *25*, 1039-1048.

[128] Mansilla, S., Bataller, M. and Portugal, J., Mitotic catastrophe as a consequence of chemotherapy, *Anticancer Agents Med Chem*. 2006, *6*, 589-602.

[129] Bernhard, D., Schwaiger, W., Crazzolara, R., Tinhofer, I., Kofler, R. and Csordas, A., Enhanced MTT-reducing activity under growth inhibition by resveratrol in CEM-C7H2 lymphocytic leukemia cells, *Cancer Lett.* 2003, *195*, 193-199.

[130] Pagliacci, M.C., Spinozzi, F., Migliorati, G., Fumi, G., Smacchia, M., Grignani, F., Riccardi, C. and Nicoletti, I., Genistein inhibits tumour cell growth in vitro but enhances mitochondrial reduction of tetrazolium salts: a further pitfall in the use of the MTT assay for evaluating cell growth and survival, *Eur J Cancer.* 1993, *29A*, 1573-1577.

[131] Ulrich, S., Loitsch, S.M., Rau, O., von Knethen, A., Brune, B., Schubert-Zsilavecz, M. and Stein, J.M., Peroxisome Proliferator-Activated Receptor {gamma} as a Molecular Target of Resveratrol-Induced Modulation of Polyamine Metabolism, *Cancer Res.* 2006, *66*, 7348-7354.

[132] Lu, J., Ho, C.H., Ghai, G. and Chen, K.Y., Resveratrol analog, 3,4,5,4'-tetrahydroxystilbene, differentially induces pro-apoptotic p53/Bax gene expression and inhibits the growth of transformed cells but not their normal counterparts, *Carcinogenesis.* 2001, *22*, 321-328.

[133] Clement, M.V., Hirpara, J.L., Chawdhury, S.H. and Pervaiz, S., Chemopreventive agent resveratrol, a natural product derived from grapes, triggers CD95 signaling-dependent apoptosis in human tumor cells, *Blood.* 1998, 92, 996-1002.

In: Encyclopedia of Vitamin Research
Editor: Joshua T. Mayer

ISBN: 978-1-61761-928-1
© 2011 Nova Science Publishers, Inc.

Chapter 43

Effect of a Diet Rich in Cocoa Flavonoids on Experimental Acute Inflammation[*]

M. Castell[†1,4], A. Franch[1,2,4], S. Ramos-Romero[1], E. Ramiro-Puig[3], F. J. Pérez-Cano[1,4] and C. Castellote[1,2,4]

[1]Department of Physiology, Faculty of Pharmacy,
University of Barcelona, Barcelona, Spain
[2]CIBER *Epidemiología y Salud Pública*, Barcelona, Spain
[3]INSERM U793, Faculté Necker-Enfants Malades, Paris, France
[4]Members of *Institut de Recerca en Nutrició i Seguretat Alimentària*
(INSA, University of Barcelona)

Abstract

Cocoa has recently become an object of interest due to its high content of flavonoids, mainly the monomers epicatechin and catechin and various polymers derived from these monomers called procyanidins. Previous *in vitro* studies have shown the ability of cocoa flavonoids to down-regulate inflammatory mediators produced by stimulated macrophages, but there are no studies that consider the effects of *in vivo* cocoa intake on inflammatory response. In the present article, we report the *in vivo* cocoa inhibitory effect on the acute inflammatory response. Female Wistar rats received Natural Forastero cocoa containing 21.2 mg flavonoids/g for 7 days (2.4 or 4.8 g per rat kg, p.o.). Then, acute inflammation was induced by means of carrageenin, histamine, serotonin, bradykinin or PGE_2 hind-paw injection. Rats fed 4.8 g/kg/day cocoa showed a significant reduction in the hind-paw edema induced by carrageenin from the first hour after induction ($P<0.05$).

---

[*] A version of this chapter was also published in *Flavonoids: Biosynthesis, Biological Effects and Dietary Sources, edited by Raymond B. Keller* published by Nova Science Publishers, Inc. It was submitted for appropriate modifications in an effort to encourage wider dissemination of research.
[†] E-mail: margaridacastell@ub.edu

However, cocoa intake did not modify the edema induced by histamine, serotonin or PGE_2. Only a certain protective effect was observed at the lowest dose of cocoa in the bradykinin model. Moreover, peritoneal macrophages from rats that received 4.8 g/kg/day cocoa for 7 days showed a reduced ability to produce radical oxygen species (ROS), nitric oxide (NO), tumor necrosis factor α (TNFα) and interleukin 6 (IL-6). This fact could justify, at least partially, the beneficial effect of cocoa on carrageenin-induced inflammation. In summary, a diet rich in cocoa flavonoids was able to down-regulate the acute inflammatory response by decreasing the inflammatory potential of macrophages.

1. Introduction

One of the foods with a relatively high content of flavonoids is cocoa, which is obtained from the beans of the *Theobroma cacao* tree (Lee, 2003). The beneficial effects of cocoa were known as early as 600 BC: the Mayans and Aztecs roasted and ground cocoa beans to prepare a divine beverage called *xocolatl*, which was mainly used to cure fatigue, fever, infections, and heart pain (Hurst et al., 2002). Although most people presently see cocoa and its derivatives only as snacks, scientific evidence of the health benefits of cocoa known by the ancients is emerging now.

In addition to being a rich source of fiber (26–40%), proteins (15–20%), carbohydrates (~15%), and lipids (10–24%), cocoa powder contains minerals, vitamins (A, E, B and folic acid) and a high amount of flavonoids. However, cocoa flavonoid content is difficult to establish because it depends on geographic origin, climate, storage methods and manufacturing processes (Manach et al., 2004; McShea et al., 2008). Cocoa powder mainly contains the flavanols (-)-epicatechin, (+)-catechin and polymers derived from these monomers called procyanidins; it is reported to contain up to 70 mg/g of polyphenols (Vinson et al., 1999). Epicatechin and catechin are biologically active, but epicatechin is more efficiently absorbed than catechin (Baba et al., 2001). Procyanidins are the major flavonoids in cocoa and chocolate products ranging from 2.16 to 48.70 mg/g (Gu et al., 2006). Short procyanidins (dimers and trimers) are absorbed in the small intestine and rapidly detected in plasma (Baba et al., 2000). However, large procyanidins are less efficiently absorbed in its polymeric form, but can be metabolized by colon microflora to phenolic acids and then absorbed (Manach et al., 2004). Quercetin and its derivatives, naringenin, luteolin and apigenin, are also present in smaller quantities (Sanchez-Rabaneda et al., 2003).

Experimental and clinical data suggest that the consumption of cocoa flavonoids can produce positive clinical benefits in the cardiovascular system (review by Buijsse et al., 2006 and Cooper et al., 2008) and also in brain function (reviewed by McShea et al., 2008). Cocoa intake reduces the risk of cardiovascular disease by modulating blood pressure (Grassi et al., 2005; Taubert et al., 2007) as well as decreasing blood cholesterol (Baba et al., 2007), moreover it produces vasodilatation and inhibits platelet activation and aggregation (Hermann et al., 2006). *In vitro* assays and studies in animal models suggest that cocoa has beneficial effects on neurodegenerative disorders such as Alzheimer's disease and Parkinson's disease (Datla et al., 2007; Ramiro-Puig et al., 2009a). However, it remains to establish doses and length of treatment because a recent trial in healthy adults does not find neuropsychological effects after a short-term dark chocolate intake (Crews et al., 2008). Biological effects of cocoa are mainly attributed to the high content of antioxidant polyphenols (reviewed in

Ramiro-Puig et al., 2009b). Cocoa has a potent antioxidant capacity compared to products traditionally considered high in antioxidants (Lee et al., 2003; Vinson et al., 2006). Flavonoids act as antioxidants by directly neutralizing free radicals, chelating Fe^{2+} and Cu^+ which enhance highly aggressive ROS, inhibiting xanthine oxidase that is responsible for ROS production, and up-regulating or protecting antioxidant defense (Cotelle, 2001). Epicatechin and catechin are very effective in neutralizing several types of free radicals (Hatano et al., 2002; Yilmaz et al., 2004). Procyanidins account for the highest percentage of antioxidants in cocoa products (Gu et al., 2006) and they also scavenge radicals with an activity that is proportional to the number of monomeric units they contain (Counet et al., 2003). In addition, quercetin and other compounds such as methylxanthines contribute to cocoa's antioxidant activity (Lamuela-Raventos at al., 2001; Azam et al., 2003). The antioxidant properties of flavonoids in cocoa lead us to consider it as a potential beneficial ingredient able to down-regulate the inflammatory response. *In vitro* studies showed that cocoa flavonoids modulate cytokines and eicosanoids produced during inflammation (Mao et al., 2000; Schramm et al., 2001). In response to inflammatory stimulus, macrophages produce nitric oxide (NO) and cytokines, mainly tumor necrosis factor-α (TNFα) and interleukin (IL-) 1, IL-6, and IL-12, and chemokines, such as monocyte chemoattractant protein 1 (MCP-1) (reviewed by Medzhitov, 2008). *In vitro* studies have demonstrated the regulatory effects of cocoa on secretion of inflammatory mediators (reviewed by Ramiro-Puig et al., 2009b). Flavonoid-rich cocoa extract added to LPS-stimulated macrophages decreases secretion of TNFα, MCP-1, and NO (Ono et al., 2003; Ramiro et al., 2005). However, other studies with purified cocoa flavonoid fractions show an enhanced secretion of TNFα, IL-1, IL-6 and IL-10 from stimulated human peripheral blood mononuclear cells (Kenny et al., 2007). Although these *in vitro* studies concerning the anti-inflammatory ability of cocoa flavonoids, alone or in the whole product, few studies focus on the *in vivo* effect. It has been described that supplementation with cocoa products in humans did not affect markers of inflammation (Mathur et al., 2002); however, a recent cross-sectional analysis shows that the regular intake of dark chocolate by a healthy population from southern Italy is inversely related to serum C-reactive protein concentration (di Giuseppe et al., 2008).

The aim of this study was, firstly, to ascertain the potential anti-inflammatory activity induced by cocoa intake and, secondly, to test this potential on several rat models of acute inflammation. The first goal was developed in peritoneal macrophages obtained from rats that had received daily cocoa for a week, and was focused on the production of oxidants (ROS and NO) and cytokines (TNFα and IL-6). Secondly, in rats with the same cocoa diet, the development of acute inflammation was determined after induction with carrageenin, histamine, serotonin, bradykinin and prostaglandin E_2 (PGE_2).

2. Material and Methods

2.1. Animals

Eight-week-old female Wistar rats were obtained from Harlan (Barcelona, Spain). Rats were housed 3 per cage in controlled conditions of temperature and humidity in a 12:12 light:dark cycle. Rats had free access to food (chow ref. 2014, Harlan Teklad, Madison, WI,

USA) and water. Animals were randomly distributed in 3-4 experimental groups in each experimental design (n = 8-10/group). Two of them were daily administered, by oral gavage, with cocoa in mineral water at doses of 2.4 g/kg/day and 4.8 g/kg/day for 7 days. We used Natural Forastero cocoa (Nutrexpa, Barcelona, Spain) containing 21.2 mg of total phenols/g according to the Folin-Ciocalteu method (Singleton et al., 1999). The remaining animals received the same volume of vehicle (mineral water). Handling was done in the same time range to avoid the influence of biological rhythms. At the end of the study rats were sacrificed by CO_2 inhalation. Studies were performed in accordance with the institutional guidelines for the care and use of laboratory animals established by the Ethical Committee for Animal Experimentation at the University of Barcelona and approved by the Catalonian Government.

2.2. Isolation of Peritoneal Macrophages

After 7 days of cocoa or vehicle administration p.o., rats were anaesthetized with ketamine/xylacine (i.m., 90 mg/kg and 10 mg/kg, respectively) to obtain peritoneal macrophages. 40 mL ice-cold sterile phosphate buffer solution (PBS) pH 7.2 was injected to peritoneal cavity. Abdominal massages were immediately performed to induce cell migration. Cell suspension was aspirated, centrifuged (170 g, 5 min, 4 °C) and resuspended in cold DMEM+GlutaMAX media (Invitrogen, Paisley, UK) containing 10% fetal bovine serum (PAA, Pashing, Austria), 100 IU/mL streptomycin-penicillin (Sigma-Aldrich, St Louis, MO, USA) (DMEM-FBS). Cell count and viability was determined by double staining with acridine orange and ethidium bromide (Sigma) followed by fluorescence light microscopical analysis. Cells were plated and cultured in different conditions according to the assay.

2.3. ROS Production by DCF Assay

To determine the effects of cocoa on ROS production, peritoneal macrophages (25 x 10^3 cells/100 μL in DMEM-FBS) were plated in 96 well black plates (Corning Inc, NY, USA) and allowed to attach overnight (37 °C, 5% CO_2). Macrophages were washed once with warm RPMI-1640 medium without phenol red (Sigma) containing 100 IU/mL streptomycin-penicillin and incubated with 20 μmol/L of reduced 2',7'-dichlorofluorescein diacetate (H_2DCF-DA, Invitrogen) probe for 30 min at 37 °C. H_2DCF-DA diffuses through the cell membrane and is enzymatically hydrolyzed by intracellular esterases to form non-fluorescent 2',7'-dichlorofluorescein (H_2DCF) which is oxidized by ROS to a fluorescent compound (DCF). Thus, DCF fluorescence intensity is proportional to intracellular ROS production. Fluorescence was measured every 30 min by fluorometry (excitation 538 nm, emission 485 nm) up to 3.5 h. For each animal, background from corresponding wells without fluorescent probe was subtracted.

2.4. Cytokine and NO Production

Immediately after isolation, macrophages were plated in 12-well flat-bottom plate (TPP, Trasadingen, Switzerland) at 1.2 x 10^6/mL in DMEM-FBS (37 °C, 5% CO_2) overnight to allow macrophage adhesion. Non-adherent cells were removed by washing three times with warm sterile PBS. The attached macrophages were stimulated by addition of 1 μg/mL lypopolysaccharide (LPS) from *E.coli* O55:B5 (Sigma). Supernatants were collected for quantification of TNFα after 6 h and IL-6 and NO after 24 h. Supernatants were stored at -80 °C until evaluation. Cells were harvested to determine cell viability. The concentration of TNFα and IL-6 in supernatants was quantified using rat ELISA sets from BD Pharmingen (Erembodegen, Belgium), following the manufacturer's instructions.

Stable end product of NO, NO_2^-, was quantified by a modification of Griess reaction. Briefly, macrophage supernatants (100 μL) were mixed with 60 μL sulphanilamide 1% (in 1.2 N HCl) and 60 μL N-(1-naphthyl)ethylene-diamine dihydrochloride 0.3% (in distilled water) for 10 min at room temperature. Absorbance was read spectrophotometrically at 540 nm. The concentration of NO_2^- was calculated using known concentration of $NaNO_2$.

2.5. Induction of Acute Inflammation in Rat Hind Paws

Five rat models of acute inflammation were induced by subplantar injection of carrageenin λ, histamine, serotonin, bradykinin or PGE_2, all from Sigma-Aldrich. After 7 days of cocoa or vehicle administration p.o., animals were injected with 0.1 mL carrageenin λ (10 mg/mL), histamine (5 mg/mL), serotonin (5 mg/mL), bradykinin (0.08 mg/mL) or PGE_2 (0.01 mg/mL), in saline solution. The left hind paw was injected with the same volume of saline solution. A reference treatment group was constituted by animals administered with vehicle during 7 days that received one dose of indomethacin (p.o., 10 mg/kg, Sigma in 0.1% CMC-Tween 20) 1 h prior to the induction of inflammation.

2.6. Inflammation Assessment

Paw volume was measured by using a water plethysmometer (UGO Basile, Comerlo, VA, Italy). Left and right hind paws were measured just before the induction (time 0). After carrageenin injection, paw volumes were quantified at 30 min and every hour until 6 h. In the other 4 experimental models, the measurements were performed each 15 min during the first hour, and each 30 min up to 2 h. All determinations were performed in a blinded manner. Paw volumes were expressed as percentage of increase with respect to time 0. Area under curve (AUC) was calculated between time 0 and the end of the inflammatory period evaluation.

2.7. Statistics

The software package SPSS 16.0 (SPSS Inc., Chicago, IL, USA) was used for statistical analysis. Conventional one-way ANOVA was performed, considering the experimental group as independent variable. When treatment had a significant effect on dependent variable, Scheffe's test was applied. Significant differences were accepted when $P < 0.05$.

3. Results

3.1. Peritoneal Macrophages Viability

Peritoneal macrophages were obtained from rats after cocoa intake (2.4 or 4.8 g/kg/day) or vehicle for 7 days. Cells were 98% viable when isolated. After overnight culture and washing, some cells were LPS-stimulated and 6 h later, they showed a viability of about 40% whereas non-stimulated cultures were ~50% viable. However, 24 h after LPS stimulation, macrophage viability reached ~70% and 75% in LPS-stimulated and non-stimulated macrophages, respectively. There were no differences among cells obtained from both cocoa-administered rats and those from reference animals.

3.2. ROS and NO Production by Peritoneal Macrophages

ROS production from peritoneal macrophages increased progressively along the 3.5 h assay (Figure 1A). Cells obtained from 2.4 g/kg cocoa animals produced the same ROS levels as reference macrophages. Macrophages isolated from animals that received 4.8 g/kg/day of cocoa synthesized lower ROS than reference cells already at 0.5 h and all along the studied period. Differences between both groups were higher as later measurements were made but they did not reach statistically significant results because of the high variability.

NO production was detected in macrophage culture medium after 24 h of LPS-stimulation or in resting conditions (Figure 1B).

Macrophages obtained from rats that received 2.4 g/kg/day of cocoa showed NO levels similar to those from reference group, both in LPS-stimulation and in resting conditions. Nevertheless, NO secretion by macrophages isolated from animals with an intake of 4.8 g/kg/day of cocoa was lower than that quantified in the reference group in any culture condition (P<0.05, Figure 1B).

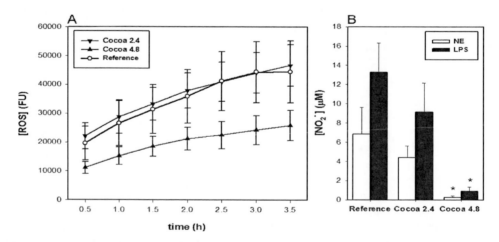

Figure 1. ROS and NO production by peritoneal macrophages. Time-course of ROS production from peritoneal macrophages (A) was determined by means of DCF assay. NO cell production, quantified as NO_2^- concentration (B), was measured by modified Griess assay in LPS-stimulated and resting macrophages. Values are summarized as mean ± SEM (n = 8-9). * P<0.05 compared with reference group.

3.3. TNFα and IL-6 Secretion from Peritoneal Macrophages

TNFα secretion was quantified in LPS-stimulated and resting macrophages. Macrophages from animals administered with 4.8 g/kg/day of cocoa produced lower TNFα levels than those of reference cells (P<0.05, Figure 2A). The reduction of TNFα levels was about 75% and 82% in both non-stimulated and LPS-stimulated conditions, respectively. Conversely, macrophages from animals that received 2.4 g/kg/day of cocoa did not modify the secretion of this cytokine.

In addition, 4.8 g/kg/day of cocoa intake diminished the IL-6 secretion by non-stimulated and LPS-stimulated macrophages (P<0.01, Figure 2B). In this case, the IL-6 inhibition got up to 94% in non-stimulated macrophages and to 88% in LPS-stimulated ones with respect to reference cells. No significant differences in IL-6 levels were found in macrophage cultures from animals administered with 2.4 g/kg cocoa.

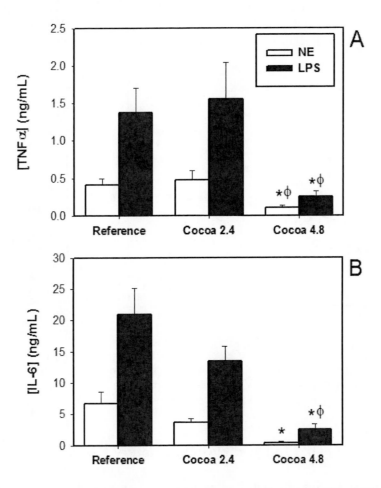

Figure 2. TNFα and IL-6 secretion from peritoneal macrophages. TNFα (A) and IL-6 (B) concentration (ng/mL) in cell culture supernatants was determined by means of ELISA assay. Values are summarized as mean ± SEM (n = 8-9). * P<0.05 compared with reference group. ϕ P<0.05 compared with 2.4 g/kg cocoa group.

3.4. Paw Edema Induced by Carrageenin

The time-course of hind-paw volume increase after carrageenin injection is summarized in Figure 3A. Paw edema was detected in the reference group from 30 min after carrageenin injection. Thereafter, it rose reaching a maximum increase of ~80% with respect to time 0 at 5-6 h post-injection. Indomethacin showed its anti-inflammatory effect from 1 h post-induction ($P<0.05$) and during all the study ($P<0.01$). Animals from 2.4 g/kg cocoa group displayed a lower paw volume increase than reference group during the first hour ($P<0.05$); thereafter, however, their paw edema fit the reference pattern. Animals that had taken 4.8 g/kg/day of cocoa showed a significant paw edema improvement which was already detected 2 h after carrageenin injection ($P<0.05$), and remained until the end of the study ($P<0.05$). At this time, the inflammation developed in the 4.8 g/kg cocoa group was the 68% of that of the reference group.

AUC from paw edema time-course was calculated between 0 and 6 h post-induction (Figure 3B). AUC from 4.8 g/kg cocoa animals was 30% lower than that in reference group ($P<0.001$), whereas, indomethacin inhibition was of about 44% ($P<0.001$).

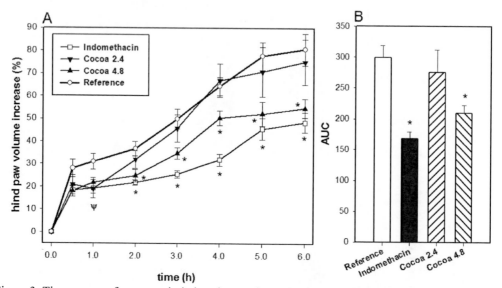

Figure 3. Time-course of carrageenin-induced paw edema. Percentage of hind-paw volume increase respect to time 0 (A) along 6 h from carrageenin-injection. Area under the curve (B) determined between time 0 and 6 h post-induction. Values are summarized as mean ± SEM (n = 8-10). * $P<0.05$ compared with reference group. ψ $P<0.05$ all treated groups compared with reference group.

3.5. Acute Paw Edema Induced by Inflammatory Mediators

Time-course of acute inflammation induced by histamine, serotonin, bradykinin and PGE_2 are showed in Figure 4. Paw edema induced by histamine (Figure 4A) or bradykinin (Figure 4C) was maximum at 0.5 h after injection, rising up to 40%. Paw edema induced by serotonin (Figure 4B) reached increase of 55% at 2 h of induction and hind-paw volumes increased until 30% for animals injected with PGE_2 solution (Figure 4D).

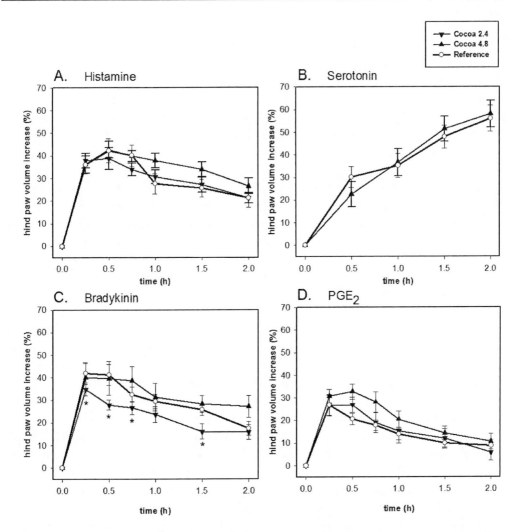

Figure 4. Time-course of paw edema in acute inflammatory models. Time-course of histamine- (A), serotonin- (B), bradykinin- (C), and PGE_2-induced acute inflammation (D) in the studied groups. Values are summarized as mean ± SEM (n = 8-10). * P<0.05 compared with reference group.

Cocoa-enriched diet did not protect from the development of histamine-, serotonin- and PGE_2-induced paw edema. Nevertheless, a significant reduction of paw volume increase was detected in 2.4 g/kg cocoa group in the bradykinin model. These animals showed lower inflammation at 15 min post-injection (P<0.05) and during all studied period (P<0.01). Daily intake of 2.4 g/kg cocoa reduced up to 28% the AUC of hind paw volume evolution (P<0.05, data not shown). Indomethacin did not show anti-inflammatory effects in these models of acute inflammation (data not shown).

Discussion

This study shows the *in vivo* anti-inflammatory power of a high cocoa intake for a week. Although several studies demonstrate the regulatory effect of cocoa flavonoids *in vitro* on cells under inflammatory stimulus (Mao et al., 2000; Ono et al., 2003; Ramiro et al., 2005), there are few evidences of the effect of cocoa on inflammatory response in physiological conditions. Here we show two *in vivo* evidences that allow suggesting the inflammation inhibition by a cocoa diet.

The first part of this study shows that a high cocoa intake for a week reduces the inflammatory potential of macrophages. During an inflammatory response, macrophages are crucial cells participating in the secretion of mediators that eventually induce vasodilatation, vascular permeability increase and leukocyte migration (Medzhitov, 2008). Moreover, macrophages produce a battery of reactive oxygen, nitrogen and halogen species which are proposed to cause damage to surrounding tissues (Son et al., 2008). In the present study, macrophages from animals that had taken a high dose of cocoa produced lower levels of reactive nitrogen species and also had a tendency to synthesize lower reactive oxygen species. These results agree with *in vitro* studies showing that cells from different origins treated with cocoa fractions or flavonoids alone decrease the production of ROS in a dose-dependent manner (Sanbongi et al., 1997, Erlejman et al., 2006; Granado-Serrano et al., 2007; Ramiro-Puig et al., 2009a). Moreover, cocoa fractions are reported to reduce the levels of NO when produced in inflammatory conditions (Ono et al., 2003; Lyu et al., 2005; Ramiro et al., 2005). These results seem to be contradictory with the effects of cocoa flavonoids in vascular tissue where they are reported to promote NO bioactivity and then to cause vasodilatation and decrease blood pressure (Sies et al., 2005; Taubert et al., 2007). These opposite effects seem to be related to the enzyme isoform involved in NO synthesis: eNOS in the endothelial region, or iNOS after an aggressive stimulus (Karim et al., 2000; Ono et al., 2003). Therefore, cocoa compounds would have contrary effects depending on these enzyme isoforms.

In a similar way, macrophages isolated from animals that had taken a high dose of cocoa for a week showed a lower ability to secrete two essential cytokines in the inflammatory process, TNFα and IL-6. These results agree with those previously obtained after adding a cocoa extract on a macrophage cell line (Ramiro et al., 2005), although there are controversial results when cocoa flavonoid fractions were used on blood mononuclear cells (Mao et al., 2000; Kenny et al., 2007). In any case, an important difference between these *in vitro* studies and those showed here consists in the compounds that achieve cells. In a more physiological approach, the present study suggests that metabolites derived from cocoa absorbed fractions have anti-inflammatory properties. How macrophages down-regulate their inflammatory response in the presence of cocoa metabolites remains to be established. However, some *in vitro* studies show that flavonoids such as epicatechin, catechin, dimeric procyanidins and quercetin can modify the NF-κB pathway (Mackenzie et al., 2004; Comalada et al., 2005) involved in the production of inflammatory products. Therefore, it can be suggested that the cocoa absorbed fraction, flavonoids or even other compounds, can also interact with this transduction pathway.

After demonstrating the effect of cocoa in reducing some inflammatory mediators *ex vivo*, the second part of this study was focused on ascertaining whether a cocoa enriched diet was able to directly modulate a local inflammation *in vivo*. Specifically, we examined the effect of cocoa on the local inflammatory response induced by carrageenin in the rat hind paw (Winter et al., 1962). This model is widely applied for the screening of anti-inflammatory drugs which provokes a progressive local edema during 4–6 h, that remains even up to 24 h. Carrageenin-induced edema is accompanied with prostanoids and pro-inflammatory cytokines increase in paw tissues, mainly consisting in an early increase of TNFα followed by elevations in IL-1β and IL-6 (Guay et al., 2004; Rocha et al., 2006; Loram et al., 2007). As shown here, rats that received cocoa for a week developed a lower carrageenin-induced paw edema than reference animals. This regulatory effect was seen at the first hour of induction by both cocoa doses (2.4 and 4.8 g/kg/day) and, in those animals with the high cocoa dose, remained until the end of the study. These results confirm preliminary studies using a higher dose (Ramos-Romero et al., 2008). Although the cocoa compounds responsible for this effect remain to be established, flavonoids are good candidates because two s.c. or i.v. injections of catechin and epicatechin produced a significant reduction of paw edema in the carrageenin model (Matsuoka et al., 1995). Moreover, quercetin, also present in small quantities in cocoa, inhibited the carrageenin-induced paw edema when administered i.p. to mice (Rotelli et al., 2003), and also diminished the carrageenin-induced air pouch when administered locally to rats (Morikawa et al., 2003). In addition, other isolated flavonoids (Ferrándiz et al., 1991) or plant extracts (Autore et al., 2001; Chakradhar et al., 2005; Ghule et al., 2006) have shown an inhibitory effect on carrageenin-induced edema.

The anti-inflammatory effect of cocoa on carrageenin-induced edema may be due to its action on different events during the inflammatory response. In the carrageenin model, it has been described that histamine and serotonin released from local mast cells are responsible for the inflammation in the first phase, followed by kinins and therefore by the local production of prostaglandins (Morris, 2003). To analyze which mechanism/s could be influenced by cocoa, we have tested the effect of cocoa intake on acute inflammatory models induced by several single mediators. Cocoa intake had no protective effect in edema induced by histamine or serotonin. These results allow us to suggest that cocoa compounds did not counteract the actions of vasoactive amine. This fact could be explained by the vasodilator effect of cocoa (Hermann et al., 2006) that would add to the vasoactive inflammatory mediators. In contrast, other flavonoid-enriched plant extracts or isolated flavonoids have shown anti-inflammatory effect in histamine- and serotonin-induced acute inflammation. In these cases, however, there are different routes of administration and a short period between administration and inflammation induction (Sala et al., 2003; Gupta et al., 2005; Zhou et al., 2006; Paulino et al., 2006). On the other hand, cocoa intake could modulate the release of these inflammatory mediators because the down-regulatory role of some flavonoids on mast cell activation and histamine release has been recently described (Park et al., 2008; Shimoda et al., 2008).

In the present study, cocoa intake also produced no inhibition on PGE_2-induced inflammation. Despite these results, it has been described that some flavonoids may inhibit cyclooxygenase pathways and PGE_2 synthesis (de Pascual-Teresa et al., 2004; Delporte et al., 2005). Therefore, although cocoa could not counteract PGE_2 effects when it was injected, it remains to know if it could regulate its synthesis.

Interestingly, rats receiving the lowest dose of cocoa (2.4 g/kg/day) developed a significant reduction of paw edema induced by bradykinin. This effect may be partially attributed to the fact that flavonoids are able to bind bradykinin (Richard et al., 2006) and then antagonize its effects (Yun-Choi et al., 1993). Moreover, it has been suggested that bradykinin stimulate TNFα release from macrophages (Loram et al., 2007), a process that can be down-modulated by cocoa intake as shown here. On the other hand, bradykinin acts on endothelial cells causing vasodilatation, and on non-myelinated afferent neurons, mediating pain (Marceau et al., 2004). These actions would not be affected by a cocoa diet and then would explain the mild effect of cocoa on the bradykinin model. In addition, the beneficial properties of cocoa on this model were not observed at the highest dose. This lack of effect could be explained by the vasodilator consequences of cocoa intake, which at high concentration would predominate over the antagonistic action of flavonoids on bradykinin.

Therefore, from the experimental models induced by single inflammatory mediators, it could be suggested that the anti-inflammatory effect of 2.4 g/kg/day cocoa was due at least partially by regulating bradykinin actions. This effect could explain the inhibition observed with this dose during the first hour in the carrageenin model. Later, the same dose would not be able to counteract the macrophage activation phase, which agrees with results from peritoneal macrophages. On the contrary, higher doses of cocoa inhibit carrageenin-induced edema longer, which could be the result of the down-regulation of mediators produced by macrophages as reactive oxygen and nitrogen species and cytokines.

In summary, a high intake of cocoa could produce anti-inflammatory effects *in vivo*, as shown *in vitro*. Although it remains to be ascertained the precise mechanism of action of cocoa and its effectiveness in other inflammatory processes, cocoa seems a good candidate to be considered as a functional food.

Acknowledgments

S.R. is the recipient of fellowships from the Ministerio de Educación y Ciencia (BES-2006-13640). The present study was supported by the Ministerio de Educación y Ciencia, Spain (AGL2005-002823) and from SGR 2005-0083 of the Generalitat de Catalunya.

References

Autore, G., Rastrelli, L., Lauro, M.R., Marzocco, S., Sorrentino, R., Sorrentino, U., Pinto, A., and Aquino, R. (2001). Inhibition of nitric oxide synthase expression by a methanolic extract of *Crescentia alata* and its derived flavonols. *Life Sci., 70,* 523-534.

Azam, S., Hadi, N., Khan, U. N., and Hadi, S. M. (2003). Antioxidant and prooxidant properties of caffeine, theobromine and xanthine. *Med. Sci. Monit., 9,* 325-330.

Baba, S., Natsume, M., Yasuda, A., Nakamura, Y., Tamura, T., Osakabe, N., Kanegae, M., and Kondo K. (2007). Plasma LDL and HDL cholesterol and oxidized LDL concentrations are altered in normo- and hypercholesterolemic humans after intake of different levels of cocoa powder. *J. Nutr., 137,* 1436-1441.

Baba, S., Osakabe, N., Natsume, M., Muto, Y., Takizawa, T., and Terao, J. (2001). Absorption and urinary excretion of (-)-epicatechin after administration of different levels of cocoa powder or (-)-epicatechin in rats. *J. Agric. Food Chem., 49,* 6050-6056.

Baba, S., Osakabe, N., Natsume, M., Yasuda, A., Takizawa, T., Nakamura, T., and Terao, J. (2000). Cocoa powder enhances the level of antioxidative activity in rat plasma. *Br. J. Nutr., 84,* 673-680.

Buijsse, B., Feskens, E. J. M., Kok, F. J., and Kromhout, D. (2006). Cocoa intake, blood pressure, and cardiovascular mortality. *Arch. Intern. Med., 166,* 411-417.

Chakradhar, V., Babu, Y. H., Ganapaty, S., Prasad, Y. R., Rao, N. K. (2005) Anti-inflammatory activity of a flavonol glycoside from *Tephrosia spinosa. Nat. Prod. Sci., 11,* 63-66.

Comalada, M., Camuesco, D., Sierra, S., Ballester, I., Xaus, J., Gálvez, J., and Zarzuelo, A. (2005). In vivo quercitrin anti-inflammatory effect involves release of quercetin, which inhibits inflammation through down-regulation of the NF-κB pathway. *Eur. J. Immunol., 35,* 584-592.

Cooper, K. A., Donovan, J. L., Waterhouse, A. L., and Williamson, G. (2008). Cocoa and health: a decade of research. *Br. J. Nutr., 99,* 1-11.

Cotelle, N. (2001). Role of flavonoids in oxidative stress. *Curr. Top Med. Chem., 1,* 569-590.

Counet, C., and Collin, S. (2003). Effect of the number of flavanol units on the antioxidant activity of procyanidin fractions isolated from chocolate. *J. Agric. Food Chem., 51,* 6816-6822.

Crews, W. D. Jr., Harrison, D. W., and Wright, J. W. (2008). A double-blind, placebo-controlled, randomized trial of the effects of dark chocolate and cocoa on variables associated with neuropsychological functioning and cardiovascular health: clinical findings from a sample of healthy, cognitively intact older adults. *Am. J. Clin. Nutr., 87,* 872-880.

Datla KP, Zbarsky V, Rai D, Parkar, S., Osakabe, N., Aruoma, O. I., and Dexter, D. T. (2007). Short-term supplementation with plant extracts rich in flavonoids protect nigrostriatal dopaminergic neurons in a rat model of Parkinson's disease. *J. Am. Coll. Nutr., 26,* 341-349.

de Pascual-Teresa, S., Johnston, K. L., DuPont, M. S., O'Leary, K. A., Needs, P. W., Morgan, L. M., Clifford, M. N., Bao, Y., and Williamson, G. (2004). Quercetin metabolites downregulate cyclooxygenase-2 transcription in human lymphocytes ex vivo but not in vivo. *J. Nutr., 134,* 552-557.

Delporte, C., Backhouse, N., Erazo, S., Negrete, R., Vidal, P., Silva, X., López-Pérez J. L., Feliciano, A. S., and Muñoz, O. (2005). Analgesic-antiinflammatory properties of *Proustia pyrifolia. J. Ethnopharmacol., 99,* 119-124.

di Giuseppe, R., di Castelnuovo, A., Centritto, F., Zito, F., de Curtis, A., Costanzo, S., Vohnout, B., Sieri, S., Krogh, V., Donati, M. B., de Gaetano, G., and Iacoviello, L. (2008). Regular consumption of dark chocolate is associated with low serum concentrations of C-reactive protein in a healthy Italian population. *J. Nutr., 138,* 1939-1945.

Erlejman, A. G., Fraga, C. G., and Oteiza, P. I. (2006). Procyanidins protect Caco-2 cells from bile acid- and oxidant-induced damage. *Free Radic. Biol. Med., 41,* 1247-1256.

Ferrándiz, M. L. and Alcaraz, M. J. (1991). Anti-inflammatory activity and inhibition of arachidonic acid metabolism by flavonoids. *Agents Actions, 32,* 283-288.

Ghule, B. V., Ghante, M. H., Saoji, A. N. and Yeole, P. G. (2006). Hypolipidemic and antihyperlipidemic effects of *Lagenaria siceraria* (Mol.) fruit extracts. *Indian J. Exp. Biol., 44,* 905-909.

Granado-Serrano, A. B., Martín, M. A., Izquierdo-Pulido, M., Goya, L., Bravo, L., and Ramos, S. (2007). Molecular mechanisms of (-)-epicatechin and chlorogenic acid on the regulation of the apoptotic and survival/proliferation pathways in a human hepatoma cell line. *J. Agric. Food Chem., 55,* 2020-2027.

Grassi, D., Necozione, S., Lippi, C., Croce, G., Valeri, L., Pasqualetti, P., Desideri, G., Blumberg, J. B., and Ferri, C. (2005) Cocoa reduces blood pressure and insulin resistance and improves endothelium-dependent vasodilation in hypertensives. *Hypertension, 46,* 398–405.

Gu, L., House, S. E., Wu, X., Ou, B., and Prior, R. L. (2006) Procyanidin and catechin contents and antioxidant capacity of cocoa and chocolate products. *J. Agric. Food Chem., 54,* 4057-4061.

Guay, J., Bateman, K., Gordon, R., Manzini, J., and Riendeau, D. (2004). Carrageenan-induced paw edema in rat elicits a predominant prostaglandin E_2 (PGE_2) response in the central nervous system associated with the induction of microsomal PGE_2 synthase-1. *J. Biol. Chem., 279,* 24866-24872.

Gupta, M., Mazumder, U. K., Kumar, R. S., Gomathi, P., Rajeshwar, Y., Kakoti, B. B., and Selven, V. T. (2005). Anti-inflammatory, analgesic and antipyretic effects of methanol extract from *Bauhinia racemosa* stem bark in animal models. *J. Ethnopharmacol., 98,* 267-273.

Hatano, T., Miyatake, H., Natsume, M., Osakabe, N., Takizawa, T., Ito, H., and Yoshida, T. (2002). Proanthocyanidin glycosides and related polyphenols from cacao liquor and their antioxidant effects. *Phytochemistry, 59,* 749-758.

Hermann, F., Spieker, L. E., Ruschitzka, F., Sudano, I., Hermann, M., Binggeli, C., Lüscher, T. F., Riesen, W., Noll, G., and Corti, R. (2006). Dark chocolate improves endothelial and platelet function. *Heart, 92,* 119-120.

Hurst, W. J., Tarka, S. M. Jr., Powis, T. G., Valdez, F. Jr. and Hester, T. R. (2002). Cacao usage by the earliest Maya civilization. *Nature, 418,* 289-290.

Karim, M., McCormick, K., and Kappagoda, C. T. (2000). Effects of cocoa extracts on endothelium-dependent relaxation. *J. Nutr., 130,* S2105–S2108.

Kenny, T. P., Keen, C. L., Schmitz, H. H., and Gershwin, M. E. (2007). Immune effects of cocoa procyanidin oligomers on peripheral blood mononuclear cells. *Exp. Biol. Med. (Maywood), 232,* 293-300.

Lamuela-Raventos R. M., Andres-Lacueva, C., Permanyer, J., and Izquierdo-Pulido, M. (2001). More antioxidants in cocoa. *J. Nutr., 131,* 834-835.

Lee, K. W., Kim, Y. J., Lee, H. J. and Lee, C. Y. (2003). Cocoa has more phenolic phytochemicals and a higher antioxidant capacity than teas and red wine. *J. Agric. Food Chem., 51,* 7292-7295.

Loram, L. C., Fuller, A., Fick, L. G., Cartmell, T., Poole, S., and Mitchell, D. (2007). Cytokine profiles during carrageenan-induced inflammatory hyperalgesia in rat muscle and hind paw. *J. Pain, 8,* 127-136.

Lyu, S., Rhim, J., and Park, W. (2005) Antiherpetic activities of flavonoids against herpes simplex virus type 1 (HSV-1) and type 2 (HSV-2) in vitro. *Arch. Pharm. Res., 28,* 1293-1301.

Mackenzie, G. G., Carrasquedo, F., Delfino, J. M., Keen, C. L., Fraga, C. G., and Oteiza, P. I. (2004) Epicatechin, catechin, and dimeric procyanidins inhibit PMA-induced NF-κB activation at multiple steps in Jurkat T cells. *FASEB J., 18,* 167-169.

Manach, C., Scalbert, A., Morand, C., Remesy, C. and Jimenez, L. (2004). Polyphenols: food sources and bioavailability. *Am. J. Clin. Nutr., 79,* 727-747.

Mao, T., Van De Water, J., Keen, C. L., Schmitz, H. H., and Gershwin, M. E. (2000). Cocoa procyanidins and human cytokine transcription and secretion. *J. Nutr., 130,* S2093–S2099.

Marceau, F., and Regoli, D. (2004). Bradykinin receptor ligands: therapeutic perspectives. *Nat. Rev. Drug Discov., 3,* 845-852.

Mathur, S., Devaraj, S., Grundy, S. M., and Jialal, I. (2002). Cocoa products decrease low density lipoprotein oxidative susceptibility but do not affect biomarkers of inflammation in humans. *J. Nutr., 132,* 3663–3667.

Matsuoka, Y., Hasegawa, H., Okuda, S., Muraki, T., Uruno, T., and Kubota, K. (1995). Ameliorative effects of tea catechins on active oxygen-related nerve cell injuries. *J. Pharmacol. Exp. Ther.,* 274, 602-608.

McShea, A., Ramiro-Puig, E., Munro, S. B., Casadesus, G., Castell, M., and Smith, M. A. (2008). Clinical benefit and preservation of flavonols in dark chocolate manufacturing. *Nutr. Rev., 66,* 630-641.

Medzhitov, R. (2008). Origin and physiological roles of inflammation. *Nature, 454,* 428-435.

Morikawa, K., Nonaka, M., Narahara, M., Torii, I., Kawaguchi, K., Yoshikawa, T., Kumazawa, Y., and Morikawa, S. (2003). Inhibitory effect of quercetin on carrageenan-induced inflammation in rats. *Life Sci., 74,* 709-721.

Morris, C. J. (2003). Carrageenan-induced paw edema in the rat and mouse. *Method. Mol. Biol., 225,* 115-121.

Ono, K., Takahashi, T., Kamei, M., Mato, T., Hashizume, S., Kamiya, S., and Tsutsumi, H. (2003). Effects of an aqueous extract of cocoa on nitric oxide production of macrophages activated by lipopolysaccharide and interferon-gamma. *Nutrition, 19,* 681-685.

Park, H. H., Lee, S., Son, H. Y., Park, S. B., Kim, M. S., Choi, E. J., Singh, T. S., Ha, J. H., Lee, M. G., Kim, J. E., Hyun, M. C., Kwon, T. K., Kim, Y. H., and Kim, S. H. (2008) Flavonoids inhibit histamine release and expression of proinflammatory cytokines in mast cells. *Arch. Pharm. Res., 31,* 1303-1311.

Paulino, N., Teixeira, C., Martins, R., Scremin, A., Dirsch, V. M., Vollmar, A. M., Abreu, S. R., de Castro, S. L., and Marcucci, M. C. (2006). Evaluation of the analgesic and anti-inflammatory effects of a Brazilian green propolis. *Planta Med., 72,* 899-906.

Ramiro, E., Franch, A., Castellote, C., Perez-Cano, F., Permanyer, J., Izquierdo-Pulido, M., and Castell, M. (2005). Flavonoids from *Theobroma cacao* down-regulate inflammatory mediators. *J. Agric. Food Chem., 53,* 8506-8511.

Ramiro-Puig, E., Casadesús, G., Lee, H. G., Zhu, X., McShea, A., Perry, G., Pérez-Cano, F. J., Smith, M. A., and Castell, M. (2009a) Neuroprotective effect of cocoa flavonoids on *in vitro* oxidative stress. *Eur. J. Nutr., 48,* 54-61.

Ramiro-Puig, E., and Castell, M. (2009b) Cocoa: antioxidant and immunomodulator. *Br. J. Nutr., 101,* 931-40.

Ramos-Romero, S., Ramiro-Puig, E., Pérez-Cano, F. J., Castellote, C., Franch, A. and Castell, M. (2008). Anti-inflammatory effects of cocoa in rat carrageenin-induced paw oedema. *Proc. Nutr. Soc., 67,* E65.

Richard, T., Lefeuvre, D., Descendit, A., Quideau, S., and Monti, J. P. (2006). Recognition characters in peptide-polyphenol complex formation. *Biochim. Biophys. Acta, 1760,* 951-958.

Rocha, A. C., Fernandes, E. S., Quintao, N. L., Campos, M. M., and Calixto, J. B. (2006). Relevance of tumour necrosis factor-alpha for the inflammatory and nociceptive responses evoked by carrageenan in the mouse paw. *Br. J. Pharmacol., 5,* 688-695.

Rotelli, A. E., Guardia, T., Juarez, A. O., de la Rocha, N. E., and Pelzer, L. E. (2003). Comparative study of flavonoids in experimental models of inflammation. *Pharmacol. Res., 48,* 601-606.

Sala, A., Recio, M. C., Schinella, G. R., Máñez, S., Giner, R. M., Cerdá-Nicolás, M., and Rosí, J. L. (2003). Assessment of the anti-inflammatory activity and free radical scavenger activity of tiliroside. *Eur. J. Pharmacol. 461,* 53-61.

Sanbongi, C., Suzuki, N., and Sakane, T. (1997). Polyphenols in chocolate, which have antioxidant activity, modulate immune functions in humans in vitro. *Cell Immunol., 177,* 129-136.

Sanchez-Rabaneda, F., Jáuregui, O., Casals, I., Andres-Lacueva, C., Izquierdo-Pulido, M., and Lamuela-Raventos, R. M. (2003). Liquid chromatographic/ electrospray ionization tandem mass spectrometric study of the phenolic composition of cocoa (*Theobroma cacao*). *J. Mass Spectrom., 38,* 35-42.

Schramm, D. D., Wang, J. F., Holt, R. R., Ensunsa, J. L., Gonsalves, J. L., Lazarus, S. A., Schmitz, H. H., German, J. B., and Keen, C. L. (2001) Chocolate procyanidins decrease the leukotriene-prostacyclin ratio in humans and human aortic endothelial cells. *Am. J. Clin. Nutr., 73,* 36–40.

Shimoda, K., Kobayashi, T., Akagi, M., Hamada, H., and Hamada H. (2008) Synthesis of Oligosaccharides of Genistein and Quercetin as Potential Anti-inflammatory Agents. *Chem. Let., 37,* 876-877.

Sies, H., Schewe, T., Heiss, C., and Kelm, M. (2005). Cocoa polyphenols and inflammatory mediators. *Am. J. Clin. Nutr., 81,* S304-12.

Singleton, V. L., Orthofer R., and Lamuela-Raventós, R. M (1999). Analysis of total phenols and other oxidation substrates and antioxidants by means of Folin-Ciocalteu reagent. *Method. Enzymol., 299,* 152-178.

Son, J., Pang, B., McFaline, J. L., Taghizadeh, K., and Dedon, P. C. (2008). Surveying the damage: the challenges of developing nucleic acid biomarkers of inflammation. *Mol. Biosyst., 4,* 902-908.

Taubert, D., Roesen, R., Lehmann, C., Jung, N., and Schomig, E. (2007) Effects of low habitual cocoa intake on blood pressure and bioactive nitric oxide: a randomized controlled trial. *JAMA., 298,* 49-60.

Vinson, J. A., Proch, J., and Zubik, L. (1999). Phenol antioxidant quantity and quality in foods: cocoa, dark chocolate, and milk chocolate. *J. Agric. Food Chem., 47,* 4821-4824.

Vinson, J. A., Proch, J., Bose, P., Muchler, S., Taffera, P., Shuta, D., Samman, N., and Agbor, G. A. (2006). Chocolate is a powerful ex vivo and in vivo antioxidant, an antiatherosclerotic agent in an animal model, and a significant contributor to antioxidants in the European and American Diets. *J. Agric. Food Chem., 54,* 8071-8076.

Winter, C. A., Risley, E. A., and Nuss, G. W. (1962). Carrageenan-induced edema in hind paw of the rat as an assay for anti-inflammatory drugs. *Proc. Soc. Exp. Biol., 111,* 544-547.

Yilmaz, Y., and Toledo, R. T. (2004). Major flavonoids in grape seeds and skins: antioxidant capacity of catechin, epicatechin, and gallic acid. *J. Agric. Food Chem., 52,* 255-260.

Yun-Choi H. S., Chung, H. S., and Kim, Y. J. (1993) Evaluation of some flavonoids as potential bradykinin antagonist. *Arch. Pharm. Res., 16,* 283-288.

Zhou, H., Wong, Y. F., Cai, X., Liu, Z. Q., Jiang, Z. H., Bian, Z. X., Xu, H. X., and Liu, L. (2006). Suppressive effects of JCICM-6, the extract of an anti-arthritic herbal formula, on the experimental inflammatory and nociceptive models in rodents. *Biol. Pharm. Bull., 29,* 253-260.

In: Encyclopedia of Vitamin Research
Editor: Joshua T. Mayer

ISBN: 978-1-61761-928-1
© 2011 Nova Science Publishers, Inc.

Chapter 44

Mechanisms at the Root of Flavonoid Action in Cancer: A Step Toward Solving the Rubik's Cube[*]

Maria Marino[†] and Pamela Bulzomi

Department of Biology, University Roma Tre, Viale G. Marconi,
446, I-00146 Roma, Italy

Abstract

The biological activity of flavonoids was first recognized when the antiestrogenic principle present in red clover that caused infertility in sheep in Western Australia was discovered. These adverse effects of flavonoids placed these substances in the class of endocrine-disrupting chemicals. On the other hand, flavonoids are recently claimed to prevent several cancer types and to reduce incidence of cardiovascular diseases, osteoporosis, neurodegenerative diseases, as well as chronic and acute inflammation. Despite these controversial effects, a huge number of plant extracts or mixtures, containing varying amounts of isolated flavonoids, are commercially available on the market as dietary supplements and healthy products. The commercial success of these supplements is evident, even though the activity and mechanisms of flavonoid action are still unclear.

Owing to their chemical structure, the most obvious feature of flavonoids is their ability to quench free radicals. However, in the last few years many exciting new indication in elucidating the mechanisms of flavonoid actions have been published. Flavonoids inhibit several signal transduction-involved kinases and affect protein functions via competitive or allosteric interactions. Among others, flavonoids interact with and affect the cellular responses mediated by estrogen receptors (ERα and ERβ). In

---

[*] A version of this chapter was also published in *Flavonoids: Biosynthesis, Biological Effects and Dietary Sources, edited by Raymond B. Keller* published by Nova Science Publishers, Inc. It was submitted for appropriate modifications in an effort to encourage wider dissemination of research.

[†] Tel. 0039-06-57336345; fax 0039-06-57336321. e-mail address: m.marino@uniroma3.it (M. Marino)

particular, our recent data indicate that some flavonoids (i.e., naringenin and quercetin) decouple specific ERα action mechanisms, important for cell proliferation, driving cells to the apoptosis. Therefore, distinct complex mechanisms of actions, possibly interacting one another, for nutritional molecules on cell signalling and response can be hypothesized.

Aim of this review is to provide an updating picture about mechanisms by which flavonoids play a role in cellular response and in preventing human pathologies such as cancer. In particular, their direct interaction with nuclear receptors and/or by their ability to modulate the activity of key enzymes involved in cell signaling and antioxidant responses will be presented and discussed.

1. Introduction

Flavonoids, phenylbenzo-pyrones (phenylchromones), are a large group of non nutrient compounds naturally produced from plants as part of their defence mechanisms against stresses of different origins. They are present in all terrestrial vascular plants; whereas, in mammals, flavonoids occur only through dietary intake (Birt et al., 2001). Flavonoids, have an assortment of structures based on a common three-ring nucleus (Middleton et al., 2000) in which primary substituents (eg, hydroxyl, methoxyl, or glycosyl groups) can be further substituted (e.g., additionally glycosylated or acylated) sometimes yielding highly complex structures (Cheynier, 2005) (Figure 1). More than 4,000 different flavonoids, have been described and categorized into 6 subclasses as a function of the type of heterocycle involved: flavonols, flavones, flavanols, flavanonols, flavanones, and isoflavones (Figure 1) (Birt et al., 2001; Manach et al., 2004).

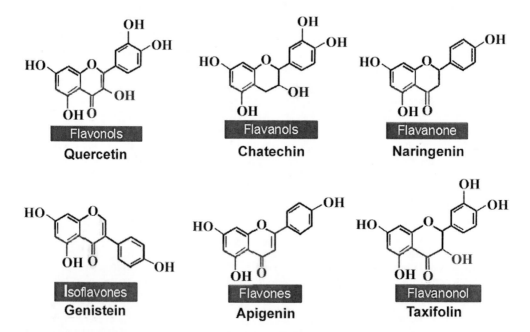

Figure 1. Chemical structures of commonly occurring plant flavonoids.

First recognized in '40 as the antiestrogenic principle present in red clover that caused infertility in sheep in Western Australia (Bennetts et al., 1946; Galluzzo and Marino, 2006), more recently, the use of flavonoids to curb menopausal symptoms and provide a "natural" and presumably cancer risk-free estrogenic replacement (Ling et al., 2004) has become popular in Western countries.

Thus, a huge number of preparations are now commercially available on the market as health food products. As dietary supplements they are obtainable as plant extracts or mixtures, containing varying amounts of isolated or concentrate flavonoids in bakery, dairy, infant formulas (Tomar and Shiao, 2008). The commercial success of these supplements is evident and the consumption of these compounds in Western countries is increasing even if different and opposite flavonoid effects have been reported.

In particular, epidemiological data show that in pre-menopausal women, assuming daily soy, follicle stimulating and luteinizing hormone levels significantly decreased, increasing menstrual cycle length (Jacobs and Lewis, 2002). Hyperplasia of mammary glands in both sexes, aberrant or delayed spermatogenesis, histological changes in the vagina and ovary, mineralization of renal tubules in males, modulation of natural killer cell activity, and myelotoxicity had been observed in rats exposed to isoflavone genistein through placental transfer or lactational exposure, or ingestion (Flynn et al., 2000; Delclos et al., 2001; Guo et al., 2005; Doerge et al., 2006). On the other hand, a positive association between the increased intake of phytoestrogen and reduced amount of neurodegenerative diseases, improvement of cognition and learning (Kirk et al., 1998), and fewer tendency to osteoporosis (Zhang et al., 2003; Adlercreutz et al., 2004) have also been reported. In addition, diets rich in flavonoids also lead to lower serum cholesterol levels, low-density lipoproteins, and triglycerides (Delclos et al., 2001), thus reducing the incidence of cardiovascular diseases (Doerge et al., 2006). Finally, the close relationship between flavonoids and cancer is suggested by the large variation in rates of specific cancers in different countries and by the spectacular changes observed in the incidence of cancer in migrating populations (Guo et al., 2005; Béliveau and Gingras, 2007; Benavente-García and Castillo, 2008). These observations are strengthened by many experimental data obtained from studies using cellular and animal models (Caltagirone et al., 2000; Fenton and Hord, 2004; Albini et al., 2005; Béliveau and Gingras, 2007; Espìn et al., 2007; Benavente-García and Castillo, 2008).

Flavonoids have been considered able to modulate this wide spectrum of responses due to their chemical structure compatible with putative antioxidant properties which can interact with reactive oxygen-nitrogen species (RONS)-mediated intracellular signaling (Virgili and Marino, 2008). However, different cellular effects not directly related to flavonoid antioxidant capacity have been recently reported. Flavonoids could modulate the activity of several kinases and could affect protein functions (e.g. receptors) via competitive or allosteric interactions. Thus, flavonoids should be considered pleiotropic substances which possess distinct mechanisms of action possibly interacting each other.

Aim of this review is to provide an update about mechanisms by which flavonoids play a role in cellular response and in preventing cancer.

2. Prooxidant/Antioxidant Activity of Flavonoids

RONS, including nitric oxide (NO) and hydrogen peroxide (H_2O_2), are endogenously synthesized in several cells were participate, as second messengers, in cytokine and/or growth factor signals (Stone and Jang, 2006). On the other hand, RONS are the principal responsible of oxidative stress initiation when their production exceeds cellular antioxidant defenses. The consequence of RONS action is the damage of membrane lipids, proteins, and DNA with the subsequent onset of various diseases (Moskaug et al., 2005).

RONS, either directly or indirectly, regulates the activity of some of the most well-known signaling enzymes including guanylyl cyclase, phospholipase C, phospholipase A2, phospholipase D, activating protein-1 (AP-1), nuclear factor κB (NF-κB), insulin receptor, c-Src, Jun N-terminal kinase, and p38 kinase (MAPK) (Hehner et al., 2000). Moreover, a significant inhibition of phosphatase activity, paralleled by the net increase of phosphorylation level, has been reported (O'Loghlen et al., 2003, Hao et al., 2006).

Due to their chemical structure, flavonoids are able to quench free radicals by forming resonance-stabilized phenoxyl radicals *in vitro*, in cell cultures, and in cell free systems (Hanasaki et al., 1994, Ursini et al., 1994, Birt et al., 2001). In addition, these compounds have been considered able to impair the RONS-mediated intracellular signaling by directly inhibiting the involved enzymes or by chelating trace elements involved in free radical production or up-regulating the antioxidant cellular response (Surh, 2003, Lee et al., 2005, Chiang et al., 2006, Kweon et al., 2006). Thus, an high intake of flavonoids should be associated with a reduced risk of degenerative diseases such as cardiovascular disease and cancer. Experimental data have shown that flavonoids block the progression of latent microtumors (Béliveau and Gingras, 2007) and this effect could be elicited via the modulation of the enzymatic systems responsible for neutralizing free radicals (Conney, 2003; Ioannides and Lewis 2004) and/or by directly inducing cancer cell death by apoptosis. For example, phenethyl isothiocyanate from cruciferous vegetables, curcumin from turmeric, resveratrol from grapes, and naringenin from oranges have all been shown to possess strong pro-apoptotic activity against cells isolated from a variety of tumors (Totta et al., 2004; Karunagaran et al., 2005; Totta et al., 2005). Thus, the antioxidant activity of flavonoids could represent the close relationship between flavonoids and cancer chemoprevention.

However, flavonoids also possess pro-oxidant properties which could contribute to their anti-cancer activity (Galati et al., 2000). Flavonoid pro-oxidant activity seems to be involved in the inhibition of mitochondrial respiration and is related to their *in vitro* ability to undergo to auto-oxidation to produce superoxide anions. On the other hand, transition metals, which catalyze auto-oxidation, result linked to proteins *in vivo* and it is unlikely they could significantly participate in the auto-oxidation of polyphenols. As alternative mechanism flavonoids pro-oxidant activity could be dependent from the activity of peroxidases (O'Brien, 2000). As an example, the apigenin in the presence of myeloperoxidase forms a peroxyl radical *in vitro* (Galati et al., 2001) which leads to the intracellular production of ROS and contributes to the apoptotic and necrotic cell death (Wang et al., 1999; Morrissey et al., 2005; Vargo et al., 2006; Miyoshi et al., 2007). Baicalin-apoptosis induction is also accompanied with the generation of intracellular ROS and the increase of the cytochrome c release (Ueda et al., 2002). Cytochrome c release and mitochondrial transmembrane potential disruption precedes the apoptosoma activation in MCF-7 cell treated with 200μM of the stilbene trans-resveratrol (Filomeni et al., 2007). Contrasting results have been obtained treating cells with quercetin. This flavonoid possess an high antioxidant activity preventing the H_2O_2-induced ROS production in a dose-dependent manner not related with its pro-apoptotic effect. In addition, the cell treatment with 50 μM quercetin induces an increase of ROS production in a cell context dependent way (Galluzzo et al., 2008 and literature cited therein). Thus, other action mechanism(s) independent from antioxidant/pro-oxidant effects of flavonoids should be evoked to explain the potential chemopreventive and chemoprotective effect of these substances.

3. Flavonoids as Kinase Inhibitors

Cancer progression arrest and tumor cell growth inhibition have been associated with the strong affinity of flavonoid for proteins involved in a variety of cellular processes.

The flavonoid-induced inhibition of the epidermal growth factor receptor (EGF-R), protein kinase C (PKC), phosphatydil inositol 3 kinase (PI3K) and extracellular regulated kinase (ERK) have been described (Hagiwara et al., 1988; Spencer et al., 2003; Kim et al., 2008). As a possible mechanism their competition with ATP for the binding to the protein catalytic site has been evoked (Chao, 2000; Manthey, 2000). However, in most reports, direct demonstration of such inhibition was not shown. Indeed, although EGF stimulation of EGF-R tyrosine auto-phosphorylation in prostate and breast cancer cells was blocked by tyrphostins (synthetic tyrosine kinase inhibitors), genistein had no effect (Peterson and Barnes, 1996). In rats treated with genistein, the reduced reactivity of EGF-R with anti-phosphotyrosine antibodies was shown instead to result from a reduction in the amount of EGF-R protein (Dalu et al., 1998). These data suggest that genistein elicits its effects through transcriptional processes rather than directly on tyrosine kinase activity.

Moreover, flavonoids can block enzyme activity modulating redox-sensitive transcription factors. Curcumin (diferuloylmethane) and epigallocatechin-3-gallate (EGCG) induce hemeoxygenase-1 (HO-1), an enzyme with antioxidant properties which influences the apoptosis, promoting nuclear translocation of the nuclear factor (erythroid-derived 2)-related factor (Nrf2) (Andreadi et al., 2006).

There is growing evidence that phytoestrogens could have a protective effect on the initiation or progression of breast cancer by inhibiting the local production of estrogens from circulating precursors in breast tissue. Indeed *in vitro* experiments have shown that phytoestrogens, mainly flavones and flavonones, inhibit the activity of key steroidogenic enzymes (i.e., aromatase and 17β-hydroxysteroid dehydrogenase) involved in the synthesis of estradiol from circulating androgens and estrogen sulphate (Rice and Whitehead, 2006).

Flavonoid ability to prevent cell invasion and matrix degradation, as well as alterations of cellular metabolism, has been associated to their effect on cancer progression reduction (Manna et al., 2000; Pellegatta et al., 2003; El Bedoui et al., 2005; Wung et al., 2005). In particular, the alteration of glucose homeostasis by the inhibition of glycogen phosphorylase activity has been reported (Jakobs et al., 2006). The glucose uptake could be also inhibited directly by flavonoid binding to the glucose transporter 4, or indirectly by inhibiting PI3K/AKT pathway-induced by insulin receptor (IR) phosphorylation (Nomura et al., 2008).

However, flavonoids-dependent kinases inhibition is present at high flavonoid concentration (>50 μM). At present the relative importance of each of these pathways and their putative cross-talk remains to be established as well as the clinical significance in nutritionally relevant flavonoid concentration (i.e., 0.1-10 μM) remain unsolved.

4. Flavonoids as Nuclear Receptor Ligands

Nuclear receptors (NR) are ligand-activated transcription factors sharing a common evolutionary history (Gronemeyer et al., 2004), having similar sequence features at the protein level (Figure 2). A specific corresponding endogenous ligand for some of the NRs is not known, and therefore these receptors have been named "orphan receptors." This group includes the lipid-regulating peroxisome proliferator-activated receptors (PPARs), the liver X receptor, the farnesoid X receptor, and the pregnane nuclear receptor (PXR). Fibrates or glitazones, oxysterols, bile acids, and xenobiotics could activate the orphan receptors of the NR1 subfamily and produce effects that resemble some of the actions caused by flavonoid intake (Virgili ad Marino, 2008).

Resveratrol, has been found to selectively activate PPARα and PPARγ transcriptional activity by 15- to 30-fold above control levels. This activation was dose dependent at quite high concentrations (10, 50, and 100 μM) in endothelial cells (Shay and Banz, 2005). Experimental data demonstrate that genistein could act as a ligand for PPARγ with a K_i comparable to that of some known PPARγ ligands (Iqbal et al., 2002; Dang et al., 2003). In particular genistein seems to be an PPARα agonists. In fact female obese Zucker rats consuming a high isoflavone diet improved their glucose tolerance and displayed liver triglyceride and cholesterol and plasma cholesterol levels significantly lower than controls (Mezei et al., 2003).

This data is consistent with the hypothesis that soy isoflavones improve lipid metabolism and have an antidiabetic effect by activating PPAR receptors and is in agreement with observations in humans treated with antidiabetic PPARα agonists (e.g. GW501516) used to treat hyperlipidemia and type 2 diabetes (Elisaf et al., 2002).

Mixtures of isoflavones and isolated isoflavones have been reported to induce PXR transcriptional activity (Ricketts et al., 2005) which has been shown to be activated by a chemically and structurally diverse set of xenobiotic and endogenous compounds and to regulate gene expression pathways involved in metabolism and transport of these same classes of compounds (Moore and Kliewer, 2000; Wang et al., 2007). Notably, PXR has been shown to directly regulate the cytochrome P450 3A gene, a phase I drug metabolism gene, whose product is responsible for the metabolism of drugs (Moore and Kliewer, 2000; Wang et al., 2007). Other authors reported that genistein, formononetin, kaempferol, and apigenin did not exhibit PXR ligand activity (Mnif et al., 2007). Thus, at present the contribution of PXR signaling to the flavonoid effects on human health remains elusive. Contrasting data have also been reported about flavonoids effects on AhR. Quercetin, galangin, diosmin, and diosmetin increase the expression of phase I enzymes, important for the prevention of cancer, by binding to AhR receptor (Kang et al., 1999).

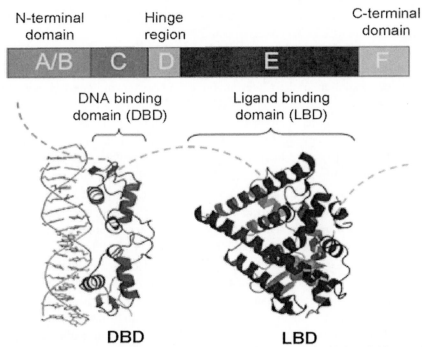

Figure 2. NRs share an evolutionarily conserved structure consisting of the high variable *N*-amino-terminal region involved in transactivation (A and B domains), the conserved DNA binding region (DBD, C domain), the hinge region, the ligand binding domain (LBD; E domain), and the *C*-terminal region (F domain). For details, see text.

Computer docking analyses and mammalian two-hybrid experiments indicate that isoflavones (i.e., genistein, daidzein, and biochanin A) and one flavone (trihydroxyflavone) are relatively poor ligands of estrogen related receptor γ (ERRγ, NR3) but they can act as agonists of ERRα and ERRβ activity (Suetsugi et al., 2003).

4.1. Flavonoids as Estrogen Receptor Ligands

At concentrations more physiologically achievable in the plasma (from 0.1 μM to 10 μM) after the consumption of meals rich in flavonoids (Manach et al., 2004), flavonoids can bind to and, consequently, modulate ER activity (Birt et al., 2001; Totta et al., 2004) leading to estrogenic or antiestrogenic effects. Because of their ability to interfere with E2 action, flavonoids are actually defined as dietary phytoestrogen (Saarinen et al., 2006).

Flavonoids interfere with organ and tissue responses to 17β-estradiol (E2) by binding to estrogen receptors ERα and ERβ. ERα and ERβ are encoded by two different genes and belong to the nuclear receptor superfamily (NR3A1 and NR3A2, respectively) (Figure 2) (Nilsson et al., 2001). E2 binding to its receptors causes ER dissociation from heat shock proteins, ER dimerization (omo/eterodimerization) and binding to specific DNA sequences [estrogen response element (ERE)] thus triggering to the transcription of responsive genes (Ascenzi et al., 2006). Moreover, ERα, but not ERβ, can regulate gene transcription through its indirect interaction with the transcription factors stimulating protein 1 (Sp-1) and AP-1 (Ascenzi et al., 2006). Both in the direct and indirect action modes, ERs need to interact with coregulatory proteins (coactivators or corepressors) which provide a platform upon which additional proteins are assembled (Ascenzi et al., 2006).

A growing number of reports indicate E2 effects in living cells are mediated by various pathways rather than by a single uniform mechanism. E2 rapid effects have been attributed in most cells to a population of ERs present on the plasma membranes (Levin 2005). We recently demonstrated that ERα undergoes *S*-palmitoylation on a cysteine residue (Cys447) present in the ligand binding domain (LBD) which allows receptor anchoring to plasma membrane, association to caveolin-1, and which accounts for the ability of E2 to activate different signaling pathways (Acconcia et al., 2005a). The Cys399 residue present in the LBD of ERβ is also subjected to *S*-palmitoylation (Galluzzo et al., 2007) indicating that a similar mechanism also works for ERβ localization to the plasma membrane and association to caveolin-1. Thus, ERα and ERβ have to be considered as a population of protein(s) which localization in the cell can dynamically change, shuttling from membrane to cytosol and to the nucleus on the dependence of E2 binding (Acconcia et al., 2005a; Levin, 2005). As a consequence, rapid and more prolonged E2 actions could be more finely coordinated. The physiological significance of ERs-dependent rapid pathways is quite clarified, at least for some E2 target tissues. The mechanism by which E2 exerts proliferative properties has been assumed to be exclusively mediated by ERα-induced rapid membrane-starting actions (Marino et al., 2005; Ascenzi et al., 2006), whereas E2 induces cell death through ERβ non-genomic signaling (Acconcia et al., 2005b). In the nervous system, E2 influences neural functions (e.g., cognition, behavior, stress responses, and reproduction) in part inducing such rapid responses (Farach-Carson and Davis, 2003). In the liver, rapid E2-induced signals are deeply linked to the expression of LDL-receptor and to the decreased cholesterol-LDL levels in the plasma (Distefano et al., 2002). An important mode of E2-mediated atheroprotection is linked to E2 capability to rapidly activate endothelial NOS and NO production (Chambliss et al., 2002).

These rapid effects (E2 extranuclear signals) include the activation of mitogen-activated protein kinase (MAPK) (i.e., p38, extranuclear regulated kinases [ERK]), PI3K, signal transducer and activator of transcription, epidermal growth factor receptor, Src kinase, Shc kinase, protein kinase C, adenylate cyclase, GTP-binding proteins, and NOS (Dang and Lowik, 2005). Microarray analysis of gene expression in vascular endothelial cells treated with E2 for 40 min showed that 250 genes were up-regulated; this could be prevented by Ly294002, a PI3K inhibitor. Interestingly, the transcriptional activity of the E2-ERα complex could be inhibited by pre-treating cells with PD98059 and U0126, two ERK inhibitors (Ascenzi et al., 2006). These findings support the idea that E2-induced rapid signals synergize with genomic events to maintain the pleiotropic hormone effects in the body (Galluzzo and Marino, 2006).

A plethora of papers indicates the ability of flavonoids to bind both ER isoforms maintaining the ERs gene transcriptional ability, nevertheless several epidemiological and experimental data show that flavonoid effects can be both estrogen mimetic and antiestrogenic. Several groups have demonstrated that flavonoid affinity to ERs is lower than E2 (Kuiper et al., 1997). Competition binding studies confirm that nutritional molecules (e.g., genistein, coumestrol, daidzein, and equol) show a distinct preference for ERβ (Kuiper et al., 1997; Mueller et al., 2004; Escande et al., 2006), although the prenylated chalcone occurring in hops, 8-prenylnaringenin, has been found to be a potent ERα agonist, but a weak agonist of ERβ in E2 competition assays (Stevens and Page, 2004). Phytochemicals as the isoflavonoids daidzein and genistein, the flavanone naringenin, and the flavonol quercetin increase the activity of ERE-luciferase reporter gene construct in cells expressing ERα or ERβ (Mueller, 2002; Totta et al., 2004; Virgili et al., 2004; Totta et al., 2005), but impair ERα interaction with Sp-1 and AP-1 (Peach et al., 1997; Liu et al., 2002; Virgili et al., 2004). Cluster analysis of DNA microarray in MCF-7 cells show a very similar profiles between estrogen responding genes and 10 μM genistein (Terasaka et al., 2004) while the expression of only five genes is affected by daidzein with respect to E2 in TM4 Sertoli cells. These five genes were related to cell signaling, cell proliferation, and apoptosis, suggesting a possible correlation with the inhibition of cell viability reported after treatment with daidzein (Adachi et al., 2005).

The capability of flavonoids to influence E2 rapid actions in both reproductive and non-reproductive E2-target tissues and how such effects may impact the normal development and physiological properties of cells largely have not been tackled until very recently (Somjen, 2005; Watson, 2005). In fact, scarce information is available on the non genomic signal transduction pathways activated after the formation of flavonoids:ERα and flavonoids:ERβ complexes. Recent evidence favors the idea that besides coactivator association, the ER-LBD is essential and sufficient also for activation of rapid E2-induced signals (Marino et al., 2005). Thus, it is possible that flavonoids could induce different conformational changes of ER, also precluding the activation of rapid signaling cascades (Galluzzo et al., 2008). As support of this hypothesis our group have recently demonstrated that quercetin and naringenin hamper ERα-mediated rapid activation of signaling kinases (i.e., ERK/ MAPK and PI3K/AKT) and cyclin D1 transcription only when HeLa cells, devoid of any ER isoforms, were transiently transfected with a human ERα expression vector (Virgili et al., 2004). In particular, naringenin, inducing conformational changes in ER, provokes ERα depalmitoylation faster than E2, which results in receptor rapid dissociation from caveolin-1, impairing ERα binding to molecular adaptor and signaling proteins (e.g., modulator of non genomic actions of the ER, c-Src) involved in the activation of the mitogenic signaling cascades (i.e., ERK/MAPK and PI3K/AKT) (Galluzzo et al., 2008). Moreover, naringenin induces the ERα-dependent, but palmitoylation-independent, activation of p38/MAPK, which in turn is responsible for naringenin-mediated antiproliferative effects in cancer cells. Naringenin, decoupling ERα action mechanisms, prevents the activation ERK/MAPK and PI3K/AKT signal transduction pathways thus, drives cells to apoptosis (Galluzzo et al., 2008). On the other hand, naringenin does not impair the ERα-mediated transcriptional activity of an ERE-containing promoter (Totta et al., 2004; Virgili et al., 2004). As a whole, this flavanone modulates specific ERα mechanisms and can be considered as 'mechanism-specific ligands of ER' (Totta et al., 2004).

In the same cell system, we recently demonstrated that quercetin activates the rapid ERα-dependent phosphorylation of p38/MAPK and, in turn, the induction of a proapoptotic cascade (i.e., caspase-3 activation and PARP cleavage) (Galluzzo et al., 2008a). This result proves that quercetin- and naringenin-induced apoptosis in cancer cells depends on the flavonoid interference with ERα-mediated rapid actions suggesting a role of endocrine disruptor for these flavonoids (Galluzzo et al 2008a).

As previously described, E2 mediates a wide variety of complex biological processes including skeletal muscle differentiation via ERα-dependent signals (Marino, personal communication). Our recent data show that Nar stimulation of rat skeletal muscle cells (L6), decoupling ERα mechanism of action, impedes the E2-dependent differentiation further sustaining the antiestrogenic role played by flavonoids (Marino, personal communication).

Thus, flavonoids have a very complex spectrum of activities: they can function as mechanism-specific ligands of ERα (Totta et al., 2004) due to their ability to decouple ERα activities, eliciting estrogenic or antiestrogenic effects downstream of these pathways (Galluzzo et al., 2008).

Conclusions

Interest on dietary compounds has evolved since their therapeutic properties has been discovered. Flavonoids are documented to play a major role amongst the hormonally agents in food, nonetheless the importance of their role in human health has not yet unequivocally established.

Flavonoids have a chemical structure compatible with a strong putative antioxidant. Neverthless, flavonoids antioxidant/pro-oxidant properties could be considered a simplified approach to the function of molecules of nutritional interest due to the fact that their antioxidant and/or pro-oxidant capacities are chemical properties which are not necessarily associated to an equivalent biological function (Virgili and Marino, 2008). Remarkably, flavonoids have also a strong affinity for protein so they can modulate cellular function inhibiting or modulating protein functions (Figure 3).

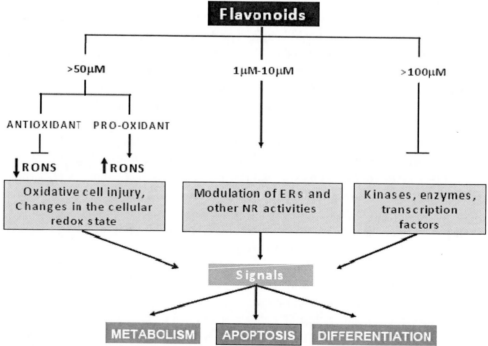

Figure 3. Schematic model illustrating the multiple effects of flavonoids on cell functions.

Normally, human flavonoid plasma concentrations are in the low nanomolar range, but upon flavonoid supplementation they may increase to the high nanomolar or low micromolar range (Boots et al., 2008).

Thus, flavonoids do not appear to be present in the circulation at high enough concentrations to contribute significantly to total antioxidant capacity (concentration of circulating endogenous antioxidant, ascorbate or urate, has been estimated to be in the range of 159-380 µmol/l for a normal individual) (Stevenson and Hurst, 2007) or inhibition kinases activity.

At concentrations more physiologically achievable in the plasma (from 0.1 µM to 10 µM) after the consumption of meals rich in flavonoids (Manach et al., 2004), these compounds can bind to and, consequently, modulate ER activities leading to estrogenic or antiestrogenic effects (Figure 3). As before reported, the long-term estrogenic effects of flavonoids have been extensively studied, whereas there is a lack of experimental data concerning the influence of natural estrogenic compounds on rapid E2-mediated mechanism (Galluzzo and Marino, 2006). Our recent data have highlighted the ability of these compounds to influence also rapid actions of E2 in both reproductive and non reproductive E2-target tissues (Totta et al., 2004; Galluzzo et al., 2008; Galluzzo et al., 2008a).

Thus more attention have to be focus on estrogenicity or antiestrogenicity of these compounds. Estrogenicity *per se* is not an adverse effect, it is a natural mechanism of hormone action controlled via homeostatic mechanisms. However, a chemical with estrogenic properties acting out of context within the endocrine system, or at a vulnerable developmental time-point may have the potential to induce an adverse effect (Fisher et al., 2004). As well as estrogenicity, compounds with antiestrogenic effects could exert both protective or adverse effects depending on cellular context (Galluzzo and Marino, 2006). A current mounting evidence also show that *in utero* and early life phytoestrogen exposure, may promote the onset of breast cancer later in life (Tomar and Shiao, 2008). Thus, more studies are necessary to assess how flavonoid effects impact the normal development and physiological properties of cells at different phases of human life (Somjen et al., 2005; Watson et al., 2005). In particular, their effects in early infant age still deserves special consideration (Virgili and Marino, 2008). Moreover, while several studies are underway to understand how these compounds modulate ER activity, flavonoid interaction and modulation of androgen receptor (AR) is poorly understood. Because of the importance of AR activity in male physiology, also flavonoid interaction and modulation of AR should be considered.

Flavonoids act trough several and distinct action mechanisms (Figure 3). Understanding the cross-talk within these different pathways and the elaborate feedback mechanisms will provide an opportunity to obtain a full picture, which may be relevant to various physiological or pathological states. Assessing phytoestrogen effects at multiple levels, both *in vitro* and *in vivo*, could represent a step towards the employ of these compounds as nutriceuticals able to exert specific responses in target cells or to modulate selectively ER activities in specific target tissues and organs (Galluzzo et al., 2008a).

Acknowledgments

The Authors wish to thank past and present members of their laboratories who contributed to the ideas presented here through data and discussions.

References

Acconcia, F., Ascenzi, P., Bocedi, A., Spisni, E., Tomasi, V., Trentalance, A., Visca, P., and Marino, M. (2005a). Palmitoylation-dependent estrogen receptor α membrane localization: regulation by 17β-estradiol. *Mol. Biol. Cell*, 16, 231-238.

Acconcia, F., Totta, P., Ogawa, S., Cardillo, I., Inoue, S., Leone, S., Trentalance, A., Muramatsu, M., and Marino, M. (2005b). Survival versus apoptotic 17β-estradiol effect: role of ERα and ERβ activated non-genomic signaling. *J. Cell. Physiol.*, 203, 193-201.

Adachi, T., Okuno, Y., Takenaka, S., Matsuda, K., Ohta, N., Takashima, K., Yamazaki, K., Nishimura, D., Miyatake, K., Mori, C., and Tsujimoto, G. (2005). Comprehensive analysis of the effect of phytoestrogen, daidzein, on a testicular cell line, using 1210 mRNA and protein expression profile. *Food Chem. Toxicol.*, 43, 529-535.

Adlercreutz, H., Heinonen, S.M., and Penalvo-Garcia, J. (2004). Phytoestrogens, cancer and coronary heart disease. *Biofactors*, 22, 229-236.

Albini, A., Tosetti, F., Benelli, R., and Noonan, D.M. (2005). Tumor inflammatory angiogenesis and its chemoprevention. *Cancer Res.*, 65, 10637-10641.

Andreadi, C. K., Howells, L.M., Atherfold, P.A., and Manson, M.M. (2006). Involvement of Nrf2, p38, B-Raf, and nuclear factor-κB, but not phosphatidylinositol 3-kinase, in induction of hemeoxygenase-1 by dietary polyphenols. *Mol. Pharmacol.*, 69, 1033-1040.

Ascenzi, P., Bocedi, A., and Marino, M. (2006). Structure-function relationship of estrogen receptor α and β: impact on human health. *Mol. Aspects Med.*, 27, 299-402.

Béliveau, R., and Gingras, D. (2007). Role of nutrition in preventing cancer. *Can. Fam. Physician*, 53, 1905-1911.

Benavente-García, O., and Castillo, J. (2008). Update on uses and properties of citrus flavonoids: new findings in anticancer, cardiovascular, and anti-inflammatory activity. *J. Agric. Food Chem.*, 56, 6185-6205.

Bennetts, H.W., Underwood, E.J., and Shier, F.L. (1946). A specific breeding problem of sheep on subterranean clover pasture in western Australia. *Austr. Vet. J.*, 22, 2-12.

Birt, D.F., Hendrich, S., and Wang, W. (2001). Dietary agents in cancer prevention: flavonoids and isoflavonoids. *Pharmacol. Ther.*, 90, 157-177.

Boots, A.W., Haenen, G.R., and Bast, A. (2008). Health effects of quercetin: from antioxidant to nutraceutical. *Eur. J. Pharmacol.*, 585, 325-337.

Caltagirone, S., Rossi, C., Poggi, A., Ranelletti, F.O., Natali, P.G., Brunetti, M., Aiello, F.B., and Piantelli, M. (2000). Flavonoids apigenin and quercetin inhibit melanoma growth and metastatic potential. *J. Cancer*, 87, 595-600.

Chambliss, K.L., Yuhanna, I.S., Anderson, R.G., Mendelsohn, M. E., and Shaul, P.W. (2002). ERbeta has nongenomic action in caveolae. *Mol. Endo.*, 16, 938-946.

Chao, S.H., Fujinaga, K., Marion, J.E., Taube, R., Sausville, E.A., Senderowicz, A.M., Peterlin B.M., and Price D.H. (2000). Flavopiridol inhibits P-TEFb and blocks HIV-1 replication. *J. Biol. Chem.*, 275, 28345-28348.

Cheynier, V. (2005). Polyphenols in foods are more complex than often thought. *Am. J. Clin. Nutr.*, 81, 223-229.

Chiang, A.N., Wu, H.L., Yeh, H.I., Chu, C.S., Lin, H.C., and Lee, W.C. (2006). Antioxidant effects of black rice extract through the induction of superoxide dismutase and catalase activities. *Lipids*, 41, 797-803.

Conney, A.H. (2003). Enzyme induction and dietary chemicals as approaches to cancer chemoprevention: the seventh DeWitt S. Goodman lecture. *Cancer Res.*, 63, 7005-7031.

Dalu, A., Haskell, J.F., Coward, L., and Lamartiniere, C.A. (1998). Genistein, a component of soy, inhibits the expression of the EGF and ErbB2/Neu receptors in the rat dorsolateral prostate. *Prostate*, 37, 36-43.

Dang, Z.C., Audinot, V., Papapoulos, S.E., Boutin, J.A., and Lowik, C.W. (2003). PPARγ as a molecular target for the soy phytoestrogen genistein. *J. Biol. Chem.*, 278, 962-967.

Dang, Z.C., and Lowik, C. (2005). Dose-dependent effects of phytoestrogens on bone. *Trends Endocrinol. Metab.*, 16, 207-213.

Delclos, K.B., Bucci, T.J., Lomax, L.G., Latendresse, J.R., Warbritton, A., Weis, C.C., and Newbold, R.R. (2001). Effects of dietary genistein exposure during development on male and female CD (Sprague–Dawley) rats. *Reprod. Toxicol.*, 15, 647-663.

Distefano, E., Marino, M., Gillette, J.A., Hanstein, B., Pallottini, V., Bruning, J., Krone, W., and Trentalance, A. (2002). Role of tyrosine kinase signaling in estrogen-induced LDL receptor gene expression in HepG2 cells. *Biochim. Biophys. Acta*, 1580, 145-149.

Doerge, D.R., Twaddle, N.C., Churchwell, M.I., Newbold, R.R., and Delclos, K.B. (2006). Lactational transfer of the soy isoflavone, genistein, in Sprague-Dawley rats consuming dietary genistein. *Reprod. Toxicol.*, 21, 307-312.

El Bedoui, J., Oak, M.H., Anglard, P., and Schini-Kerth, V.B. (2005). Catechins prevent vascular smooth muscle cell invasion by inhibiting MT1-MMP activity and MMP-2 expression. *Cardiovasc. Res.*, 67, 317-325.

Elisaf, M. (2002). Effects of fibrates on serum metabolic parameters. *Curr. Med. Res. Opin.*, 18, 269-276.

Escande, A., Pillon, A., Servant, N., Cravedi, J.P., Larrea, F., Muhn, P., Nicolas, J.C., Cavailles, V., and Balaguer, P. (2006). Evaluation of ligand selectivity using reporter cell lines stably expressing estrogen receptor alpha or beta. *Biochem. Pharmacol.*, 71, 1459-1469.

Espìn, J.C., Garcìa-Conesa, M.T., and Tomàs-Barberàn, F.A. (2007). Nutraceuticals: facts and fiction. *Phytochemistry*, 68, 2986-3008.

Farach-Carson, M.C., and Davis, P.J. (2003). Steroid hormone interactions with target cells: cross talk between membrane and nuclear pathways. *J. Pharmacol. Experimen. Ther.*, 307, 839- 845.

Fenton, J.I., and Hord, N.G. (2004). Flavonoids promote cell migration in nontumorigenic colon epithelial cells differing in Apc genotype: implications of matrix metalloproteinase activity. *Nutr. Cancer*, 48, 182-188.

Filomeni, G., Graziani, I., Rotilio, G., and Ciriolo, M.R. (2007). Trans-resveratrol induces apoptosis in human breast cancer cells MCF-7 by the activation of MAP kinases pathways. *Genes Nutr.*, 2, 295-305.

Fisher, J.S. (2004). Are all EDC effects mediated via steroid hormone receptors? *Toxicol.*, 205, 33-41.

Flynn, K.M., Ferguson, S.A., Delclos, K.B. and Newbold, R.R. (2000). Effects of genistein exposure on sexually dimorphic behaviors in rats. *Toxicol. Sci.*, 55, 311-319.

Galati, G., Moridani, M.Y., Chan, T.S., and O'Brien, P.J. (2001). Peroxidative metabolism of apigenin and naringenin versus luteolin and quercetin: glutathione oxidation and conjugation. *Free Radic. Biol. Med.*, 30, 370-382.

Galati, G., Teng, S., Moridani, M.Y., Chan, T.S., and O'Brien, P.J. (2000). Cancer chemoprevention and apoptosis mechanisms induced by dietary polyphenolics. *Drug Metabol. Drug Interact.*, 17, 311-349.

Galluzzo, P., Ascenzi, P., Bulzomi, P., and Marino, M. (2008). The nutritional flavanone naringenin triggers antiestrogenic effects by regulating estrogen receptor α-palmitoylation. *Endocrinology*, 149, 2567-2575.

Galluzzo, P., Martini, C., Bulzomi, P., Leone, S., Bolli, A., Pallottini, V., and Marino, M. (2008a). Quercitin-induced apoptotic cascade in cancer cells: antioxidant versus estrogen receptor-dependent mechanisms. *Mol. Nutr. Food Res.*, In Press.

Galluzzo, P., Caiazza, F., Moreno, S., and Marino, M. (2007). Role of ERbeta palmitoylation in the inhibition of human colon cancer cell proliferation. *Endocr. Relat. Cancer,* 359, 102-107.

Galluzzo, P., and Marino, M. (2006). Nutritional flavonoid impact on nuclear and extranuclear estrogen receptor activities. *Genes Nutr.* 1, 161-176.

Gronemeyer, H., Gustafsson, J.-Å., and Laudet, V. (2004). Principles for modulation of the nuclear receptor superfamily. *Nat. Rev.,Drug Discovery*, 3, 950–964.

Guo, T.L., Germolec, D.R., Musgrove, D.L., Delclos, K.B., Newbold, R.R., Weis, C.C. and White, K.L.Jr. (2005). Myelotoxicity in genistein-, nonylphenol-, methoxychlor-, vinclozolin- or ethinyl estradiol-exposed F1 generations of Sprague-Dawley rats following developmental and adult exposures. *Toxicology,* 211, 207-219.

Hagiwara, M., Inoue, S., Tanaka, T., Nunoki, K., Ito, M., and Hidaka, H. (1988). Differential effects of flavonoids as inhibitors of tyrosine protein kinases and serine/threonine protein kinases. *Biochem. Pharmacol.*, 37, 2987-2992.

Hanasaki, Y., Ogawa, S., and Fukui, S. (1994). The correlation between active oxygens scavenging and antioxidative effects of flavonoids. *Free Rad. Biol. Med.,* 16, 845-850.

Hao, Q., Rutherford, S. A., Low, B., and Tang, H. (2006). Selective regulation of hydrogen peroxide signaling by receptor tyrosine phosphatase-α. *Free Radic. Biol. Med.,* 41, 302-310.

Hehner, S.P., Hofmann, T.G., Dienz, O., Droge, W., and Schmitz, M. L. (2000). Tyrosine-phosphorylated Vav1 as a point of integration for T-cell receptor-and CD28- mediated activation of JNK, p38, and interleukin-2 transcription. *J. Biol. Chem,.* 275, 18160–18171.

Ioannides, C., and Lewis, D. F. (2004). Cytochromes P450 in the bioactivation of chemicals. *Curr. Top. Med. Chem.,* 4, 1767-1788.

Iqbal, M. J., Yaegashi, S., Ahsan, R., Lightfoot, D.A., and Banz, W. J. (2002). Differentially abundant mRNAs in rat liver in response to diets containing soy protein isolate. *Physiol. Genomics,* 11, 219-226.

Jacobs, M.N., and Lewis, D.F. (2002). Steroid hormone receptors and dietary ligands: a selected review. *Proc. Nutr. Soc.*, 61, 105-122.

Jakobs, S., Fridrich, D., Hofem, S., Pahlke, G., and Eisenbrand, G. (2006). Natural flavonoids are potent inhibitors of glycogen phosphorylase. *Mol. Nutr. Food Res.,* 50, 52-57.

Kang Z.C., Tsai S.J., and Lee H. (1999). Quercetin inhibits benzo[*a*]pyrene-induced DNA adducts in human Hep G2 cells by altering cytochrome P-450 1A1 expression. *Nutr. Cancer*, 35, 175-179.

Karunagaran, D., Rashmi, R., and Kumar, T.R. (2005). Induction of apoptosis by curcumin and its implications for cancer therapy. *Curr. Cancer Drug Targets*, 5, 117-129.

Kim, E.J., Choi, C.H., Park, J.Y., Kang, S.K., and Kim, Y.K. (2008). Underlying mechanism of quercetin-induced cell death in human glioma cells. *Neurochem. Res.*, 33, 971-979.

Kirk, E.A., Sutherland, P., Wang, S.A., Chait, A., and LeBoeuf, R.C. (1998). Dietary isoflavones reduce plasma cholesterol and atherosclerosis in C57BL/6 mice but not LDL receptor-deficient mice. *J. Nutr.*, 128, 954-959.

Kuiper, G.G., Carlsson, B., Grandien, K., Enmark, E., Häggblad, J., Nilsson. S., and Gustafsson, J.A. (1997). Comparison of the ligand binding specificity and transcript tissue distribution of estrogen receptors α and β. *Endocrinology*, 138, 863-870.

Kweon, M.H., In Park, Y., Sung, H.C., and Mukhtar, H. (2006). The novel antioxidant 3-O-caffeoyl-1-methylquinic acid induces Nrf2-dependent phase II detoxifying genes and alters intracellular glutathione redox. *Free Radic. Biol. Med.*, 40, 1349-1361.

Lee, J. S., and Surh, Y. J. (2005). Nrf2 as a novel molecular target for chemoprevention. *Cancer Lett.* 224, 171-184.

Levin, E.R. (2005). Integration of the extranuclear and nuclear actions of estrogen. *Mol. Endocrinol.*, 19, 1951-1959.

Ling, S., Dai, A., Williams, M.R., Husband, A.J., Nestel, P.J., Komesaroff, P.A., and Sudhir, K. (2004). The isoflavone metabolite cis-tetrahydrodaidzein inhibits ERK-1 activation and proliferation in human vascular smooth muscle cells. *J. Cardiovasc. Pharmacol.*, 435, 622-628.

Liu, M. M., Albanese, C., Anderson, C. M., Hilty, K., Webb, P., Uht, R. M., Price, R. H., Pestell, R. G., and Kushner, P. J. (2002). Opposing action of estrogen receptors a and b on cyclin D1 gene expression. *J. Biol. Chem.*, 277, 24353-24360.

Manach, C., Scalbert, A., Morand, C., Remesy, C., and Jimenez L. (2004). Polyphenols: food sources and bioavailability. *Am. J. Clin. Nutr.*, 79, 727-747.

Manna, S.K., Mukhopadhyay, A. and Aggarwal, B.B. (2000). Resveratrol suppresses TNFα-induced activation of nuclear transcription factors NF-κB, activator protein-1, and apoptosis: potential role of reactiveoxygen intermediates and lipid peroxidation. *J. Immunol.*, 164, 6509-6519.

Manthey, J.A. (2000). Biological properties of flavonoids pertaining to inflammation, *Microcirculation*, 6, 29-34.

Marino, M., Acconcia, F., and Ascenzi P. (2005). Estrogen receptor signalling: bases for drug actions. *Curr Drug Targets Imm. Endo. Metabol. Disorder.*, 5, 305-14.

Mezei, O., Banz, W.J., Steger, R.W., Peluso, M.R., Winters, T.A., and Shay, N. (2003). Soy isoflavones exert antidiabetic and hypolipidemic effects through the PPAR pathways in obese Zucker rats and murine RAW 264.7 cells. *J. Nutr.*, 133, 1238-1243.

Middleton, E.Jr., Kandaswami, C., and Theoharides, T.C. (2000). The effects of plant flavonoids on mammalian cells: implications for inflammation, heart disease, and cancer. *Pharmacol. Rev.*, 52, 673-751.

Miyoshi, N., Naniwa, K., Yamada, T., Osawa, T., and Nakamura, Y. (2007). Dietary flavonoid apigenin is a potential inducer of intracellular oxidative stress: The role in the interruptive apoptotic signal, *Arch. Biochem. Biophys.*, 466, 274-82.

Mnif, W., Pascussi, J. M., Pillon, A., Escande, A., Bartegi, A., Nicolas, J. C., Cavaillès, V., Duchesne, M.J., and Balaguer, P. (2007). Estrogens and antiestrogens activate hPXR. *Toxicol. Lett.*, 170, 19-29.

Moore, J.T., and Kliewer, S.A. (2000).Use of the nuclear receptor PXR to predict drug interactions. *Toxicol.*, 153, 1-10.

Morrissey C., O'Neill A., Spengler B., Christoffel V., Fitzpatrick J.M., and Watson R.W. (2005). Apigenin drives the production of reactive oxygen species and initiates a mitochondrial mediated cell death pathway in prostate epithelial cells. *Prostate*, 63, 131-142.

Moskaug, J.O., Carlsen, H., Myhrstad, M.C., and Blomhoff, R. (2005). Polyphenols and glutathione synthesis regulation. *Am. J. Clin. Nutr.*, 81, 277-283.

Mueller, S. O. (2002). Overview of in vitro tools to assess the estrogenic and antiestrogenic activity of phytoestrogens. *J. Chromatogr.*, 777, 155-165.

Mueller, S.O., Simon, S., Chae, K., Metzler, M., and Korach, K.S. (2004). Phytoestrogens and their human metabolites show distinct agonistic and antagonistic properties on estrogen receptor alpha (ERalpha) and ERbeta in human cells. *Toxicol. Sci.*, 80, 14-25.

Nilsson, S., Makela, S., Treuter, E., Tujague, M., Thomsen, J., Andersson, G., Enmark, E., Pettersson, K., Warner, M., and Gustafsson, J.-Å. (2001). Mechanism of estrogen action, *Physiol. Rev.*, 81, 1535-1565.

Nomura, M., Takahashi, T., Nagata, N., Tsutsumi, K., Kobayashi, S., Akiba, T., Yokogawa, K., Moritani, S., and Miyamoto, K. (2008). Inhibitory mechanisms of flavonoids on insulin-stimulated glucose uptake in MC3T3-G2/PA6 adipose cells. *Biol. Pharm. Bull.*, 31, 1403-9.

O'Brien P.J. (2000). Peroxidases, *Chem. Biol. Interact.*, 129, 113-139.

O'Loghlen, A., Perez-Morgado, M.I., Salinas, M., and Martin, M.E. (2003). Reversible inhibition of the protein phosphatase 1 by hydrogen peroxide: potential regulation of eIF2α phosphorylation in differentiated PC12 cells. *Arch. Biochem. Biophys.*, 417, 194-202.

Pellegatta, F., Bertelli, A.A.E., Staels, B., Duhem, C., Fulgenzi, A., and Ferrero, M.E. (2003). Different short- and long-term effects of resveratrol on nuclear factor-kappaB phosphorylation and nuclear appearance in human endothelial cells. *Am. J. Clin. Nutr.*, 77, 1220-1228.

Peterson, G., Barnes, S. (1993). Genistein and biochanin A inhibit the growth of human prostate cancer cells but not epidermal growth factor receptor tyrosine autophosphorylation. *Prostate*, 22, 335-345.

Peterson, G., Barnes, S. (1996). Genistein inhibits both estrogen and growth factor-stimulated proliferation of human breast cancer cells. *Cell Growth Differ.*, 7, 1345-1351.

Rice, S., and Whitehead, S.A. (2006). Phytoestrogens and breast cancer-promoters or protectors?, *Endocr. Relat. Cancer*, 13, 995-1015.

Ricketts, M.L., Moore, D.D., Banz, W.J., Mezei, O., and Shay, N.F. (2005). Molecular mechanisms of action of the soy isoflavones includes activation of promiscuous nuclear receptors. *J. Nutr. Biochem.*, 16, 321-330.

Saarinen, N.M., Mäkelä, S., Penttinen, P., Wärri, A., Lorenzetti, S., Virgili, F., Mortensen, A., Sørensen, I.K., Bingham, C., Valsta, L.M., Vollmer, G., and Zierau, O. (2006). Tools to evaluate estrogenic potency of dietary phytoestrogens: a consensus paper from the EU Thematic Network "Phytohealth" (QLKI-2002-2453). *Genes Nutr.*, 1, 143-158.

Shay, N. F., and Banz, W. J. (2005). Regulation of gene transcription by botanicals: novel regulatory mechanisms. *Ann. Rev. Nutr.*, 25, 297-315.

Somjen, D., Kohen, E., Lieberherr, M., Gayer, B., Schejter, E., Katzburg, S., Limor, R., Sharon, O., Knoll, E., Posner, G.H., Kaye, A.M., and Stern, N. (2005). Membranal effects of phytoestrogens and carboxy derivatives of phytoestrogens on human vascular and bone cells: new insights based on studies with carboxy-biochanin. *A. J. Steroid Biochem. Mol. Biol.,* 93, 293-303.

Spencer, J.P., Rice-Evans, C., Williams, R.J. (2003). Modulation of pro-survival Akt/protein kinase B and ERK1/2 signaling cascades by quercetin and its in vivo metabolites underlie their action on neuronal viability. *J. Biol. Chem.,* 278, 34783-34793.

Stevens, J.F., and Page, J. E. (2004). Xanthohumol and related prenylflavonoids from hops and beer: to your good health!, *Phytochem.,* 65, 1317-1330.

Stevenson, D.E., and Hurst, R.D. (2007). Polyphenolic phytochemicals-just antioxidants or much more?, *Cell Mol. Life Sci.,* 64, 2900-2916.

Stone, J.R., and Yang, S. (2006). Hydrogen peroxide: a signaling messenger. *Antioxid. Redox Signaling,* 8, 243-270.

Suetsugi, M., Su, L., Karlsberg, K., Yuan, Y.C., and Chen, S. (2003). Flavone and isoflavone phytoestrogens are agonists of estrogen-related receptors. *Mol. Cancer Res.,* 1, 981-991.

Surh, Y.J. (2003). Cancer chemoprevention with dietary phytochemicals. *Nat. Rev. Cancer,* 3, 768-780.

Terasaka, S., Aita, Y., Inoue, A., Hayashi, S., Nishigaki, M., Aoyagi, K., Sasaki, H., Wada-Kiyama, Y., Sakuma, Y., Akaba, S., Tanaka, J., Sone, H., Yonemoto, J., Tanji, M., and Kiyama, R.U. (2004). Using a customized DNA microarray for expression profiling of the estrogen-responsive genes to evaluate estrogen activity among naturalestrogens and industrial chemicals. *Environ. Health Perspect.,* 112, 773-781.

Tomar, R.S,. and Shiao, R. (2008). Early Life and Adult Exposure to Isoflavones and Breast Cancer Risk. *J. Environ. Sci. Health C. Environ. Carcinog. Ecotoxicol. Rev.,* 26, 113-73.

Totta, P., Acconcia, F., Leone, S., Cardillo, I., and Marino, M. (2004). Mechanisms of naringenin-induced apoptotic cascade in cancer cells: involvement of estrogen receptor α and β signalling. *IUBMB Life,* 56, 491-499.

Totta, P., Acconcia, F., Virgili, F., Cassidy, A., Weinberg, P.D., Rimbach, G., and Marino, M. (2005). Daidzein-sulfate metabolites affect transcriptional and antiproliferative activities of estrogen receptor-beta in cultured human cancer cells. *J. Nutr.,* 135, 2687-2693.

Ueda, S., Nakamura, H., Masutani, H., Sasada, T., Takabayashi, A., Yamaoka, Y., and Yodoi, J. (2002). Baicalin induces apoptosis via mitochondrial pathway as prooxidant, *Mol. Immunol.,* 38, 781-91.

Ursini, F., Maiorino, M., Morazzoni, P., Roveri, A., and Pifferi, G. (1994). A novel antioxidant flavonoid (IdB 1031) affecting molecular mechanisms of cellular activation. *Free Rad. Biol. Med.,* 16, 547-553.

Vargo M.A., Voss O.H., Poustka F., Cardounel A.J., Grotewold E., and Doseff A.I. (2006). Apigenin-induced-apoptosis is mediated by the activation of PKCδ and caspases in leukemia cells. *Biochem. Pharmacol.,* 72, 681-692.

Virgili, F., and Marino, M. (2008). Regulation of cellular signals from nutritional molecules: a specific role for phytochemicals, beyond antioxidant activity. *Free Radic. Biol. Med.,* 45, 1205-1216.

Virgili, F., Acconcia, F., Ambra, R., Rinna, A., Totta, P., and Marino, M. (2004). Nutritional flavonoids modulate estrogen receptor α signaling. *IUBMB Life,* 56, 145-151.

Wang I.K., Lin-Shiau S.Y., and Lin J.K. (1999). Induction of apoptosis by apigenin and related flavonoids through cytochrome c release and activation of caspase-9 and caspase-3 in leukaemia HL-60 cells. *Eur. J. Cancer,* 35, 1517-1525.

Wang, H., Huang, H., Li, H., Teotico, D.G., Sinz, M., Baker, S.D., Staudinger, J., Kalpana, G., Redinbo, M.R., and Mani, S. (2007). Activated pregnenolone X-receptor is a target for ketoconazole and its analogs. *Clin. Cancer Res.,* 13, 2488-2495.

Watson, C.S., Bulayeva, N.N., Wozniak, A.L., and Finnerty, C.C. (2005). Signaling from the membrane via membrane estrogen receptor-alpha: estrogens, xenoestrogens and phytoestrogens. *Steroids,* 70, 364-371.

Wung B.S., Hsu M.C., Wu C.C., and Hsieh C.W. (2005). Resveratrol suppresses IL-6-induced ICAM-1 gene expression in endothelial cells: Effects on the inhibition of STAT3 phosphorylation. *Life Sciences,* 78, 389-397.

Zhang, X., Shu, X.O., Gao, Y., Yang, G., Li, Q., Li, H., Jin, F., and Zheng, W. (2003). Soy food consumption is associated with lower risk of coronory heart disease in Chinese women. *J. Nutr.,* 133, 2874-2878.

In: Encyclopedia of Vitamin Research
Editor: Joshua T. Mayer

ISBN: 978-1-61761-928-1
© 2011 Nova Science Publishers, Inc.

Chapter 45

Antiophidian Mechanisms of Medicinal Plants[*]

Rafael da Silva Melo[1], Nicole Moreira Farrapo[1],
Dimas dos Santos Rocha Junior[1,4], Magali Glauzer Silva[1],
José Carlos Cogo[2], Cháriston André Dal Belo[3],
Léa Rodrigues-Simioni[4], Francisco Carlos Groppo[5]
and Yoko Oshima-Franco[†1,4]

[1]Universidade de Sorocaba, UNISO, Sorocaba, São Paulo, Brazil
[2]Universidade do Vale do Paraiba, UNIVAP, São José dos Campos, São Paulo, Brazil
[3]Universidade Federal do Pampa, São Gabriel, RS, Brazil
[4]Universidade Estadual de Campinas, UNICAMP, Campinas, São Paulo, Brazil
[5]Universidade Estadual de Campinas, UNICAMP, Piracicaba, São Paulo, Brazil

Abstract

Vegetal extracts usually have a large diversity of bioactive compounds showing several pharmacological activities, including antiophidian properties. In this study, both coumarin and tannic acid (100 µg/mL) showed no changes in the basal response of twitches in mouse nerve phrenic diaphragm preparations. In opposite, *Crotalus durissus terrificus* (Cdt 15 µg/mL) or *Bothrops jararacussu* (Bjssu 40 µg/mL) venoms caused irreversible neuromuscular blockade. Tannic acid (preincubated with the venoms), but not coumarin, was able to significantly inhibit ($p < 0.05$) the impairment of the muscle strength induced by Cdt ($88 \pm 8\%$) and Bjssu ($79 \pm 7.5\%$), respectively. A remarkable precipitation was observed when the venoms were preincubated with tannic acid, but not

---

[*] A version of this chapter was also published in *Flavonoids: Biosynthesis, Biological Effects and Dietary Sources, edited by Raymond B. Keller* published by Nova Science Publishers, Inc. It was submitted for appropriate modifications in an effort to encourage wider dissemination of research.
[†] Phone: +55 15 2101 7000 - Fax: +55 15 2101 7112, E-mail: yofranco@terra.com.br

with coumarin. *Plathymenia reticulata* is a good source of tannins and flavonoids whereas *Mikania laevigata* contain high amounts of coumarin. *P. reticulata* (PrHE, 0.06 mg/mL) and *M. laevigata* (MlHE, 1 mg/mL) hydroalcoholic extracts were assayed with or without Bjssu or Cdt venoms. Both PrHE and MlHE showed protection against Bjssu (79.3 ± 9.5% and 65 ± 8%, respectively) and Cdt (73.2 ± 6.7% and 95 ± 7%, respectively) neuromuscular blockade. In order to observe if the protective mechanism could be induced by protein precipitation, tannins were eliminated from both extracts and the assay was repeated. MlHE protected against the blockade induced by Bjssu (57.2 ± 6.7%), but not against Cdt. We concluded that plants containing tannins could induce the precipitation of venoms' proteins and plants containing coumarin showed activity against *Bothrops* venoms, but not against *Crotalus* venoms. We also concluded that the use of isolated bioactive compounds could not represent the better strategy against ophidian venoms, since the purification may exclude some bioactive components resulting in a loss of antivenom activity. In addition, *M. laevigata* showed better antiophidian activity than *P. reticulata*.

Keywords: Bothrops jararacussu, Crotalus durissus terrificus, medicinal plant.

Introduction

The use of medicinal plants has been practiced for many generations. In addition, plants had contributed for the development of many valuable substances such as morphine, the principal alkaloid in opium and the prototype opiate analgesic and narcotic; vincristine, the antitumor alkaloid isolated from *Vinca Rosea*; rutin, a flavonol glycoside found in many plants, used therapeutically to decrease capillary fragility [4].

The animal kingdom constitutes another interesting source of investigation, mainly venomous animals, first due to its pathological effects caused by envenomation and second by the therapeutical possibilities of their constituents. For example, bradykinin, a nonapeptide messenger enzymatically produced from kallidin in the blood, is derived from *Bothrops jararaca* venom [21].

Many people have been seeking complementary and alternative medicines as an adjunct to conventional therapies. There is a renewed interest in the therapeutic potential of venoms from bees, snakes and scorpions or sea-anemones toxins [23]. Salmosin, a desintegrin derived from snake venom that contains the Arg-Gly-Asp (RGD) sequence, was reported to be both antiangiogenic and anti-tumorigenic [18].

The natural resources are the largest reservoir of drugs [29], and the investigation of substances with therapeutic effects has been performed by isolation, extraction and/or purification of new compounds of vegetable origin [1]. Nowadays, there are many sophisticated - but yet very expensive, laborious and long-time demanding – methods to obtain these new compounds from plant or animal origin.

One of the most used experimental models to test pharmacological and antivenom properties of new compounds is the nerve phrenic diaphragm preparations isolated from rats [3], which was also modified for mice. Anatomically and physiologically this preparation represents the nerve-muscle synapse and the muscular contraction, respectively. Pharmacological effects can be showed by blockade, facilitation or contracture, among other possibilities. *B. jararacussu* venom, for example, causes both neuromuscular blockade and severe local myonecrosis.

Mikania laevigata, popularly known as "guaco", is related to *Mikania glomerata* Sprengel, being both used to treat respiratory diseases. Both have pharmacological activities attributed to coumarin [5, 12, 20, 24]. The main difference between the two species is the flowering period: *M. laevigata* flourishes in September and *M. glomerata* in January [24]. Some authors have also attributed an antiophidian property against brazilian snake venoms to *M. glomerata* [20, 28], but this property was not studied in *M. laevigata*.

Plathymenia reticulata Benth, popularly known as "vinhático", is a plant from Brazilian "cerrado" that has anti-inflammatory properties, and a previous phytochemical study identified tannins and flavonoids as its principal constituents [11].

The aim of the present study was to investigate the neutralizing ability of two commercial phytochemicals (tannic acid and coumarin) against the neuromuscular blockade induced by two crude snake venoms - *Bothrops jararacussu* and *Crotalus durissus terrificus*. In addition, hydroalcoholic extracts from plants containing tannic acid (*Plathymenia reticulata* Benth) and coumarin (*Mikania laevigata* Schultz Bip. ex Baker) were assayed against *B. jararacussu* venom.

Materials and Methods

Animals

Male Swiss white mice (26-32 g) were supplied by Anilab - Animais de Laboratório (Paulínia, São Paulo, Brazil). The animals were housed at $25 \pm 3°C$ on a 12-h light/dark cycle and had access to food and water *ad libitum*. This project (protocol number A078/CEP/2007) was approved by the institutional Committee for Ethics in Research of Vale do Paraiba University (UNIVAP), and the experiments were carried out according to the guidelines of the Brazilian College for Animal Experimentation.

Venoms

Crude venoms were obtained from adults *Bothrops jararacussu* (Bjssu) and *Crotalus durissus terrificus* (Cdt) snakes (Serpentário do Centro de Estudos da Natureza) and certified by Prof. Dr. José Carlos Cogo, Vale do Paraíba University (UNIVAP, São José dos Campos, SP, Brazil).

Phytochemicals

Tannic acid and coumarin were purchased from Sigma-Aldrich (USA) and used as standard phytochemicals.

M. Laevigata Extract

The leaves of *M. laevigata* (1 kg) were harvested from plants at the University of Sorocaba (UNISO) herbarium. A voucher specimen was deposited in the UNISO herbarium. The powder (1 kg) obtained from *M. laevigata* leaves were percolated during 10 days in 50% hydroalcoholic solution. After this period, the solution was dried at 40°C by using forced air circulation (dryer Marconi, São Paulo, Brazil) and crushed (10 Mesh, 1.70 mm) by using a macro mill (type Wiley, MA 340 model, Marconi, São Paulo, Brazil). After this procedure, 50% hydroalcoholic solution (Synth, São Paulo, Brazil) was added until complete extraction (when the solution was incolor). Then, the extract was evaporated until dryness by using a rotatory evaporator (Tecnal, São Paulo, Brazil) at 50 °C. The resulting powder (131.68g) was stored at room temperature and protected from light and humidity until the assays.

P. Reticulata Extract

The barks from *P. reticulata* were collected in October 2006 in Miracema city, Tocantins State, Brazil. A specimen was deposited (protocol NRHTO 3327) at the herbarium of Federal University of Tocantins (UFT). The barks were dehydrated in a stove at 37°C during 48 hours, powdered, ground in a mill, macerated with alcohol (70%) during 24 hours and percolated in order to obtain a 20% (m/v) hydroalcoholic extract [27].

Protein Precipitation Assay and Tannins Determination

The proteins in the extract solutions were precipitated [14] with 1.0 mg/mL bovine serum albumine (BSA, fraction V, Sigma) solution in 0.2 M acetate buffer (pH 4.9). After centrifugation, the precipitate was dissolved in sodium dodecyl sulfate (Sigma)/ triethanolamine (Merck) solution and the tannins were complexed with $FeCl_3$. The supernatant of each extract (containing free tannins) was used for venom neutralizing assays, and the coloring complex was spectrophotometrically read at 510 nm for tannins determination [13, 14]. The tannin concentration in the samples was measured through a standard curve obtained by a polynomial regression y=1.754x–0.1253 (R^2=0.9971). Tannic acid was used for the standard curve. All solutions were analyzed in triplicate.

Thin Layer Chromatography

Aliquots of the *M. laevigata* and *P. reticulata* hydroalcoholic extracts (MlHE and PrHE, respectively) were spotted in thin-layer silica gel plates (0.3 mm thick, Merck, Germany) with appropriate standards [15, 30]. The solvent system consisted of acetone:chloroform:formic acid (10:75:8, v/v). The phytochemical groups used as standards (1% methanol - m/v, Sigma-Aldrich, USA) were coumarin and tannic acid. The separated spots were visualized with NP/PEG as following: 5% (v/v) ethanolic NP (diphenylboric acid 2-aminoethyl ester, Sigma, Switzerland) followed by 5% (v/v) ethanolic PEG 4000 (polyethylene glycol 4000, Synth, Brazil), being visualized under U.V. light at 360 nm. The retention factor (Rf) of each standard was compared with those spots exhibited by both extracts obtained from *M. laevigata* and *P. reticulata*.

Mouse Phrenic Nerve-Diaphragm Muscle (PND) Preparation

The phrenic nerve-diaphragm muscle [3] was obtained from mice previously anesthetized with halotane and sacrificed by exsanguination. The diaphragm was removed and mounted under a tension of 5 g in a 5 mL organ bath containing aerated Tyrode solution (control). After equalization with 95% O_2 and 5% CO_2, the pH of this solution was 7.0. The preparations were indirectly stimulated with supramaximal stimuli (4 x threshold, 0.06 Hz, 0.2 ms) delivered from a stimulator (model ESF-15D, Ribeirão Preto, Brazil) to the nerve by bipolar electrodes. Isometric twitch tension was recorded with a force displacement transducer (cat. 7003, Ugo Basile), coupled to a 2-Channel Recorder Gemini physiograph device (cat. 7070, Ugo Basile) via a Basic Preamplifier (cat. 7080, Ugo Basile). PND preparations were allowed to stabilize for at least 20 min before the addition of one of the following solutions: Tyrode solution (control, n=7); phytochemicals (tannic acid or coumarin, 100 mg/mL, n=6 each); venoms (Bjssu 40 µg/mL, n=10; Cdt 15 µg/mL, n=7); *P. reticulata* hydroalcoholic extract (PrHE, 0.06 mg/mL, n=8) or *M. laevigata* hydroalcoholic extract (MlHE, 1 mg/mL, n=5). The neutralization assays were carried out after preincubating the PND preparations with the Tyrode solution during 30 min. After preincubation, the following substances were added to the bath: phytochemicals + Cdt or Bjssu (n=6, each); MlHE + Bjssu ou Cdt venoms (n=19 and 6, respectively); PrHE + Bjssu or Cdt venoms (n=8 and 5, respectively). In order to verify the influence of tannins on the venoms neutralization, extracts free of tannins (-) were also assayed against the crude venoms.

Experimental Design

The rationale experimental design is bellow presented (Figure 1).

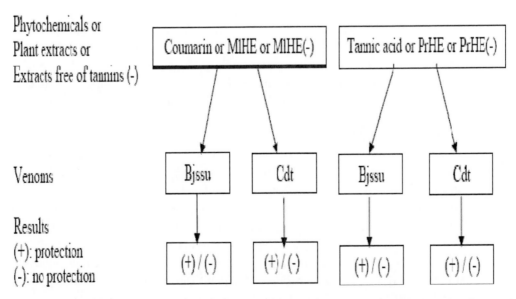

Figure 1. Experimental design showing the rationale steps of the study on the isolated preparation.

Statistical Analysis

Each pharmacological protocol was repeated at least five times. The results were expressed as the mean ± S.E.M. Student's *t*-test was used for statistical comparison of the data and the significance level was set at 5%.

Results and Discussion

Medicinal plants with inhibitory properties against snake venoms have been extensively studied and excellent reviews have been published [19, 32]. Searches focusing the source (leaves, branches, stems, roots, rhizomes, seeds, barks, aerial parts or whole) that concentrates the major bioactive compound, which is able to neutralizing the toxicological effects of venomous snake, have been received special attention [10, 25, 33].

The isolation of bioactive compound usually involves extensive and laborious work using high amount of solvents and expensive techniques such as *nuclear magnetic resonance coupled to mass spectrum that is only available in big research facilities.*

When a plant extract shows some pharmacological action, it has been required the same evidence by its bioactive compound. Cintra-Francischinelli et al. [8] showed that the methanolic extract from Casearia sylvestris Sw. has inhibitory effect against the in vitro neurotoxicity and myotoxicity of Bothrops jararacussu venom and its major toxin, bothropstoxin-I. Although the authors showed rutin as an important component in the methanol extract of C. sylvestris, the isolated rutin in its commercial form did not protect against the toxic effects of both venom and toxin.

Based on these observations, a reverse strategy was hypothesized using initially two commercial phytochemical standards (tannic acid and coumarin) against two snake venoms: *Bothrops jararacussu* (Bjssu) and *Crotalus durissus terrificus* (Cdt). The same protocol was also repeated with selected hydroalcoholic extracts from *Plathymenia reticulata*, which has tannins and flavonoids [11], and *Mikania laevigata*, which has coumarin [9]. The standard phytochemicals at concentration of 100 μg/mL caused no change on the basal response of neuromuscular preparation, and this concentration was chosen for further neutralization assays against the characteristic blockade induced by Bjssu (Figure 2A) and Cdt (Figure 2B) venoms.

Only tannic acid was able to neutralizing the paralysis of both venoms (*$p<0.05$, compared to the respective venoms). During the incubation time only tannic acid showed a precipitate formation (Figure 3), which was more intense when incubated with Cdt than with Bjssu venom, which in turn showed a certain turbidity level. The formation of a precipitate due to a protein complex formation caused by tannic acid maybe could cause loss of venom toxicity. Kuppusamy and Das [17] also found evidences of the protective effects of tannic acid, when injected subcutaneously, against lethal activity, haemorrhage and creatine kinase release that are induced in mice submitted to poisoning with *Crotalus adamanteus* venom. Pithayanakul et al. [26] investigated the *in vitro* venom neutralizing capacity of tannic acid against the activities of *Naja kaouthia* (*Naja naja kaouthia* Lesson - Elapidae).

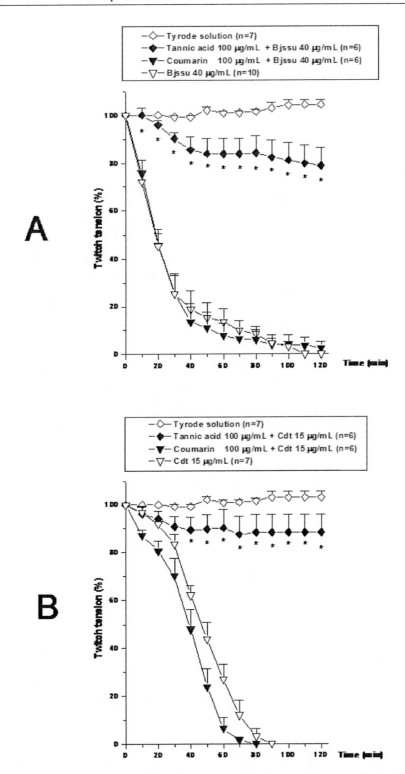

Figure 2. Pharmacological assays on mouse phrenic nerve-diaphragm preparations (indirect stimuli). Neutralization of *Bothrops jararacussu* venom (A, Bjssu), and *Crotalus durissus terrificus* venom (B, Cdt) by tannic acid and coumarin. Each point represents the mean ± S.E.M. of the number of experiments (n) showed in the legend. *$p<0.05$ compared to venom.

Preincubation Procedure

Cdt venom   Bjssu venom

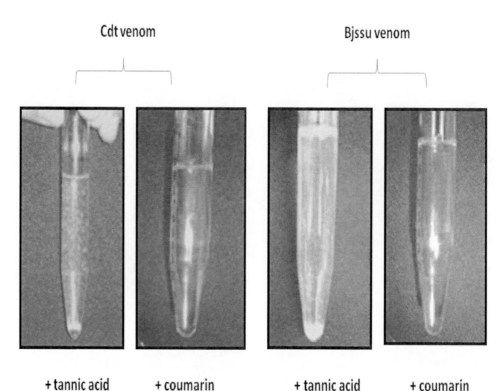

+ tannic acid   + coumarin   + tannic acid   + coumarin

Figure 3. Preincubation procedure. *Crotalus durissus terrificus* venom (Cdt) or *Bothrops jararacussu* venom (Bjssu) were preincubated with tannic acid or coumarin, 30 min prior the pharmacological assays. Note that tannic acid causes a visible protein precipitation, but not coumarin.

PrHE (1) showed two different substances with retention factor (Rf) of 1.8 cm and 5.2 cm. Tannic acid (2) showed substances with Rf of 1.9 cm and 4.5 cm. MlHE (6) showed four substances with Rf 4.3 cm, 5.5 cm, 8.5 cm and 9.0 cm. Under the solvent and revelator systems used, commercial coumarin was not visualized (5). When tannins were complexed with bovine serum albumin (BSA), no substance was visualized in 3, 4 and 7, respectively free of tannins (-), PrHE (-) and MlHE (-).

The pharmacological results using extracts free of tannins (-) are showed in Figure 6. Note that only MlHE (-) partially protected against the paralysis of Bjssu venom (Figure 6A), but not against Cdt venom (Figure 6B). It is known that *in vivo* Cdt venom triggers different mechanism of action than Bjssu. The neurotoxicity induced by the *Crotalus* genus is attributed to crotoxin, the main toxin from this venom [2, 7, 31], whereas the *Bothrops* genus is mainly myotoxic [22], due its main toxin, bothropstoxin-I [16]. Maybe plants having coumarin could inhibit phospholipases with no catalytic activity (Lys49PLA$_2$), as those found in Bjssu venom, but they are not able to avoid the action of Asp49PLA$_2$ triggered by Cdt venom. Similar understanding was related by Cavalcante et al. [6] regarding to the ability of aqueous extract of *Casearia sylvestris* against snake venoms phospholipase A$_2$ toxins.

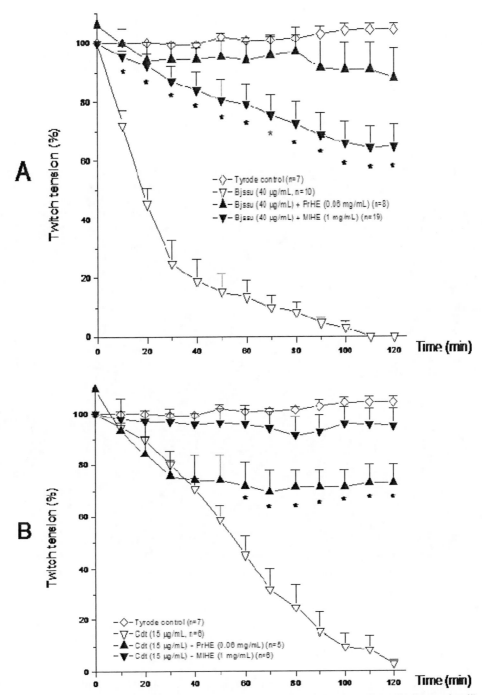

Figure 4. Pharmacological assays on mouse phrenic nerve-diaphragm preparations (indirect stimuli). Neutralization of Bothrops jararacussu venom (A, Bjssu), and Crotalus durissus terrificus venom (B, Cdt) by P. reticulata (PrHE) and M. laevigata (MlHE) hydroalcoholic extracts. Each point represents the mean ± S.E.M. of the number of experiments (n) showed in legend. *$p<0.05$ compared to venom.

The isolation of substances from potential medicinal plants, even at high costs, to try to keep their pharmacological effect at the end of the process is a modern tendency. We presented a rationale experimental design, which tests probably phytochemicals before their commercial availability. Our results showed that isolated compounds not always preserve the same pharmacological efficacy as that seen with total extract.The results allowed proposing the following different mechanisms by which plants can neutralize crude venoms: 1) complexing proteins *in vitro* (as verified in tannic acid) or 2) mechanistically by a phytocomplex formation.

We also observed the interference of phytochemicals free of tannins (-) such as the ones showed in the chromatoplaque (Figure 5).

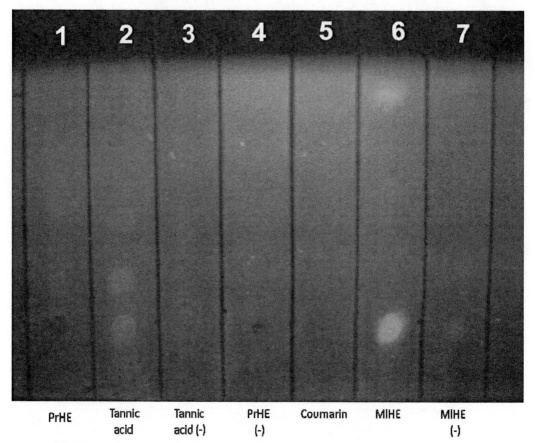

PrHE	Tannic acid	Tannic acid (-)	PrHE (-)	Coumarin	MlHE	MlHE (-)

Figure 5. Thin layer chromatography. Extracts + phytochemicals with ou without tannins (-).
Chromatographic profile of (1) or *M. laevigata* (6) hydroalcoholic extracts. Phytochemicals are showed in 2 (tannic acid) and 5 (coumarin). The withdrawal of tannins (-) from the tannic acid and *P. reticulata* and *M. laevigata* hydroalcoholic extracts and are showed in 3, 4 and 7, respectively.

The isolation of substances from potential medicinal plants, even at high costs, to try to keep their pharmacological effect at the end of the process is a modern tendency. We presented a rationale experimental design, which tests probably phytochemicals before their commercial availability. Our results showed that isolated compounds not always preserve the same pharmacological efficacy as that seen with total extract.The results allowed proposing the following different mechanisms by which plants can neutralize crude venoms: 1) complexing proteins *in vitro* (as verified in tannic acid) or 2) mechanistically by a phytocomplex formation.

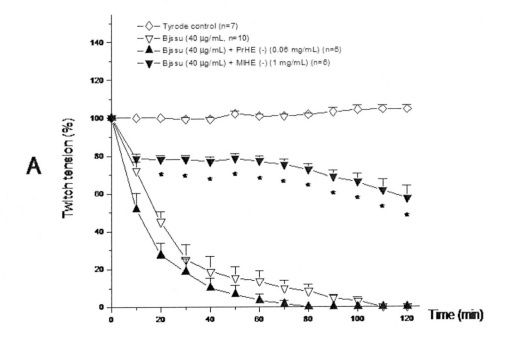

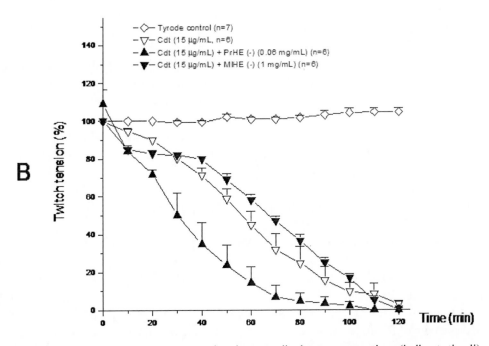

Figure 6. Pharmacological assays on mouse phrenic nerve-diaphragm preparations (indirect stimuli). Neutralization of *Bothrops jararacussu* venom (A, Bjssu), and *Crotalus durissus terrificus* venom (B, Cdt) by *P. reticulata* free of tannins [PrHE (-)] and *M. laevigata* free of tannins [MlHE (-)] hydroalcoholic extracts. Each point represents the mean ± S.E.M. of the number of experiments (n) showed in legend. *$p<0.05$ compared to venom.

Acknowledgments

This work was supported by a research grant from Fundação de Amparo à Pesquisa do Estado de São Paulo (Proc. FAPESP 04/09705-8) and PROBIC/UNISO. R.M.S. was granted a scholarship (I.C.) from PIBIC/CNPq.

References

[1]　Bezerra, JA; Campos, AC; Vasconcelos, PR; Nicareta, JR; Ribeiro, ER; Sebastião, AP; Urdiales, AI; Moreira, M; Borges, AM. Extract of *Passiflora edulis* in the healing of colonic anastomosis in rats: tensiometric and morphologic study. *Acta Cir. Bras.* 2006, 21, 16-25.

[2]　Bon, C. Multicomponent neurotoxic phospholipases A₂. In: Kini RM editor. *Venom phospholipase A₂ enzymes: structure, function and mechanism.* Chichester, England: John Wiley and Sons; 1997; 269-285.

[3]　Bülbring, E. Observation on the isolated phrenic nerve diaphragm preparation of the rat. *Br. J. Pharmacol.* 1946, 1, 38-61.

[4]　Calixto, JB; Beirith, A; Ferreira, J; Santos, AR; Filho, VC; Yunes, RA. Naturally occurring antinociceptive substances from plants. Phytother. Res. 2000, 14, 401-418.

[5]　Castro, EV de; Pinto, JEBP; Bertolucci, SKV; Malta, MR; Cardoso, M das G; , FA de M; Coumarin contents in young *Mikania glomerata* plants (guaco) under different radiation levels and photoperiod. *Acta Farm. Bonaerense* 2006, 25, 387-392.

[6]　Cavalcante, WLG; Campos, TO; Dal Pai-Silva, MD; Pereira, OS; Oliveira, CZ; Soares, AM; Gallaci M. Neutralization of snake venom phospholipase A₂ toxins by aqueous extract of *Casearia sylvestris* (Flacourtiaceae) in mouse neuromuscular preparation. *J. Ethnopharmacol.* 2007, 112, 490-497.

[7]　Chang, CC; Lee, JD. Crotoxin, the neurotoxin of South American rattlesnake venom, is a presynaptic toxin acting like beta-bungarotoxin. *Naunyn Schmiedebergs Arch. Pharmacol.* 1977, 296, 159-168.

[8]　Cintra-Francischinelli, M; Silva, MG; Andréo-Filho, N; Gerenutti, M; Cintra, ACO; Giglio, JR; Leite, GB; Cruz-Höfling, MA; Rodrigues-Simioni, L; Oshima-Franco, Y. *Phytother. Res.* 2008, 6, 784-790.

[9]　Dos Santos, SC; Krueger, CL; Steil, AA; Kreuger, MR; Biavatti, MW; Wisniewski Junior, A. LC characterisation of guaco medicinal extracts, *Mikania laevigata* and *M. glomerata*, and their effects on allergic pneumonits. *Planta Med.* 2006, 72, 679-684.

[10]　Esmeraldino, LE; Souza, AM; Sampaio, SV. Evaluation of the effect of aqueous extract of *Croton urucurana* Baillon (Euphorbiaceae) on the hemorrhagic activity induced by the venom of *Bothrops jararaca*, using new techniques to quantify hemorrhagic activity in rat skin. *Phytomedicine* 2005, 12, 570-576.

[11]　Fernandes, TT; Fernandes, ATS; Pimenta, SC. Atividade antimicrobiana das plantas *Plathymenia reticulata*, *Hymenea courbaril* e *Guazuma ulmifolia*. *Rev. Patol. Trop.* 2005, 34, 113-122.

[12]　Fierro, IM; da Silva, AC; Lopes, C da S; de Moura, RS; Barja-Fidalgo, C. Studies on the anti-allergic activity of *Mikania glomerata*. J. Ethnopharmacol. 1999, 66, 19-24.

[13] Hagerman, AE; Butler, LG. Choosing appropriate methods and standards for assaying tannins. *J. Chem. Ecol.* 1989, 15, 1795-1810.

[14] Hagerman, AE; Butler, LG. Protein precipitation method for the quantitative determination of tannins. *J. Agr. Food Chem.* 1978, 26, 809-812.

[15] Harborne, JB. *Phytochemical Methods: A Guide to Modern Techniques of Plants Analysis*, 3rd Edition, London: Chapman and Hall, 1998.

[16] Homsi-Brandeburgo, MI; Queiroz, LS; Santo-Neto, H; Rodrigues-Simioni, L; Giglio, JR. Fractionation of *Bothrops jararacussu* snake venom: partial chemical characterization and biological activity of bothropstoxin. *Toxicon* 1988, 26, 615-627.

[17] Kuppusamy, UR; Das, NP. Protective effects of tannic acid and related natural compounds on *Crotalus adamanteus* subcutaneous poisoning in mice. *Pharmacol. Toxicol.* 1993, 72, 290-295.

[18] Kim, SI; Kim, KS; Kim, HS; Choi, MM; Kim, DS; Chung, KH; Park, YS. Inhibition of angiogenesis by salmosin expressed *in vitro*. Oncol. Res. 2004, 14, 227-233.

[19] Lizano, S; Domont, G; Perales, J. Natural phospholipase A(2) myotoxin inhibitor proteins from snakes, mammals and plants. *Toxicon* 2003, 42, 963-977.

[20] Maiorano, VA; Marcussi, S; Daher, MAF; Oliveira, CZ; Couto, LB; Gomes, AO; França, SZ; Soares, AM; Pereira, PS. Antiophidian properties of the aqueos extract of *Mikania glomerata. J. Ethnopharmacol.* 2005, 102, 364-370.

[21] MeSH – Medical Subject Headings (2008) Bradykinin. Available in: <http://www.ncbi.nlm.nih.gov/entrez/query.fcgi?CMD=searchandDB=mesh>, Pubmed, 25 June 2008.

[22] Ministério da Saúde do Brasil. *Manual de diagnóstico e tratamento de acidentes por animais peçonhentos*, 2nd Edition, Brasília: Fundação Nacional da Saúde; 2001.

[23] Mirshafiey, A. Venom therapy in multiple sclerosis. Neuropharmacology 2007, 53, 353-361.

[24] Moraes, MD. A família Asteraceae na planície litorânea de Picinguaba – Município de Ubatuba (master thesis), São Paulo, Brazil: Universidade Estadual de Campinas, 1997.

[25] Mors, WB; Nascimento, MC; Pereira, BM; Pereira, NA. Plant natural products active against sanke bite – the molecular approach. Phytochemistry 2000, 55, 627-642.

[26] Pithayanukul, P; Ruenraroengsak, P; Bavovada, R; Pakmanee, N; Suttisri, R. *In vitro* investigation of the protective effects of tannic acid against the activities of *Naja kaouthia* venom. *Pharmaceutical Biol.* 2007, 45, 94-97.

[27] Portuguese Farmacopeia. Instituto Nacional da Farmácia e do Medicamento. 7th Edition, Lisboa: Infarmed, 2002, 2792p.

[28] Ruppelt, BM; Pereira, EF; Gonçalves, LC; Pereira, NA. Pharmacological screening of plants recommended by folk medicine as anti-snake venom--I. Analgesic and anti-inflammatory activities. *Mem. Inst. Oswaldo Cruz* 1991, 86, 203-205.

[29] Sévenet, T. Looking for new drugs: what criteria? J. Ethnopharmacol. 1991, 32, 83-90.

[30] Simões, CMO; Schenkel, EP; Gosmann, G; Mello, JCP; Mentz, LA; Petrovick, PR. *Farmacognosia: da Planta ao Medicamento*, 5th Edition, Porto Alegre/Florianópolis: UFRGS/UFSC, 2004.

[31] Slotta, KH; Fraenkel-Conrat, H. Schlangengiffe, III: Mitteilung Reiningung und crystallization des klappershclangengiffes. Ber. Dtsch. Chem. Ges. 1938, 71, 1076-1081.

[32] Soares, AM; Ticli, FK; Marcussi, S; Lourenço, MV; Januário, AH; Sampaio, SV; Giglio, JR; Lomonte, B; Pereira, PS. Medicinal plants with inhibitory properties against snake venoms. *Curr. Med. Chem.* 2005, 12, 2625-2641.

[33] Veroneše, EL; Esmeraldino, LE; Trombone, AP; Santana, AE; Bechara, GH; Kettelhut, I; Cintra, AC; Giglio, JR; Sampaio, SV. Inhibition of the myotoxic activity of *Bothrops jararacussu* venom and its two major myotoxins, BthTX-I and BthTX-II, by the aqueous extract of *Tabernaemontana catharinensis* A. DC. (Apocynaceae). *Phytomedicine* 2005, 12, 123-130.

In: Encyclopedia of Vitamin Research
Editor: Joshua T. Mayer

ISBN: 978-1-61761-928-1
© 2011 Nova Science Publishers, Inc.

Chapter 46

Molecular Targets of Flavonoids during Apoptosis in Cancer Cells[*]

Kenichi Yoshida[†]

Department of Life Sciences, Meiji University, 1-1-1 Higashimita,
Tama-ku, Kawasaki, Kanagawa 214-8571, Japan

Abstract

There are serious concerns about the increasing global cancer incidence. As currently used chemotherapeutics agents often show severe toxicity in normal cells, anti-carcinogenic compounds included in the dietary intakes of natural foods are expected to be applicable to a novel approach to preventing certain types of cancer without side effects. Polyphenolic compounds, such as flavonoids, are ubiquitous in plants and are presently considered to be the most promising in terms of having anti-carcinogenic properties probably due to their antioxidant effect. To gain further insights into how flavonoids exert anti-carcinogenic actions on cancer cells at the molecular level, many intensive investigations have been performed. Currently, the common signaling pathways elicited by flavonoids are recognized as tumor suppressor p53 and survival factor AKT. These factors are potential effectors of flavonoid-induced apoptosis via activation of Bax and caspase family genes. The present chapter emphasizes pivotal molecular mechanisms underlying flavonoid-induced apoptosis in human cancer cells. In particular, this chapter focuses on representative flavonoids such as soy isoflavone, green tea catechin, quercetin, and anthocyanin.

---

[*] A version of this chapter was also published in *Flavonoids: Biosynthesis, Biological Effects and Dietary Sources, edited by Raymond B. Keller* published by Nova Science Publishers, Inc. It was submitted for appropriate modifications in an effort to encourage wider dissemination of research.
[†] Tel. and Fax.: +81-44-934-7107, e-mail: yoshida@isc.meiji.ac.jp

Introduction

A major part of cancer incidence is thought to be related to life style factors such as dietary intake tendencies. Considerable attention has been paid to bioactive polyphenols, especially flavonoids, in dietary intake of many fruits and vegetables for the sake of cancer prevention, because human population or epidemiologic studies have suggested that flavonoid intake may reduce the risk of specific types of cancer [1-3]. Flavonoids have been extensively investigated in terms of how they act on various signal transduction pathways and their influences on the processes of cell fate determination [4, 5]. Induction of apoptosis in cancer cells by flavonoids is one of the most promising lines of evidence. Apoptosis induced by flavonoids usually involves modulating p53, nuclear factor-kappaB (NF-kappaB), activator protein-1 (AP-1), or mitogen-activated protein kinases (MAPK) [6-8]. Natural products are being investigated that can antagonize the anti-apoptotic effects of Bcl-2 family proteins such as Bcl-xL and Bcl-2 [9].

The changes which transform normal cells into cancer cells have been characterized as successive molecular events including activation of oncogenes and inactivation of antioncogenes, and all of these genes are known to be essential components of cellular signal transduction pathways and effectors of the cell cycle and apoptosis control. Basically, loss of anti-oncogenes results in the fragility of chromosomes and oncogenic activation renders cells more resistant to apoptosis and metastatic phenotypes. Needless to say, in considering cancer cell control via inhibition of metastasis and angiogenesis, inducing immune response and inflammatory cascade specific for cancer cells, and modulation of drug resistance are all promising approaches. In this chapter, we summarize recent progress in molecular studies of major flavonoids acting on apoptotic cancer cells.

1. Tea Polyphenol Catechins

Polyphenolic compounds contained in tea leaves are called as catechins, the most abundant of which is (-)-epigallocatechin-3-gallate (EGCG). EGCG has been known to regulate the cell cycle and apoptosis, and this is achieved in part by modulating the RAS/RAF/MAPK, phosphoinositide 3-kinase (PI3-K)/AKT, protein kinase C (PKC), NF-kappaB, AP-1 signaling pathways, and ubiquitin/proteasome degradation pathways [10-21]. Among these, inhibition of AKT signaling and modulation of pro-apoptotic factors by EGCG are well known. For example, EGCG has been shown to increase Bax and decrease Bcl-2 and AKT Ser473 phosphorylation in MDA-MB-231 human breast cancer cells [22]. Induction of pro-apoptotic proteins such as Bax, Bid and Bad, and suppression of Bcl-xL and Bcl-2 by EGCG in human gastric cancer cells MKN45 has also been described [23]. In hepatocellular carcinoma cells HLE, EGCG-induced apoptosis down-regulated Bcl-xL and Bcl-2 via inactivation of NF-kappaB [24]. These line of evidence suggest a mitochondrial-dependent pathway to be pivotal for EGCG-induced apoptosis. EGCG-induced apoptosis in MCF-7 breast cancer cells involves down-regulation of surviving expression via suppression of the AKT signaling pathway [25]. In MCF-7 breast cancer cells as well, JNK activation and Bax expression were reported in EGCG-induced apoptosis [26]. In human bladder cancer cells

T24, inhibition of PI3-K/AKT activation and the resultant modulation of Bcl-2 family proteins during EGCG-induced apoptosis has been reported [27].

EGCG can affect two important transcription factors, p53 and NF-kappaB, during apoptosis in cancer cells. Involvement of the NF-kappaB pathway has been shown in EGCG-mediated apoptosis of human epidermoid carcinoma cells, A431 [28, 29]. EGCG can stabilize p53 and inhibit NF-kappaB, and this leads to a change in the ratio of Bax/Bcl-2 in a manner that favors apoptosis in human prostate carcinoma cells, LNCaP [30]. The importance of p53 and Bax during EGCG-induced apoptosis has also been shown in human breast cancer cells MDA-MB-468 [31]. Using different prostate cancer cell lines, p53 downstream targets p21 and Bax have been shown to be essential for EGCG-induced apoptosis [32]. There is also a controversial report about p53, but this is not the case for p21, being dispensable for apoptosis in human prostate carcinoma cells [33]. Other than p53, EGCG has been shown to affect many cell cycle regulators such as the cyclin-dependent kinase (CDK) inhibitor and the retinoblastoma gene product (pRb)-E2F in different cancer cells [34-37]. Recent findings on EGCG-induced apoptosis in cancer cells favor an essential role of p53 in EGCG-induced apoptosis. Additionally, survival factor AKT tends to be suppressed by EGCG in many cancer cells. These two pathways appear to synergistically induce cell cycle deregulation and alteration of Bcl-2/Bax balance, thereby leading to the induction of apoptosis in cancer cells.

2. Soy Isoflavones

Genistein, which is structurally related to 17beta-estradiol, is one of the predominant soybean isoflavones. Genistein has been shown to inhibit protein tyrosine kinase activity, especially those of epidermal growth factor receptor and Src tyrosine kinase [38, 39], and is implicated in protection against different cancers [40]. By regulating a wide array of genes, genistein regulates the cell cycle and apoptosis. The common signaling pathways inhibited by genistein for the prevention of cancer have been extensively examined and are known as the NF-kappaB and AKT signaling pathways [41-45]. For example, apoptosis in many cancer cells including the breast cancer cell line MDA-MB-231, prostate cancer cell line PC3, and head and neck cancer cells treated with genistein has been shown to be executed partly through the down-regulation of NF-kappaB and AKT pathways [46-48].

In contrast to apoptosis induced by EGCG in cancer cells, accumulating evidence suggests that p53 does not appear to play a significant role during apoptosis in cancer cells. Genistein induced apoptosis in a variety of human cancer cells regardless of p53 status [49]. A p53-independent pathway of genistein-induced apoptosis in non-small cell lung cancer cells H460 has also been reported [50]. Although Puma, a p53-induced apoptosis regulator, has been identified as an up-regulated gene in genistein-induced apoptosis of A549 cells, its down-regulation had no effects on genistein-induced apoptosis [51]. p21, p53-target gene, has been shown to be an important candidate molecule in determining the sensitivity of normal and malignant breast epithelial cells to genistein and also in genistein-induced apoptosis in prostate adenocarcinoma and non-small lung cancer cell line H460 [52-55]. Notably, p21 induction by genistein was reported to function in a p53-independent manner in human breast carcinoma cells and prostate carcinoma cells [56, 57]. Genistein-induced apoptosis in primary gastric cancer cells is partly explained by down-regulation of Bcl-2 and up-regulation of Bax

[58]. Along with p21, Bax was detected in genistein-induced apoptosis of the breast cancer cell line MDA-MB-231 through a p53-independent pathway [59]. Taken together, these observations indicate that genistein induces apoptosis in variety of cancer cells largely via inhibition of AKT and NF-kappaB pathways, and that p53 involvement in genistein-induced apoptosis may well be minor while p21 and Bax play certain roles in genistein-induced apoptosis.

3. Quercetin

Quercetin is a ubiquitous bioactive plant flavonoid found in onions, grapes, green vegetables, etc., which has been shown to inhibit the proliferation of a variety of human cancer cells. Quercetin is thought to induce apoptosis possibly through regulating MAPK such as by suppressing extracellular signal-regulated kinase (ERK) and c-Jun N-terminal kinase (JNK) phosphorylation [60]. Tumor necrosis factor (TNF) alpha-induced apoptosis in osteoblastic cells, MC3T3-E1, was shown to be promoted by quercetin when JNK and AP-1 were activated [61]. TNF-related apoptosis-inducing ligand (TRAIL)-induced apoptosis and the resultant caspase activation was also promoted by quercetin in human prostate cancer cells with accompanying suppression of AKT phosphorylation [62]. In human prostate cancer cells, LNCaP, quercetin-induced apoptosis was accompanied by a decrease in the inhibitory AKT Ser473 phosphorylation and its downstream Bad Ser136 phosphorylation. These processes can promote dissociation of Bax from Bcl-xL and then Bax translocation to the mitochondrial membrane, and induce activation of caspase family genes [63]. In a human hepatoma cell line HepG2, quercetin induced apoptosis possibly by direct activation of the caspase cascade and by inhibiting survival signaling such as AKT [64]. These results indicate that quercetin-directed suppression of AKT phosphorylation could be the major molecular axis for quercetin-induced apoptosis in cancer cells.

p53 has been thought to have an important role in apoptosis in quercetin-treated=cells [65]; however, there is a discrepancy regarding the p53 requirement in quercetin-induced apoptosis. Regardless of p53 status, quercetin was able to induce Bad and caspase family genes and this resulted in apoptosis of nasopharyngeal carcinoma cell lines [66]. Quercetin induced apoptosis in the human prostate cancer cell line PC-3 with increased levels of insulin-like growth factor-binding protein-3 (IGFBP-3), Bax, and p21 protein and with decreased levels of Bcl-xL and Bcl-2 proteins, suggesting that quercetin-induced apoptosis may occur in a p53-independent manner because PC-3 lack p53 [67, 68]. In contrast to the above reports, quercetin has been shown to induce cell cycle arrest and apoptosis in human hepatoma cells, HepG2, in a p53-dependent manner, and this resulted in an increased ratio of Bax/Bcl-2 [69]. Moreover, p53-dependent up-regulation of p21 has been shown to attenuate apoptosis in quercetin-treated A549 and H1299 lung carcinoma cells [70]. An important role of p21 in quercetin-induced apoptosis of MCF-7 human breast cancer cells has been reported [71]. Taken together, these findings indicate that quercetin-induced apoptosis in cancer cells requires both inactivation of survival factor AKT and modulation of the expression of the Bcl-2 family of proteins, especially for Bax activation. Recent findings suggest that quercetin-induced apoptosis does not apparently requir p53, though more extensive studies are needed.

Results obtained to date indicate that quercetin can be applied to a wide variety of cancer cells that lack p53.

4. Anthocyanins

Anthocyanins, reddish pigments, are abundant in many fruits and vegetables such as blueberries and red cabbage. As is well known for other flavonoids, anthocyanins have the ability to act as antioxidants and are expected to be of potential clinical relevance as evidenced by animal models [72]. Moreover, berry phenolics, in which the major components are anthocyanins, have been known to show anti-carcinogenic properties mainly through the induction of apoptosis in multiple types of cancer cells [73-76]. Among anthocyanins, malvidin, has been shown to be the most potent apoptosis inducer by modulating specifically MAPK in the human gastric adenocarcinoma cell line AGS [77]. Anthocyanins, derived from potato, induced apoptosis in the prostate cancer cell line LNCaP and PC-3 accompanied by MAPK and JNK activation, but caspase-dependent apoptosis was observed only in LNCaP cells [78]. Hibiscus anthocyanins induced apoptosis in human promyelocytic leukemia cells, HL-60, and this was critically regulated specifically by p38 kinase in MAPK and PI3-K [79]. In the human hepatoma cell line HepG2, delphinidin, components of anthocyanins induced apoptosis with increased JNK phosphorylation and Bax and decreased Bcl-2 protein [80]. Molecular targets of anthocyanins likely include two regulatory axes: 1) MAPK activation followed by JUN phosphorylation and 2) p53 activation followed by Bax protein activation. These two pathways are known to contribute equally to apoptosis in normal cells [81]. The contribution of p53 status in anthocyanin-induced apoptosis should be further verified by studying a series of cancer cells.

Conclusion

Flavonoids are rich sources of potentially useful medical compounds, because they have been well characterized as reducing cancer risk. Indeed, flavonoids are known to exhibit antioxidant and anti-inflammatory actions as well as anti-carcinogenic effects on many types of cancer cells. Cell culture-based experiments have revealed numerous candidate molecules for development of flavonoids for drug targeting; however, the results of assays with very high concentrations of flavonoids do not necessarily support the adaptablility of these compounds to clinical treatments. The results cell culture-based experiments should be verified and confirmed first using animal models and then in epidemiological studies. Molecular mechanisms of flavonoid actions on cellular targets are not fully characterized and many features remain to be elucidated. For example, the synergistic actions of flavonoids should be carefully investigated, because we usually ingest multiple flavonoids simultaneously from dietary sources, such as fruits, and beverages. Moreover, combination effects between flavonoids and cancer preventive chemotherapeutic agents are a promising approach to reducing side effects. Exploring the actual molecular targets of flavonoids would presumably be a very promising road to the control cancer cells.

References

[1] Neuhouser ML. Dietary flavonoids and cancer risk: evidence from human population studies. Nutr. Cancer. 2004. 50 (1): 1-7.

[2] Schabath MB, Hernandez LM, Wu X, Pillow PC, Spitz MR. Dietary phytoestrogens and lung cancer risk. JAMA. 2005. 294 (12): 1493-1504.

[3] Theodoratou E, Kyle J, Cetnarskyj R, Farrington SM, Tenesa A, Barnetson R, Porteous M, Dunlop M, Campbell H. Dietary flavonoids and the risk of colorectal cancer. Cancer Epidemiol Biomarkers Prev. 2007. 16 (4): 684-693.

[4] Ramos S. Effects of dietary flavonoids on apoptotic pathways related to cancer chemoprevention. J. Nutr. Biochem. 2007. 18 (7): 427-442.

[5] Ramos S. Cancer chemoprevention and chemotherapy: dietary polyphenols and signalling pathways. Mol. Nutr. Food Res. 2008. 52 (5): 507-526.

[6] Dong Z. Effects of food factors on signal transduction pathways. Biofactors. 2000. 12 (1-4): 17-28.

[7] Kong AN, Yu R, Chen C, Mandlekar S, Primiano T. Signal transduction events elicited by natural products: role of MAPK and caspase pathways in homeostatic response and induction of apoptosis. Arch. Pharm. Res. 2000. 23 (1): 1-16.

[8] Fresco P, Borges F, Diniz C, Marques MP. New insights on the anticancer properties of dietary polyphenols. Med. Res. Rev. 2006. 26 (6): 747-766.

[9] Pellecchia M, Reed JC. Inhibition of anti-apoptotic Bcl-2 family proteins by natural polyphenols: new avenues for cancer chemoprevention and chemotherapy. Curr. Pharm. Des. 2004. 10 (12): 1387-1398.

[10] Yang CS, Chung JY, Yang GY, Li C, Meng X, Lee MJ. Mechanisms of inhibition of carcinogenesis by tea. Biofactors. 2000. 13 (1-4): 73-79.

[11] Lin JK. Cancer chemoprevention by tea polyphenols through modulating signal transduction pathways. Arch Pharm Res. 2002. 25 (5): 561-571.

[12] Lambert JD, Yang CS. Mechanisms of cancer prevention by tea constituents. J. Nutr. 2003. 133 (10): 3262S-3267S.

[13] Park AM, Dong Z. Signal transduction pathways: targets for green and black tea polyphenols. J. Biochem. Mol. Biol. 2003. 36 (1): 66-77.

[14] Chen D, Daniel KG, Kuhn DJ, Kazi A, Bhuiyan M, Li L, Wang Z, Wan SB, Lam WH, Chan TH, Dou QP. Green tea and tea polyphenols in cancer prevention. Front Biosci. 2004. 9: 2618-2631.

[15] Beltz LA, Bayer DK, Moss AL, Simet IM. Mechanisms of cancer prevention by green and black tea polyphenols. Anticancer Agents Med. Chem. 2006. 6 (5): 389-406.

[16] Khan N, Afaq F, Saleem M, Ahmad N, Mukhtar H. Targeting multiple signaling pathways by green tea polyphenol (-)-epigallocatechin-3-gallate. Cancer Res. 2006. 66 (5): 2500-2505.

[17] Na HK, Surh YJ. Intracellular signaling network as a prime chemopreventive target of (-)-epigallocatechin gallate. Mol. Nutr. Food Res. 2006. 50 (2): 152-159.

[18] Chen L, Zhang HY. Cancer preventive mechanisms of the green tea polyphenol (-)-epigallocatechin-3-gallate. Molecules. 2007. 12 (5): 946-957.

[19] Shankar S, Ganapathy S, Srivastava RK. Green tea polyphenols: biology and therapeutic implications in cancer. Front Biosci. 2007. 12: 4881-4899.

[20] Shukla Y. Tea and cancer chemoprevention: a comprehensive review. Asian Pac. J. Cancer Prev. 2007. 8 (2): 155-166.

[21] Chen D, Milacic V, Chen MS, Wan SB, Lam WH, Huo C, Landis-Piwowar KR, Cui QC, Wali A, Chan TH, Dou QP. Tea polyphenols, their biological effects and potential molecular targets. Histol Histopathol. 2008. 23 (4): 487-496.

[22] Thangapazham RL, Passi N, Maheshwari RK. Green tea polyphenol and epigallocatechin gallate induce apoptosis and inhibit invasion in human breast cancer cells. Cancer Biol. Ther. 2007. 6 (12): 1938-1943.

[23] Ran ZH, Xu Q, Tong JL, Xiao SD. Apoptotic effect of Epigallocatechin-3-gallate on the human gastric cancer cell line MKN45 via activation of the mitochondrial pathway. World J. Gastroenterol. 2007. 13 (31): 4255-4259.

[24] Nishikawa T, Nakajima T, Moriguchi M, Jo M, Sekoguchi S, Ishii M, Takashima H, Katagishi T, Kimura H, Minami M, Itoh Y, Kagawa K, Okanoue T. A green tea polyphenol, epigalocatechin-3-gallate, induces apoptosis of human hepatocellular carcinoma, possibly through inhibition of Bcl-2 family proteins. J. Hepatol. 2006. 44 (6): 1074-1082.

[25] Tang Y, Zhao DY, Elliott S, Zhao W, Curiel TJ, Beckman BS, Burow ME. Epigallocatechin-3 gallate induces growth inhibition and apoptosis in human breast cancer cells through survivin suppression. Int. J. Oncol. 2007. 31 (4): 705-711.

[26] Hsuuw YD, Chan WH. Epigallocatechin gallate dose-dependently induces apoptosis or necrosis in human MCF-7 cells. Ann. N Y Acad Sci. 2007. 1095: 428-440.

[27] Qin J, Xie LP, Zheng XY, Wang YB, Bai Y, Shen HF, Li LC, Dahiya R. A component of green tea, (-)-epigallocatechin-3-gallate, promotes apoptosis in T24 human bladder cancer cells via modulation of the PI3K/Akt pathway and Bcl-2 family proteins. Bioche.m Biophys Res. Commun. 2007. 354 (4): 852-857.

[28] Ahmad N, Gupta S, Mukhtar H. Green tea polyphenol epigallocatechin-3-gallate differentially modulates nuclear factor kappaB in cancer cells versus normal cells. Arch. Biochem. Biophys. 2000. 376 (2): 338-346.

[29] Gupta S, Hastak K, Afaq F, Ahmad N, Mukhtar H. Essential role of caspases in epigallocatechin-3-gallate-mediated inhibition of nuclear factor kappa B and induction of apoptosis. Oncogene. 2004. 23 (14): 2507-2522.

[30] Hastak K, Gupta S, Ahmad N, Agarwal MK, Agarwal ML, Mukhtar H. Role of p53 and NF-kappaB in epigallocatechin-3-gallate-induced apoptosis of LNCaP cells. Oncogene. 2003. 22 (31): 4851-4859.

[31] Roy AM, Baliga MS, Katiyar SK. Epigallocatechin-3-gallate induces apoptosis in estrogen receptor-negative human breast carcinoma cells via modulation in protein expression of p53 and Bax and caspase-3 activation. Mol. Cancer Ther. 2005. 4 (1): 81-90.

[32] Hastak K, Agarwal MK, Mukhtar H, Agarwal ML. Ablation of either p21 or Bax prevents p53-dependent apoptosis induced by green tea polyphenol epigallocatechin-3-gallate. FASEB J. 2005. 19 (7): 789-791.

[33] Gupta S, Ahmad N, Nieminen AL, Mukhtar H. Growth inhibition, cell-cycle dysregulation, and induction of apoptosis by green tea constituent (-)-epigallocatechin-3-gallate in androgen-sensitive and androgen-insensitive human prostate carcinoma cells. Toxicol Appl. Pharmacol. 2000. 164 (1): 82-90.

[34] Ahmad N, Cheng P, Mukhtar H. Cell cycle dysregulation by green tea polyphenol epigallocatechin-3-gallate. Biochem. Biophys Res. Commun. 2000. 275 (2): 328-334.

[35] Masuda M, Suzui M, Weinstein IB. Effects of epigallocatechin-3-gallate on growth, epidermal growth factor receptor signaling pathways, gene expression, and chemosensitivity in human head and neck squamous cell carcinoma cell lines. Clin. Cancer Res. 2001. 7 (12): 4220-4229.

[36] Ahmad N, Adhami VM, Gupta S, Cheng P, Mukhtar H. Role of the retinoblastoma (pRb)-E2F/DP pathway in cancer chemopreventive effects of green tea polyphenol epigallocatechin-3-gallate. Arch. Biochem. Biophys. 2002. 398 (1): 125-131.

[37] Gupta S, Hussain T, Mukhtar H. Molecular pathway for (-)-epigallocatechin-3-gallate-induced cell cycle arrest and apoptosis of human prostate carcinoma cells. Arch. Biochem. Biophys. 2003. 410 (1): 177-185.

[38] Peterson G. Evaluation of the biochemical targets of genistein in tumor cells. J. Nutr.. 1995. 125 (3 Suppl): 784S-789S.

[39] Bektic J, Guggenberger R, Eder IE, Pelzer AE, Berger AP, Bartsch G, Klocker H. Molecular effects of the isoflavonoid genistein in prostate cancer. Clin. Prostate Cancer. 2005. 4 (2): 124-129.

[40] Valachovicova T, Slivova V, Sliva D. Cellular and physiological effects of soy flavonoids. Mini Rev. Med. Chem. 2004. 4 (8): 881-887.

[41] Sarkar FH, Li Y. Mechanisms of cancer chemoprevention by soy isoflavone genistein. Cancer Metastasis Rev. 2002. 21 (3-4): 265-280.

[42] Sarkar FH, Li Y. Soy isoflavones and cancer prevention. Cancer Invest. 2003. 21 (5): 744-757.

[43] Sarkar FH, Li Y. The role of isoflavones in cancer chemoprevention. Front Biosci. 2004. 9: 2714-2724.

[44] Li Y, Ahmed F, Ali S, Philip PA, Kucuk O, Sarkar FH. Inactivation of nuclear factor kappaB by soy isoflavone genistein contributes to increased apoptosis induced by chemotherapeutic agents in human cancer cells. Cancer Res. 2005. 65 (15): 6934-6942.

[45] Sarkar FH, Adsule S, Padhye S, Kulkarni S, Li Y. The role of genistein and synthetic derivatives of isoflavone in cancer prevention and therapy. Mini. Rev. Med. Chem. 2006. 6 (4): 401-407.

[46] Gong L, Li Y, Nedeljkovic-Kurepa A, Sarkar FH. Inactivation of NF-kappaB by genistein is mediated via Akt signaling pathway in breast cancer cells. Oncogene. 2003. 22 (30): 4702-4709.

[47] Li Y, Sarkar FH. Inhibition of nuclear factor kappaB activation in PC3 cells by genistein is mediated via Akt signaling pathway. Clin. Cancer Res. 2002. 8 (7): 2369-2377.

[48] Alhasan SA, Aranha O, Sarkar FH. Genistein elicits pleiotropic molecular effects on head and neck cancer cells. Clin. Cancer Res. 2001. 7 (12): 4174-4181.

[49] Li M, Zhang Z, Hill DL, Chen X, Wang H, Zhang R. Genistein, a dietary isoflavone, down-regulates the MDM2 oncogene at both transcriptional and posttranslational levels. Cancer Res. 2005. 65 (18): 8200-8208.

[50] Lian F, Li Y, Bhuiyan M, Sarkar FH. p53-independent apoptosis induced by genistein in lung cancer cells. Nutr. Cancer. 1999. 33 (2): 125-131.

[51] Tategu M, Arauchi T, Tanaka R, Nakagawa H, Yoshida K. Puma is a novel target of soy isoflavone genistein but is dispensable for genistein-induced cell fate determination. Mol. Nutr. Food Res. 2008. 52 (4): 439-446.

[52] Davis JN, Singh B, Bhuiyan M, Sarkar FH. Genistein-induced upregulation of p21WAF1, downregulation of cyclin B, and induction of apoptosis in prostate cancer cells. Nutr. Cancer. 1998. 32 (3): 123-131.

[53] Lian F, Bhuiyan M, Li YW, Wall N, Kraut M, Sarkar FH. Genistein-induced G2-M arrest, p21WAF1 upregulation, and apoptosis in a non-small-cell lung cancer cell line. Nutr. Cancer. 1998. 31 (3): 184-191.

[54] Shao ZM, Wu J, Shen ZZ, Barsky SH. Genistein exerts multiple suppressive effects on human breast carcinoma cells. Cancer Res. 1998. 58 (21): 4851-4857.

[55] Upadhyay S, Neburi M, Chinni SR, Alhasan S, Miller F, Sarkar FH. Differential sensitivity of normal and malignant breast epithelial cells to genistein is partly mediated by p21(WAF1). Clin. Cancer Res. 2001. 7 (6): 1782-1789.

[56] Shao ZM, Alpaugh ML, Fontana JA, Barsky SH. Genistein inhibits proliferation similarly in estrogen receptor-positive and negative human breast carcinoma cell lines characterized by P21WAF1/CIP1 induction, G2/M arrest, and apoptosis. J. Cell Biochem. 1998. 69 (1): 44-54.

[57] Choi YH, Lee WH, Park KY, Zhang L. p53-independent induction of p21 (WAF1/CIP1), reduction of cyclin B1 and G2/M arrest by the isoflavone genistein in human prostate carcinoma cells. Jpn J. Cancer Res. 2000. 91 (2): 164-173.

[58] Zhou HB, Chen JJ, Wang WX, Cai JT, Du Q. Apoptosis of human primary gastric carcinoma cells induced by genistein. World J. Gastroenterol. 2004. 10 (12): 1822-1825.

[59] Li Y, Upadhyay S, Bhuiyan M, Sarkar FH. Induction of apoptosis in breast cancer cells MDA-MB-231 by genistein. Oncogene. 1999. 18 (20): 3166-3172.

[60] Ahn J, Lee H, Kim S, Park J, Ha T. The anti-obesity effect of quercetin is mediated by the AMPK and MAPK signaling pathways. Biochem. Biophys Res. Commun. 2008. 373 (4): 545-549.

[61] Son YO, Kook SH, Choi KC, Jang YS, Choi YS, Jeon YM, Kim JG, Hwang HS, Lee JC. Quercetin accelerates TNF-alpha-induced apoptosis of MC3T3-E1 osteoblastic cells through caspase-dependent and JNK-mediated pathways. Eur. J. Pharmacol. 2008. 579 (1-3): 26-33.

[62] Kim YH, Lee YJ. TRAIL apoptosis is enhanced by quercetin through Akt dephosphorylation. J. Cell Biochem. 2007. 100 (4): 998-1009.

[63] Lee DH, Szczepanski M, Lee YJ. Role of Bax in quercetin-induced apoptosis in human prostate cancer cells. Biochem. Pharmacol. 2008. 75 (12): 2345-2355.

[64] Granado-Serrano AB, Martín MA, Bravo L, Goya L, Ramos S. Quercetin induces apoptosis via caspase activation, regulation of Bcl-2, and inhibition of PI-3-kinase/Akt and ERK pathways in a human hepatoma cell line (HepG2). J. Nutr. 2006. 136 (11): 2715-2721.

[65] Plaumann B, Fritsche M, Rimpler H, Brandner G, Hess RD. Flavonoids activate wild-type p53. Oncogene. 1996. 13 (8): 1605-1614.

[66] Ong CS, Tran E, Nguyen TT, Ong CK, Lee SK, Lee JJ, Ng CP, Leong C, Huynh H. Quercetin-induced growth inhibition and cell death in nasopharyngeal carcinoma cells

are associated with increase in Bad and hypophosphorylated retinoblastoma expressions. Oncol Rep. 2004. 11 (3): 727-733.

[67] Vijayababu MR, Kanagaraj P, Arunkumar A, Ilangovan R, Dharmarajan A, Arunakaran J. Quercetin induces p53-independent apoptosis in human prostate cancer cells by modulating Bcl-2-related proteins: a possible mediation by IGFBP-3. Oncol Res. 2006. 16 (2): 67-74.

[68] Vijayababu MR, Kanagaraj P, Arunkumar A, Ilangovan R, Aruldhas MM, Arunakaran J. Quercetin-induced growth inhibition and cell death in prostatic carcinoma cells (PC-3) are associated with increase in p21 and hypophosphorylated retinoblastoma proteins expression. J. Cancer Res. Clin. Oncol. 2005. 131 (11): 765-771.

[69] Tanigawa S, Fujii M, Hou DX. Stabilization of p53 is involved in quercetin-induced cell cycle arrest and apoptosis in HepG2 cells. Biosci. Biotechnol. Biochem. 2008. 72 (3): 797-804.

[70] Kuo PC, Liu HF, Chao JI. Survivin and p53 modulate quercetin-induced cell growth inhibition and apoptosis in human lung carcinoma cells. J. Biol. Chem. 2004. 279 (53): 55875-55885.

[71] Choi JA, Kim JY, Lee JY, Kang CM, Kwon HJ, Yoo YD, Kim TW, Lee YS, Lee SJ. Induction of cell cycle arrest and apoptosis in human breast cancer cells by quercetin. Int. J. Oncol. 2001. 19 (4): 837-844.

[72] Fimognari C, Lenzi M, Hrelia P. Chemoprevention of cancer by isothiocyanates and anthocyanins: mechanisms of action and structure-activity relationship. Curr. Med. Chem. 2008. 15 (5): 440-447.

[73] Hou DX. Potential mechanisms of cancer chemoprevention by anthocyanins. *Curr. Mol. Med.* 2003. 3 (2): 149-159.

[74] Yi W, Fischer J, Krewer G, Akoh CC. Phenolic compounds from blueberries can inhibit colon cancer cell proliferation and induce apoptosis. J. Agric. Food Chem. 2005. 53 (18): 7320-7329.

[75] Seeram NP, Adams LS, Zhang Y, Lee R, Sand D, Scheuller HS, Heber D. Blackberry, black raspberry, blueberry, cranberry, red raspberry, and strawberry extracts inhibit growth and stimulate apoptosis of human cancer cells in vitro. J. Agric. Food Chem. 2006. 54 (25): 9329-9339.

[76] Neto CC. Cranberry and its phytochemicals: a review of in vitro anticancer studies. J. Nutr. 2007. 137 (1 Suppl): 186S-193S.

[77] Shih PH, Yeh CT, Yen GC. Effects of anthocyanidin on the inhibition of proliferation and induction of apoptosis in human gastric adenocarcinoma cells. Food Chem. Toxicol. 2005. 43 (10): 1557-1566.

[78] Reddivari L, Vanamala J, Chintharlapalli S, Safe SH, Miller JC Jr. Anthocyanin fraction from potato extracts is cytotoxic to prostate cancer cells through activation of caspase-dependent and caspase-independent pathways. Carcinogenesis. 2007. 28 (10): 2227-2235.

[79] Chang YC, Huang HP, Hsu JD, Yang SF, Wang CJ. Hibiscus anthocyanins rich extract-induced apoptotic cell death in human promyelocytic leukemia cells. Toxicol Appl. Pharmacol. 2005. 205 (3): 201-212.

[80] Yeh CT, Yen GC. Induction of apoptosis by the Anthocyanidins through regulation of Bcl-2 gene and activation of c-Jun N-terminal kinase cascade in hepatoma cells. J. Agric Food Chem. 2005. 53 (5): 1740-1749.

[81] Lo CW, Huang HP, Lin HM, Chien CT, Wang CJ. Effect of Hibiscus anthocyanins-rich extract induces apoptosis of proliferating smooth muscle cell via activation of P38 MAPK and p53 pathway. Mol. Nutr. Food Res. 2007. 51 (12): 1452-1460.

In: Encyclopedia of Vitamin Research
Editor: Joshua T. Mayer

ISBN: 978-1-61761-928-1
© 2011 Nova Science Publishers, Inc.

Chapter 47

Flavan-3-ol Monomers and Condensed Tannins in Dietary and Medicinal Plants[*]

Chao-Mei Ma[†] and Masao Hattori

Institute of Natural Medicine, University of Toyama, 2630 Sugitani,
Toyama 930-0194, Japan

Abstract

Flavan-3-ols with the most well known members being catechin and epicatechin are a group of phenolic compounds widely distributed in nature. The oligomers and polymers of flavan-3-ols are known as condensed tannins which used to be considered as anti-nutritional components. In recent years, more and more evidences proved that these compounds were beneficial to human health as nutrition and lifestyle have fundamentally changed in modern society. These phenolic compounds showed great potential for the treatment of lifestyle related diseases, such as type 2 diabetes, obesity, and metabolic syndrome. They were also reported to have effects on slowing down the aging progress as well as on prevention of Alzheimer's disease, cardiovascular disease, and cancer. This chapter describes the structures, chemical properties, isolation and identification methods, bioactivity and distribution of flavan-3-ol monomers and condensed tannins in dietary sources and medicinal plants. Case studies such as the chemical and biological investigations of tannins in the stems of *Cynomorium songaricum* (a well known tonic in China) and in other plants are provided.

---

[*] A version of this chapter was also published in *Flavonoids: Biosynthesis, Biological Effects and Dietary Sources, edited by Raymond B. Keller* published by Nova Science Publishers, Inc. It was submitted for appropriate modifications in an effort to encourage wider dissemination of research.

[†] Corresponding authors: Phone: (81)-76-4347633. Fax: (81)-76-4345060. Email: saibo421@inm.u-toyama.ac.jp (M. Hattori); ma@inm.u-toyama.ac.jp or mchaomei@hotmail.com (CM. Ma).

Introduction

Flavan-3-ols with the most well known members being catechin and epicatechin are a group of phenolic compounds widely distributed in nature. The oligomers and polymers are known as proanthocyanidins or in another word, condensed tannins, characterized by their typical astringency taste. This sensory property causes the dry and puchery feeling in the mouth following the consumption of tea, red wine and some unripened fruits (http://en.wikipedia.org/wiki/Tannin). Tannins used to be considered as anti-nutritional components due to their ability to bind with proteins. However, as nutrition and lifestyle have fundamentally changed in modern society, more and more evidences proved that these compounds have beneficial effects to human health (*Ren and Chen,* 2007; Shahidi, 1997*). As polyphenol compounds with potent anti-oxidative activity,* they showed effects on slowing down the aging progress as well as on prevention of Alzheimer's disease, cardiovascular disease, and cancer. These phenolic compounds also showed potential for the treatment of lifestyle-related diseases, such as type 2 diabetes, obesity, and metabolic syndrome. There is an excellent review well discussed the bioactivities of tannins from edible sources, especially their antioxidant and radical scavenging activities, their prevention effects of cancer and cardiovascular diseases, inhibition of LDL oxidation and platelet aggregation effects (Santos-Buelga and Scalbert, 2000). The present chapter describes more about the chemical aspect of these compounds, including the structures, chemical properties, isolation and identification methods of flavan-3-ol monomers and condensed tannins in dietary sources. Their updated bioactivities will also be discussed. Case studies such as the chemistry and bioactivity of tannins in teas, peanut skins, grapes, wine and in the stems of *Cynomorium songaricum* (a well known tonic in China) are presented.

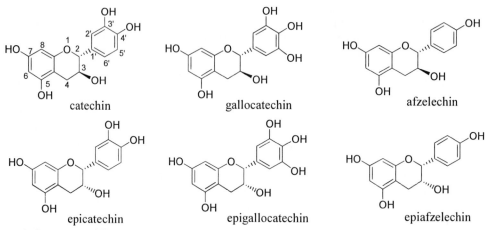

Figure 1. Structures of flavan-3-ol monomers.

Chemical Structures of Flavan-3-ol Monomers

The most widely spread flavan-3-ols, (-)-epicatechin and (+)-catechin, are a pair of epimers, both possessing a catechol group in their structures with the difference only on the stereo chemistry of C-3. Other flavan-3-ol monomers include epigallocatechin/gallocatechin and epiafzelechin/afzelechin, each pair of them having the same stereo-chemical difference as that of epicatechin/catechin. Epigallocatechin/gallocatechin have a galloyl group (one more hydroxyl group in the structure of catechol) in their structures while epiafzelechin/afzelechin have one less phenolic hydroxyl group in the structures of catechol (Figure 1).

Flavan-3-ol monomers are the basic component units of oligomers and polymers (often called condensed tannin). Epicatechin/catechin are the most frequently used extending flavan-3-ol units in tannin structures. Sometimes epicallocatechin/gallocatechin and epiafzelechin/afzelechin are also found as the extending flavan-3-ol units.

Oligomers of Flavan-3-ols (Harborne FRS JB and Baxter H, 1999)

Dimers of flavan-3-ols linked through one C-C bond are named as procyanidin Bs. There are many isomers of procyanidin Bs differed by the nature of their component monomer units, order of the monomers, configurations of the linkage bonds and the linkage positions. The most common linkages are C4→C8 (such as procyanidins B_1-B_4, figure 2) or C4→C6 (such as procyanidins B_5 and B_6, figure 2). Most prodelphinidins are flavan 3-ol dimers using one or two gallocatechin/epigallocatechin as their monomer unit(s), such as prodephinidin B_1. A-type procyanidins are flavan-3-ol dimers linked through one ether bond in addition to a C-C bond. The most common procyanidin As are procyanidins A_2 and A_1 (Figure 3). Procyanidin Cs are flavan-3-ol trimers (Figure 4). The following figures show the structures of some representative flavan-3-ol oligomers. Please note that though in most cases procyanidin Bx is the same compound of proanthocyanidin Bx (where x is a certain number), sometimes they are different compounds. For example, procyanidin B_6 and proanthocyanidin B_6 are different, the former being a catechin (4→6) catechin dimer while the latter containing a galloyl group conjugated with an epicatechin dimer (Scifinder). Most flavan 3-ols link with C4→C8/C4→C6 bonds in larger oligomers and polymers (Figure 5). Some times procyanidin A units can also be found in the structures of oligomers and polymers of condensed tannins.

Procyanidin B$_1$
Epicatechin-(4β-8)-catechin
Proanthocyanidin B1
Procyanidol B1

Procyanidin B$_2$
Epicatechin-(4β-8)-epicatechin
Proanthocyanidin B2
Procyanidol B2

Figure 2. (Continued).

Procyanidin B₃
Catechin-(4α-8)-catechin
Proanthocyanidin B3
Procyanidol B3

Procyanidin B₄
Catechin-(4α-8)-epicatechin
(-)-Procyanidin B4
Procyanidol B4

Procyanidin B₅
Epicatechin-(4β-6)-epicatechin
Proanthocyanidin B5
Procyanidol B5

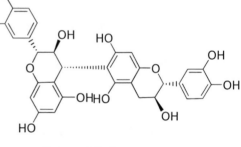

Procyanidin B₆
Catechin-(4α-6)-catechin
Procyanidol B6

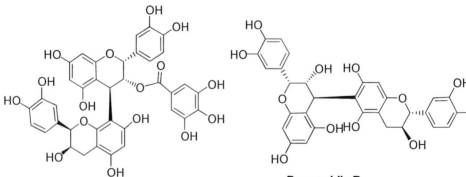

Proanthocyanidin B₆

Procyanidin B₇
Epicatechin-(4β-6)-catechin
Proanthocyanidin B7

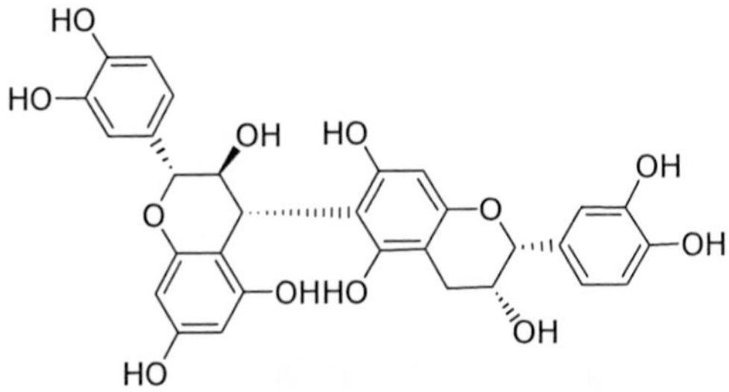

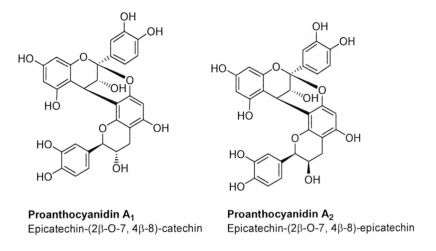

Procyanidin B$_8$
Catechin-(4α-6)-epicatechin
Procyanidol B$_8$

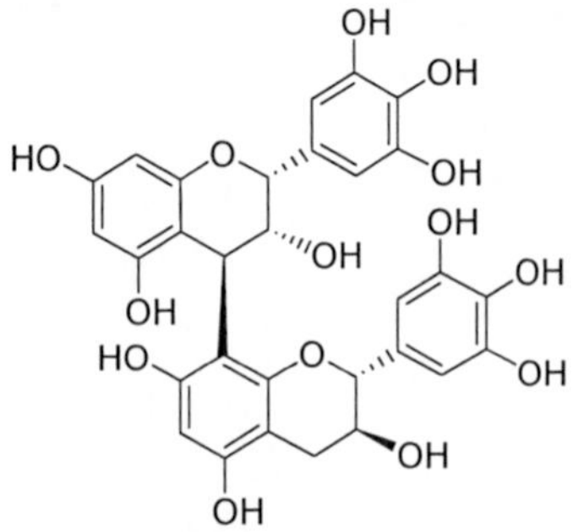

Prodelphinidin B$_1$
Epigallocatechin-(4β-8)-gallocatechin

Figure 2. Structures of some procyanidin Bs and prodelphinidin B$_1$.

Proanthocyanidin A$_1$
Epicatechin-(2β-O-7, 4β-8)-catechin

Proanthocyanidin A$_2$
Epicatechin-(2β-O-7, 4β-8)-epicatechin

Figure 3. Structures of two representative procyanidin As.

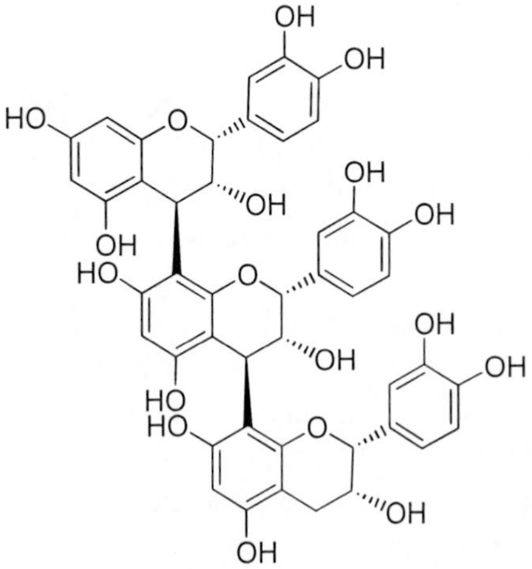

Procyanidin C1

Figure 4. Structures of one representative procyanidin Cs.

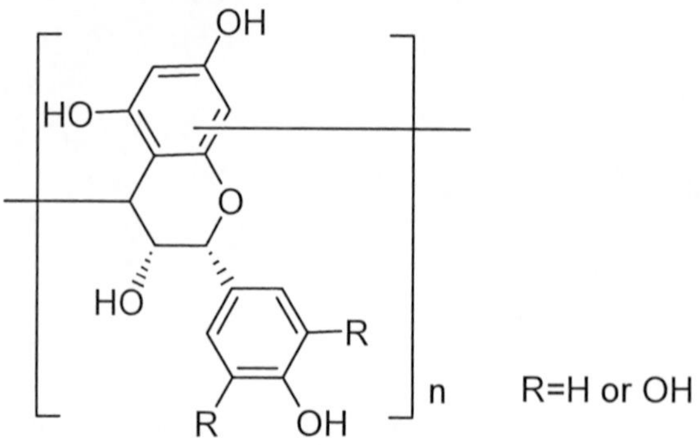

Figure 5. Structures of flavan-3-ol oligomers and polymers.

Astringency and Bitterness

Astringency and bitterness are the characteristic tastes of tannins. A study has showed that these sensory properties are related to the structures especially for flavan-3-ol monomers, dimers and trimers. The monomers were significantly higher in bitterness than the dimers, which were significantly higher than the trimers. Astringency of the monomers was lower than the dimers or trimers. The linkages between the monomeric units also influence both of the sensory properties. Catechin-(4→6)-catechin was more bitter than catechin-(4→8)-catechin/epicatechin. Astringency was affected by both the linkage and the identity of the monomeric units. Catechin-(4→8)-catechin had lower astringency than either catechin-(4→6)-catechin or catechin-(4→8)-epicatechin (Peleg *et al.*, 1999).

Chemical Properties

Flavan-3-ols are chemically unstable, being especially liable to undergoing numerous enzymatic and chemical oxidation or condensation. Adequate use of the oxidation and condensation process can produce foods of special color and taste. For example, oolong tea (semi-fermented), and black tea (fermented) can be produced by controlling the fermentation degree catalyzed by the enzyme. Due to the phenolic hydroxyl and ether groups in the para and ortho-positions, C8 and C6 are highly nucleophilic. In the contrast, C4 is electrophilic due to its aliphatic nature and near to some eletro-withdraw groups. As a result, the linkages between monomers in condensed tannins are usually C4→C8 or C4→C6. These linkage bonds are sensitive to acids and alkaline and this property can be used to induce degradation of the oligomers and polymers to study their monomer components. This property can also be used to produce water soluble smaller oligomers or their derivatives by acid treatment of the insoluble polymers in the presence of other reagents. A successful example is the preparation of oligomeric proanthocyanidin-cysteine complexes (Figure 6) which showed higher bioavailability and antioxidant capacity and prolonged survival time in the animal test groups (Fujii *et al.*, 2007). Other interesting bioactive compounds can also be synthesized using flavan-3-ols as starting materials. For example, under acid catalyst, catechin reacts with ketone compounds via an Oxa-Pictet-Spengler reaction to yield planer derivatives with a bridge between the 3-*O* group on ring C and C6′ on ring B (Figure 6). The planer catechin derivatives showed potent anti-oxidative activity and strong α-glucosidase inhibitory activity, suggesting the potential of using these planer catechin derivatives as lead compounds for the development of anti-diabetic agents [Hakamata *et al.*, 2006; Fukuhara *et al.*, 2002]. The highly nucleophilic C-8 position makes it possible to react with some electrophilic reagents to yield the C-8 substituted catechin derivatives (Figure 6). These compounds were synthesized upon protection of the phenolic OH groups with benzyl groups and de-protection with hydrogenation after the reaction finished (Nour-Eddine *et al.*, 2007).

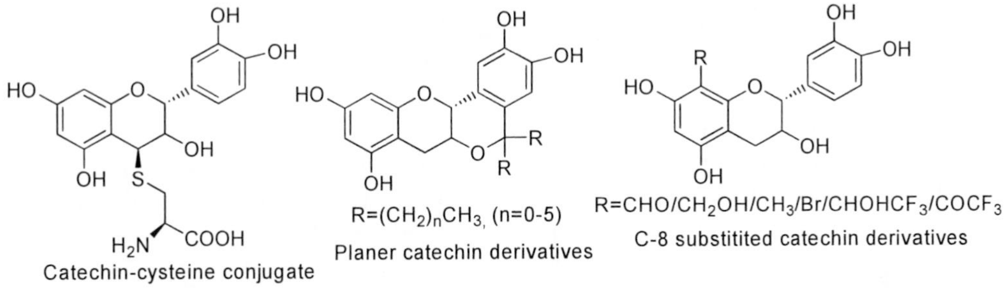

Figure 6. Structures of some synthesized catechin derivatives.

Isolation and Identification Methods

Acetone-water 7:3 is an effective solvent to extract flavan-3-ol monomers and oligomers. The procedure is usually carried out at room temperature and ultrasound can improve the extraction rate. After evaporation of the acetone under reduced pressure, the residual aqueous phase is extracted with ethyl acetate to eliminate some lipophilic non-tannin compounds. The aqueous solution containing tannin is applied to a Sephadex LH_{20} column, eluted with water containing increasing amount of methanol/ethanol to separate the flavan 3-ol oligomers. To obtain pure flavan 3-ol oligomers, repeated chromatography on Sephadex LH_{20} and in combination with Diaion HP-20 column chromatography are needed. Thin-layer chromatography on SiO_2 gel with an acidic solvent system gives better separation than on ODS. Benzene-ethyl formate-formic acid (2/1:7:1), chloroform-ethyl acetate-formic acid (1:7:1) and chloroform-ethyl acetate-formic acid-isopropanol (1:7:1:1) are some examples of the solvent systems used for separation of these compounds on normal phase TLC (Ezaki-Furuichi *et al.*, 1986). In the case of HPLC, normal-phase is better than ODS in separation and purification of flavan 3-ol oligomers. One example of the mobile phase for normal-phase HPLC composed of A: chloromethane/methanol/water (42:7:1) and B: dichloromethane/ methanol/water (5:44:1). The elution program was set by slowly increasing solvent B from 0% to100% in 5 h (Hellström *et al.*, 2007).

The structures of flavan 3-ol monomers and oligomers are usually determined by careful analysis of their NMR and MS data and by comparing with reported data. Sometimes chemical degradation is needed to determine the structures of new flavan 3-ol oligomers. Professor Nishioka and his group in Japan have isolated and determined the structures of many new flavan 3-ol oligomers from various plants. Their published papers displayed detailed spectral data of the condensed tannins. These spectral data can be used to assistant structure determination of pure tannin compounds isolated from other plant sources (Hwang *et al.*, 1989; Morimoto *et al.*, 1987; Morimoto *et al.*, 1988; Kashiwada *et al.*, 1986; Hsu *et al.*, 1985).

Determination of Polyphenol Contents

Flavan-3-ol oligomers of low molecular weight can be detected and estimated by chromatographic techniques. As the polymerization degree increases, the number of isomers increases rapidly, which result in a broad peak for the complex mixture of isomers. For this reason, some non-chromatographic methods were developed for measuring total phenolic compounds, total tannins, or condensed tannins. Non-extractable tannin are measured by degradation of the polymers to monomers first.

Folin-Ciocalteu colorimetric method or its modified method relies on the property that phenolic compounds inhibit the oxidation of the reagent. As a result, the method is not specific for tannins but for all reducing substances. This method is used to determine the total reducing capacity of the samples and sometimes used to estimate the contents of total phenolic compounds. Briefly, 50 μl of sample solution, 250 μl of Folin-Diocalteu's reagent and 750 μl of 10% Na_2CO_3 were mixed and incubated at rt for 2 h. The absorbance at 756 nm was measured and the results were expressed as milligrams of catechin (or gallic acid equivalent or other compounds) equivalent per gram of dry plant (Mai *et al.*, 2007).

Aromatic aldehydes, such as vanillin or 4-dimethylaminocinnamaldehyde (DMACA) method is based on the property that tannins react with aldehyde compound to form colored products. This method is more specific to condensed tannins than the Folin-Ciocalteu method, but some other phenolic compounds may also react with the reagent (Herderich *et al.*, **2008**).

The n-BuOH-HCl-Fe[III] method is to de-polymerize condensed tannins and oxidize the released units to colored anthocyanidins under the strong reaction condition. The reaction mixture consists of a methanol solution of tested sample, n-BuOH-conc.HCl (95:5, v/v) and the ferric reagent (2% of $NH_4Fe(SO_4)_2$ $12H_2O$ in 2M HCl) in a ratio of 1:6:0.2. The solution is thoroughly mixed and the container is tightly closed before being heated at 95° C for 40 min. Absorbance at 520-580 nm (560 nm for example) is measured and the content is calculated by comparing with catechin solutions of known concentrations underwent the same reaction. The results are expressed as catechin equivalent (Porter LJ *et al.*, 1986.)

Protein precipitate assay can be used to estimate the amount of total tannins. Other compounds that precipitate with proteins such as, hydrolysable tannins and some other phenolic compounds will be included. The degree of polymerization and the number and position of phenolic hydroxyl groups influence the precipitate ability. The results are usually expressed as tannic acid equivalent. Using the property that tannin-protein complexes dissolve in sodium dodecylsulfate solution to liberate the proteins and tannins. A dot-blot assay for protein determination based on the reversible binding of benzoxanthene yellow to the protein spots can be used for the quantification (Hoffmann *et al.*, 2002.).

Thiolysis de-polymerization of condensed tannins in the presence of benzylmercaptan releases monomer derivatives such as benzylthioepicatechin. HPLC analysis of the degradation products could qualitatively and quantitatively determine the extender units of condensed tannins (Matthews *et al.*, 1997; Santos-Buelga and Scalbert 2000).

ESI and API-MS are also used to study flavan-3-ol oligomers. TOFMS can be used to analyze flavan-3-ol oligomers/polymers with higher molecular weights. The MS method can provide information about the polymerization degree and the type of the component monomer units. However, it is hard to determine the exact structures of these condensed tannins only by MS and accurate quantification of these compounds by MS is difficult to achieve, especially for larger oligomers or polymers.

Tannins in Some Dietary Materials

Peanut Skins

Peanut skins are used to treat chronic haemorrhage and bronchitis in Chinese traditional medicine. The skins contain both B-type and A-type proanthocyanidins. The B-type dimers include B2, B3 and B4.

The A-type dimers, with one C-C bond and one ether bond linkages, include proanthocyanidin A_1 (p1), proanthocyanidine A_2 (p2), epicatechin-(2β-*O*-7, 4β-8)-*ent*-epicatechin (p3), epicatechin-(2β-*O*-7, 4β-6)-catechin (p4), epicatechin-(2β-*O*-7, 4β-6)-*ent*-catechin (p5) and epicatechin-(2β-*O*-7, 4β-6)-*ent*-epicatechin (p6). Peanut skins also contain some oligomers having A-type proanthocyanidin unit, such as p7 and p8 (Figure 7). These compounds may be responsible for the bitter taste of the peanut skins. Like other phenolic compounds, these compounds showed free radical-scavenging effects, which could protect the fatty acids in the peanut seeds from oxidation (Lou *et al.*, 2004; Lou *et al.*,1999).

Tea Polyphenols

Teas contain large quantity of polyphenols with gallocatechins and their gallate esters being among the main constituents. During fermentation process, the colorless (gallo) catechins in fresh tea leaves are oxidized to theaflavins and thearubigins in the presence of tea polyphenol oxidase and peroxidase and under the influence of pH. Theaflavins display a bright orange-red color and thearubigins display a red-brown or dark-brown color in solution. The chemical structures of theaflavins contain a substituted benzotropolone moiety formed from two flavan 3-ol units (Figure 8). Thearubigins are heterogeneous polymers whose chemical structures have not yet been completely characterized (Davis *et al.*, 1997; Takino *et al.*, 1965).

Tea flavan 3-ols exhibited a wide range of health beneficial effects. Professor Yokozawa and her group in University of Toyama, Japan, have worked on pharmacological evaluation of green teas and the components for decades. Their research group proved that the flavan-3-ols had effects on scavenging of nitric oxide and superoxide and that gallic acid conjugates of flavan-3-ols were more active than the un-conjugated ones. (-)-Epigallocatechin 3-*O*-gallate, (-)-gallocatechin 3-*O*-gallate and (-)-epicatechin 3-*O*-gallate exhibited higher scavenging activity on both nitric oxide and superoxide than (-)-epigallocatechin, (+)-gallocatechin, (-)-epicatechin and (+)-catechin did (Nakagawa and Yokozawa, 2002).

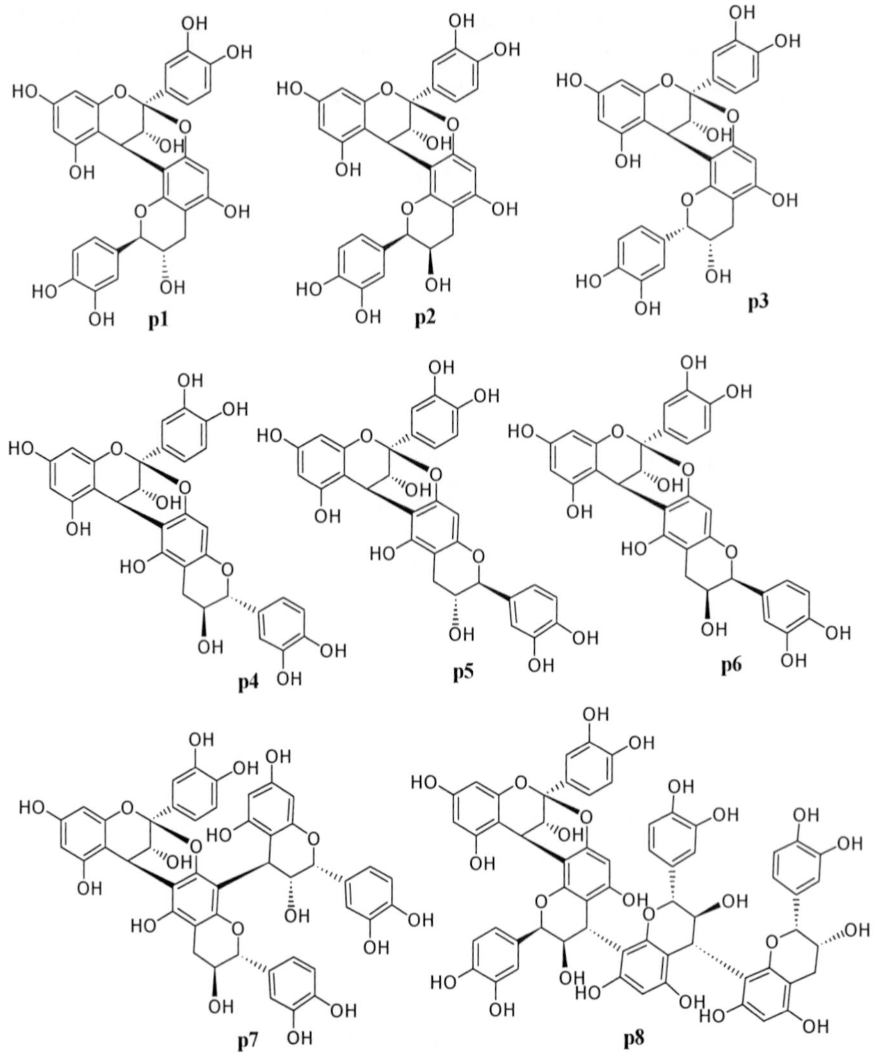

Figure 7. Structures of some flavan-3-ol dimers and trimers isolated from peanut skins.

These compounds also showed protective effect on 2,2'-azobis(2-amidinopropane) dihydro-chloride (AAPH)-induced cellular damage. Again, the gallic acid conjugates of flavan-3-ols were more effective than the un-conjugated ones (Yokozawa *et al.*, 2000).This group also examined the effect of green tea polyphenols on diabetic nephropathy, using rats that had been subjected to subtotal nephrectomy and injection of streptozotocin. After 50 days administration of the tea polyphenols, improved kidney function was observed in the rats with diabetic nephropathy by measuring the following parameters: urinary protein excretion, kidney weight, morphological changes, serum levels of urea nitrogen, creatinine clearance and hyperglycaemia. Administration of tea polyphenols also increased the activity of superoxide dismutase in the kidney to a significant extent. Based on these results, the researchers suggested that tea polyphenols may be beneficial for patients with diabetic nephropathy (Yokozawa *et al.*, 2005). In addition, oral administration of (-)-epigallocatechin 3-*O*-gallate, one of the major constituents of teas, had protective effect for rats with chronic renal failure (Nakagawa *et al.*, 2004).

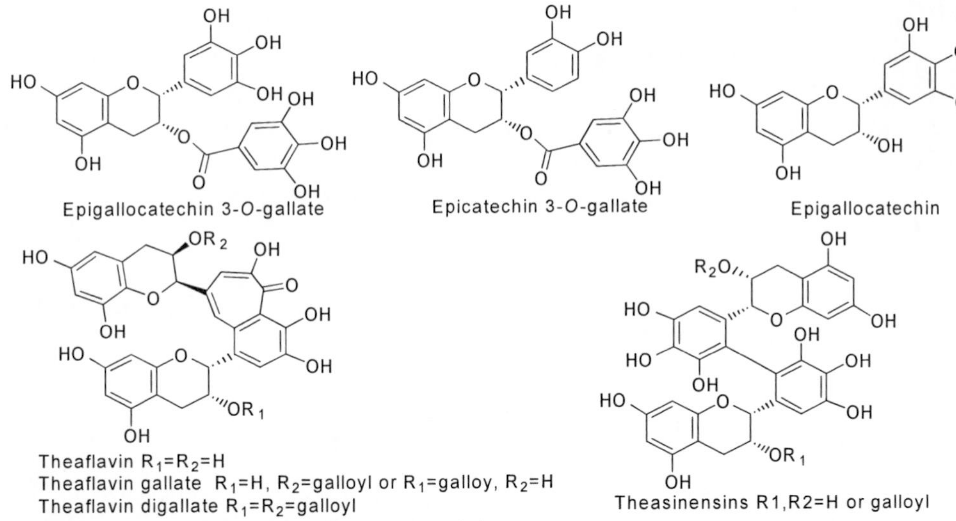

Epigallocatechin 3-O-gallate

Epicatechin 3-O-gallate

Epigallocatechin

Theaflavin R₁=R₂=H
Theaflavin gallate R₁=H, R₂=galloyl or R₁=galloy, R₂=H
Theaflavin digallate R₁=R₂=galloyl

Theasinensins R1,R2=H or galloyl

Figure 8. Structures of some phenolic compounds in teas.

Flavan-3-ols in Wine

Phenolic compounds, mainly flavan-3-ols and anthocyanins play important roles in the quality of wines. Their structures and amounts affect the color and sensory property such as astringency of the wines. The type and quantity of flavan-3-ols in wines depend not only on the kinds of the original fruits but also on the manufacture method, storage time and storage temperature. Due to their high chemical reactivity, the phenolic compounds polymerize and condense with other compounds in the wine solution to produce some special compounds for individual wines. The condensation causes a change of color from light to dark during the storage and aging process. The reaction of catechin condensed with glyoxylic acid, a compound may be derived from tartaric acid, is such an example (Figure 9). This reaction is generally observed during the aging of wines and other grape-derived foods (Es-Safi et al., 2000.)

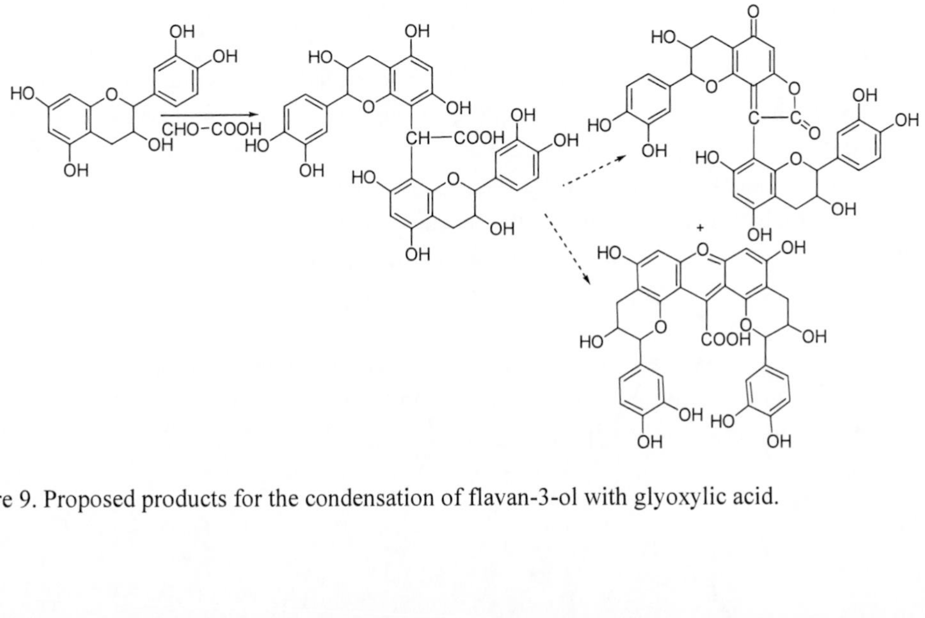

Figure 9. Proposed products for the condensation of flavan-3-ol with glyoxylic acid.

Flavan-3-ol related compounds, anthocyanins (Figure 10), can also undergo similar condensation, such as with pyruvic acid, an end-product of the glycolysis cycle during fermentation, to form stable red pigments as shown in Figure 11. Other yeast metabolites other than pyruvic acid were also found to react with grape anthocyanins, suggesting that this type of condensation may be an important route of conversion grape anthocyanins into stable pigments during the maturation and ageing of wine, thus increase the color stability of aged wines (Fulcrand *et al.*,1998).

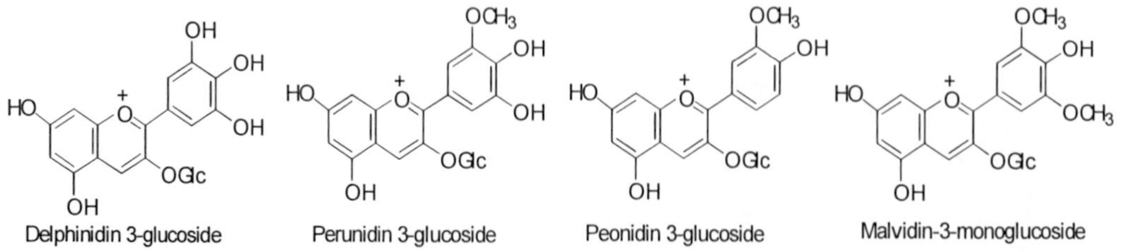

Figure 10. Some anthocyanins in grape.

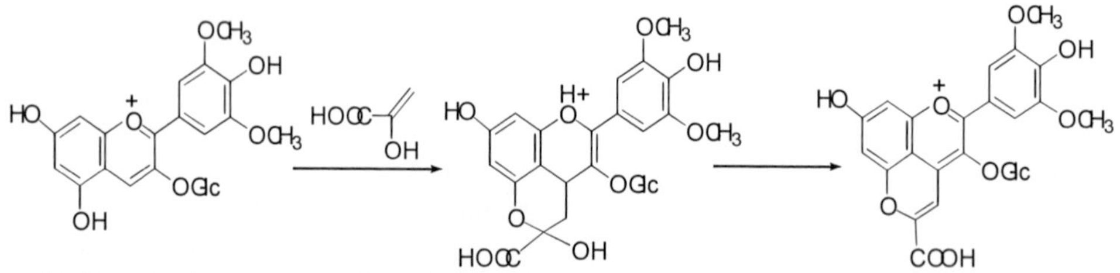

Figure 11. Reaction between pyruvic acid and malvidin 3-monoglucoside.

Grape Tannins

Recent years have witnessed increasing interest in using grape seed extracts as active ingredients in health promotion products. Grape seed tannins are a complex mixture of oligomers and polymers composed of catechin, epicatechin and epicatechin-3-gallate. Oligomers are mainly B-type linked through the C4→C6 or C4→C8 bond (Nu′ n˜ez *et al.*, 2006). Epicatechin was the major component in the extended chain while catechin was more abundant in terminal units than in extension units. The proportion of galloyllated units varied from 13% to 29% as the M_r, increased. Degrees of polymerization ranged from 2.3 to 15.1 or from 2.4 to 16.7 as measured by two different methods (Prieur *et al.*, 1994).

Grape skins also contain tannins with epicatechin representing 60% of the extension units, whereas 67% of the terminal units consisting of catechin. The degree of polymerization ranged from 3 to 80. The proportion of galloyllated units was 3% to 6% (Souquet *et al.*, 1996).

Tannins in grape seeds are shorter and have more epicatechin gallate as the monomer units. Tannins in grapes skin are generally larger and comprise more epigallocatechin as the monomer units (Herderich and Smith, **2008**).

Cynomorium Tannins

Cynomorium songaricum Rupr (Cynomoriaceae) (Figure 12) is a parasitic plant living on the roots of *Nitraria sibirica,* mainly growing in the northern part of China, such as Inner Mongolia Autonomous Region. The stems of *C. Songaricum* is a well known traditional Chinese medicine reputed to have tonic effect. In addition to medicinal applications, extracts of this plant are frequently added to wines and teas. The fresh stems are also consumed by the local people as food or vegetable. Our research results showed that this plant contained large amount of condensed tannins (in catechin equivalent: nearly 20% of the dried stems).

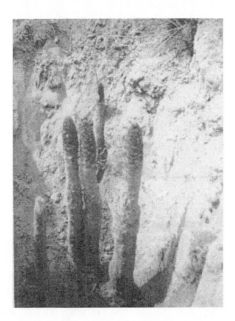

Figure 12. *C. songaricum* growing in the half-deserted areas of Inner Mongolia, China.

By separating the tannin fractions on Sephadex LH-20 and MCI gel CHP20P columns, both with H_2O-MeOH as mobile phases, we isolated procyanidins B_1 and B_6, flavan 3-ol trimers, tetramers, pentamers and a mixture of higher oligomers and polymers. The two isomers (procyanidins B_1 and B_6) of dimeric flavan 3-ols were separated as pure compounds. The trimers, tetramers and pentamers were obtained as mixtures of isomers containing epicatechin/catechin as the flavan 3-ol unit as indicated by their API-MS spectra. The polymer fraction was further divided to sub-fractions by ultrafiltration using centripre-10, centriprep-30 and cintricon plus-20 biomax-100, corresponding to 10, 30 and 100 kDa molecular-weight cutoffs. Although, for tannin, these cutoffs may not reflect the molecular sizes accurately, they may reflect the correct order of molecular sizes. Thiolytic degradation of the tannin polymers yielded benzylthioepicatechin as the predominant product, indicating that the extender flavan unit of the polymers in *C. songaricum* is mainly epicatechin. The *C. songaricum* tannins showed inhibitory activity on HIV-1 protease and the potency increased as the molecular sizes increased. The most potent activity was found in the sub-fraction with the largest molecular weights (IC_{50}=2 µg/ml) (Ma *et al.*, 1999).

Our recent study demonstrated that the methanol extract of this herb had potent anti-oxidative activity and moderate α-glucosidase inhibitory activity. Flavan-3-ol monomer and oligomers were found to be the active components by activity guided fractionation and isolation. The results suggested that that *C. songaricum* might be beneficial for patients with lifestyle related diseases, such as type 2 diabetes, obesity, and metabolic syndrome (Ma *et al.*, 2009).

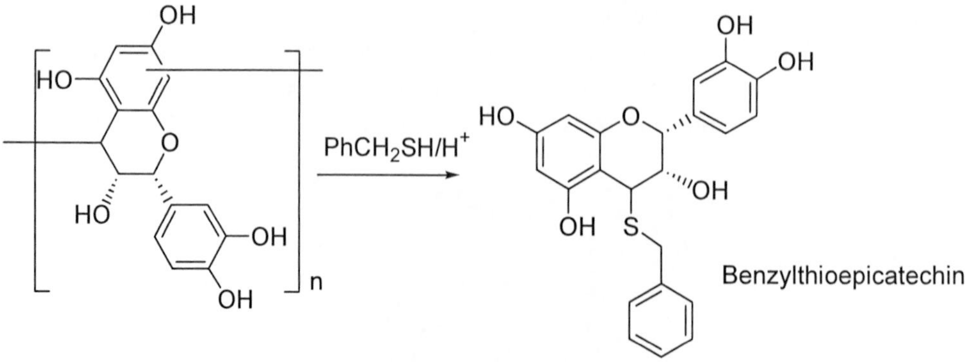

Figure 13. Thiolytic degradation of *C. songaricum* tannins.

Distribution in Other Dietary Sources

The contents of the phenolic compounds play important role in the antioxidant activity and other related bioactivities of fruits and vegetables. Cai et al. have studied a large number of plants about the relationship between their antioxidant activity and the contents of phenolic compounds. It was found that the antioxidant activity and the total phenolic contents for the tested herbs (112 species) were positively and significantly linearly correlated (methanolic/ aqueous: R^2 = 0.964/0.953). Plants with higher total phenolic contents showed higher antioxidant capacity. The study showed that the contents of phenolic compounds in common fruits and vegetables were in the order of followings (from high to low phenolic contents): eggplant, spinach, Chinese lettuce, Washington red apple, broccoli, orange, Fuji apple, tomato, spring onion, kiwifruit, carrot, garlic, cucumber and pear. Tannins are among the main components of the phenolic compounds in these plants (Cai *et al.*, 2004).

Mai et al. investigated the α-glucosidase inhibitory and antioxidant activities of Vietnamese edible plants and discussed their relationships with the polyphenol contents. The results showed that the extracts from plants used for making drinks showed the highest activities, followed by edible wild vegetables, herbs, and dark green vegetables. Positive relationships among α-glucosidase inhibitory activities, antioxidant activities and polyphenol contents of these plants were found. All the 5 plants (*Camellia sinensis* (Che Xanh), *Cleistocalyx operculatus* (Voi), *Psidium guajava* (Oi), *Nelumbo nucifera* (Sen), *Sophora japonica* (Hoe)) used for making drinks had high enzyme inhibitory activities and high antioxidant activities (Mai *et al.*, 2007).

Conclusion

Flavan 3-ols consumed in our daily foods and beverages play important roles in helping us to keep healthy. *As potent antioxidants,* they have effects on slowing down the aging progress as well as on prevention of Alzheimer's disease, cardiovascular disease, and cancer. These compounds also have inhibitory activity on α-glucosidase, suggesting they may have effect to prevent some modern diseases, such as type 2 diabetes, obesity, and metabolic syndrome.

Chemically, these compounds are unstable. Their C8 and C6 are highly nucleophilic, while C4 is electrophilic. Due to these chemical properties, these compounds are easy to polymerize and to condense with other compounds co-existing in the dietary materials. Specific controls of these reactions can produce dietary materials with special color, sensory property and biological activity.

Separation and identification work for the flavan 3-ol conjugates are considerably more difficult than for other types of small natural products, and thus the identification and biological activity of pure tannin compounds have not been fully investigated.

While the healthy beneficial effects of tannins are emphasized in this paper and in many other articles in recent years, caution will also be taken not to consume too much tannin mixtures as the non-specific interactions of tannin mixtures with proteins may cause some adverse effects. However, the current situation is that people, especially those in developed countries, do not take enough phenolic compounds, which lead to increasing cases of obesity and other modern diseases, thus, higher intake of tannin-containing vegetables and fruits in daily diets is recommended.

References

Cai Y, Luo Q, Sun M, Corke H. 2004. Antioxidant activity and phenolic compounds of 112 traditional Chinese medicinal plants associated with anticancer. *Life Sci* 74: 2157-2184.

Davis AL, Lewis JR, Cai Y, Powell C, Davies AP, Wilkins JPG, Pudney P, Clifford MN. 1997. A polyphenolic pigment from black tea. *Phytochemistry* 46:1397-1402.

Es-Safi N-E, Le Guerneve C, Cheynier V, Moutounet M. 2000. New phenolic compounds formed by evolution of (+)-catechin and glyoxylic acid in hydroalcoholic solution and their implication in changes of grape-derived foods. *J Agric Food Chem* 48: 4233-4240.

Ezaki-Furuichi E, Nonaka G, Nishioka I, Hayashi K. 1986. Tannins and related compounds. Part XLIII. Isolation and structures of procyanidins (condensed tannins) from Rhaphiolepis umbellata. *Agric Biol Chem* 50: 2061-2067.

Fujii H, Nakagawa T, Nishioka H, Sato E, Hirose A, Ueno Y, Sun B, Yokozawa T, Nonaka G. 2007. Preparation, characterization, and antioxidative effects of oligomeric proanthocyanidin−l-cysteine complexes. *J Agric Food Chem* 55: 1525-1531.

Fukuhara K, Nakanishi I, Kansui H, Sugiyama E, Kimura M, Shimada T, Urano S, Yamaguchi K, Miyata N. 2002. Enhanced radical-scavenging activity of a planar catechin analogue. *J Am Chem Soc* 124: 5952-5953.

Fulcrand H, Benabdeljalil C, Rigaud J, Cheynier V, Moutounet M. 1998. A new class of wine pigments generated by reaction between pyruvic acid and grape anthocyanins. *Phytochemistry*: 47: 1401-1407.

Hakamata W, Nakanishi I, Masuda Y, Shimizu T, Higuchi H, Nakamura Y, Saito S, Urano S, Oku T, Ozawa T, Ikota N, Miyata N, Okuda H, Fukuhara K. 2006. Planar catechin analogues with alkyl side chains: a potent antioxidant and an ▣-glucosidase inhibitor. *J Am Chem Soc* 128: 6524 -6525.

Harborne FRS JB, Baxter H. 1999. The handbook of natural flavonoids. 2: 2016-2067.

Hellström J, Sinkkonen J, Karonen M, Mattila P. 2007. Isolation and structure elucidation of procyanidin oligomers from Saskatoon berries (*Amelanchier alnifolia*). *J Agric Food Chem* 55: 157–164.

Herderich MJ, Smith PA. 2008. Analysis of grape and wine tannins: Methods, applications and challenges. *Aust J Grape Wine Res* 11: 205-214.

Hoffmann E M, Muetzel S, Becker K. 2002. A modified dot-blot method of protein determination applied in the tannin-protein precipitation assay to facilitate the evaluation of tannin activity in animal feeds. *Br J Nutr* 87: 421–426.

Hsu FL, Nonaka G, Nishioka I. 1985. Tannins and related compounds. XXXI. Isolation and characterization of proanthocyanidins in Kandelia candel (L.) Druce. *Chem Pharm Bul* 33: 3142-3152.

http://en.wikipedia.org/wiki/Tannin. access date: Nov 25, 2008.

Hwang T H, Kashiwada Y, Nonaka G, Nishioka I. 1989. Tannins and related compounds. Part 74. Flavan-3-ol and proanthocyanidin allosides from Davallia divaricata. *Phytochemistry* 28: 891-896.

Kashiwada Y, Nonaka G, Nishioka I. 1986. Tannins and related compounds. XLVIII. Rhubarb. (7). Isolation and characterization of new dimeric and trimeric procyanidins. *Chem Pharm Bull* 34: 4083-4091.

Lou H, Yamazaki Y, Sasaki T, Uchida M, Tanaka H, Oka S. 1999. A-type proanthocyanidins from peanut skins. *Phytochemistry* 51: 297-308.

Lou H, Yuan H, Ma B, Ren D, Ji M, Oka S. 2004. Polyphenols from peanut skins and their free radical-scavenging effects. *Phytochemistry* 65: 2391-2399.

Ma CM, Nakamura N, Miyashiro H, Hattori M, Shimotohno K. 1999. Inhibitory effects of constituents from *Cynomorium songaricum* and related triterpene derivatives on HIV-1 protease. *Chem Pharm Bull* 47: 141-145.

Ma CM, Sato N, Li XY. Nakamura N, Hattori M. 2009. Flavan-3-ol contents, anti-oxidative and α-glucosidase inhibitory activities of *Cynomorium songaricum*. *Food Chem* in press, *Available online 4 May 2009.*

Mai TT, Thu NN, Tien PG , Chuyen NV. 2007. alpha-glucosidase inhibitory and antioxidant activities of Vietnamese edible plants and their relationships with polyphenol contents. *J Nutr Sci Vitaminol* 53: 267-276.

Matthews S, Mila I, Scalbert A, Pollet B, Lapierre C, HerveÂ duPenhoat CLM, Rolando C, Donnelly DMX. 1997. Method for estimation of proanthocyanidins based on their acid depolymerization in the presence of nucleophiles. *J Agric Food Chem* 45:1195-1201.

Morimoto S, Nonaka G, Nishioka I. 1987. Tannins and related compounds. LIX. Aesculitannins, novel proanthocyanidins with doubly-bonded structures from Aesculus hippocastanum L. *Chem Pharm Bull* 35: 4717-29.

Morimoto S, Nonaka G, Nishioka I. 1988. Tannins and related compounds. LX. Isolation and characterization of proanthocyanidins with a doubly-linked unit from Vaccinium vitis-idaea L. *Chem Pharm Bull* 36: 33-38.

Nakagawa T, Yokozawa T. 2002. Direct scavenging of nitric oxide and superoxide by green tea. *Food Chem Toxicol* 40: 1745-1750.

Nakagawa T, Yokozawa T, Sano M, Takeuchi S, Kim Mujo, Minamoto S. 2004. Activity of (-)-Epigallocatechin 3-O-Gallate against Oxidative Stress in Rats with Adenine-Induced Renal Failure. *J Agric Food Chem* 52: 2103-2107.

Nour-Eddine E, Souhila G, Henri D P. 2007. Flavonoids: hemisynthesis, reactivity, characterization and free radical scavenging activity. *Molecules* 12: 2228-58.

Nu´n˜ez V, Go´mez-Cordove´s C, Bartolome´ B, Hong Y-J, Mitchell A E. 2006. Non-galloylated and galloylated proanthocyanidin oligomers in grape seeds from *Vitus vinifera* L. cv. Graciano, Tempranillo and Cabernet Sauvignon. *J Sci Food Agric* 86:915–921.

Peleg H, Gacon K, Schlich P, Noble AC. 1999. Bitterness and astringency of flavan-3-ol monomers, dimers and trimers. *J Sci Food Agric* 79:1123-1128.

Porter LJ, Hrstich LN, Chan BG. 1986. The conversion of procyanidins and prodelphinidins to cyanidin and delphinidin. *Phytochemistry* 25:223-230.

Prieur C, Rigaud J, Cheynier V, Moutounet M. 1994. Oligomeric and polymeric procyanidins from grape seeds. *Phytochemistry* 36, 781–784.

Ren Y, Chen X. 2007. Distribution, Bioactivities and therapeutical potentials of pentagalloylglucopyranose. *Curr Bioact Compd* 3: 81-88.

Santos-Buelga C, Scalbert A. 2000. Proanthocyanidins and tannin-like compounds– nature, occurrence, dietary intake effects on nutrition and health. *J Sci Food Agric* 80:1094-1117.

Scifinder, access date: Dec.7, 2008.

Shahidi F. 1997. Beneficial health effects and drawbacks of antinutrients and phytochemicals in foods. In F. Shahidi, *Antinutrients and phytochemicals in food (ACS symposium series 662)* (pp. 1-9). American Chemical Society, Washington, D.C.

Souquet JM, Cheynier V, Brossaud F, Moutounet M. 1996. Polymeric proanthocyanidins from grape skins. *Phytochemistry* 43: 509–512.

Takino Y, Ferretti A, Flanagan V, Gianturco M, Vogel M. 1965. Structure of theaflavin, a polyphenol of black tea. *Tetrahedron Lett* 6: 4019±4025.

Yokozawa T, Cho E, Hara Y, Kitani K. 2000. Antioxidative Activity of Green Tea Treated with Radical Initiator 2,2'-Azobis(2-amidinopropane) Dihydrochloride. *J Agric Food Chem* 48: 5068-5073.

Yokozawa T, Nakagawa T, Oya T, Okubo T, Juneja LR. 2005. Green tea polyphenols and dietary fibre protect against kidney damage in rats with diabetic nephropathy. *J Pharm Pharmac* 57: 773-780.

In: Encyclopedia of Vitamin Research
Editor: Joshua T. Mayer

ISBN: 978-1-61761-928-1
© 2011 Nova Science Publishers, Inc.

Chapter 48

Chemotaxonomic Applications of Flavonoids*

Jacqui M. McRae[†1,2], *Qi Yang*[2], *Russell J. Crawford*[1] *and Enzo A. Palombo*[1]

[1] Environment and Biotechnology Centre, Faculty of Life and Social Sciences, Swinburne University of Technology, Hawthorn, VIC,
[2] CSIRO Molecular and Health Technologies, Clayton, VIC

Abstract

Accurate taxonomic groupings are important for many applications, especially for medicinal plants. For example, structural analogues of the antitumour agent, paclitaxel, found in common *Taxus* species have increased the availability of this life-saving medicine without relying on the slow growing and comparatively uncommon, *T. brevifolia* [1]. Flavonoids have a long history of use as chemotaxonomic markers and have assisted in resolving many taxonomic disputes that have arisen as a result of morphological classification. In recent times, there has been increased interest in using molecular systematics and bioinformatics as alternatives to traditional chemotaxonomic techniques, however the investigation of the types flavonoids present in plants is still a useful technique to rapidly assess plant taxonomy.

Planchonia careya is a medicinal plant that contains a range of antibacterial compounds. Species of this genus are morphologically related to *Barringtonia* and *Careya* species and there have been several changes of nomenclature to reflect the uncertainty of these relationships.

Our recent investigation of some of the comprising flavonoids from *Planchonia careya* has revealed similar distinctive compounds to those found in *Planchonia grandis*

* A version of this chapter was also published in *Flavonoids: Biosynthesis, Biological Effects and Dietary Sources, edited by Raymond B. Keller* published by Nova Science Publishers, Inc. It was submitted for appropriate modifications in an effort to encourage wider dissemination of research.
† Email: epalombo@swin.edu.au

that are notably absent from *Barringtonia* and *Careya* taxa. Therefore the comparatively simple analysis of the flavonoid component of plant extracts can confirm or contest phenetic groupings to help resolve taxonomic discrepancies.

1. Introduction

Current taxonomic classifications group species into genera or families based on morphological similarities. Although this method has proven to be satisfactory in most cases, multiple revisions in the classification of many species highlight the inadequacies of phenetic taxonomy [2]. A more precise method of classification is often required to accurately group species, and molecular systematics and chemical taxonomy (also referred to as chemotaxonomy or biochemical systematics) have been used in these applications. Molecular systematics, including bioinformatics and DNA barcoding, is used to detect the presence of certain genetic markers in related plant species, while chemotaxonomy focuses on the similarities of compounds produced when a particular gene is expressed in related taxa [3, 4]. The utilization of both taxonomic methods can therefore provide a great deal of data for understanding the functions of secondary metabolites in plants [2, 5].

Secondary metabolites commonly have restricted distribution patterns in plants, with many occurring only in particular families or within species of a particular genus [1]. Morphologically-related plants are known to produce similar secondary metabolites and this observation led to the development of chemotaxonomy. This concept was in its infancy in the 1950s and grew in prominence over the following two decades [6, 7]. The advent of DNA sequencing technology in the 1990s eclipsed the enthusiasm for chemotaxonomy for a time, however it has since been shown that both techniques are required to provide adequate data for the phenetic and classification of a plant species [5, 7].

Chemotaxonomy ideally relies on the systematic analysis of particular phytochemicals in all known species of each family or genus. Specific types of compounds that are present in members of a particular genus and absent from representatives of a related genus (referred to as chemotaxonomic indicators or markers), can be used to prove if the morphological grouping is accurate. These compounds can also assist in the classification of new species. Chemotaxonomic markers must have particular characteristics to be of value in systematic investigations, including chemical complexity and structural variability, stability, and widespread distribution in plant species [6].

Alkaloids are a structurally diverse class of compounds and have therefore been used as chemotaxonomic markers [8, 9]. However, this class is limited in this application since these compounds occur in less than 20% of angiosperm families [10]. Flavonoids are less diverse than the alkaloids, with over 8 150 known structures reported up to the year 2006 [2] compared with the 12 000 known alkaloids, although they appear to be almost universally distributed among plant families. This makes them more widespread than other classes of secondary metabolites and therefore flavonoids have been used extensively as chemotaxonomic markers [2, 11].

Distribution patterns of flavonoid glycosylation and acylation in plant species have shown strong correlations with morphologically related species. Chemotaxonomic investigations of flavonoid glycosides have demonstrated that complex glycosidic patterns occur in many plant families and these usually correlate with morphological classifications

[12]. For example, investigations of the flavonol tri- and tetraglycosides of *Styphnolobium* and *Cladrastis* genera indicated that the morphological sub-grouping of some species may be inaccurate [13]. Further, the closely related genera, *Pergularia* and *Gomphocarpus* (Asclepiadaceae), were confirmed as being distinct based on the presence or absence of certain quercetin O-diglycosides and acylated kaempferol glycosides [14].

Chemotaxonomy has also resolved some issues that had arisen due to the difficulty of morphological classifications. The controversial distinction between the genera *Malus* (apple) and *Pyrus* (pear) was resolved by the presence of dihydrochalcones in all known species of *Malus*, and the absence of such compounds from *Pyrus* species [6]. Further, the recent creation of a separate grouping for some *Ateleia* species (Leguminosae) has been supported by the discovery of unusual flavonoid glycosides in only some of these species. This study also confirmed the placement of the *Ateleia* genus in the subfamily Papilionoideae, based on the glycosylation pattern of the comprising flavonols, thus validating the morphological classification [15]. Chemotaxonomic investigations of the types of anthocyanins present in certain species of Lecythidaceae and Myrtiflorae have also supported the morphological division of these families [16].

These correlations validate the use of phytochemicals in plant taxonomy and also the use of flavonoids as chemotaxonomic indicators. In addition, the ongoing discovery of novel flavonoid glycosides is a testament to their structural diversity and may yet reveal many novel compounds.

2. Extraction and Analysis of Flavonoid Glycosides for Chemotaxonomy

Current phytochemical investigations of flavonoid distribution in plant samples often utilizes liquid chromatography-mass spectrometry (LC-MS) and ultraviolet (UV) spectroscopy with photodiode array (PDA) detection [17, 18]. Previous investigations often used thin layer chromatography (TLC) and spot tests, which could not fully characterize the compound structure [19]. Further investigation of unknown flavonoids requires high performance liquid chromatography (HPLC)-piloted separation and isolation of the compounds of interest for structural elucidation.

Flavonoid glycosides and conjugates are water soluble and therefore can be extracted from the plant material with aqueous solutions [20]. Initial separation of the flavonoids from the hydrophilic carbohydrates and proteins present in the crude extract is best achieved with a polymeric chromatographic media such as Amberlite™ XAD resin. This media adsorbs relatively hydrophobic compounds and is particularly useful in capturing phenolic compounds from aqueous solutions [21]. Further HPLC-piloted separation and isolation is best achieved with reversed phase C18 media and size-exclusion chromatography, generally with Sephadex™ LH20 gel, using the distinctive UV profiles produced by flavonoids and their conjugates as a separation guide [20].

Identification of an isolated flavonoid may involve infra-red (IR) spectroscopy to determine the functional groups present, and MS for determining the molecular weight and the distinctive fragmentation patterns of the compound [22, 23]. The most commonly used technique for structural elucidation of unknown isolated compounds is nuclear magnetic resonance (NMR) spectroscopy. This is the most powerful tool available to natural products chemists as it allows the characterization of an unknown compound without destroying the sample. Improvements in the sensitivity of the instrument (greater than 500 MHz) as well as the development of multibond heteronuclear experiments have enabled the complete characterization of complex compound structures with less than one milligram of sample [24].

NMR technology is continually being improved and recent developments include the use of cryoprobes, which greatly increase the signal to noise ratio and therefore reduce the experiment time or the amount of sample [25]. The use of submicro-inverse-detection gradient NMR probes and other inverse detection techniques has also led to increases in the sensitivity of NMR spectroscopy enabling the elucidation of compounds of less than 0.05 μmol [26]. The use of NMR spectroscopy has enabled the full structural elucidation of many thousands of novel flavonoid glycosides that may have otherwise remained only partially characterized.

3. Application of Chemotaxonomic Techniques

This laboratory recently investigated the presence of potential chemotaxonomic indicators in the tropical Australian tree, *Planchonia careya* (F. Muell) R. Knuth (Lecythidaceae) [27]. The morphological similarities of *P. careya* with many *Barringtonia* species (Figure 1) resulted in the original classification of *P. careya* as *Barringtonia careya* F. Muell. (Barringtonaceae) (1866). This classification was later changed to *Careya arborea* Roxb. var. *australis* Benth. (alternatively referred to as *C. australis* F. Muell.) in 1882, due to the morphological similarities with the *Careya* genus, also of the Lecythidaceae family [28].

The leaves and bark of *P. careya* are used medicinally in the treatment of sores and skin infections. For cleaning a wound and preventing infection, an infusion was made from the inner bark of *P. careya*, and this was used to bathe the affected area, before applying a bandage made from the fibrous root bark [29]. Alternatively, the leaves of *P. careya* were crushed and applied directly to wounds and ulcers to prevent or treat infections [30, 31]. This traditional medicinal use has been validated by the isolation of several antibacterial compounds from the leaves [32].

Approximately 14 *Planchonia* species are found across Australasia from the Andaman Islands to Papua New Guinea and Australia [28].

Many of these species have experienced similar taxonomic contention to *P. careya* so the exact number of species remains uncertain. Chemotaxonomy is therefore a more useful method of clarifying the classification of *Planchonia* taxa as distinct from other species. Crublet et al. [33] isolated three novel acylated kaempferol hexaglycosides from the leaves of *P. grandis* (1-3, Figure 2), yet no similar compounds have been isolated from *Careya* or *Barringtonia* species. The presence of related compounds in *P. careya* would indicate that acylated flavonol polyglycosides were effective chemotaxonomic markers for the *Planchonia* genus [27].

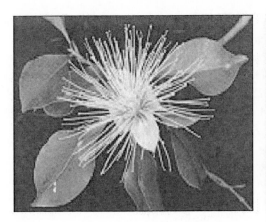 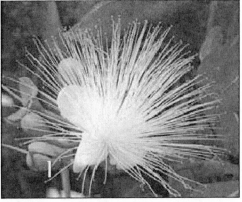

Figure 1. Comparison of the flowers from *Planchonia careya* and *Barringtonia racemosa* [39, 40].

	R₁	R₂	R₃
1	*trans-p*-Coumaroyl	α-L-Rhamnosyl	β-D-Glucosyl
2	*cis-p*-Coumaroyl	α-L-Rhamnosyl	β-D-Glucosyl
3	*trans-p*-Coumaroyl	α-L-Rhamnosyl	α-L-Rhamnosyl
4	*trans-p*-Coumaroyl	H	H

Figure 2. Compounds isolated from *Planchonia* sp.: 1-3, Acylated kaempferol hexaglycosides isolated from *P. grandis*; 4, Acylated kaempferol tetraglycoside isolated from *P. careya.*

To assess this premise, a collection of fresh *P. careya* leaves were crushed and extracted with water by immersion in the solvent. After a total of three 24 hour extractions, the flavonoid component of the crude aqueous extract was concentrated on XAD-16 resin and eluted with methanol. Separation was achieved with reversed phase C18 (100-200 mesh) media followed by Medium Pressure C18 (15 µm) media and isolation with preparative reversed phase HPLC (5 µm) gave the novel acylated flavonol tetraglycoside, kaempferol 3-O-[α-rhamnopyranosyl(1→3)-(2-O-p-coumaroyl)]-β-glucopyranoside, 7-O-[α-rhamnopyranosyl-(1→3)-(4-O-p-coumaroyl)]-α-rhamnopyranoside (4, Figure 2). Structural elucidation was achieved with 1D and 2D (homonuclear and heteronuclear) NMR experiments and mass spectrometry, and TLC of the acid hydrolysis products enabled the verification of the comprising sugar units [34, 35].

Other acylated kaempferol glycosides, such as a 3-O-coumaroylglucopyranoside from the leaf hairs of *Quercus ilex* (Fagaceae), reportedly have a strong UV-B absorbing capacity, a property that is attributable to many flavonoids although stronger in those with acylating acids [36, 37]. This and the possible regulation of plant growth may the reasons for the biosynthesis of such large molecules in the leaves of plants [37, 38].

The similarity in structure and glycosylation pattern of the compounds isolated from two *Planchonia* taxa suggest that other derivatives are likely to be found in related taxa. The presence of these acylated kaempferol polyglycosides can thus be considered as a reliable taxonomic indicator for members of the *Planchonia* genus and can therefore prevent taxonomic disputes based on morphological assessment.

Conclusion

The advent of molecular systematics techniques has led to a significant reduction in chemotaxonomic investigations in recent years. However, the capacity of chemotaxonomy as a comparatively simple and reliable method of plant classification ensures the continued validity of this technique.

Acknowledgments

The authors would like to thank the Sunshine Foundation for providing financial support for this research and Andrew Ford of the CSIRO Tropical Rainforest Centre for collecting the plant material. We also thank Dr. Noel Hart for his expertise in methods of compound separation and Dr. Roger Mulder for assistance with the NMR elucidation.

References

[1] Wildman, H. G. In *Pharmaceutical bioprospecting and its relationship to the conservation and utilization of bioresources*, International conference on biodiversity and bioresources: Conservation and utilization, 1997, Phuket, Thailand, 1999; IUPAC, Ed. Phuket, Thailand, 1999.

[2] Williams, C. A., Flavone and flavonol O-glycosides. In: *Flavonoids: Chemistry, biochemistry and applications*, Andersen, O. M.; Markham, K. R., Eds. Taylor and Francis Group: Florida, USA, 2006; pp 749-855.

[3]   Kress, W. J.; Wurdack, K. J.; Zimmer, E. A.; Weigt, L. A.; Janzen, D. H., Use of DNA barcodes to identify flowering plants. *Proceedings of the National Academy of Science*, 2005, 105, (23), 8369-8374.

[4]   Lahaye, R.; van der Bank, M.; Bogarin, D.; Warner, J.; Pupulin, F.; Gigot, G.; Maurin, O.; Duthoit, S.; Barraclough, T. G.; Savolainen, V., DNA barcoding the floras of biodiversity hotspots. *Proceedings of the National Academy of Science*, 2008, 105, (8), 2923-2928.

[5]   Albach, D. C.; Grayer, R. J.; Kite, G. C.; Jensen, S. R., *Veronica*: Acylated flavone glycosides as chemosystematic markers. *Biochemical Systematics and Ecology*, 2005, 33, 1167-1177.

[6]   Harborne, J. B., *Comparative biochemistry of the flavonoids*. Academic Press Inc Ltd.: London, England, 1967; p 304-314.

[7]   Waterman, P. G., The current status of chemical systematics. *Phytochemistry*, 2007, 68, 2896-2903.

[8]   Ober, D., Chemical ecology of alkaloids exemplified with the pyrrolizidines. In: *Recent advances in phytochemistry, Volume 37: Intergrative phytochemistry from ethnobotany to molecular ecology*, Romeo, J. T., Ed. Pergamon (Elsevier Science Ltd): Oxford, England, 2003; pp 204-206.

[9]   Waterman, P. G., The chemical systematics of alkaloids: A review emphasising the contribution of Robert Hegnauer. *Biochemical Systematics and Ecology*, 1999, 27, 395-406.

[10]   Facchini, P. J.; Bird, D. A.; MacLeod, B. P.; Park, S.; Samanani, N., Multiple levels of control in the regulation of alkaloid biosynthesis. In: *Recent advances in phytochemistry, Volume 37: Intergrative phytochemistry from ethnobotany to molecular ecology*, Romeo, J. T., Ed. Pergamon (Elsevier Science Ltd): Oxford, England, 2003; pp 144-145.

[11]   Ibrahim, R. K.; Anzellotti, D., The enzymatic basis of flavonoid biodiversity. In: *Recent advances in phytochemistry, Volume 37: Intergrative phytochemistry from ethnobotany to molecular ecology*, Romeo, J. T., Ed. Pergamon (Elsevier Science Ltd): Oxford, England, 2003; pp 2-12.

[12]   Harborne, J. B.; Williams, C. A., Flavone and flavonol glycosides. In: *The flavonoids: Advances in research*, Harborne, J. B.; Mabry, T. J., Eds. Chapman and Hall Ltd: London, UK, 1982; pp 261-311.

[13]   Kite, G. C.; Stoneham, C. A.; Veitch, N. C., Flavonoid tetraglycosides and other constituents from the leaves of *Styphynolobium japonicum* (Leguminosae) and related taxa. *Phytochemistry*, 2007, 68, 1407-1416.

[14]   Heneidak, S.; Grayer, R. J.; Kite, G. C.; Simmonds, M. S. J., Flavonoid glycosides from Egyptian species of the tribe Ascelpiadaceae (Apocynaceae, subfamily Asclepiadoideae). *Biochemical Systematics and Ecology*, 2006, 34, 575-584.

[15]   Veitch, N. C.; Tibbles, L. L.; Kite, G. C.; Ireland, H. E., Flavonol tetraglycosides from *Atelia chicoasinensis* (Leguminosae). *Biochemical Systematics and Ecology*, 2005, 33, 1274-1279.

[16]   Lowry, J. B., Anthocyanins of the Melastomataceae, Myrtaceae and some allied families. *Phytochemistry*, 1976, 15, (4), 513-516.

[17] de Rijke, E.; Out, P.; Niessen, W. M. A.; Ariese, F.; Gooijer, C.; Brinkman, U. A. T., Analytical separation and detection methods for flavonoids. *Journal of Chromatography A*, 2006, 1112, 31-63.

[18] Mabry, T. J.; Markham, K. R.; Thomas, M. B., *The systematic identification of the flavonoids*. Springer-Verlag New York Inc: Berlin, Germany, 1970.

[19] Gluchoff-Fiasson, K. G.; Fiasson, J. L.; Waton, H., Quercetin glycosides from European aquatic *Ranunculus* species of subgenus *Batrachium*. *Phytochemistry*, 1997, 45, (5), 1063-1067.

[20] Marsten, A.; Hostettmann, K., Separation and quantification of flavonoids. In: *Flavonoids: Chemistry, biochemistry and applications*, Andersen, O. M.; Markham, K. R., Eds. Taylor and Francis Group: Florida, USA, 2006; pp 8-31.

[21] Hostettmann, K.; Hostettmann, M., Isolation techniques for flavonoids. In: *The flavonoids: Advances in research*, Harborne, J. B.; Mabry, T. J., Eds. Chapman and Hall Ltd: London, UK, 1982; pp 6-10.

[22] Foo, L. Y., Proanthocyanidins: Gross chemical structures by infra-red spectra. *Phytochemistry*, 1981, 20, (6), 1397-1402.

[23] Ajees, A. A.; Balakrishna, K., Arjunolic acid. *Acta Crystallographica*, 2002, E58, o682-o684.

[24] Breitmeyer, E., *Structure elucidation by NMR in organic chemistry*. 3rd ed.; John Wiley and Sons, LTD: West Sussex, England, 2002.

[25] Fossen, T.; Andersen, O. M., Spectroscopic techniques applied to flavonoids. In: *Flavonoids: Chemistry, biochemistry and applications*, Andersen, O. M.; Markham, K. R., Eds. Taylor and Francis Group: Florida, USA, 2006; pp 40-98.

[26] Martin, G. E.; Guido, J. E.; Robins, R. H.; Sharaf, M. H. M.; Schiff, J., P.L.; Tackie, A. N., Submicro Inverse-detection gradient NMR: A powerful new way of conducting structure elucidation studies with <0.05 μmol samples. *Journal of Natural Products*, 1998, 61, (5), 555-559.

[27] McRae, J. M.; Yang, Q.; Crawford, R. J.; Palombo, E. A., Acylated flavonoid tetraglycoside from Planchonia careya leaves. *Phytochemistry Letters*, 2008, 1, 99-102.

[28] Barrett, R. L., A review of Planchonia (Lecythidaceae) in Australia. *Australian Systematic Botany*, 2006, 19, 147-153.

[29] Barr, A.; Chapman, J.; Smith, N.; Beveridge, M., *Traditional bush medicines: An Aboriginal pharmacopoeia*. Greenhouse Publications Pty Ltd: Northern Territory, Australia, 1988; p 178-179.

[30] Cribb, A. B.; Cribb, J. W., *Wild medicine in Australia*. William Collins Pty Ltd.: Sydney, Australia, 1983.

[31] Lassak, E. V.; McCarthy, T., *Australian medicinal plants*. Reed New Holland Publishers (Australia) Pty Ltd: Sydney, Australia, 2001.

[32] McRae, J. M.; Yang, Q.; Crawford, R. J.; Palombo, E. A., Antibacterial compounds from *Planchonia careya* leaf extracts. *Journal of Ethnopharmacology*, 2008, 116, 554-560.

[33] Crublet, M. L.; Long, C.; Sevenet, T.; Hadi, H. A.; Lavaud, C., Acylated flavonol glycosides from leaves of *Planchonia grandis*. *Phytochemistry*, 2003, 64, 589-594.

[34] Brasseur, T.; Angenot, L., Six flavonol glycosides from leaves of *Strychnos variabilis*. *Phytochemistry*, 1988, 27, (5), 1487-1490.

[35] Malhorta, O. P.; Dey, P. M., Specificity of sweet-almond α-galactose. *Biochemistry Journal*, 1967, 103, (3), 739-743.

[36] Skaltsa, H., UV-B protective potential and flavonoids content of leaf hairs of *Quercus ilex*. *Phytochemistry*, 1994, 37, 987.

[37] Gould, K. S.; Lister, C., Flavonoids function in plants. In: *Flavonoids: Chemistry, biochemistry and applications*, Andersen, O. M.; Markham, K. R., Eds. Taylor and Francis Group: Florida, USA, 2006; pp 397-425.

[38] Furuya, M.; Galston, A. W., Flavonoid complexes in Pisum sativum L. - I: Nature and distribution of the major components *Phytochemistry*, 1965, 4, 285-296.

[39] van Heygen, G. http://www.vanheygen.com/Silhouette/images/baringtonia.jpg.

[40] TSOE Townsville city council state of the environment report. http://www.soe-townsville.org/nat_days/tree_day/images/PlanchoniaCareyaFlower.jpg.

In: Encyclopedia of Vitamin Research
Editor: Joshua T. Mayer

ISBN: 978-1-61761-928-1
© 2011 Nova Science Publishers, Inc.

Chapter 49

Bioanalysis of the Flavonoid Composition of Herbal Extracts and Dietary Supplements[*]

Shujing Ding[1] and Ed Dudley[2]
[1]MRC Human Nutrition Research,
Elsie Widdowson Laboratory, Fulbourn Road, Cambridge CB1 9NL, UK
[2]Biochemistry and Biomolecular Mass Spectrometry,
Swansea University, Singleton Park, Swansea, SA2 8PP, UK

Abstract

Flavonoids are one of the most diverse and widespread groups of natural products. They ubiquitously occur in all parts of plants including the fruit, pollen, roots and heartwood. Plant extracts rich in flavonoids such as: Ginkgo biloba extract, soy bean extract and green tea extract are popular dietary supplements. Numerous physiological activities have been attributed to them and their potential roles in the prevention of hormone-dependent cancers have been investigated. Over 5000 different flavonoids have been described to date and they are classified into at least 10 chemical groups. Flavonoid compounds usually occur in plants as glycosides in which one or more of the phenolic hydroxyl groups are combined with sugar residues.

Quality control of these plant-extract products is problematic due to the many varying factors in herbal medicine. Unlike synthetic drugs (in which the concentration and activity of a single known bio-molecule is monitored), there are many uncertainties in terms of species variation, geographical source, cultivation, harvest, storage and processing techniques which may lead to a product of different quality and efficacy. To evaluate the quality of flavonoids contained within plant extracts it is therefore very important to develop an analytical method which can monitor the quantity and variety of

---

[*] A version of this chapter was also published in *Flavonoids: Biosynthesis, Biological Effects and Dietary Sources, edited by Raymond B. Keller* published by Nova Science Publishers, Inc. It was submitted for appropriate modifications in an effort to encourage wider dissemination of research.

flavonoids efficiently. Also the study of the absorption and retention of these compounds within individuals is more problematic as more than one active compound is ingested from the plant extracts.

The challenge presented by such extracts is therefore to determine the different flavonoid species present in any given extract and also to determine any modification or fortification of the extract. Furthermore, Administration, Distribution, Metabolism and Excretion (ADME) studies require the quantitative analysis of multiple components rather than a single drug compound. The increase in the number of new flavonoid reports is due to two main factors: the advances in methods of separation and the rapid development and application of modern mass spectrometry (MS). Mass spectrometry proved to be the most effective technique in flavonoids research both in plant extract and in biological samples. In this expert commentary we will review the methods available for studying this wide-ranging class of compounds and also how modern techniques have been applied in order to "mine" the data obtained for flavonoid specific information from a complex metabolomic analysis.

Flavonoids: Source, Clinical Properties and Structures

The flavonoids represent a very diverse group of natural products with more than 6500 known flavonoid structures having been identified [1]. They ubiquitously occur in all parts of plants and plant extracts rich in flavonoids such as *Ginkgo biloba* extracts are among the most popular dietary supplements taken by the general public. The flavonoids are structurally similar to steroid hormones, particularly estrogens, and have been studied extensively.

Table 1. Herbal extracts, their flavonoid content and medical proterties

Plant name	Flavonoid content	Major flavonoids	Medical properties	Ref
Lycium Barbarum	0.16% wt/vol	myricetin quercetin Kaempferol	Benefiting the liver and kidney, replenishing vital essence and improving eyesight	[3]
Hawthorn	0.1-2% wt/vol	rutin, hyperoside, Vitexin	Gastroprotective, stimulating Digestion, anti-microbial and anti-inflammatory activities	[4]
Ginkgo Biloba extract	240mg/g	Quercetin kaempferol Isorhamnetin	Improving peripheral blood flow, reducing cerebral insufficiency	[5]
Hippophae rhamnoides extract	10-439µg/g	Quercetin kaempferol Isorhamnetin	A cough relief, aiding digestion, invigorating blood circulation, and alleviating pain	[6]
Tea	4.9-136.3mg/g	Catechins theaflavins	Anti-oxidant activity, free radical scavengers	[7]
Soy bean	0.56-3.81mg/g	Daidzein genistein glycitein	Reduced risk of some diseases moderated by oestrogen (e.g.) breast cancer and osteoporosis	[8]

These studies have shown that flavonoids exhibit many biological activities, including anti-allergenic, anti-viral, anti-inflammatory and vasodilating actions. Numerous physiological activities have also been attributed to these compounds and their potential role in the prevention of hormone-dependent cancers has also been investigated [2]. A summary of some of the herbal remedies that contain flavonoids and the benefits associated with them is shown in Table 1. Flavonoids are largely planar molecules and their structural variation arises in part from the pattern of substitutions within this basic molecule such as: hydroxylation, methoxylation, prenylation or glycosylation.

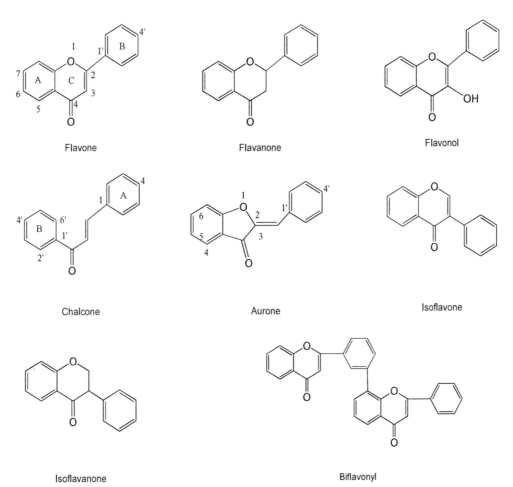

Figure 1. Basic structure of common subclasses of flavonoids.

The flavonoids are classified into at least 10 chemical groups. Figure 1 lists common subclasses of flavonoids and also demonstrates the chemical numbering system applied to both the atoms and rings (A, B and C) when comparing the structures of different flavonoids. Flavonoid compounds usually occur in plants as glycosides in which one or more of the phenolic hydroxyl groups are combined with sugar residues, forming an acid-labile glycoside O-C bond. There are also other forms of conjugated sugars (e.g. D-glucose, L-rhamnose) which contribute to the complex and diverse nature of the individual molecules that have been identified.

Analysis of Flavonoids – A Review

Due to the complex nature of the herbal remedies available (compared to usual pharmaceutical drugs which are composed mainly of a single active agent and formulation chemicals) the application of strict and stringent regulatory rules governing the "purity" of such a mixture is more complicated than those applied to drug moieties by the Food and Drug Administration Authority (FDA). Despite this, the World Health Organisation (WHO) have accepted that the "fingerprint" analysis of the levels of flavonoids and natural products in herbal remedies which claim the benefits of the presence of such compounds, is an acceptable methodology for monitoring the validity of any new or existing "natural product" [9]. This requirement was included in the European Economic Council guideline 75/318 "Quality of Herb Drugs" [10]. Taking *Gingko Biloba* extracts as an example, the flavonoids content is an important parameter in terms of quality control. The applied threshold for commercial standardized extracts of *Ginkgo* is that flavonoids constitute no less than 24% of the material and terpene lactones no less than 6% [11]. However in North America such extracts are considered to be a "dietary supplement" rather than a medicinal product and hence they do not attract the same level of scrutiny compared to Europe. The analysis of the levels of the flavonoids (considered to be – at least one of many – bioactive agents present in herbal extracts) is therefore useful in order to demonstrate that the individual taking the extract is obtaining the expected benefits from these herbal remedies. Furthermore, such analyses are also invaluable for the purpose of identifying any artificial fortification of extracts which are claimed to be "pure". Any such analysis can be used to study the entire flavonoid content of an extract and quantitate the levels of "active" flavonoids in a given sample (similar to any drug quality control assay). Alternatively "fingerprint" assays compare the entire profile of these compounds in a given sample to that of a "pure", unfortified extract in order to ensure that the extract has the properties associated with the herb. Such "fingerprint" analyses are however complicated due to the fact that the flavonoid composition of any herbal extract may be altered due to natural environmental or conditions in which the herb is grown prior to harvesting and so identifying an "ideal" flavonoid profile for comparison with commercial herbal extracts can be problematic. Despite these potential complications, these two major routes of bio-analysis of the flavonoid content of herbal extracts are commonly employed. Fingerprint analysis allows the evaluation of the quality of plant extracts and is able to provide comprehensive (including flavonoids and other components determination) and semi-quantitative information for complicated plant extract samples. More recently bioinformatic programs (e.g. fuzzy influence diagrams) have become available and may be applied in order to minimise subjective judgments when studying such data [12]. This development is a very important step when the active component is unknown in such complex biological extracts.

Fingerprint analysis of flavonoids can be achieved by using several chromatographic techniques including thin-layer chromatography (TLC) [13], high-performance liquid chromatography (HPLC) [14], gas chromatography (GC) [15] high-performance capillary electrophoresis (HPCE) [16] and high-speed counter-current chromatography (HSCCC) [17]. More recently, GC [18] and HPLC [19] in combination with mass spectrometry (MS) have become a popular alternative for fingerprint analysis as they have the advantage of providing more information compared to the previously applied techniques. Traditional quantitation of flavonoids has been achieved by spectrophotometry [20] and HPLC [21]. Both of these techniques require an acid hydrolysis step of the plant extract in order to convert the conjugated flavonoids into flavonoid aglycones. For spectrophotometry, rutin is normally chosen as the reference standard and only total flavonoid can be quantified as "rutin equivalent". HPLC is able to quantify individual flavonoids provided that their aglycone counterparts are available as standard reference compounds and flavonoids are quantified as aglycone equivalents in such assays. A 2-4 hours soxhlet extraction is required to convert the flavonoid glycosides to aglycones for the above two analytical methods. There are also reports of the quantitation of flavonoids in herbal remedies using GC/MS [22], offering better separation and specificity than spectrophotometry and HPLC. However, a time-consuming trimethylsilylate derivatisation step is required prior to GC/MS analysis.

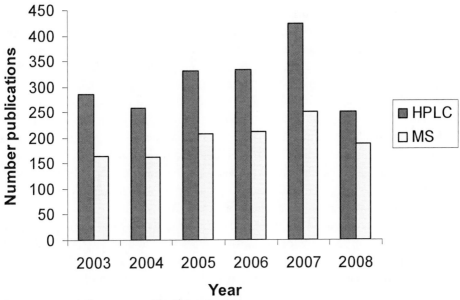

*Note 2008 data from 1st January until 31st October only.

Figure 2. Article title search results for flavonoid analysis by HPLC and MS between 2003 and 2008.

Capillary electrophoresis separation coupled with UV or ESI-MS detectors has also been applied to the study of flavonoids, offering an interesting alternative to HPLC separation [23]. In addition, UPLC is regarded as one way to achieve faster, more efficient separations with liquid chromatography by using smaller particle size stationary phase materials, and this separation technique has also applied to flavonoid analysis [24]. However, as a separation technique, HPLC is the more widely applicable and offers a larger range of choices (in terms of solid phases and column sizes) and when coupled to mass spectrometry detection it can provide structure-selective information concerning the analytes. This is very important in matrices as complicated as plant extracts. Hence, whilst HPLC-UV detection analysis remains well used for flavonoid analysis, mass spectrometry is becoming increasingly used also for such studies as can be seen Figure 2. Reports of the application of HPLC/MS for flavonoid analysis have more than doubled in the recent five years comparing to the previous five years. In this review therefore, we propose to focus on the mass spectrometric properties of flavonoids and mass spectrometric analysis of flavonoids in both plant extract and biological samples.

Mass Spectrometry and Its' Application to the Analysis of Flavonoids in Plant Extract and Metabolites *In Vivo*

Prior to mass spectrometry analysis, an extraction protocol is required in order to extract the flavonoids from the samples under study. This can be simply done by ultrasonic extraction or pressurised liquid extraction [25]. The sample is freeze-dried or crushed up (using a simple pestle and mortar) and methanol added to the resulting material. The solvent will solubilise the flavonoids whilst leaving other components of the sample undissolved and so either filtration or centrifugation can then be applied to the sample to remove this undissolved material and the "purified" flavonoid-methanol extract taken for analysis. Mass spectrometry allows the study of a mixture of compounds (with or without online separation by techniques such as HPLC) and analyses the flavonoids as ions generated from the neutral molecules. For a compound to be analysed by mass spectrometry, the first requirement is that the molecule must form such an ion- usually by formation of a proton adduct with a positive charge or the loss of a proton forming a negative ion. The most commonly utilised technique for forming ions from flavonoids to date is electrospray (ESI) which has been successfully applied to a large number of biological molecules ranging from small entities such as amino acids to peptides, proteins and oligonucleotides. The electrospray process requires that the ion is formed in solution and has the distinct advantage of being easily hyphenated to modern separation techniques such as HPLC. The ESI mode of mass spectrometry is often used for the analysis of flavonoids, since it is a kind of soft ionisation mode (i.e. the ionisation process does not fragment the compound being ionised). The ionised analytes are either protonated or depronated depnding on the solution chemistry. We have studied the flavonoids ability to form ions in an electrospray source and compared the ability of the technique to form both positive and negative ions. In ESI MS, the signal intensity of an individual flavonoid is much stronger (10^{2-3}) in negative mode than positive mode, and in positive mode, the pseudomolecular ion signal is very weak and sodium and potassium adducts are dominant, hence most flavonoid analysis is carried out in negative mode. In this mode, the deprotonated molecular ions will generally be the most abundant ion, and the agycone counterpart can be observed in all flavonoid glycoside mass spectra as an in-source derived fragment. The results, summarised in Figure 3, demonstrate that a negative ionisation approach is substantially more sensitive compared to the formation of positive ions when analysing flavonoids as the intensity of the ions formed is far greater. Given the structure of the flavonoids, this is a sensible conclusion as there are few atoms within the structure with the pre-requisite basic properties to attract a positive proton as would be required to form a positive adduct ion. Once formed, several different mass spectrometric experiments may be performed in order to gain information regarding the flavonoids present in a given sample. The first such method discussed here is accurate mass analysis.

Accurate mass analysis, analogous to modern "metabolomic" analyses, often utilises the direct infusion of the sample of interest. A large number of ions are generated as a result and catalogued. The mass of each ion is measured to a high degree of accuracy and the empirical formula of the compounds present is suggested from the *m/z* value of the ion. This technique requires high resolution mass spectrometers, usually fourier transform mass spectrometers, capable of generating the required degree of mass accuracy. An example spectrum of this type of analysis is indicated in Figure 4. The highlighted ions (indicated by an *) correspond to the flavonoids and in addition to these ions many terpene lactone ions are observed. The mass accuracy of the detected ions is presented in Table 2.

Such analysis allows the rapid analysis of complex samples with quick analysis times (Figure 4 analysis time was 1 minute), however there are a number of disadvantages related to the technique. Firstly, isobaric flavonoids cannot be distinguished as no separation of the compounds present is performed prior to their analysis. Hence, flavonoids with identical glycoside groups attached in a different orientation will give only one signal, for example, 3-O-[6-O- (α-L-rhamnosyl)-β-D-glucosyl] kaempferol and 3-O-[2-O-(β-D-glucosyl)-α-L-rhamnosyl] kaempferol, both of which exist in *Ginkgo biloba* extracts [26].

Ion intensity of positive and negative mode

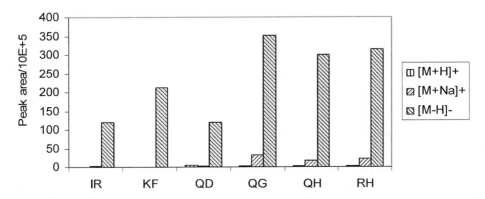

Figure 3. Comparison of ion intensity in positive and negative mode for some flavonoid components in *Ginkgo biloba*.

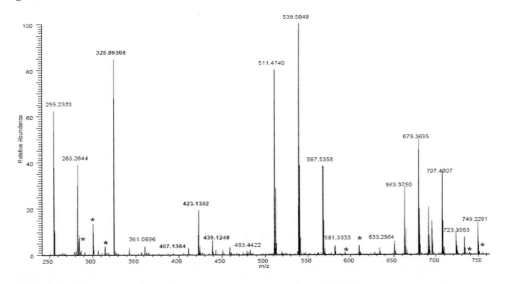

Figure 4. Mass spectrum of a direct infusion of a *G. biloba* extract on an accurate mass – mass spectrometer. (provided by Dr C. Williams, EPSRC National Mass Spectrometry Service Centre, Swansea University)

Table 2. Accurate mass analysis of a *Ginkgo biloba* extract

m/z	Theo. mass	Delta (ppm)	RDB equiv.	Formula	Identification
325.0930	325.0929	1.21	7.5	$C_{15}H_{17}O_8$	Bilobalide
423.1302	423.1297	1.25	9.5	$C_{20}H_{23}O_{10}$	Ginkgolide B/J
439.1248	439.1246	0.49	9.5	$C_{20}H_{23}O_{11}$	Ginkgolide C
407.1348	407.1348	0.11	9.5	$C_{20}H_{23}O_9$	Ginkgolide A
301.0355	301.0354	0.41	11.5	$C_{15}H_9O_7$	Quercetin
285.0406	285.0405	0.49	11.5	$C_{15}H_9O_6$	Kaempferol
315.0512	315.0510	0.55	11.5	$C_{16}H_{11}O_7$	Isorhametin
609.1461	609.1461	-0.01	13.5	$C_{27}H_{29}O_{16}$	Quercetin glycoside
593.1509	593.1512	-0.49	13.5	$C_{27}H_{29}O_{15}$	Kaempferol glycoside
739.1863	739.1880	-2.26	19.5	$C_{36}H_{35}O_{17}$	Kaempferol glycoside
755.1807	755.1829	-2.19	19.5	$C_{36}H_{35}O_{18}$	Quercetin glycoside

The *m/z* of both is 593Th as they exhibit identical empirical formulae, and hence these compounds cannot be distinguished by this method. As a result it is impossible to specify the exact nature of individual moieties as different arrangements of the sugars attached to the agylcone would generate identical data.

A further complication during accurate mass analysis arises due to the possibility of ion suppression. This occurs due to the fact that a specific amount of "charge" is available for the ionisation of the sample and hence the compounds present in the mixture "compete" for this charge. The presence of an easily ionised compound within the mixture may therefore limit the ionisation of others and hence the absence (or reduction in intensity) of a flavonoid ion may not represent an absence (or decrease in level) of the compound but may arise due to this factor. From this spectrum it can be noticed that *Ginkgo biloba* terpene lactone signals significantly suppressed the ionisation of flavonoids, despite the fact that the content of flavonoids is much higher than terpene lactones in the extract.

In order to address both of these issues, the application of a separation technique – preferably directly linked to the mass spectrometer – can be utilised. HPLC analysis is again applied with reverse phase (C18) stationary phases being the most commonly used. Recent developments in the miniaturisation of HPLC columns, and the systems used to run them, have led to lower mobile phase flow rates being applied in HPLC-MS analyses. This miniaturisation, due to the concentration sensitive nature of electrospray ionisation source of the mass spectrometer, leads to a significant increase in sensitivity. The reduction of the internal diameter of the HPLC from 4.6 mm to 0.3 mm (and reduction in required mobile phase flow rate from 1mL/min to 4µL/min) has been shown to result in a 80-100 fold increase in sensitivity of the HPLC-MS assay [27, 28]. The HPLC separation prior to analysis allows isobaric flavonoids to be separated and hence individually analysed and also removes the potential inaccuracy of the data obtained due to ion suppression effects. In order to further alleviate the problem of isobaric flavonoids in the extract, the combination of the HPLC separation of flavonoids with tandem mass spectrometry (MS/MS and MS[n] analysis) - in which the ions are fragmented with an inert "collision" gas and the fragment ions determined – allows an information rich analysis to be performed without bias towards any particular flavonoid.

MS/MS requires the isolation of the ion of interest - the precursor ion- which is then fragmented to generate "product ions". These product ions can themselves be individually isolated and fragmented further in an MS^3 experiment. This type of analysis can be done in a "data dependent" fashion in which the mass spectrometer "decides" which ion to fragment (based on ion abundance and how often the ion is detected) and which of its product ions to fragment further. This type of analysis – most commonly applied to trypsin digests of proteins in proteomic analyses [29] – takes the most abundant ion in a given mass spectrum and fragments this ion, next the most abundant product ion is further fragmented generating further structural data.

As the flavonoids are eluted from the HPLC column, they each -for a given time window- become the most abundant such ion and so information on the majority of the flavonoids can be obtained in an automated fashion.

Under MS/MS conditions, flavonoids are fragmented into a series of product ions. For a flavonoid glycoside, the loss of the sugar moiety is commonly seen, producing the corresponding aglycone as the main fragment ion. This is a very important characteristic and can be used to facilitate the bioanalysis of individual flavonoid species in a mixture. For flavonoid aglycones, the diagnostic product ions produced by further fragmentation are illustrated in Figure 5.

Many of the modern mass spectrometers e.g. triple quadrupoles, Q-TOFs can carry out MS/MS analysis since there have two tandem analysers, however ion trap mass spectrometers have a unique capability in that it stores ions. Once an ion is stored, it can be manipulated in many different ways to perform multistage MS/MS experiments (MS^n), hence it is frequently used for the structural elucidation of unknown flavonoids.

The application of this fragmentation process to the identification of a flavonoid separated by the miniaturised HPLC separation and analysed by ESI-MS, MS/MS and MS^3 is shown in Figure 6 and Figure 7.

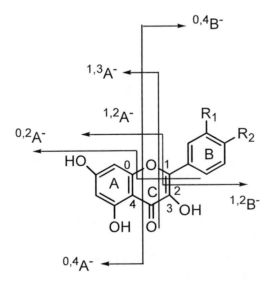

Figure 5. Nomenclature and diagnostic product ions of deprotonated flavonols formed by ESI-ion trap mass spectrometer, the symbols $^{i,j}A^+$ and $^{i,j}B^+$ are used to designate primary product ions containing intact A and B rings, respectively. The superscripts i and j refer to the bonds of the C-ring that have been broken [30].

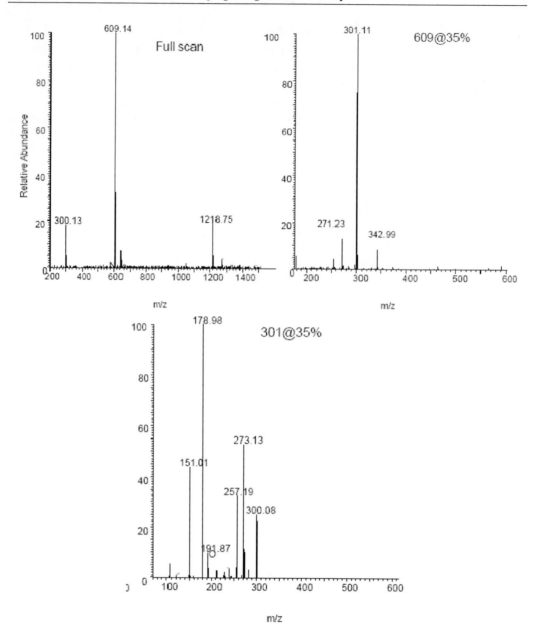

Figure 6. Data-dependent analysis rutin by HPLC-MS showing the full scan mass spectrum, the MS/MS spectrum of *m/z* 609 and the MS³ spectrum of *m/z* 301 via m/z 609.

The information obtained from the data dependent fragmentation analysis can also be re-searched in order to study selectively specific types of flavonoid glycosides. This process is based on the knowledge that under MS/MS conditions, the loss of the sugar moiety is the first fragmentation event observed. The two most commonly bound sugars in these glycosides are a glucosyl group and a rhamnosyl group.

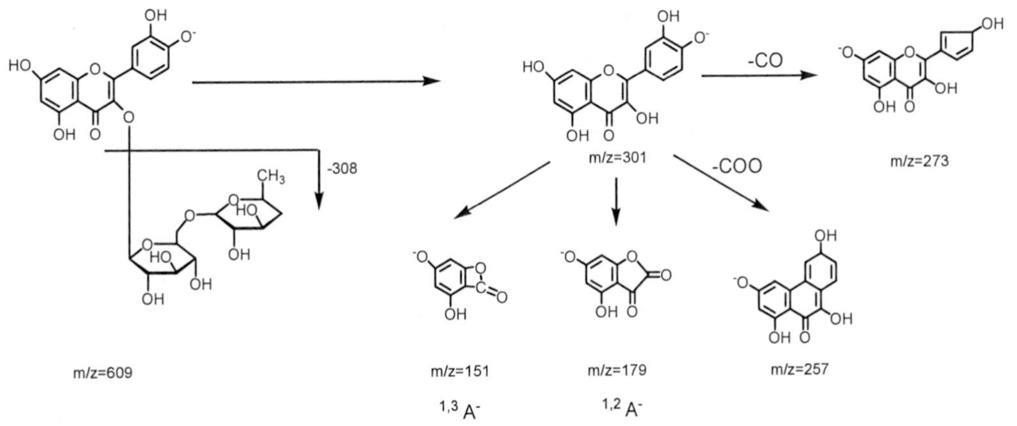

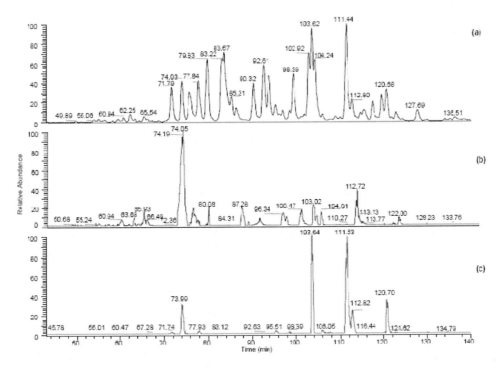

Figure 7. Illustration of the MS/MS and MS^3 fragmentation pathways observed during the fragmentation of rutin in an ion trap mass spectrometer (see Figure 6).

When these are lost in MS/MS experiments the product ion formed represents the loss of 162Da and 146Da respectively. Therefore a useful approach is to highlight in the complex dataset (obtained during the data dependent acquisition) all ions that exhibited these mass losses during fragmentation analysis. Figure 8 indicates the total ion chromatogram for a herbal extract indicating all ions monitored in the mass spectrometer compared to the selecting highlighting of those that lose 162 and 146Da.

Figure 8. Capillary HPLC/MS total ion chromatogram (TIC) of *Gingko biloba* extract (a) base peak full scan (b) neutral loss of *m/z* 162 (c) neutral loss of *m/z* 146.

It can clearly be seen that this filtering process allows the specific study of such compounds and further study of these peaks confirmed their status as flavonoids.

Flavonoids show biological properties through their free radical-scavenging antioxidant activities and metal-ion-chelating abilities [31]. Despite the benefits of these components, their bioavailability after oral administration is considered to be a limiting factor [32]. Mass spectrometry has therefore also been more recently applied to the analysis of flavonoids in the urine of subjects who have taken herbal extracts in order to determine the time taken for the compounds to be eliminated from the body. After ingestion, flavonoid glycosides are thought to be first hydrolyzed by micro-organisms in the gastrointestinal tract to aglycones. The liberated aglycones can be absorbed through the intestinal wall and are eventually excreted in the urine and bile as glucuronides and sulphate conjugates [33]. The analysis of components excreted in urine is complicated due to their lower levels and the large number of other high abundant species also excreted. Therefore, the urine samples are generally incubated with the enzyme β-glucuronidase/sulfatase to convert flavonoids into their aglycones as a first step of the analysis. In doing so, aglycone concentrations are increased to a detectable level and the analysis is simplified. A number of analytical techniques have been utilized in order to evaluate the metabolism and bioavailability of flavonoids *in vitro* and *in vivo*. The methods utilised previously for the study of urinary and other biologically important flavonoids levels include HPLC [34-36] and mass spectrometry (GC/MS [37, 38] and HPLC/MS [39]). There are also reports of online solid phase extraction using a reverse phase trap column (the outline of such an experiment is shown in Figure 9 [40]) and this methodology was shown to allow the quick and efficient clean up of the injected urine sample.

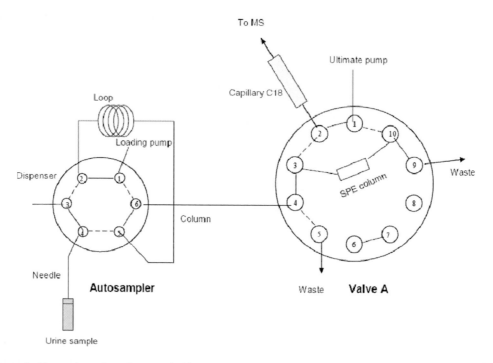

Figure 9. Illustration of a column-switching HPLC/MS system. The components to be analysed were retained on the C_{18}-Trap precolumn while the salt in the sample went to waste. After 3 minutes, Valve A was switched and components trapped on the precolumn were eluted to C_{18} analytical column and detected by mass spectrometry.

The comparison of the on-line clean-up method with off-line purification methodologies demonstrated that the on-line purification protocol does not suffer from any significant loss of analyte or interference from other matrix materials, and this method required minimal prior sample preparation and thereby facilitating higher throughput and greater automation.

Conclusion

Flavonoids are a diverse, yet important, group of chemical entities in many herbal extracts and their analysis in such materials is essential in order to gauge the appropriateness of different commercially available extracts. However, such an undertaking is complicated by the varied nature of these compounds. Fingerprint analysis – the comparison of the global metabolite profile of an extract compared to a "pure" standard - offers the ability to monitor such products and has been suggested as being beneficial by major regulatory organisations. Whilst many different techniques have been applied to such analyses in the past, the application of mass spectrometry offers an improvement in the quality of the data that can be obtained in an automated fashion. Furthermore, the ease by which the flavonoid-specific data can be extracted from the information (representing the total metabolite profile determined by such analyses) is improved by such experiments.

Mass spectrometry has a further application in the quantitation of flavonoid elimination via urinary excretion after the consumption of such herbal extracts and can therefore be of use in determining the longevity of the flavonoid. The application of the on-line clean-up and concentration of the flavonoids has been investigated and shown to allow accurate quantitation whilst minimising sample pre-treatment and work-up prior to analysis.

References

[1]   J.B.Harborne and C,A, Williams, *Phytochemistry*, 55 (2000) 481-504.

[2]   F. Teillet, A. Boumendjel, J. Boutonnat and X. Ronot, *Med. Res. Rev.*, 28 (2008) 715-745.

[3]   L. Kim, C. Francis and N. Ken, *Food Chemistry*,105 (2007) 353–363.

[4]   V.M. Tadić, S. Dobrić and G.M. Marković , *et al. J Agric. Food Chem.*, 56 (2008) 700-7709.

[5]   X. Mouren, P. Caillard, and F. Schwartz, *Angiology,* 45 (1994) 413-417.

[6]   Q. Zhang and H. Cui, *J. Sep. Sci.,* 28 (2005) 1171–1178.

[7]   M. Friedman, C.E. Levin, S.H. Choi, E. Kozukue and N. Kozukue, *Food Sci.*, 71 (2006) C328-C337.

[8]   R.J. Fletcher, *British J. Nutrition,* (2003) S39-S43.

[9]   World Health Organization, *Guidelines for the Assessment of Herbal Medcines*, Munich, 28.6.1991, WHO, Geneva, (1991).

[10] UNICEF/UNDP/World Bank/WHO, *Handbook of non-clinical safety testing*, (2004).

[11] T.A.van Beek, *J. Chromatogr. A*, 967 (2002) 21-55.

[12] H.Y.Kao, C.H. Huang,   T.C.Kao and H.C. Kao, *International. J. Innovational Computing and Information Control*, 4 (2008) 2057-2067.

[13] C.D. Birk, G. Provensi, G. Gosmann, F.H. Reginatto and E.P. Schenkel, *J. Liq Chromatogr. Relat. Tech.*, 28 (2005) 2285-2291.

[14] C. Chen, H. Zhang, W. Xiao , Z.P.Yong and N. Bai, *J Chromatogr. A* , 1154 (2007) 250-259.

[15] P.Drasar and J. Moravcova, *J. Chromatogr. B*, 812 (2004) 3–21.

[16] C.B. Fang, X.C.Wan, C.J. Jiang, H.R. Tan, Y.H. Hu and H.Q. Cao, *J. Planar Chromatogr. Modern TLC*, 19 (2006) 348-354.

[17] M. Gu, Z.G. Su and O.Y. Fan, *J. Liq. Chromatogr. Relat. Tech.,* 29 (2006) 1503-1514.

[18] Y.P. Li, Z. Hu and L.C. He, *J. Pharmaceut. Biomed. Anal.*, 43 (2007) 1667-1672.

[19] S. Ding, E. Dudley, S. Plummer, J. Tang, R.P. Newton and A.G. Brenton, *Phytochemistry*, 69 (2008) 1555-1564.

[20] A. Rolim, C.P.M. Maciel, T.M. Kaneko, V.O. Consigilieri, I.M.N. Salgado- Santos and M.V.R. Velasco, *J. AOAC International*, 88 (2005)1015-1019.

[21] A.Kakasy, Z. Füzfai, L.Kursinszki, I. Molnár-Perl and E. Lemberkovics, *Chromatographia*, 63 (2006) S17-S22.

[22] Z. Füzfai and I. Molnár-Perl, , *J. Chromatogr. A*, 1149 (2007) 88-101.

[23] J.D. Henion, A.V. Mordehai, and J. Cai, *Anal. Chem.*, 66 (1994) 2103-2109.

[24] X.X. Ying, X.M. Lu, X.H. Sun, X.Q. Li and F.M. Li,Talanta, 72 (2007)1500-1506.

[25] X.J. Chen, B.L. Guo, S.P. Li, Q.W. Zhang, P.F. Tu and Y.T. Wang, *J. Chromatogr A*, 1163 (2007) 96-104.

[26] A. Hasler and O. Sticher, *J. Chromatogr.*, 605 (1992) 41-48.

[27] J. Liu, K.J. Volk, M.J. Mata, E.H. Kerns and M.S. Lee, *J. Pharm. Biomed. Anal.*, 15 (1997)1729.

[28] K. Lanckmans, A. Van Eeckhaut, S. Sarre, I. Smolders and Y.Michotte, *J. Chromatogr. A*, 1131 (2006) 166-175.

[29] B.R. Wenner and B.C. Lynn, *J. Am. Soc. Mass Spectrometry*, 15 (2004)150-157.

[30] Y.L. Ma, Q.M. Li, H. Van den Heuvel and M. Claeys, *Rapid Commun. Mass Spectrom.*, 11 (1997) 1357-1364.

[31] C.A. Rice-Evans, N.J. Miller and G. Paganga, *Trends Plant Sci.*, 2 (1997)152-159.

[32] F.V. DeFeudis and K. Drieu, *Current Drug Targets*, 1 (2000) 25-58.

[33] J.K. Prasain, C.C. Wang and S. Barnes, *Free Radical Biol. Med.*, 37 (2004) 1324 -1350.

[34] S.E. Nielsen and L.O. Dragsted, *J. Chromatogr. B*, 707 (1998) 81-89.

[35] I. Erlund, G. Alfthan, H. Siren, K. Ariniemi and A. Aro, *J. Chromatogr. B*, 727 (1999)179.

[36] F.M. Wang, , T.W. Yao and S. Zeng, *J. Pharm. Biomed. Anal.*, 33 (2003) 317-321.

[37] D.G. Watson and E.J. Oliveira, *J. Chromatogr. B*, 723 (1999) 203-210.

[38] D.G. Watson and A.R. Pitt, R*apid Commun. Mass Spectrom.*, 12 (1998) 153 -156.

[39] E.J. Oliveira and D.G. Watson, *FEBS letters*, 471 (2000) 1-6.

[40] S. Ding, E. Dudley, L. Chen, S. Plummer, J. Tang, R.P. Newton and A.G. Brenton, *Rapid Commun. Mass Spectrom.*, 20 (2006) 3619 – 3624.

In: Encyclopedia of Vitamin Research
Editor: Joshua T. Mayer

ISBN: 978-1-61761-928-1
© 2011 Nova Science Publishers, Inc.

Chapter 50

Antibacterial Effects of the Flavonoids of the Leaves of *Afrofittonia Silvestris*[*]

Kola' K. Ajibesin

Department of Pharmacognosy, Olabisi Onabanjo University, Ogun State

Abstract

Afrofittonia silvestris Lindau, commonly known as the hunter's weed, is a procumbent herb trailing on moist ground. The leaves of the plant are used to heal sore feet, skin infections and as laxative. The leaves were macerated in 50 % ethanol and the liquid extract concentrated to dryness. The dry extract was evaluated for antibacterial activity by adopting agar diffusion method. The extract was partitioned between water, ethyl acetate and butanol successively and further subjected to antibacterial testing. The most active extract, ethyl acetate extract, was purified through various chromatographic methods to obtain pure compounds identified by spectroscopic methods as kaempferide 3–O–β–D–glucopyranoside and kaempferol 5,4'-dimethoxy-3,7-O- α-L-dirhamnoside. These compounds produced significant antibacterial effects, while the minimum inhibitory concentrations of the fractions and the pure compounds ranged between 25 and 250 µg/mL. These flavonoids are reported for the first time in this plant, while kaempferol 5,4'-dimethoxy-3,7-O- α-L-dirhamnoside is a new compound.

Keyword: *Afrofittonia silvestris*, antibacterial activity, kaempferide 3–O–β–D–glucopy ranoside, kaempferol 5,4'-dimethoxy-3,7-O- α-L-dirhamnoside.

---

[*] A version of this chapter was also published in *Flavonoids: Biosynthesis, Biological Effects and Dietary Sources, edited by Raymond B. Keller* published by Nova Science Publishers, Inc. It was submitted for appropriate modifications in an effort to encourage wider dissemination of research.

Introduction

Afrofittonia silvestris is a procumbent herb trailing on moist ground and commonly known as the hunter's weed (Hutchinson and Dalziel, 1958). The plant grows throughout the year (Taylor, 1966). The leaves of the plant are employed in traditional medicine in the treatment of diseases such as digestive tract disorders, sores, skin diseases and constipation (Burkill, 1985; Etukudo, 2003; Ajibesin et al., 2008). Although no chemical report of this plant is in literature, its nutritional values have been established (Odoemena et al., 2002).

This study was designed to isolate and identify the antibacterial principles of *Afrofittonia silvestris*.

Materials and Methods

General Experimental Procedures

The NMR spectra were recorded on a Brucker DR – 500 MHz (^{1}H 1) and 50 MHz (^{13}C), in CD_3OD using TMS as internal standard. Mass spectroscopy was determined using Electro spray ionization (ESI) Full MS and Finnigan LCQ Deca-MS, Agilent series 1100-LC. UV spectroscopy was determined by Dionex, UVD 340 S Dionex. Melting points were determined on a Kofler hot-stage microscope (uncorrected). TLC was carried out on silica gel 60 F_{254} (Merck). Solvent systems such as EtOAc-CH_3OH; 8:2 (A), CH_2Cl_2-MeOH; 9:1 (B), CH_2Cl_2-MeOH; 4:1 (C), CH_2Cl_2-MeOH; 7:3 (D), CH_2Cl_2-MeOH-H_2O; (7:3:1) were employed. UV light (λ max 254 nm and 366 nm), $FeCl_3$ spray, vanillin/H_2SO_4 and conc. H_2SO_4 sprays followed by activating at $100°C$ for 5 min., were used for detection of spots.

Plant Material

The leaves (6 kg) of *Afrofittonia silvestris* were collected in July, 2000, at Ikot Ekpene in Akwa Ibom State, Nigeria. The plant was identified and authenticated by Dr. U. Essiett of the Department of Botany, University of Uyo, Uyo, Nigeria. Voucher specimen (KKA 2) was deposited in the Department of Pharmacognosy and Natural Medicine herbarium, Faculty of Pharmacy, University of Uyo, Uyo, Nigeria.

Extraction of *A. Silvestris* Leaves

The dried leaf powder (4 kg) of *A. silvestris* was extracted by maceration using 50 % EtOH (10 L). It was filtered and the marc re-extracted with the fresh solvent mixture for 12 h (x2) and filtered. The filtrates were pooled together and concentrated to dryness *in vacuo* at $40°C$.

Antibacterial Test

The extracts and the fractions were reconstituted in MeOH-H$_2$O (1:1) to obtain a stock solution of 20 mg/mL. 50 µl of this solution was introduced into each of the equidistant wells (8 mm) bored on the agar plate surface previously inoculated with each of the test organisms. A control well containing Gentamicin (5 µg/mL) was placed in each of the plates seeded with bacteria. The bacteria were incubated at 37 ^{O}C for 24 h (Alade and Irobi, 1993). Antibacterial activity was expressed as average diameter of the zones of inhibition calculated as a difference in diameter of the observed zones and those of the wells.

Minimum Inhibitory Concentration

The minimum inhibitory concentration (MIC)was determined by incorporating various amounts (250 – 6.25 µg/mL) of the solution of extracts and fractions into sets of test tubes containing the culture media.50 µl of the standard test bacterial broth cultures were added into each of the test tubes. The set of tubes containing a mixture of bacteria and the sample (extracts and fractions) were incubated at 37 ^{O}C for 24 h (Cos et al., 2006).

A positive control tube containing only the growth medium of each of the organisms was also set up. The MIC was regarded as the lowest concentration of the extract or fraction that did not permit any visible growth when compared with that of the control tubes.

Activity-Guided Fractionation of A. *Silvestris*

The dry extract was dissolved in water and successively shaken with EtOAc (6x300 mL) and BuOH (6x300 mL) to afford ethylacetate (20 g), butanol (25 g) and aqueous extracts (35 g) respectively.

The resultant 3 fractions were evaluated against the test organisms at 20 mg/mL in aqueous methanol (MeOH:H$_2$O; table 2). The antibacterial principles were partitioned more largely into ethyl acetate fraction followed by butanol and aqueous fractions respectively.

Isolation and Characterization

The EtOAc, butanol and aqueous fractions of the plant species were subjected to TLC analysis, using solvent systems A, D and E respectively, visualized under the UV light (λ 254 nm) before using 100 % H$_2$SO$_4$ and FeCl$_3$ solution as detecting spray reagents. The most active EtOAc fraction (16 g) showed flavonoid components and was chromatographed on silica (Merck, 0.040-0.063 mm particle size) by accelerated gradient chromatography (AGC) column and eluted with C$_6$H$_{14}$ containing increasing amount of CH$_2$Cl$_2$, followed by increasing amount of CH$_3$OH (4:1, 9:1). Four flavonoid fractions coded A, B, C, D were obtained, two (B, C) of which showed significant antibacterial effects. The more active (C) of the two flavonoid fractions was further fractionated on silica by vacuum liquid chromatography (VLC), using EtOAc in gradient with CH$_3$OH and H$_2$O (7:2:1). Final purification was carried out on silica by preparative thin layer chromatography (prep. TLC), using EtOAc-CH₃OH (4:1) as mobile phase to give **1** (30 mg). The less active flavonoid fraction was purified by repeated AGC (silica) to yield **2** (21 mg). The two compounds along with the fractions were subjected to antibacterial test.

kaempferol 5,4'-dimethoxy-3,7-O- α-L-dirhamnoside **1**. Yellow powder, mp 220 ^{0}C (MeOH), UV CH₃OH λ max nm: 272, 334, ESI Full MS – m/z (rel. int.): 607 [M+H]$^+$ (100), 461 [M+H-Rham.]$^+$ (25), 299 [M+H-2Rham.]$^+$ (5). ^{1}HNMR (CD₃OD): δ 6.70 (1h, d, J= 2.2 Hz, H-6), 6.77 (1H, d, J= 2.2 Hz, H-8), 7.10 (1H, d, J= 8.8 Hz, H-3', 5'), 7.98 (1H, dd, J= 8.8 Hz, H-2', 6'), 5.48 (1h, d, J= 1.4 Hz, H-1'''), 5.24 (1H, d, J= 1.4 Hz, H-1'''), 0.72 (3H, d, J= 6.2 Hz, H-6'''), 0.64 (3H, d, J= 6.2 Hz, H-6''), 3.29 (3H, s, -OMe), 3.95 (3H, s, -OMe), 2.40-4.92 (8H, sugar protons).
^{13}CNMR: see table 1.

Table 1. ^{13}CNMR spectral data for compounds 1 and kaempferol 3,7- dirhamnoside

Aglycone			sugar moiety		
C	1	K	C	1	K
2(C)	157.0	156.4	1''(CH)	102.3	102.2
3(C)	134.8	134.8	1'''(CH)	100.0	99.8
4(C)	180.0	178.2	2''(CH)	70.5	70.5
5(C)	163.5	161.2	2'''(CH)	70.4	70.4
6(CH)	93.5	98.7	3''(CH)	71.7	71.0
7(C)	164.0	162.0	3'''(CH)	71.1	70.6
8(CH)	93.0	94.9	4''(CH)	72.0	71.9
9(C)	157.1	157.1	4'''(CH)	71.5	71.4
10(C)	106.0	106.0	5''(CH)	70.4	70.4
1'(C)	122.0	120.6	5'''(CH)	70.1	70.1
2',6' (C)	131.2	131.0	6''(CH3)	18.0	18.2
3',5' (C)	112.3	115.8	6'''(CH3)	17.9	17.8
4'(C)	163.2	160.5			
MeO	57.8				
	58.0				

K= kaempferol 3,7- dirhamnoside.

Known compound **2** was identified by comparing its spectroscopic data with those in literature (Lahtinen et al., 2005).

Results and Discussion

Two flavonoids were isolated from the leaves of *A. silvestris*. Kaempferol-5,4'-dimethoxy–3,7–O–α–L–dirhamnoside 1, a yellow powder, was isolated with the aid of accelerated gradient chromatography (AGC), vacuum liquid chromatography (VLC) and preparative thin layer chromatography (prep. TLC), while kaempferide 3–O–β–D–glucopyranoside 2 was separated with AGC alone. Compound 1 gave a UV spectrum which showed absorption maxima at 271 (band II) and 335 nm (band I) which indicated a flavonoid structure skeleton (Toker et al., 2004). The ESI Full mass spectrum showed a $[M+H]^+$ peak at m/z 607 consistent with the molecular formula $C_{29}H_{34}O_{14}$. The peak at m/z 461 was due to the loss of one rhamnose unit. The fragment ion corresponding to m/z 299 indicated the successive loss of two rhamnose units.

In the ^{1}HNMR spectrum, the meta-coupled protons of H-6 and H-8 appeared separately as doublets at δ6.70 and δ6.77 (J = 4.9Hz) respectively. In the B ring, the protons at C-3'/5' showed a doublet at δ7.10 (1H, J = 8.8 Hz), while their coupled protons at ortho position C-2'/6' occurred as two doublets at δ7.98 (1H, J = 8.8 Hz). Two singlets at δ3.29 and δ3.95 integrating for 3H respectively represented two methoxy groups. The signals at δ0.64 and δ0.72 (d, J = 6.2 Hz), each integrated for 3-protons, assigned rhamnose-CH_3 protons (Mabry et al., 1970). In addition, two anomeric protons assigned to H-1 of the two rhamnose moieties were observed at δ5.24 and δ5.48 as narrow doublets for α configuration of the glycosidic linkage (Toker et al., 2004).

The structure indicated by the ^{1}HNMR was supported by ^{13}CNMR spectrum. The two methoxy groups attached at positions 5 and 4' were indicated by the signals at 57.8 and 58.0 ppm respectively. The ^{13}C NMR spectra gave many similarities with kaempferol 3,7-O- α-dirhamnoside (Gohar and Elmazar, 1997) in the benzopyrone ring and sugar moiety. However, the position of the 1st methoxy group of 1 was indicated by the downfield shift of C-4' by 2.7 ppm and the upfield shift of the ortho carbons (C-3'/5') by 3.5 ppm with respect to the same signals in the ^{13}C NMR spectra of kaempferol 3, 7-O- α-dirhamnoside. Furthermore, the position of the other methoxy group on C-5 was shown by the downfield shift of C-5 by 2.3 ppm when compared with the ^{13}C NMR signal of the same kaempferol 3,7-O- α- dirhamnoside, while the ortho carbon C-6 shifted much upfield by 5.2 ppm. Thus, the main distinction between kaempferol 3,7-O- α- dirhamnoside and 1 appears to be the methoxy groups present in the latter, which was further confirmed by its larger molar mass. Similar distinctions were made when 1 was compared with another kaempferol 3,7- O-α-L-dirhamnoside isolated from *Tilia argentea* (Toker et al., 2004). Also, 1 shared some resonance characteristics when compared with the aglycone of kaempferide 3 rhamnoside where only one methoxy was attached at C-4' to form kaempferide (Bilia et al. 1993). The glycosylation at C-3 and C-7 was shown by their ^{13}CNMR signals at 134.8 ppm (s) and 164.0 ppm (s) respectively. The MS fragmentation of 1 also suggested O-glycosilation at C-3 and C-7. The sugar region gave eight sugar carbon signals at ca. 70.1-72.0 ppm, with the anomeric carbons resonating at 102.3 ppm (s, C-1'') and 100.0 ppm (s, C-1''') respectively. The presence of two characteristic rhamnose methyl signals at 17.9 and 18.0 ppm further confirmed the presence of two rhamnose residues (Agrawal, 1989; Neeru et al., 1990). Consequently, the data for compound 1 are uniquely consistent with the structure of kaempferol -5,4'-dimethoxy-3,7-O- α-L-dirhamnoside, a compound hitherto not reported in literature. The data showed that 1 is different from kaempferol-3,7- O- α-L-dirhamnoside earlier isolated from *Chenopodium* species and *Tilia argentea* in that it has two extra methoxyl groups (Gohar and Elmazar, 1997; Toker et al., 2004).

Kaempferide 3-O-β-glucoside 2, earlier detected in the larval faeces of sawfly species (Lahtinen et al., 2005), was also present in the plant.

The antibacterial effects of A. silvestris have been determined to be due mainly to kaempferol -5,4'-dimethoxy-3,7-O- α-L-dirhamnoside, while Kaempferide 3-O-β-glucoside was also isolated as antibacterial principle showing less inhibitory activity. It is noteworthy that kaempferol -5,4'-dimethoxy-3,7-O- α-L-dirhamnoside elicited better antibacterial effect than Gentamicin, the standard drug used. Antimicrobial activity of phenolics has been similarly established in Acalypha species (Adesina et al., 2000).

Conclusion

No previous report of the antibacterial effects of kaempferol -5,4'-dimethoxy-3,7-O- α-L-dirhamnoside and Kaempferide 3-O-β-glucoside was found in literature. The two conpounds are responsible for the antibacterial effects of the plant, and this validates its uses in traditional medicine for treating infections.

Table 2. Antibacterial activity of the extracts of *A. silvestris*

Zone of inhibition of organisms(mm)[a]						
Microorganism	L	E	B	Aq	Gen	MeOH:H2O
E. coli NCIB 86	9±1.00*	7±1.41*	4±0.00	3±0.00	12±1.58*	0
B. cereus						
NCIB 6349	10±1.00 *	7±1.73*	5±2.12	4±2.20	13±1.41*	0
S. aureus						
NCIB 8588	12±1.41*	10±1.58*	7±1.00*	4±0.00	13±1.00*	0
Ps. aeruginosa						
NCIB 950	10±2.20*	8±0.00*	5±1.00	3±1.00	15±2.12*	0

L: leaf extract, E: ethyl acetate extract, B: butanol extract, Aq: aqueous extract, Gen: gentamicin, values are mean±SD(n=4), *: p<0.01 with respect to control.

Table 3. Antibacterial activity of fractions and flavonoids isolated from *A. silvestris*

Microorganism	A	B	C	D	1	2	Gen	MeOH: H2O (1:1)
E.coli NCIB 86	5±0.00	8±1.40*	9±1.00*	4±2.12	15±2.20*	13±1.00*	12±1.58*	0
B. cereus								
NCIB 6349	6±0.00	9±1.00*	11±1.00*	5±0.00	16±2.12*	13±1.41*	13±1.41*	0
S. aureus								
NCIB 8588	6±2.45	8±1.41*	12±2.82*	5±1.00	18±1.41*	14±2.82*	13±1.00*	0
Ps. aeruginosa								
NCIB 950	5±1.00	7±2.45	11±1.41*	4±0.00	20±1.00*	15±2.45*	15±2.12*	0

Values are mean±SD (n=4), *: p<0.01 with respect to control, Gen: gentamicin.

Table 4. MIC of the fractions and flavonoids isolated from *A. silvestris* (μg/mL)

Microorganism	A	B	C	D	1	2	Gen
E.coli NCIB 86	>250	250	200	>250	50	100	200
B. cereus							
NCIB 6349	>250	200	100	>250	25	100	100
S. aureus							
NCIB 8588	>250	250	100	>250	25	50	50
Ps. aeruginosa							
NCIB 950	>250	250	100	>250	25	50	50

Gen: gentamicin.

References

Adesina, S K, Idowu, O, Ogundaini, A O, Oladimeji, H, Olugbade, T A, Onawunmi, G O and Pais, M (2000). Antimicrobial constituents of the leaves of *Acalypha wilkesiana* and *Acalypha hispida*. *Phytother. Res.* 14: 371-374.

Agrawal, P K (1989). Carbon-13 NMR of Flavonoids. Armsterdam, Elsevier.

Ajibesin, K K, Ekpo, B A, Bala, D N, Essien, E E and Adesanya, S A (2008). Ethnobotanical survey of Akwa Ibom State of Nigeria. *J. Ethnopharmacol.* 115(3): 387-408.

Alade, P I and Irobi, O N (1993). Antimicrobial activities of crude leaf extracts of *Acalypha wilkesiana*. *J. Ethnopharmacol.* 39: 171-174.

Bilia, A R, Palmae, E, Marsili, A, Pistelli, I and Morelli, I (1993) A flavonol glycoside from *Agrimonia eupatoria*. *Phytochemistry.* 32 (4): 1078-1079.

Burkill, H M (1985). The Useful Plants of West Tropical Africa (Edition 2), Vol. 1, Families A-D. Kew: Royal Botanic Gardens.

Cos, P, Vlietnick, A J, Berghe, D V and Maes, L (2006). Anti-infective potential of natural products: How to develop a stronger in vitro 'proof-of-concept'. *J. Ethnopharmacol.* 106: 290-302.

Etukudo, I (2003). Ethnobotany: convention and traditional uses of plants. Nigeria: Verdict press.

Gohar, A A and Elmazar, M M A (1997). Isolation of hypotensive flavonoids from *Chenopodium* species growing in Egypt. *Phytother. Res.* 11: 564-567.

Hutchinson, J and Dalziel, J M (1958). Flora of West Tropical Africa, Vol. 1, part II, Vol. II. London: Crown Agents for Overseas Government.

Lahtinen, M, Kapari, L, Ossipov, V, Salminen, J, Haukioja, E and Pihlaja, K (2005). Biochemical transformation of birch leaf phenolics in larvae of six species of sawflies. *Chemoecology.* 15 (3): 153-159.

Neeru, J, Sarwar, Alam M, Kamil, M, Ilyas, M, Niwa, M and Sakae, A (1990). Two flavonoid glycosides from *Chenopodium ambrosoides*. *Phytochemistry.* 29 (12): 3988-3991.

Odoemena, C S, Sampson, E A, Bala, D N and Ajibesin, K K (2002). Phytochemical study and nutritive potential of *Afrofritomia sylevestris* leaf. *Nig. J. Nat. Prod. and Med.* 6: 42-43.

Taylor, S R (1966). Investigation on plants of West Africa III, phytochemical studies of some plants of Sierra Leone. Africa Noire 28: 5.

Toker, G, Memisoglu, M, Yesilada, E and Aslan, M (2004). Main flavonoids of *Tilia argentea* DESF. ex DC. Leaves. *Turk. J. Chem.* 28: 745-749.

In: Encyclopedia of Vitamin Research
Editor: Joshua T. Mayer

ISBN: 978-1-61761-928-1
© 2011 Nova Science Publishers, Inc.

Chapter 51

Why Is Bioavailability of Anthocyanins So Low?[*]

Sabina Passamonti[†]
Department of Life Sciences, University of Trieste
Via L. Giorgieri 1, 34127 Trieste

1. Chemistry, Dietary Intake and Bioavailability of Anthocyanins

Following ingestion, anthocyanins are detected intact in blood [5, 6] in a time lapse considerably shorter than that observed with other dietary flavonoids [7]. However, the anthocyanins concentrations in plasma barely exceed 10^{-7} M, which translates into less than 0.1% absorption, including anthocyanin metabolites [8]. These features are indicative of various biochemical issues underlying the quite limited bioavailability of anthocyanins in mammalian organisms.

2. General Mechanistic Aspects of Limited Anthocyanin Bioavailability

2.1. Transporter-Mediated Absorption at the Cellular Level

Being found in plasma as intact glycosylated compounds, anthocyanins must have diffused across the gastro-intestinal barrier via membrane transporters catalysing their

---

[*] A version of this chapter was also published in *Flavonoids: Biosynthesis, Biological Effects and Dietary Sources, edited by Raymond B. Keller* published by Nova Science Publishers, Inc. It was submitted for appropriate modifications in an effort to encourage wider dissemination of research.

[†] Email: spassamonti@units.it

specific, sequential translocation from the gastro-intestinal lumen into the epithelial cells and from the cells into the blood. Molecules as polar as dietary anthocyanins cannot permeate epithelial barriers without the involvement of specific membrane transporters [9], unless epithelial barriers are disrupted, in which case para-cellular transport can occur [10].

2.1.1. Consequences of Transporter-Mediated Absorption: Rapidity

In turn, transporter-mediated absorption of anthocyanin provides the kinetic mechanism for their rapid absorption. Similarly to enzymes that are powerful enhancers of the rate of chemical transformations, membrane transporters are powerful enhancers of the rate of transport of solute molecules across membrane-bordered compartments [11].

2.1.2. Consequences of Transporter-Mediated Absorption: Saturability

Transporter-mediated absorption of anthocyanin implies that the rate of their absorption must display saturation with respect to their concentration. Similarly to enzymes, transporters kinetics obeys the Michaelis-Menten law, which is based on the existence of a transporter-substrate complex, featured by a Michaelis-Menten constant, Km, and a maximal velocity of transport, Vmax. Transport kinetics may deviate from the Michaeli-Menten law, yielding a sigmoidal dependence of transport rate as a function of the substrate concentration; also in such case Vmax is predicted to occur at infinite substrate concentrations. High-affinity transporters are quite efficient at transporting solutes at low solute concentrations, but are also inevitably saturated at relatively low solute concentrations. As a consequence, a high-affinity transporter specific for anthocyanins and expressed in the gastro-intestinal epithelium will also be a low-capacity transporter and therefore will enable low absorption.

2.1.3. Bilitranslocase: An Anthocyanin-Specific Membrane Transporter

Bilitranslocase is a membrane transporter originally identified in the liver [12] and extensively characterised for its transport function [13]. It is assayed in vitro using rat liver plasma membrane vesicles, which contain bilitranslocase, and the phthalein dye bromosulfophthalein as the transport substrate [14, 15]. This synthetic dye displays pH-dependent tautomerism, shifting between the phenolic, colourless species and the quinoidal, purple one. In this respect, BSP and anthocyanins are quite similar and this provided the rationale for the investigation of the interaction of these pigments with bilitranslocase. It was found that all six aglycones, their mono- as well as their di-glucosides behaved as competitive inhibitors of bilitranslocase transport activity [16]. Subtle changes in the glycosyl moiety were found to be associated with decreased affinity or with a change of the inhibition modality, i.e. from competitive to non-competitive inhibition [16]. The transporter seems to be quite selectively specific for anthocyanins, since related flavonols with the same pattern of glycosylation do not interact with bilitranslocase [17], presumably because they are not able to fit to the transport site, that accepts only planar molecules [17, 18]. The affinity of bilitranslocase for anthocyanins is described by their inhibition constants, ranging 2-22 µM. For these values, bilitranslocase should reasonably play a role in the uptake of anthocyanins from plasma, where they occur at very low concentrations, into the liver. Indeed, transport of anthocyanins into human hepatic cells is bilitranslocase-mediated, as shown by the strong inhibition of uptake caused by specific anti-bilitranslocase antibodies [19]. No other anthocyanin-specific membrane transporter has yet been identified, but certainly will be discovered, since membrane transport is rarely determined by just a single type of carrier.

2.2. Environment-Dependent Absorption at the Supra-Cellular Level

At the level of supra-cellular structures, like the gastro-intestinal tract, more complex factors combine to yield profound impacts on both the rate and extent of absorption of anthocyanins.

2.2.1. Distribution and Density of Anthocyanin-Specific Transporters

The first factor to be considered is the distribution and density of anthocyanin-specific transporters along the cranio-caudal axis of the gastro-intestinal tract. Consequently, the more upstream the transporter localisation, the fastest will be the absorption of anthocyanins, and vice-versa. Furthermore, critical is the sub-cellular localisation of transporters in absorptive epithelia, made by polarised cells that are distinctively equipped with influx and efflux transporters, so to favour the unidirectional trans-cellular passage of nutrients and other solutes.

2.2.2. Occurrence of Bilitranslocase in the Gastro-Intestinal Epithelium

This carrier is found in the gastric epithelium [20], more specifically at the level of two of the four main cell types lining the gastric glands, i.e. the mucus-secreting cells that are found at the luminal surface of the mucosa and the acid-secreting parietal cells, that are located more deeply in the columnar setting of the glands [21]. Moreover, it has recently been found also in the intestinal epithelium at the level of the apical (luminal) plasma membrane domain (unpublished data).

This localisation seems to adequately justify both the prediction that anthocyanins might be absorbed form the stomach [22] and its subsequent demonstration [22, 23]. A deeper mechanistic demonstration is difficult to be obtained with gastric epithelial cells, that are heterogeneous both morphologically and functionally [24].

2.2.3. Absorption of Anthocyanins into Intestinal Cell Monolayers: A Unique Role for Bilitranslocase?

The occurrence of bilitranslocase on the apical domain of intestinal cells offers an interpretation of data obtained testing anthocyanins absorption by human intestinal cell (Caco-2) monolayers [25]. The data show a striking correspondence between the extent of absorption of various anthocyanins and the affinity of anthocyanins for bilitranslocase [16]. Delphinidin 3-glucoside, the poorest anthocyanidin monoglucoside inhibitor of bilitranslocase (K_i=8.6 μM), was the least absorbed compound; the most absorbed ones, peonidin 3-glucoside and malvidin 3-glucoside, are also the best bilitranslocase ligands (K_i=1.8 and 1.4 μM, respectively). The correspondence also recurs with the glycosylated derivatives of cyanidin: cyanidin 3-glucoside is better absorbed than cyanidin 3-galactoside and the former is a better bilitranslocase ligand (K_i=5.8 μM) than the latter (K_i=35 μM).

The possible role of glucose transporters in anthocyanin translocation from the lumen into intestinal cells has been ruled out on the basis that glucose fails to decrease cyanidin 3-

glucoside absorption both *in vivo* [26] and in *in vitro* intestinal models [27]. No experimental data is currently available to put forward speculations about the possible involvement of other apical transporters in anthocyanin absorption.

2.2.4. Retention of Anthocyanins into the Intestinal Epithelium: Absence of Efflux Transporters?

In the above-mentioned study, only <4% of the dose applied in the luminal compartment appeared in the serosal one [25]. In another study [28], appearance of anthocyanins in the serosal compartment could not even be detected. However, in both investigations, retention of anthocyanins into the cell monolayer was rather extensive, up to 60%. Thus, anthocyanins might enter into Caco-2 cells via bilitranslocase, but would find a barrier for their diffusion across the basolateral (serosal) side of the cell membrane, where bilitranslocase is absent and the various other nutrient efflux transporters (e.g. the facilitative glucose transporter isoforms 2 GLUT2 [29], various aminoacid transporters [30]), seem to play no significant role in the cellular efflux of anthocyanins.

Even more surprisingly, primary active transporters, such as the Multidrug Resistance Associated Protein MRP1, MRP3, MRP4 and MRP5 [31], also seem not to promote anthocyanin efflux from intestinal cells, though their role as flavonoid transporters has been demonstrated [31].

Alternative mechanisms for the escape of intracellular anthocyanins from the enteric epithelium into the blood should be taken in consideration. A very attractive one is that already highlighted for quercetin, which is not transported directly into the mesenteric portal capillaries, but rather into the lymphatic system [32], likely in association with lipoproteins.

2.3. Anthocyanin Instability in the Intestinal Tract and in Plasma: Chemistry or Biochemistry?

Anthocyanins are said to be unstable in the intestine, because of pH conditions favouring their degradation. However, their loss in simulated intraluminal conditions is limited (<10%) and certainly not enough to account for their poor bioavailability [33, 34]; rather, when in contact with the colonic microflora, they are rapidly deglycosylated and the aglycones are then easily converted to phenolic metabolites [35, 36]. In plasma, anthocyanins are also said to be easily lost, due to their very low concentration and to their association with plasma proteins. However, further mechanisms of anthocyanin "instability" might be envisaged. In particular, the question if anthocyanins are degraded in the gut, in cells or in plasma by enzyme-catalysed mechanisms has never been addressed. This possibility is not unreasonable. In the gut, microbial flora might cause flavonoid C-ring fission by secreting a chalcone isomerase, as the latter has been shown to be a specific enzyme of the faecal anaerobe *Eubacterium ramulus* [37]. Its N-terminal amino-acid sequence does not align with any protein sequence in data bases [37], suggesting that genomic analysis is not fully predictive of phenotypes.

Conclusions

In conclusion, the poor bioavailability of anthocyanis seems to stem from the fact that they are transported into intestinal cells by a carrier-mediated mechanism, that displays high affinity though low capacity of transport. Contrary to many other organic anions, these pigments are apparently not transported by other intestinal membrane carriers besides bilitranslocase, though this issue needs to be further investigated. Surprisingly, anthocyanins are retained into the intestinal cells, being unable to be transported across the basolateral domain of the enterocyte plasma membrane. The high intracellular concentration is certainly a factor limiting sustained uptake of anthocyanin from the lumen. In the colon, anthocyanins undergo de-glycosylation and rapid C-ring fission, perhaps catalysed by bacterial chalcone isomerase. Enzyme-based degradation of anthocyanins in biological fluids is an issue that deserves investigation, in order to assess all aspects of the limited anthocyanin bioavailability in mammalian organisms.

References

[1]   Andersen MØ, Jordheim M. The Anthocyanins. In: Andersen MØ, Markham KR, Ed. Flavonoids. Boca Raton, Florida, USA, CRC Press 2006; 471-551.

[2]   Mazza G, Miniati, E. Anthocyanins in fruits, vegetables and grains. Boca Raton, Florida, CRC Press 1993; 379.

[3]   Wu X, Beecher GR, Holden JM, Haytowitz DB, Gebhardt SE, Prior RL. Concentrations of anthocyanins in common foods in the United States and estimation of normal consumption. *J. Agric Food Chem.* 2006; 54: 4069-75.

[4]   Kuhnau J. The flavonoids. A class of semi-essential food components: their role in human nutrition. *World Rev. Nutr. Diet* 1976; 24: 117-91.

[5]   McGhie TK, Walton MC. The bioavailability and absorption of anthocyanins: towards a better understanding. *Mol. Nutr. Food Res.* 2007; 51: 702-13.

[6]   Prior RL, Wu X. Anthocyanins: structural characteristics that result in unique metabolic patterns and biological activities. *Free Radic. Res.* 2006; 40: 1014-28.

[7]   Manach C, Williamson G, Morand C, Scalbert A, Remesy C. Bioavailability and bioefficacy of polyphenols in humans. I. Review of 97 bioavailability studies. *Am. J. Clin. Nutr.* 2005; 81: 230S-42S.

[8]   Mazza GJ. Anthocyanins and heart health. *Ann. Ist. Super Sanita* 2007; 43: 369-74.

[9]   Lipinski CA, Lombardo F, Dominy BW, Feeney PJ. Experimental and computational approaches to estimate solubility and permeability in drug discovery and development settings. *Adv. Drug Deliv. Rev.* 2001; 46: 3-26.

[10]   Turner JR. Molecular basis of epithelial barrier regulation: from basic mechanisms to clinical application. *Am. J. Pathol.* 2006; 169: 1901-9.

[11]   Stein WD. Kinetics of transport: analyzing, testing, and characterizing models using kinetic approaches. *Methods Enzymol.* 1989; 171: 23-62.

[12]   Sottocasa GL, Lunazzi GC, Tiribelli C. Isolation of bilitranslocase, the anion transporter from liver plasma membrane for bilirubin and other organic anions. *Methods Enzymol.* 1989; 174: 50-7.

[13] Sottocasa GL, Passamonti S, Battiston L, Pascolo L, Tiribelli C. Molecular aspects of organic anion uptake in liver. *J. Hepatol.* 1996; 24: 36-41.

[14] Passamonti, S., Sottocasa, G.L. Bilitranslocase: structural and functional aspects of an organic anion carrier. In: G.S.Pandalai, Ed. Recent Research Developments in Biochemistry. Kerala, Research Signpost, Kerala, India 2002.

[15] Baldini G, Passamonti S, Lunazzi GC, Tiribelli C, Sottocasa GL. Cellular localization of sulfobromophthalein transport activity in rat liver. *Biochim Biophys Acta* 1986; 856: 1-10.

[16] Passamonti S, Vrhovsek U, Mattivi F. The interaction of anthocyanins with bilitranslocase. *Biochem. Biophys. Res. Commun.* 2002; 296: 631-6.

[17] Karawajczyk A, Drgan V, Medic N, Oboh G, Passamonti S, Novic M. Properties of flavonoids influencing the binding to bilitranslocase investigated by neural network modelling. *Biochem. Pharmacol.* 2007; 73: 308-20.

[18] Passamonti S, Sottocasa GL. The quinoid structure is the molecular requirement for recognition of phthaleins by the organic anion carrier at the sinusoidal plasma membrane level in the liver. *Biochim. Biophys. Acta.* 1988; 943: 119-25.

[19] Passamonti S, Vanzo A, Vrhovsek U, Terdoslavich M, Cocolo A, Decorti G, et al. Hepatic uptake of grape anthocyanins and the role of bilitranslocase. *Food Res. Int.* 2005; 38: 953-60.

[20] Battiston L, Macagno A, Passamonti S, Micali F, Sottocasa GL. Specific sequence-directed anti-bilitranslocase antibodies as a tool to detect potentially bilirubin-binding proteins in different tissues of the rat. *FEBS Lett.* 1999; 453: 351-5.

[21] Nicolin V, Grill V, Micali F, Narducci P, Passamonti S. Immunolocalisation of bilitranslocase in mucosecretory and parietal cells of the rat gastric mucosa. *J. Mol. Histol.* 2005; 36: 45-50.

[22] Passamonti S, Vrhovsek U, Vanzo A, Mattivi F. The stomach as a site for anthocyanins absorption from food. *FEBS Letters* 2003; 544: 210-3.

[23] Talavera S, Felgines C, Texier O, Besson C, Lamaison JL, Remesy C. Anthocyanins Are Efficiently Absorbed from the Stomach in Anesthetized Rats. *J. Nutr.* 2003; 133: 4178-82.

[24] Karam SM, Leblond CP. Identifying and counting epithelial cell types in the "corpus" of the mouse stomach. *Anat Rec* 1992; 232: 231-46.

[25] Yi W, Akoh CC, Fischer J, Krewer G. Absorption of anthocyanins from blueberry extracts by caco-2 human intestinal cell monolayers. *J. Agric. Food Chem.* 2006; 54: 5651-8.

[26] Felgines C, Texier O, Besson C, Vitaglione P, Lamaison JL, Fogliano V, et al. Influence of glucose on cyanidin 3-glucoside absorption in rats. *Mol. Nutr. Food Res.* 2008; 52: 959-64.

[27] Walton MC, McGhie TK, Reynolds GW, Hendriks WH. The flavonol quercetin-3-glucoside inhibits cyanidin-3-glucoside absorption in vitro. *J. Agric. Food Chem.* 2006; 54: 4913-20.

[28] Steinert RE, Ditscheid B, Netzel M, Jahreis G. Absorption of black currant anthocyanins by monolayers of human intestinal epithelial Caco-2 cells mounted in ussing type chambers. *J. Agric. Food Chem.* 2008; 56: 4995-5001.

[29] Kwon O, Eck P, Chen S, Corpe CP, Lee JH, Kruhlak M, et al. Inhibition of the intestinal glucose transporter GLUT2 by flavonoids. *Faseb. J.* 2007; 21: 366-77.

[30] Broer S. Amino acid transport across mammalian intestinal and renal epithelia. *Physiol. Rev.* 2008; 88: 249-86.

[31] Brand W, Schutte ME, Williamson G, van Zanden JJ, Cnubben NH, Groten JP, et al. Flavonoid-mediated inhibition of intestinal ABC transporters may affect the oral bioavailability of drugs, food-borne toxic compounds and bioactive ingredients. *Biomed. Pharmacother.* 2006; 60: 508-19.

[32] Murota K, Terao J. Quercetin appears in the lymph of unanesthetized rats as its phase II metabolites after administered into the stomach. *FEBS. Lett.* 2005; 579: 5343-6.

[33] Talavera S, Felgines C, Texier O, Besson C, Manach C, Lamaison JL, et al. Anthocyanins are efficiently absorbed from the small intestine in rats. *J. Nutr.* 2004; 134: 2275-9.

[34] Uzunovic A, Vranic E. Stability of anthocyanins from commercial black currant juice under simulated gastrointestinal digestion. *Bosn. J. Basic. Med. Sci.* 2008; 8: 254-8.

[35] Keppler K, Humpf HU. Metabolism of anthocyanins and their phenolic degradation products by the intestinal microflora. *Bioorg Med. Chem.* 2005; 13: 5195-205.

[36] Fleschhut J, Kratzer F, Rechkemmer G, Kulling SE. Stability and biotransformation of various dietary anthocyanins in vitro. *Eur. J. Nutr.* 2006; 45: 7-18.

[37] Herles C, Braune A, Blaut M. First bacterial chalcone isomerase isolated from Eubacterium ramulus. *Arch. Microbiol.* 2004; 181: 428-34.

In: Encyclopedia of Vitamin Research
Editor: Joshua T. Mayer

ISBN: 978-1-61761-928-1
© 2011 Nova Science Publishers, Inc.

Chapter 52

Flavonoids with Antimicrobial Properties[*]

Rosa Martha Pérez Gutiérrez[†]

Punto Fijo No. 16, Col. Torres de Lindavista, C.P. 07708 Mexico, D.F. Mexico

Abstract

Medicinal plants have long been utilized as a source of therapeutic agents in many cultures. Much of the research to date on the antibacterial and antifungical activities has been motivated by the desire to find useful compounds for specific agricultural o medicinal applications. As a result, bioassay designs and choice of bioassay species has varied tremendously, which complicates any attempt to find overall patterns in the relationship between structures and their biological activity against pathogenic microorganisms that produce disease in men and animals. The present review is an up-to-date and comprehensive analysis of the source plants, chemistry, structure–activity and mechanisms of action relationship of flavonoids isolated and identified from plants that present antimicrobial activity.

Introduction

The flavonoids, constituting one of the most numerous and widespread groups of natural plant constituents, are important to humans not only because they contribute to plant colors but also because many members are physiologically active. These lowmolecular-weight

---

[*] A version of this chapter was also published in *Beta Carotene: Dietary Sources, Cancer and Cognition,* *edited by Leiv Haugen and Terje Bjornson* published by Nova Science Publishers, Inc. It was submitted for appropriate modifications in an effort to encourage wider dissemination of research

[†] Corresponding author: E mail: rmpg@prodigy.net.mx

substances, found in all vascular plants, are phenylbenzopyrones. Over 4000 structures have been identified in plant sources, and they are categorized into several groups:

Aurones, isoflavones, chalcones, flavanones, flavones, flavonols, flavanon-3-ols, anthocyanidins flavan-3-ols, proanthocyanidins (occur as dimers, trimers, tetramers and pentamers; $R = 0$, 1, 2 or 3 flavan-3-ol structures), flavans, flavan-3,4-diols and dihydrochalcones [Harborne and Baxter, 1999].

Primarily recognized as pigments responsible for the autumnal burst of hues and the many shades of yellow, orange, and red in flowers and food, the flavonoids are found in fruits, vegetables, nuts, seeds, stems, flowers, and leaves as well as tea and wine and are important constituents of the human diet [Skibola and Smith, 2000]. They are prominent components of citrus fruits and other food sources. Flavonols (quercetin, myricetin, and kaempferol) and flavones (apigenin and luteolin) are the most common phenolics in plant-based foods. The daily intake of flavonoids in humans has been estimated to be approx 25 mg/d, a quantity that could provide pharmacologically significant concentrations in body fluids and tissues, assuming good absorption from the gastrointestinal tract [Tereschuk et al., 1997].

While a considerable number of potential uses of flavonoids have been suggested, such as the role in tanning of leather, fermentation of tea, manufacture of cocoa, flavouring of foodstuffs, and forest product industry, the preponderance of research efforts has been confined to their pharmacological properties. The broad spectrum of biological activity within the group and the multiplicity of actions displayed by certain individual members make the flavonoids one of the most intriguing class of biologically active compounds, termed as "bioflavonoids" [Skibola and Smith, 2000].

Structure–Activity Relationship for Antibacterial Activity of Flavonoids

2',4'- or 2',6'-dihydroxylation of the B ring and 5,7-dihydroxylation of the A ring in the flavanone structure was important for anti-MRSA activity [Tsuchiya et al.,1996]. Substitution at the 6 or 8 position with a long chain aliphatic group such as lavandulyl (5-methyl-2-isopropenyl-hex-4-enyl) or geranyl (trans-3,7-dimethyl-2,6-octadienyl) also enhanced activity. A recent report demonstrated that substitution with C_8 and C_{10} chains also enhanced the anti-*staphylococcal* activity of flavonoids belonging to the flavan-3-ol class [Stapleton et al., 2004]. 5-hydroxyflavanones and 5-hydroxyisoflavanones with one, two or three additional hydroxyl groups at the 7, 2' and 4' positions inhibited the growth of *Streptococcus mutans* and *Streptococcus sobrinus*. 5-hydroxyflavones and 5-hydroxyisoflavones with additional hydroxyl groups at the 7 and 4' positions did not exhibit this inhibitory activity [Osawa et al.,1992]. However, when examined two isoflavones with hydroxyl groups at the 5, 2' and 4' positions using an agar dilution assay, intensive inhibitory activity was detected against a wide range of *streptococcal* species [Sato et al., 1996]. This may suggest that hydroxylation at position 2' is important for activity.

The hydroxyl groups at the 2' position are important for the anti-*staphylococcal* activity of flavanones and flavones [Tsuchiya et al., 1996]. Methoxy groups were reported to drastically decrease the antibacterial activity of flavonoids [Waage and Hedin,1985]. The importance of hydroxylation at the 2' position for antibacterial activity of chalcones is supported by earlier work from Sato and colleagues, who found that 2,4,2'-trihydroxy-5'-methylchalcone and 2,4,2'-trihydroxychalcone inhibited the growth of 15 strains of cariogenic *streptococci* [Sato et al., 1997].

Hydroxylation occurs at the C-5, C- 7 and C-2', C-4' positions in antibacterial-active flavanones, whereas this pattern is absent for the nonactive species, while the presence of methoxy groups diminishes the potential to inhibit bacterial growth. It was also found that substitution of a lipophilic functional group (e.g., geranyl) at position 6 or 8 increased the resultant antibacterial activity. The OH-5 group can form an intramolecular hydrogen bond with the C-4 carbonyl, and this can lead to a higher degree of electron delocalization within the molecule [Smejkal et al., 2008].

Substitution of the B ring with halogens was found to enhance antibacterial activity, with 3'-chloro, 4'-chloro and 4'-bromo analogues each being approximately twice as effective as their parent compound against *S. aureus*, and four times more active against *Enterococcus faecalis*. Also, the 2',4'-dichloro derivative exhibited a four- to eight-fold improvement in activity against *S. aureus* and a two- to four-fold improvement against *E. faecalis*. By contrast, 3-methylene-6-bromoflavanone was less potent than the parent compound, halogenation of the A ring may diminish activity [Ward et al., 1981]. In chalcones, neither fluorination nor chlorination at position 4 of the B ring is reported to affect antibacterial potency significantly [Sato et al., 1996].

Antibacterial Mechanisms of Action of Flavonoids

For centuries, preparations containing flavonoids as the principal physiologically active constituents have been used to treat human diseases. Increasingly, this class of natural products is becoming the subject of anti-infective research, and many groups have isolated and identified the structures of flavonoids possessing antifungal, antiviral and antibacterial activity. Moreover, several groups have demonstrated synergy between active flavonoids as well as between flavonoids and existing chemotherapeutics. Reports of activity in the field of antibacterial flavonoid research are widely conflicting, probably owing to inter- and intra-assay variation in susceptibility testing. However, several high-quality investigations have examined the relationship between flavonoid structure and antibacterial activity and these are in close agreement. In addition, numerous research groups have sought to elucidate the antibacterial mechanisms of action of selected flavonoids. The activity of quercetin, for example, has been at least partially attributed to inhibition of DNA gyrase. It has also been proposed that sophoraflavone G and (-)-epigallocatechin gallate inhibit cytoplasmic membrane function, and that licochalcones A and C inhibit energy metabolism. Other flavonoids whose mechanisms of action have been investigated include robinetin, myricetin, apigenin, rutin, galangin, 2,4,2'-trihydroxy-5'-methylchalcone and lonchocarpol A. These compounds represent novel leads, and future studies may allow the development of a pharmacologically acceptable antimicrobial agent or class of agents [Ghazal et al., 2006].

Phenolic compounds present in berries selectively inhibit the growth of human gastrointestinal pathogens. Especially cranberry, cloudberry, raspberry, strawberry and bilberry possess clear antimicrobial effects against e.g. *Salmonella* and *Staphylococcus*.

Complex phenolic polymers, such as ellagitannins, are strong antibacterial agents present in cloudberry, raspberry and strawberry. Berry phenolics seem to affect the growth of different bacterial species with different mechanisms. Adherence of bacteria to epithelial surfaces is a prerequisite for colonization and infection of many pathogens. Antimicrobial activity of berries may also be related to anti-adherence activity of the berries. Utilization of enzymes in berry processing increases the amount of phenolics and antimicrobial activity of the berry products. Antimicrobial berry compounds are likely to have many important applications in the future as natural antimicrobial agents for food industry as well as for medicine [Puupponen-Pimiä et al., 2005].

Inhibition of Nucleic Acid Synthesis

Mori and colleagues in a study using radioactive precursors, showed that DNA synthesis was strongly inhibited by flavonoids in *Proteus vulgaris*, whilst RNA synthesis was most affected in *S. aureus*. Flavonoids exhibiting this activity were robinetin, myricetin and (−)-epigallocatechin. Protein and lipid synthesis were also affected but to a lesser extent. The authors suggested that the B ring of the flavonoids may play a role in intercalation or hydrogen bonding with the stacking of nucleic acid bases and that this may explain the inhibitory action on DNA and RNA synthesis [Mori et al., 1987].

Ohemeng et al., were estudied varying structure for inhibitory activity against *Escherichia coli* DNA gyrase, and for antibacterial activity against *Staphylococcus epidermidis*, *S. aureus*, *E. coli*, *S. typhimurium* and *Stenotrophomonas maltophilia* [Ohemeng et al., 1993]. It was found that *E. coli* DNA gyrase was inhibited to different extents by some flavonoids, including quercetin, apigenin and 3,6,7,3',4'-pentahydroxyflavone. Interestingly, with the exception of 7,8-dihydroxyflavone, enzyme inhibition was limited to those compounds with B-ring hydroxylation [Hilliard et al., 1995]. However, since the level of antibacterial activity and enzyme inhibition did not always correlate, they also suggested that other mechanisms were involved [Ohemeng et al., 1993].

More recently, reported that quercetin binds to the GyrB subunit of *E. coli* DNA gyrase and inhibits the enzyme's ATPase activity [Plaper et al., 2003]. Enzyme binding was demonstrated by isolating *E. coli* DNA gyrase and measuring quercetin fluorescence in the presence and absence of the gyrase subunits. The flavonoid-binding site was postulated to overlap with those of ATP and novobiocin, since addition of these compounds interfered with quercetin fluorescence. Inhibition of GyrB ATPase activity by quercetin was also demonstrated in a coupled ATPase assay. Thus supports the suggestion that quercetin's antibacterial activity against *E. coli* may be at least partially attributable to inhibition of DNA gyrase [Plaper et al., 2003].

Bernard and co-workers found that the glycosylated rutin was inhibitor of type II topoisomerase, [Bernard et al., 1997]. This compound exhibited antibacterial activity against a permeable *E. coli* strain (a strain into which the *envA1* allele had been incorporated). Using enzyme assays and a technique known as the SOS chromotest, it was shown that rutin selectively promoted *E. coli* topoisomerase IV-dependent DNA cleavage, inhibited topoisomerase IV-dependent decatenation activity and induced the SOS response of the *E. coli* strain. The group suggested that since topoisomerase IV is essential for cell survival, the rutin-induced topoisomerase IV-mediated DNA cleavage leads to an SOS response and growth inhibition of *E. coli* cells [Normark et al., 1969].

Inhibition of Cytoplasmic Membrane Function

Recently reported attempts to elucidate the mechanism of action of flavanones in the activity of sophoraflavanone G on membrane fluidity studied using liposomal model membranes and compared with the less active flavanone naringenin, which lacks 8-lavandulyl and 2'-hydroxyl groups. At concentrations corresponding to the MIC values, sophoraflavanone G was shown to increase fluorescence polarisation of the liposomes significantly. These increases indicated an alteration of membrane fluidity in hydrophilic and hydrophobic regions, suggesting that sophoraflavanone G reduced the fluidity of outer and inner layers of membranes. Naringenin also exhibited a membrane effect but at much higher concentrations. This correlation between antibacterial activity and membrane interference was suggested to support the theory that sophoraflavanone G demonstrates antibacterial activity by reducing membrane fluidity of bacterial cells [Tsuchiya and Iinuma. 2000].

(−)-epigallocatechin gallate, a strongly antibacterial catechin found in green tea. Liposomes were used as model bacterial membranes, and it was shown that epigallocatechin gallate induced leakage of small molecules from the intraliposomal space. Aggregation was also noted in liposomes treated with the compound. Catechins may perturb the lipid bilayers by directly penetrating them and disrupting the barrier function. Alternatively, catechins may cause membrane fusion, a process that results in leakage of intramembranous materials and aggregation. Interestingly, was demonstrated that leakage induced by epigallocatechin gallate was significantly lower when liposome membranes were prepared containing negatively charged lipids. It was therefore suggested that the low catechin susceptibility of Gram-negative bacteria may be at least partially attributable to the presence of lipopolysaccharide acting as a barrier [Ikigai et al., 1993].

3-O-acyl-(-)-epicatechins and 3-O-acyl-(+)-catechins possessing various aromatic groups and aliphatic chains of varying length from C4 to C16 for increasing lipophilicity were synthesized and tested for antimicrobial activities against Gram-positive, Gram-negative bacteria and fungi. The (-)-epicatechin and (+)-catechin derivatives comprised of aromatic groups increased activity and derivatives with acyl chain groups of carbon atoms in the close vicinity of C8 to C10 showed strong antimicrobial activity (MIC = 2-8 µg/ml) against Gram-positive bacteria and weak activity against fungi. However, the activity decreased when the carbon chain length of the substituents was too short (C4 to C6) or too long (C16). These results suggest that the presence of lipophilic substituents with moderate sizes might be crucial for the optimal antimicrobial activity [Park et al., 2004].

Stapleton et al., found that substitution with C_8 and C_{10} chains increased the antibacterial activity of selected flavan-3-ols (catechins). The group went on to show that cells of an MRSA clinical isolate treated with (−)-epicatechin gallate and 3-O-octanoyl-(+)-catechin, respectively, exhibited moderately and highly increased levels of labelling with the selectively permeable fluorescent stain propidium iodide. In addition, when *S. aureus* cells were grown in the presence of either (−)-epicatechin gallate or 3-O-octanoyl-(−)-epicatechin and examined by transmission electron microscopy, they were shown to form pseudomulticellular aggregates [Stapleton et al., 2004]. It has also been demonstrated by Sato and colleagues that the chalcone 2,4,2'-trihydroxy-5'-methylchalcone induces leakage of 260 nm absorbing substances from *S. mutans*. This observation generally indicates leakage of intracellular material such as nucleotide, and the authors suggested that 2,4,2'-trihydroxy-5'-methylchalcone exerts its antibacterial effect by changing the permeability of the cellular membrane and damaging membrane function [Sato et al., 1997]. In addition, the effect of galangin upon cytoplasmic integrity in *S. aureus* has been investigated by measuring loss of internal potassium. Galangin induces cytoplasmic membrane damage and potassium leakage. Whether galangin damages the membrane directly, or indirectly as a result of autolysis or cell wall damage and osmotic lysis, remains to be established however [Sato et al., 1997].

Quercetin and naringenin caused an increase in permeability of the inner bacterial membrane and a dissipation of the membrane potential. The electrochemical gradient of protons across the membrane is essential for bacteria to maintain capacity for ATP synthesis, membrane transport and motility [Mirzoeva et al., 1997]. These flavonoids significantly inhibited bacterial motility, providing further evidence that the proton motive force is disrupted. Bacterial motility and chemotaxis are thought to be important in virulence as they guide bacteria to their sites of adherence and invasion. The cytoplasmic membrane activity detected for quercetin may represent one of the additional mechanisms of antibacterial action that was suspected to be present among the seven DNA gyrase-inhibiting flavonoid compounds tested by Ohemeng and colleagues [Ohemeng et al., 1993].

Inhibition of Rnergy Metabolism

Licochalcone A and C isolated from the roots of *Glycyrrhiza inflata* demonstrated inhibitory activity against *S. aureus* and *Micrococcus luteus* but not against *E. coli*, and in preliminary tests licochalcone A inhibited incorporation of radioactive precursors into macromolecules (DNA, RNA and protein). Licochalcones may be interfering with energy metabolism in a similar way to respiratory-inhibiting antibiotics, since energy is required for active uptake of various metabolites and for biosynthesis of macromolecules. Interestingly, the licochalcones were found to inhibit strongly oxygen consumption in *M. luteus* and *S. aureus* but not in *E. coli*, which correlated well with the observed spectrum of antibacterial activity. Licochalcones A and C inhibited NADH-cytochrome *c* reductase, but not cytochrome *c* oxidase or NADH-CoQ reductase. It was therefore suggested that the inhibition site of these retrochalcones was between CoQ and cytochrome *c* in the bacterial respiratory electron transport chain [Haraguchi et al., 1998].

Flavonoids: Occurrence, Activity and Structure

Found in the root bark of *Erythrina abyssinica* (Leguminosae). The antibacterial activity of each compound is moderate against *Bacillus subtilis* [Taniguchi and Kubo, 1993].

Abyssinone IV

Abyssinone V

Abyssinone VI

Abyssinone III

Amentoflavone

Found in *Podocarpus montanus* (Podocarpaceae). It shows antifungal activity against *Botrytis cinerea* and *Trichoderma glaucum* [Harborne and Baxter 1999].

Apiforol

Apigeninidin

Found in in seeds of *Sorghum* spp. (Graminae), inhibited the growth of *Fusarium oxysporum, Gibberella zeae. Gliocladium roseum* and *Alternaria solani* [Schutt and Netzly, 1991].

Artocarpin

Artocarpesin

Artocarpin and artocarpesin isolated from methanolic extract from *Artocarpus heterophyllus* Lam (Moraceae) showed completely inhibited the growth of primary cariogenic bacteria at 3.13-12.5 µg/ml. They also exhibited the growth inhibitory effects on plaque-forming *Streptococci*. These phytochemical isoprenylflavones would be potent compounds for the prevention of dental caries [Satoa et al., 1996].

Betagarin

Induced as a phytoalexin in sugar beet, *Beta vulgaris* (Chenopodiaceae), has antifungal activity [Saini and Ghosal, 1984].

Biochanin A

The prenylated isoflavone biochanin A, was obtained from *Swartzia polyphylla* A. DC. (Leguminosae) has antibacterial activity with activity on the protein kinase C with $IC_{50} < 50$ µg/ml [Dubois and Sneden, 1995].

Bolucarpan A

Bolucarpan B

Bolucarpan C

Bolucarpan D   Bolusanthin II   Bolusanthin III

Bolusanthin IV   Isogancaonin C

Bolusanthus spedosus (Fabaceae), commonly called Tree Wisteria, is a monotypic and endemic tree in subtropical Southern Africa. The root infusion is used as an emetic while the dried inner bark is used to treat tuberculosis and relieve abdominal pains. These flavonoids were isolated from the root wood of *B. speciosus*. The compounds showed strong antimicrobial activity against *Escherichia coli, Bacillus subtilis, Staphylococcus aureus* and *Candida mycoderma*. The isolated also showed moderate to strong radical scavenging properties against DPPH radical [Erasto et al., 2002). The isoflavanones bolusanthin II, and pterocarpan showed highest activity against Gram-positive bacteria. It seems activity here is enhanced by the presence of prenyl groups at positions 6 or 8 in the A ring and 3' or 5' in B ring. It seems also that if there is only one prenyl unit and it is in in B ring, activity is somewhat reduced. The activity of isoflavanones against Gram-negative bacteria requires a free hydroxy at position 4' (and or 3') and a prenyl group at either position 3' or 5', while that against fungi require a prenyl at position 6 or 8 in A ring and a prenyl at position 3' or 5 in B ring. The pterocarpans bolucarpan A-D, only showed moderate to weak antifungal activity [Bojasel et al., 2002].

Broussonin C   Broussonin D

Found in *Broussonetia papyriferae* (Moraceae). 7,4´-Dihydroxyflavan has fungitoxic activity against *Botrytis cinerea*. It shows antibacterial activity against plant pathogens such as *Corynobacterium betae* and *C. fascians*. Broussonin C formed as a phytoalexin of *Broussonetia papyrifera* (Moraceae), has antifungal activity [Dewick, 1988].

Cajanin   Cajanol

Induces as a phytoalexin in *Cajanus cajan* (Leguminosae). It has antifungal activity [Ingham, 1983].

Catechin

(+/-)-Catechin is a potent phytotoxin, with the phytotoxicity due entirely to the (-)-catechin enantiomer has antibacterial and antifungal activities. Tetramethoxy, pentaacetoxy, and cyclic derivatives of (+/-)-catechin retained phytotoxicity. The results indicate that antioxidant properties of catechins are not a determining factor for phytotoxicity. A similar conclusion was reached for the antimicrobial properties. *Centaurea maculosa* or spotted knapweed (Asteraceae) exudes (+/-)-catechin from its roots, but the flavanol is not re-absorbed and hence the weed is not affected. The combination of phytotoxicity and antimicrobial activity, (+/-)-catechin could be a useful natural herbicide and antimicrobial [Veluri et al., 2004].

Chalconaringenin

Occurs in *Helichrysum odoratissimum* (Asteraceae), have activity against *Bacillus subtilis* and *Staphylococcus aureus* [Puyvelde et al., 1989].

Trichitia catigua A. Juss. (Meliaceae) is a tree widely distributed in Brazil and commonly known as "Catuaba". Its bark has been used in popular medicine as physical and mental tonic and especially as a sexual stimulant. A mixture of flavalignan cinchonains Ia and Ib was isolated from the bark of *T. catigua*, which exhibited antibacterial activity against *Bacillus cereus*, *Escherichia coli*, *Pseudomonas aeruginosa* and *Staphylococcus aureus* [Pizzolattia et al., 2002].

Cinchonain Ia

Cinchonain Ib

Coluteol

Colutequinone B

Coluteol and Colutequinone B, have antifungal activity against *Candida albicans*. These isoflavonoids were isolated from *Colutea arborescens* L. var. arborescens (Leguminosae), [Grosvenor and Gray 1998].

Crotmadine

Crotmarine

Found in the leaves and stems of *Crotolaria madurensis* R. Wight (Leguminosae), an ornamental shrub that grows in the Nilgiris and Madura hill. Both compounds exhibitit antifungal activity *against Trichophyton mentagrophytes* [Bhakuni and Chaturvedi, 1984].

Daidzein

Occurs in *Ulex europaeus* (Leguminosae) It has antifungal activity [Ingham, 1983].

Desmodianone A

Desmodianone B

Desmodianone C

Pure isoflavones maintained the biological activity shown in the extracts of *Desmodium canum* (Leguminosae). Isoflavones showed antimicrobial activity against *Bacillus subtilis, Staphylococcus aureus, Mycobacterium smegmatis, Streptococcus faecalis, Escherichia coli* and *Candida albicans* at concentration of 1-100 µg/ml [Monache et al., 1996].

7,4′-Dihydroxy-8-methylflavan

Found in the resin of the dragon tree, *Dracaena draco* (Agavaceae) has activity against *Botrytis cinerea, Corynobacterium betae* and *C. fascians* [Saini and Ghosal, 1984].

2(S)-5′-(1′′′, 1′′′-Dimethylallyl)-8-(3′′,3′′-dimethylallyl)-2′,4′,5,7-tetrahydroxyflavanone

2(S)-5'-(1''', 1'''-Dimethylallyl)-8-(3'',3''-dimethylallyl)-2'methoxy-,4',5,7-trihydroxy flavanone

5'-(1''', 1'''-Dimethylallyl)-8-(3'',3''-dimethylallyl)-2',4',5,7-tretrahydroxyflavone

Found in *Dalea scandens* var. paucifolia (Fabaceae). All three compounds showed significant activity against both methicillin-susceptible and methicillin-resistant *Staphylococcus aureus* [Nanayakkara et al., 2002].

(-)-(2S)-5,3'-Dihydroxy-4'-methoxy-6'',6''-dimethylchromeno-(7,8,2'',3'')-flavanone

5,7-Dihydroxy-2'-methoxy-3',4'- methylenedioxyisoflavanone

Feronia limonia Swingle (Rutaceae) which is widely distributed throughout Bangladesh, India, Ceylon and Java. The fruits of the plant are edible and considered to be a stomachic, astringent, diuretic, cardiotonic and tonic to the liver and lungs. Pyranoflavanone possess antimicrobial properties against both gram positive and gram negative bacteria,

Staphylococcus aureus, Escherichia coli, Enterobacter cloacae and *Klebsiella erogenes* with a MICs in the range 25-100 μg/ml but did not show any antifungal activity against *Aspergillus niger*, and *Candida albicans* [Rahman and Gray 2002].

4',5,-Dihydroxy-2',3'-dimethoxy-7-(5-hydroxyoxychromen-7yl)-isoflavanone

Isoflavanones were isolated from *Uraria picta* (Papilionaceae). The minimum inhibitory concentrations (MIC) for these compounds were found to be in the range of 12.5-200 μg/ml against bacteria both Gram positive and Gram negative (*Proteus vulgaris, Staphylococcus aureus, Escherichia coli*) and fungi (*Aspergillus niger* and *Candida albicans*) [Rahman et al., 2007].

Erioschalcone A

Erioschalcone B

Isoluteolin

Erioschalcones A and B were active against, *Bacillus megaterium, Escherichia coli, Chlorella fusca* and *Microbotryum violaceum*. Quercetin and isoluteolin were only active against the green alga, *Chlorella fusca*. The dihydrochalcone erioschalcone B showed the greatest activity (13 mm), against the fungal *Microbotryum violaceum*, whereas erioschalcone A was most active against the Gram-negative bacterium, *Escherichia coli* (10 mm). Moreover, the two secondary metabolites both inhibited *Chlorella fusca*. It would appear that the prenyl group present in the A ring is presumably responsible for the significant antimicrobial activity of erioschalcones A and B [Awouafack et al., 2008]. 1446

Eriotrichin B

Eriotrichin B triacetate

Found in the root bark of *Erythrina eriotricha* (Leguminosae), showed antimicrobial activity [Nkengfack et al., 1995].

Epicatechin

Epigallocatechin

Epigallocatechin-3-gallate

Catechin, epicatechin and epicatechingallate were isolated from the stem bark of *Okoubaka aubrevillei* Rinde (Malpighiaceae), showed antibacterial activity (Wagner et al., 1985). Epigallocatechin also was found in *Elaeagnus glabra* (Simaroubaceae). It inhibited DNA synthesis in *Proteus vulgaris* and *Staphylococcus aureus* [Mori et al., 1987a]. (−)-epigallocatechin gallate, a strongly antibacterial catechin found in green tea. Catechins (flavan-3-ols) are a group of flavonoids that appear to have greater activity against Gram-positive than Gram-negative bacteria. Clinical isolates of Helicobacter *pylori*, including 19 isolates highly resistant to metronidazole (MTZ) and/or clarithromycin (CLR), were used to determine *in vitro* sensitivity to tea catechins. The MIC90 of both epigallocatechin gallate (EGCg) and epicatechin gallate (ECg) was 100 μg/ml. Highly antibiotic-resistant clinical isolates showed a similar sensitivity to both EGCg and ECg. These results indicate that EGCg may be a valuable therapeutic agent against *H. pylori* infection [Yanagawa et al., 2003].

Green tea catechins, such as epigallocatechin gallate (EGCg), may be one of the potential agents in treating of pneumonia in immunocompromised due to its possible potential immunomodulatory as well as antimicrobial activity. The studies by us showed that EGCg enhanced the *in vitro* resistance of alveolar macrophages to *Legionella pneumophila* infection by selective immunomodulatory effects on cytokine formation [Yamamoto et al., 2004].

Flemiflavanone D

Flemiflavanone D, was found in *Flemingia stricta* L. (Palmaceae) showed antimicrobial activity. [Harbone, 1989].

7-Galactoside-aromadendrin

Occurs in *Eucalyptus* spp (Myrtaceae), together with aromadendrin has antimicrobial activity against Gram negative bacteria, *Kliebsiella pneumoniae,* and against the *fungus Microsporum* gypseum [Nomura, 1988].

Galangin

Galangin constituent of Galanga root (*Alpinia officinarum*, Zingiberaceae) causes bacterial cells to clump together may implicate the cytoplasmic membrane as a target site for this compound's activity. More importantly, this observation indicates that decreases in *Staphylococcus aureus* numbers detected in time-kill and minimum bactericidal concentration assays [Cushnie et al., 2007].

Glabranin

Glepidotin A

Glepidotin B

These dehydroflavonols together with pinocembrin were isolated from Glycyrrhiza lepidota (Leguminosae), showed antimicrobial activity against Staphylococcus aureus, Mycobacterium smegmatis, Escherichia coli, Salmonella gallinarum, Kliebsiella pneumoniae and Candida albican [Mitscher et al., 1983].

7-O-β-Glucosyluteolin

The flavonoid 7-O-β-glucosyluteolin is largely responsible for the modest antimicrobial activity observed in the water-soluble extracts from *Lomatium dissectum* Nutt (Apiaceae); 0.5 mg/disk elicited a 3-mm zone of inhibition toward *Xanthomonas campestris*, a Gram-negative plant pathogen [VanWagenen et al., 1988].

Induces as a phytoalexin in *Ferreirea spectabilis* (Leguminosae). It has anti- fungal activity [Ingham, 1983].

Homoferreirin

Honyucitrin

Found in *Citrus grandis* Osbeck (Rutaceae) possess antibacterial activity [Shung et al., 1988].

5-Hydroxy-7,4′-dimethoxyflavone

Found in *Jatropha podagrica* (Euphorbiaceae), shown antibacterial activity [Odebiyi, 1985].

7-Hydroxyflavan

Found in the resin of the dragon tree, *Narcissus pseudonarcissus* (Amary llidaceae) has activity against *Botrytis cinerea, Corynobacterium betae* and *C. fascians* [Saini and Ghosal, 1984].

Hyperbrasilone

Found in *Hypericum brasiliense* (Guttiferae), showed antifungal activity [Rocha et al., 1994].

Isohamnetin-3-O-rutinoside

Found in *Artemia sublessin-giana* (Compositae) shown antibacterial activity [Tan et al., 1999].

Iryantherin K   Iryantherin L

Iryanthera megistophylla A. C. Sm. is in the Myristicaceae, a family rich in flavonoids and lignans. Amazonian natives using some *Iryanthera* species for medicinal healing. The crushed leaves of some species have been used to treat seriously infected wounds, and the latex of the bark has been mixed with water for the treatment of gastric infections. MIC against *Staphylococcus aureus* gave values of 50 µg/ml for iryantherin K and 100 µg/ml for iryantherin L [Ming et al., 2002].

Kaempferol 3-glucoside

Kaempferol 3-diglucoside

Were isolated from *Solenostemma argel* (Del). (Asclepiadaceae). These were active against *Candida albicans, Aspergillus spp. A. humicola, A. niger* and *A. sulphureous* [Abd-El-Hady and Ouf, 1993].

Kaempferol 3-(2,4-di-E-*p*-coumaroyl-rhamnoside)

Found in *Pentachondra pumila* (Epacridaceae) is active against multiresistant *Staphylococcus aureus* [Bloor, 1995].

Kaempferide-3-O-β-D-glucopyranosyl-(1→2)-O-[α-l-rhamnopyranosyl-(1→6)-]- β-D-glucopyranoside

Flavonoid occurs in *Dianthus caryophyllus* exhibited a good fungitoxic activity towards *Fusarium oxysporum* f. sp. dianthi conidia germination. Its inhibitory activity is statistically appreciable, at 50 and 100 μM on potato dextrose liquid medium [Curir, et al., 2001] .

Lotisoflavan

Induces as a phytoalexin in *Lotus angustissimus* and *L. edulis* (Leguminosae). It has anti-fungal activity [Dewick, 1988].

6,8-Di-C-methylluteolin 7-methyl ether

6-C-Methylluteolin 7-methyl ether,

Two C-methyl flavonoids, were isolated from a commercially available sample of the roots of *Hydrastis Canadensis* (Ranunculaceae). These compounds showed weaker activity against test bacteria, with MICs ranging from 250 μg/mL to >500 μg/mL. It has been reported that 5-methoxy-hydnocarpin, 5-methoxyhydnocarpin-D and silybin exhibited synergistic growth inhibitory effect against *Staphylococcus aureus* when combined with berberine. In this study, an additive effect was observed for *S. mutans* when 6,8-Di-C-methylluteolin 7-methyl ether was used in combination with berberine. The MIC of berberine alone was 125 μg/mL, compared with 62.5 μg/mL in combination with this compound. The present data suggest that it may affect cell wall components such as an efflux system to potentiate the effect of berberine [Donnelly and Sheridan, 1988].

Mucronulatol

Occurs in the wood of *Machaerium mucrunulatum* (Leguminosae), is induced as a phytoalexin, has antifungal activity [Donnelly and Sheridan, 1988].

Induced as a phytoalexin in the cotyledons of sweet pea, *Lathyrus odoratus* (Leguminosae), using the fungus *Phytophthora megasperma* var. Sojae as elicitor [Harbone and Baxter, 1993].

Odoratol

Petalostemumol   Petalostemumol G

Found in *Petalostemum purpureum* (Fabaceae), exhibited activity against Staphylococcus aureus, Bacillus subtilis, Trichophyton mentagrophytes, Mycobacterium intracellulare, Cryptococcus neoformans and Candida albicans (MIC 6.25-12.5 μg/ml), (Hufford et al., 1993). Petalostemumol the most active of the compounds isolated, showed good activity against the Gram-positive bacteria S. aureus and B. subtilis, as well as moderate activity against the Gram-negative bacterium, Escherichia coli. Petalostemumol showed only moderate activity against Candida albicans and marginal activity against Cryptococcus neoformans.

Pilosanol A

Pilosanol B

Pilosanol C

Agrimonia pilosa ledeb (Rosaceae) is widely distributed in Asia. The whole plants have been used as an antihaemorrhagic, anthelmintic and anti-inflammatory agent in Chinese herbal medicine. Several chemical investigations of this plant resulted in the isolation pilosanol A , pilosanol B and pilosanol C which show antibacterial against at concentration of 100 μg/disk (8 mm inhibition) [Kasai et al., 1992].

Pinocembrin chalcone

Pinocembrin

Found in *Helichrysum trilineatum* (Asteraceae), shown antibacterial activity against *Staphylococcus aureus* [Bremner et al., 1998].

Procyanidin

The antibacterial activity of procyanidin isolated from *Machaerium floribundum* (Leguminosae) against *P. maltophilia* and *E. cloacae* was compared with that of a condensed tannin obtained from cotton, *Gossypium hirsulum*, cyanidin chloride, (+)-catechin, and (-)-epicatechin. The bioassay results show that the procyanidin from *M. floribundum* inhibited the growth of *Pseudomonas mallophilia*, but not that of *Enterobacter cloacae*, while the cotton proanthocyanidin inhibited the growth of both bacteria. The cotton proanthocya-nidin was a group of polymers with molecular weights ranging from 1500 to 6000, a prodelphinidin: procyanidin ratio of from 1.8 to 3.7, and the stereochemistry of the heterocyclic ring system was primarily *cis*. The differences in the activities of the two proanthocyanidins may be attributed to their structural differences. Cyanidin did not inhibit the growth of either of the two bacteria, while the catechins showed activity against both bacteria [Waage et al., 1984].

Quercetagetin-7-arabinosyl-galactoside

The leaves of *Tagetes minuta* (Asteraceae) showed several degrees of antimicrobial activity against Gram positive and Gram negative microorganisms. The major component of the extract: quercetagetin-7-arabinosyl-galactoside, showed significant antimicrobial activity on *Lactobacillus, Zymomonas* and *Saccharomices* species [Tereschuk et al., 1997].

Remangiflavanone A

Remangiflavanone B

These antimicrobial flavanones from methanolic extract of *Physena madagascariensis* (Cappa raceae), were bacteriocidal against *Staphylococcus aureus, Staphylococcus epidermidis* and *Enterococcus* sp. Remangiflavanone B was also bacteriocidal against *Listeria monocytogenes*, while remangiflavanone A was found to be bacteriostatic against this microorganism. In general, remangiflavanone B was slightly more potent than A, with minimum effective concentrations (MECs) as low as 4 μM against *S. aureus, S. epidermidis, and Enterococcus* sp. [Deng et al., 2000].

Sativan

Occurs in the seeds of *Derris amazonica* (Leguminosae), and is induced as a phytoalexin, in some Lotus has antifungal activity [Harbone, 1989].

Sigmoidin B

Occurs in *Erythrina berteroana* Urb. (Leguminosae) is antifungal against *Cladosporium cucurmerinum* in a TLC bioassay at a minimum concentration of 2 μg [Maillard et al., 1987].

Silybin   Silymarin II

Flavonoids isolated from fruits of *Silybum marianum*, Asteraceae. Silybin has a potent antibacterial activity, more potent than silymarin II against gram-positive bacteria without hemolytic activity, whereas it has no antimicrobial activity against gram-negative bacteria and fungi. Silybin inhibited RNA and protein synthesis on gram-positive bacteria (Lee et al., 2003).

Sinensetin

Found in the peel of *Citrus sinensis* (Rutaceae). It has antifungal activity [Harbone, 1988].

Sophoraflavanone G (5,7,2′,4′-tetrahydroxy-8-lavandulyl-flavanone) found in *Shopora exigua* (Leguminosae) completely inhibited the growth of 21 strain of methicillin-resistant *Staphylococcus aureus* (MRSA) at concentrations of 3.13-6.25 μg/ml [Sato et al., 1995].

Sophoraflavanone G

Sulcatone A

Ouratea sulcata Van Tiegh (ex Keay), which belongs to the plant family Ochnaceae is widely distributed in West and Central Africa. Extracts of leaves, alone or combined with other plants, are used in many African countries, including Cameroon, Nigeria, Congo and Gabon to treat human ailments such as upper respiratory tract infections, dysentery, diarrhoea and toothache. Plants in this family are known to be rich in biflavonoids. Investigation of the aerial parts of *Ouratea sulcata* led to the isolation of a biflavonoid named sulcatone A. This compound showed antimicrobial activity against Gram positive (*Staphylococcus aureus*, *Bacillus subtilis)*, the activities was almost equivalent to or less than those demonstrated by streptomycin. No was active (MIC > 100) against Gram negative bacterium, *E. coli* [Pegnyemb et al., 2005].

Tectorigenin

Occurs in the rhizomes of *Iris germanica* (Iridaceae), has antifungal activity [Harbone, 1989].

2′,4,4′-Tetrahydroxydihydrochalcone   2′,3′,4′,7-Tetrahydroxyisoflavone

Found in *Zollernia paraensis* (Leguminosae) showed a marked activity against *Cladisporium cucumerinum.* Dihydrochalcone also showed antimicrobial activity against two oral bacteria *Bacteroides melaninogenicus* and *Fusobacterium nucleatum* [Ferrari et al., 1983].

5,3′,4′-Trihydroxy-7-methoxyflavone-3-O-(2′′-rhamnosyl glucoside)

Two flavonoids glycosides from *Cassia occidentalis* Pods (Leguminosae), showed considerable antibiotic activity against Gram-positive organisms [Singh and Singh 1985].

5, 4′-dihydroxy-3,6,3′-trimethoxy flavone 7-O-(2′′-rhamnosylglucoside)

An activity-guided fractionation of a methanol-dichloromethane extract obtained from the aerial parts of *Eysenhardtia texana* Kunth (Fabaceae) led to the isolation of two antibacterial and antifungal flavanones. Both compounds at a concentration of 0.1 mg/ml were shown to inhibit the growth of *Staphylococcus aureus*. 4',5,7-Trihydroxy-8-methyl-6-(3-methyl-[2-butenyl])-(2S)-flavanone inhibited the growth of *Candida albicans* in an agar-gel diffusion assay. Antibacterial and antifungal activity at this concentration is typical for a variety of prenylated flavonoids [Wachter et al., 1999].

4',5,7-Trihydroxy-8-methyl-6-(3-methyl-[2-butenyl])-(2S)-flavanone

4',5, 7-Ttrihydroxy-6-methyl-8-(3-methyl-[2-butenyl])-(2S)-flavanone

3,5,7-Trihydroxyflavone-8-O-(2-methylbutyrate)

3,5,7-Trihydroxyflavone-8-O-[(Z)-2-methyl-2-butenoate]

These acyl flavonoid have been isolated from the resinous exudate of *Gnaphalium robustum* (Asteraceae) inhibited the development of *Bacillus anthracis* [Urzua and Cuadra, 1990].

4,2',4'-Trihydroxychalcone   4,2',4'-Trihydroxy-3-prenylchalcone

Occurs in *Treculia obovoidea* (Moraceae). These compounds were tested for their antimicrobial activity against Gram-positive bacteria (six species), Gram-negative bacteria (12 species) and three *Candida* species using micro-dilution methods for the determination of the minimal inhibition concentration (MIC) and the minimal microbicidal concentration (MMC). The MIC values obtained with the crude extracts varied from 78.12 to 156.251 µg/ml against 17 (80.95%) of the 21 tested microorganisms. The isolated compounds showed selective activity [Kuete et al., 2007].

2',4,4'-'Trihydroxy-3'-geranylchalcone   2',3,4,4'-Tetrahydroxy-3'-geranylchalcone

2',4',4-Trihydroxy-3'-[6-hydroxy-3, 7-dimethyl-2(E), 7-octadienyl]ch.llcone

2', 4',4-Trihydroxy-3'-[2-hydroxy- 7-methyl-3-methylene-6-octaenyl]chalcone

2'3,4,4'-Tetrahydroxy-3'-[6-hydroxy-3, 7-dimethyl-2(E), 7-octadienyl]chalcone

These chalcones were isolated from leaves of *Artocarpus nobilis* (Moraceae). All these compounds showed good fungicidal activity against *Cladosporium cadosporiodes* and high radical scavenging activity towards the 2,2'-diphenyl-1-picrylhydrazyl (DPPH) radical [Jayasinghe et al., 2004].

3-6,7-Trimetoxy,5,4´-dihydroxyflavone

This compound was identified to be responsible for the antifungal activity against *Cladosporium cucumerinum* and *Candida albicans*, was isolated from *Baccharis pedunculata* (Mill) Cabr. (Asteraceae), [Rahalison et al., 1995].

Umuhengerin

This flavonoid isolated from Lantana trifolia L. (Verbenaceae) exhibited activity against Staphylococcus aureus, (20 μg/ml), Salmonella typhimurium, (20 μg/ml), Candida tropicalis (200 μg/ml), Aspergillus niger (200 μg/ml), A. fumigatus, Trichophyton mentagro phytes (50 μg/ml), and Microsporum canis (50 μg/ml), [Rwangabo et al., 1988].

Vestitol

Occurs in the trunk of *Machaerium vestitum* (Iridaceae), has antifungal activity (Harbone, 1989).

Vestitone

Induced as a phytoalexin in the leaves of *Onobrychis viciifolia* (Leguminosae) has antifungal activity [Harbone, 1989].

2',4',4,2"-Tetrahydroxy-3'-[3"-methylbut-3"-enyl]chalcone

Isobavachalcone

Bakuchalcone

Bavachromanol

5,7,3',4'-Tetrahydroxy-6,8-diprenylisoflavone(6,8-diprenyllorobol)

Five prenylated flavonoids, were isolated from ethanol extract of the leaves of *Maclura tinctoria* (L.) Gaud (Moraceae). The inhibitory activities (IC$_{50}$) against *Candida albicans* and *Candida neofonnans* was of 0.055 and 0.015 μg/ml. respectively [Elsohlyl et al., 2001].

Wighteone

Wighteone was isolated *Neonotonia wightii* (Fabaceae) exhibited a slightly weaker antibacterial activity against these *Staphylococcus aureus* and *Enterococci foecalis* (VRE) (MICs = 6.25 µg/mL). A few anti-*Enterococci* flavonoids (flavanone, pterocarpan, pterocarpene) with one or two prenyl groups (log p = 4.8-7.2) have been reported. It is likely that anti-VRE flavonoids require one or two hydrophobic sites (isoprenoid group, methylcyclohexene ring, or benzene ring without hydroxy groups) and hydro-philic sites (hydroxy groups) [Fukai et al., 2004]

Ermanin   5-Hydroxy-3,7,4'-trimethoxyflavone

kumatakenin

These compounds were identified as the antimycobacterial principles in *Haplopappus Sonorensis* (A. Gray) S.F. Blake (Asteraceae). Ermanin was the most active compound against *Mycobacterium tuberculosis* showing 98% inhibition at 100 µg/ml, also has been reported to be antiviral, anti-inflammatory and cytotoxic activities. It is structurally related to nevadensine, a well known antimycobacterial flavone. Both flavones have similar substitution patterns with 5,7-dihydroxy and 4'-methoxy substituents, but nevadensine is additionally methoxylated at C-6 and C-8, instead of at C-3 as ermanin. Compounds 3,7,4'-trimethoxyflavone, and kumatakenin were less active against *M. tuberculosis* showing 33 and 48% at the same concentration. Though ermanin was found to be a potent cytotoxic agent against human fibrosarcoma and murine colon carcinoma cells Kumatakenin displayed low cytotoxicity against the HCT-116 cell line with an IC_{50} value of 80.9 µg/ml. Kumatakenin was reported as an antiulcer, and antiviral drug [Murillo et al., 2003].

Chrysoeriol

Eriodictyol

Hispidulin

The flavonoids hispidulin, eriodictyiol, kaempferol, quercetin, taxifolin and chrysoeriol were isolated from leaves, stems and flowers of *Centaurea floccose* (Asteraceae), showed antibacterial and antifungal activity [Negrete et al., 1987].

α,2′-Dihydroxy-4-4′-dimethoxydihydro-chalcone   2′-Hydroxy-7,4′-dimethoxyisoflavone

Found in *Virola surinamensis* (Rol.) Warb (Myristicaceae), have antifungal activity against *Cladosporium cladosporioides.* α,2'-dihydroxy-4,4'-dimethoxydihydrochalcone, biochanin A and 2'-hydroxy-7,4'-dimethoxyisoflavone were active at minimum amount of 5 μg, while the 7-hydroxyflavanone and 7-hydroxy-4'-methoxyisoflavone showed antifungal activities 10-fold higher than the positive control nystatin (10 μg) [Lopes et al., 1999].

From the roots of *Brosimopsis oblongifolia* Ducke (Moraceae) isoprenyl flavone, were isolated, that showed antimicrobial activity against *Bacillus subtilis, Staphylococcus aureus* and *Mycobacterium smergmatis*. Also showed cytotoxic activity against KB cells [Messana et al., 1987].

Cudraflavone A

Cudraflavone B

5´-Hydroxycudraflavone

Sophoraisoflavanone A

Sophoronol

Isosophoranone

Isobavachin

These flavonoids compounds are constituents of the aerial parts of Sophora tomentosa L. (Leguminosae). Showed activities against Staphylococcus aureus,Escherichia coli, Bacillus subtilis, Aspergillus Niger, Aspergillus fumigatus, Penicillium citrinum, Candida albicans and Saccharomyces sake [Komatsu et al., 1978].

Cyclokievitone

5-Deoxykievitone

Induced as a phytoalexin in *Phaseolus vulgaris* (Leguminosae). It has antifungal activity [Ingham, 1983[a]].

Kievitone and dalbergioidin induced as aphytoalexin in many Leguminosae as *Dolichos biflorus,* have antibacterial activity against *Pseudomonas, Xanthomonas* and *Achromobacter* spp. It shows antifungal activity [Dewick, 1988, Harbone, 1989].

Dalbergioidin

Kievitone

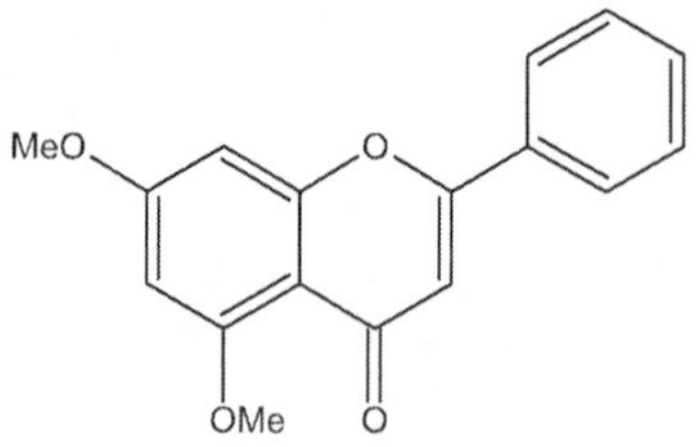

Chrysin dimethyl ether

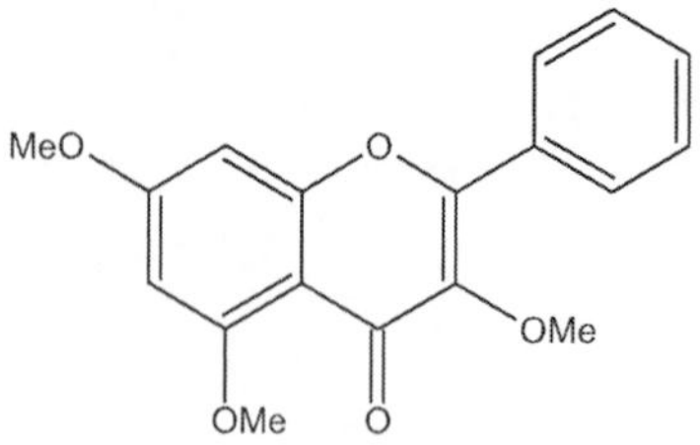

Galangin trimethyl ether

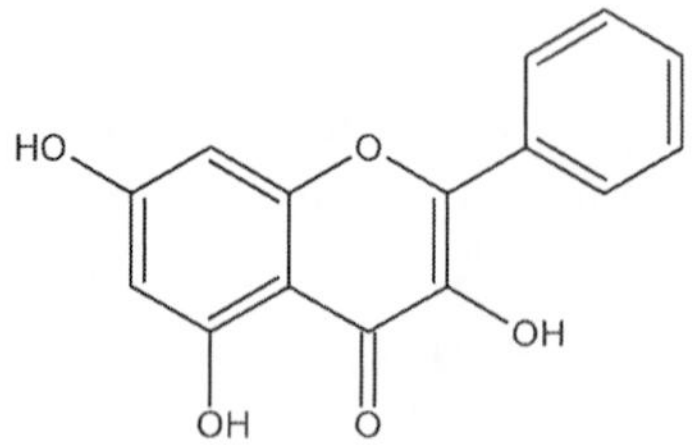

Galangin

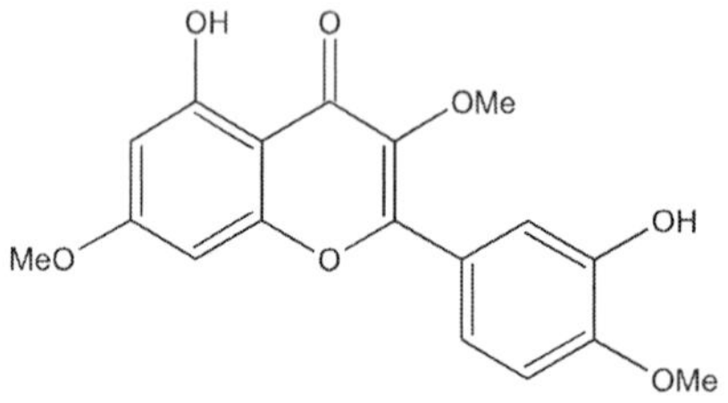

Ayanin

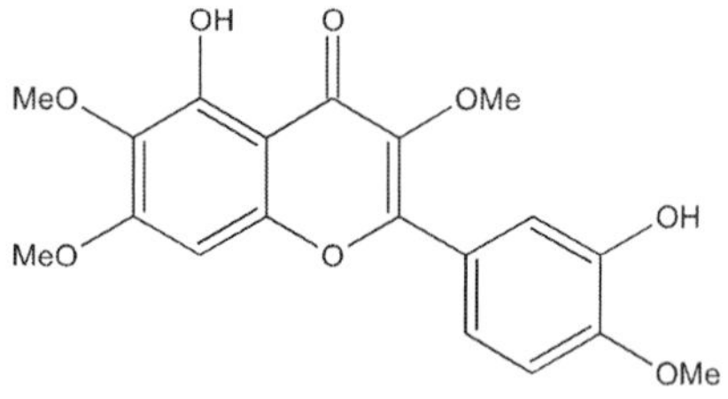

Casticin

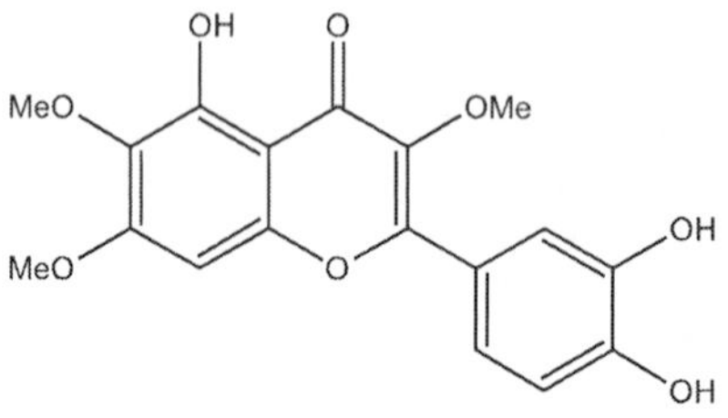

Chrysosplenol-D

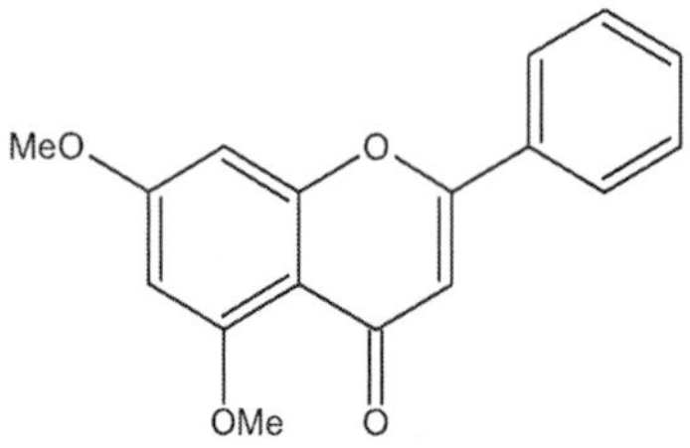

5,7-Dimethoxyflavone

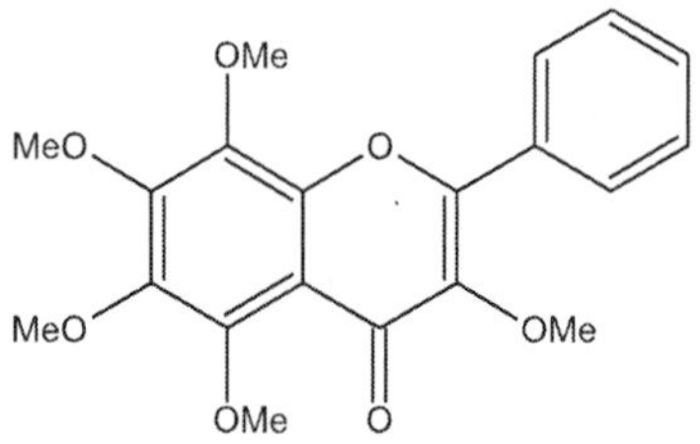

3,5,6,7,8-Pentamethoxyflavone

5,6,7-Trimethoxyflavone

3,5,7-Trimethoxyflavone

5,6,7,8-Tetramethoxyflavone

3,5,6,7-Tetramethoxyflavone

Occurs in *Helichrysum nitens* (Compositae), inhibited the growth of *Cladosporium cucumerinum* and *Deuterophoma tracheiphila* [Barberan et al., 1990].

Karanjin

Pinnatin

3′-Desmethoxy kanugin

These furanoflavones were isolated from *Pongamia glabra* (Pinata), were active against *Fusarium udum, Alternaria solani, Erysiphe polygoni* and *Ustilago tritici* [Pan et al., 1985].

Osajin   Pomiferin

Found in the fruit of *Maclura pomifera* (Moraceae) have activity against *Staphylococcus aureus* (MIC 25 µg/ml), *Escherichia coli* (MIC 12.5 µg/ml) *Salmonella gallinarum* (MIC 25 µg/ml), And *Mycobacterium smegmatis* (MIC 6.5 µg/ml) [Mahmoud, 1981].

Kaempferol   Myricetin

Quercetin

Rutin

Isoquercitrin

Quercetin, rutin, myricetin were isolated from *Desmanthus ilinoensis* (Fabaceae), showed antibacterial activity (Nicollier and Thompson, 1983). Also quercetin and kaempferol were isolated from *Peganum harmala* (Rutac eae), possess antibacterial activity [Harsh and Nag, 1984]. Butanol extract of the whole plant *Polygonum equisetiforme* showed as the major constituent quercetin. The antifungal and antibacterial activity of quercetin was compared with the antibacterial drugs gentamycin, streptomycin and ampicillin and the antifungal drug miconazole nitrate. The antifungal activity of quercetin was limited to *Candida tropicalis* and it had a narrow antibacterial spectrum of activity. However, its activities against *Enterobacter aerogenes* and *Escherichia coli* were low grade compared with ampicillin, stretomycin and gentamycin [Ghazal et al., 2006]. Isoquercitrin and rutin contribute significantly to the intensity and rango of the overall antimicrobial activity of the plant *Pelargonium radula* (Geraniaceae) (Pepeljnjak et al., 2005). Myricetin, a flavonol, inhibited ESBL-producing *Klebsiella pneumoniae* isolates at a high minimum inhibitory concentration (MIC) (MIC_{90} value 256 mg/mL), but exhibited significant synergic activity against ESBL-producing *K. pneumoniae* in separate combination with amoxicillin/clavulanate, ampicillin/sulbactam and cefoxitin. Because of the low-toxic nature of flavonoids, the combination of antibiotics and flavonoids is a potential new strategy for developing therapies for infections caused by ESBL-producing bacteria in the future [Lin et al., 2005].

7,4′-Dihydroxy-5-methoxy-flavone

4,2,4′-Trihydroxy-6′-ethoxychalcone

Quercetin-3-methyl ether

4,2,4′Trihydroxy-6-methoxychalcone

Kaempferol and quercetin (C-methylflavonols) were isolated also from *Piliostigma thonningii* (Schum.) (Caesalpiniaceae). The structure-activity relationship observed for the C-methylflavonols that the 5,7-dihydroxylation is necessary for antibacterial activity and methoxylation at C-7 significantly reduces activity, the 3′-OH may not be essential for antibacterial activity. Thus, the most active of the isolated compounds is 6-C-methylquercetin-3-methyl ether against *Staphylococcus aureus* (MIC 1.125 mM) conforms with requisite structural features [Ibewuike et al., 1997].

These flavonoids were the antimicrobial principles of the traditional medicinal plant *Achyrocline flaccida* (Compositae), [Gutkin et al., 1984].

Quercetin-3-O-glucoside

Rhamnetin-3-O-glucoside

Found in whole plant *Heterotheca camporum* (Compositae), showed antibacterial activity against bacteria (*Enterobacter cloacae* and *Pseudomonas maltophilia*), [Waage and Hedin, 1985a].

Medicarpin

Phaseollin

Pisatin

6a-Hydroxyisomedicarpin (3-methoxy-6a,9-dihydroxy

4-Hydroxydemethylmedicarpin (3,4,9-trihydroxy)

4-Hydroxymedicarpin (3,4-dihydroxy-9-methoxy)

4-Hydroxyhomopterocarpin (3,9-dimethoxy-4-hydroxy)

Pterocarpans, are characteristic of sweetclover *Melilotus alba* (Trifoleaceae) and *Trifolium pretense* L. (Trifoleaceae). Antifungal activity of compounds on mycelial growth tests indicated that medicarpin was highly inhibitory to *Helminthosporium carbonum* (ED_{50} 25 µg/ml) but much less active against *Botrytis cinerea* (ED_{50} 66 µg/ml). The latter fungus also appears to be relatively insensitive to the effects of phaseollin (ED_{50} 50µg/ml) and pisatin (ED_{50} 100 µg/ml). However, three medicarpin transformation products namely, 6a-hydroxymedicarpin, 6a-hydroxyisomedicarpin and demethylmedicarpin were essentially inactive against *B. cinerea* having ED_{50} values well in excess of 100 µg/ml. Vestitol (ED_{50} 17 µg/ml) and demethylmedicarpin (ED_{50} 50 µg/ml) were tested also against the mycelial growth of *H. carbonum* [Ingham, 1976].

(2S)-4'-Hydroxy-5,7,3'-trimethoxyflavan

(±)-5,4' -Dihydroxy -7,3'-dimethoxyflavan

(±)-3',4'-Dihydroxy-5,7-dimethoxyflavan   (±)-7,3'-Dimethoxy-4'-hydroxyflavan

(±)-7,4'-Dihydroxy-3'-methoxyflavan   (±)-5,7,3',4'-Tetrahydroxyflavanone

(±)-5,4' -Dihydroxy- 7,3'-dimethoxyflavanone   (±)-5,7,4 '-Trihydroxy -3'-methoxyflavanone

These flavonoids were isolated from *Mariscus psilostachys* (Cyperaceae) showed fungicidal activity against *Candida albicans* in the bioautographic bioassay. The minimum quantities spotted on TLC plates required to inhibit the growth of *C. albicans* were 1 μg/ml for compound (2S)-4'-Hydroxy-5,7,3'-trimethoxyflavan and 5 μg/ml for (±)-5,4' -Dihydroxy - 7,3'-dimethoxyflavan, (±)-3',4'-Dihydroxy-5,7-dimethoxyflavan, (±)-7,3'-Dimethoxy-4'-hydroxy- flavan. Compounds (±)-7,4'-Dihydroxy-3'-methoxyflavan, (±)-5,7,3',4'-Tetrahydroxyflavanone, (±)-5,4' -Dihydroxy- 7,3'-dimethoxyflavanone and (±)-5,7,4'-Trihydroxy -3'-methoxyflavanone were inactive at the limit amount of 10 μg/ml spotted on the plate.

The growth of the phytopathogenic fungus *Cladosporium cucumerinum* was inhibited by 5 μg/ml of compounds. Flavan (±)-7,3'-Dimethoxy-4'-hydroxyflavan was shown to be the most active product in the TLC bioassay with clear inhibition zones visible till 1 μg/ml [Garo et al., 1996].

Quercimeritrin   Gossypetin 8-O-rhamnoside

The flavonols glycoside together isoquercitrin and quercetin 3'-O-glucoside, were isolated from flower petals of *Gossypium arboretum* Malvaceae). These compounds showed antibacterial activity against *Pseudomonas maltophilia* and *Enterobacter cloacae* [Waage and Hedin, 1984].

2,3-Dihydroauriculatin   Auriculatin

From the root bark of *Ormosia monosperma* (Leguminosae) 10 isoflavonoids were isolated. Among these compounds only 2,3-dihydroauriculatin and auriculatin showed moderate activities against oral-microbial organisms (*Streptococcus mutans*, *Prophyromonas gingicalis* and *Actinomyces actinomycetemcomitans*) [Inuna et al., 1994].

5,7-Dihydroxy-3,8-dimethoxyflavone

Galalangin-3-methylether

Flavones isolated from Helichrysum picardii (Compositae) with a MIC of >100 µg/ml for compounds against Escherichia coli B, Salmonella LT2, Salmonella typhimurium, Proteus vulgaris, Pseudamonas aeruginosa, Citrobacter freundii, Serratia marcescens, Enterobacter aerogenes, Agrobacterium rizhogenes, Bacillus spp and Staphylococcus epidermis. Free hydroxyls at 5 and 7 positions of the flavone nucleus are necessary for antibacterial activity. The phenolic groups may interact with biological structures through hydrogen bonding and a certain degree of lipophylicity is required for the flavonoids to be active. These substances are externally located on leaf and stem surfaces, suggesting that they could act as a chemical barrier protecting plant tissues from microbial attack [Tomas-Lorente et al., 1991].

Bilobetin

4'''-O-Methylamentoflavone

7-O-Methylamentoflavone

Ginkgetin

2,3-Dihydrosciadopitysin   Sciadopitysin

Biflavones were isolated and identified from *Taxus baccata* (Taxacea) and *Ginko biloba* (Ginkgoaceae). These compounds showed antifungal activity against the fungi *Alternaria alternata, Fusarium culmorum,* and *Cladosporium oxysporum*. Bilobetin exhibited a significant antifungal activity with values of ED_{50} 14,11 and 17 μM respectively. This compound completely inhibited the growth of germinating tubes of *Cladosporium oxysporum* and *Fusarium culmorum* at a concentration 100 μM. Activity of ginkgetin and 7-O-methylamento- flavone towards *Alternaria alternata* was stronger than that of bilobetin. Moreover, slight structural changes in the cell wall of *Alternaria alternata* exposed to ginkgetin at concentration of 200 μM were observed [Krauze-Baranowskaa and Wiwart, 2003].

5,7-Dimethoxy-3',4'-methylenedioxyflavanone   Isobonducellin

2'-Hydroxy-2,3,4',6'-tetramethoxychalcone

Caesalpinia pulcherrima is used for the treatment of diarrhea and dysentery. All these compounds showved moderate to good antibacterial, activity against the gram-positive organisms *Staphylococcus aureus, Bacillus subtilis* and *Bacillus sphaericus*. Particularly isobonducellin was found to be a good antibacterial substance with an inhibition zone diameter of 11 mm at 100 μg/ml test conc. The compounds 5,7-dimethoxy-3',4'-methylenedioxyflavanone and 2'-hydroxy-2,3,4',6'-tetramethoxychalcone showed moderate activity against the gram-negative organisms. *Pseudomonas aeruginosa, Klebsiella erogenes* and *Chromobacteria violaceum*, while isobonducellin was inactive against the first two organisms and showed moderate, activity against only *Chromobacteria violaceum*. The, antifungal activity the all compounds was also moderate against the organisms, *Aspergillus niger*, and *Candida albicans* and they were inactive against *Rhizopus oryzae* [Srinivas et al., 2003].

Found in Virola surinamensis (Rol.) Warb (Myristicaceae), have antifungal activity against Cladosporium cladosporioides. Virolane and virolanol C exhibited an inhibition zone in the TLC plate at the same concentration of nystatin. ☐2'-dihydroxy-4,4'-dimethoxy-dihydrochalcone, biochanin A and 2'-hydroxy-7,4'-dimethoxyisoflavone were active at minimum amount of 5 µg, while the 7-hydroxyflavanone and 7-hydroxy-4'-methoxyisoflavone showed antifungal activities 10-fold higher than the positive control nystatin (10 µg) [Lopes et al., 1999].

α,2'-Dihydroxy-4,4'-dimethoxydihydrochalcone

7-Hydroxy-4'-methoxyisoflavone

2'-Hydroxy-7,4'-dimethoxyisoflavone

Virolanol C

Virolane

Derrisisoflavone A

Derrisisoflavone B

Derrisisoflavone C

Derrisisoflavone D

Derrisisoflavone E

Derrisisoflavone F

Erysenegalensein E

Lupalbigenin

Lupinisol A

Lupinisoflavone G   Scandinone

These diprenylisoflavones were isolated from *Derris scandens* (Leguminosae). Among the isolated compounds derrisisoflavone C, 5,7,4′-trihydroxy-6,8-diprenylisoflavone and lupalbigenin showed a relatively high activity at 250 µg/ml, against *Trichophyton mentagrophytes*, while other compounds showed lower activity at 500- 1000 µg/ml [Sekine et al., 1999].

Allolicoisoflavone A   Isopiscerythrone

Piscisoflavone A   Piscisoflavone B

These isoflavones are constituents of *Piscidia erythrina* (Leguminosae) were found be strongly antifungal when applied at 50 and 100 µg/ml against *Cladosporium herbarum* [Moriyama et al., 1992].

Quercetin-3-O-[3,4, diacetyl-α-L-rhamnopyranosyl-   Sophoronol
(1-6)-β-D-glucopyranoside]

Was isolated from aerial parts of *Tordylium apulum* (Apiaceae), are active against *Cladosporium cucumerimun,* and *Candida albicans* [Kofinas et al., 1998].

Isokurarinone   Kushecarpin A

Kushecarpin B

Kushenol A   Kushenol H

Kushenol I

Kushenol P

Kushenol Q

Kushenol R

Kushenol S

Kushenol T

Kushenol U

Kushenol X

Kuraridin

Kurarinol

Maackiain

Norkurarinone

Norkurarinol

Neokurarinol

Flavonoids from dried roots of *Sophora flavescens* Aiton (Leguminosae) were isolated. These compounds exhibited significant antiandrogen and antibacterial activities against Gram-positive bacteria *Staphylococus aureus, Propionibacterium acnes, S. epidermidis* and *Bacillus subtilis.* Minimal inhibitory concentrations (MIC) of norkurarinone, isokurarinone, norkurarinol and neokurarinol, was at concentration of 2.5-10 μg/ml. These results indicate that prenylflavanone derivatives having lavandulyl or isopentenyl moieties have potent activity, and the C-type side chain possessing a hydroxyl group reduces the antibacterial activity. A hydroxyl group at C-3 also decreased the antibacterial activity. Also, these compounds showed antibacterial activity against skin residential floras such as *S. epidermidis* and *Propionibacterium acnes* [Kuroyanagi et al., 1999].

Sakuranetin   Pectolinarigenin

Theses flavonoids, were isolated from *Hebe cupressoides* (Scrophulariaceae). pectolinarigenin is responsible for the anti-Herpes and antibacterial (against *Bacillus subtilis*) activities. Sakuranetin shown activity against *Trichophyton mentagrophytes* (Perry and Foster, 1994). Sakuranetin, showed ED_{50} against spore germination of *Pyrcularia oryzae* of 15 ppm [Kodama et al., 1992].

Licoisoflavone A   Licoisoflavone B

Lupalbigenin

Lupisoflavone

Lupinisoflavone A

Lupinisoflavone B

Lupinisoflavone C

Lupinisoflavone D

Lupinisoflavone E

Lupinisoflavone F

Luteone

Angustone A

Angustone B

Angustone C

Flavonoids found in *Lupinus albus* (Leguminosae) showed fungitoxic activity against *Cladosporium herbarum* [Tahara et al., 1984]. Isoflavonoids with antifungal activity against *Colletrotrichum gloeosporioides* and *Cladosporium cladosporioides* were isolated from the from root of *Lupinus angustifolius* Cav. (Leguminosae), [Lane et al., 1987].

Isoliquiritigenin

Isoliquiritigenin-2′-methyl ether

(2S)-7,4'-Dihydroxyflavan

(2S)-4'-Hydroxy-7-methoxyflavan

(2S)-7,3'-Dimethoxy-4'-hydroxyflavan

(25)-3',4'-Dihydroxy-7-methoxyflavan

Found in *Bauhinia Manca* (Leguminosae), these compound possess significant antifungal activity against *Botrytis cinerea, Claviceps viridis, Coprinus cinereus, Rhizoctonia solani* and *Saprolegnia asterophora* (Achenbach et al., 1988).

Aromadendrin

Dihydrokaempferide

Prunin

Taxifolin

These flavonoids together with naringenin were isolated from the wood of *Salix caprea* L. (Salicaceae), inhibited the fungi *Coniophora puteana, Sporotrichum pulverulentum* and *Trichoderma viride*. Naringenin inhibits all the fungi. Dihydrokaempferide inhibits *C. puteana*, as does aromadendrin, while taxifolin and (+)-catechin show an effect against *T. viride,* and *prunin*; has effect against *S. pulverulentum* [Malterud et al., 1985].

Isojacareubin

Sarothranol

Sarothralin

The isopentenyllated flavonol, from whole plants of *Hypericum japonicum* (Guttiferae). Their compounds exhibited antibacterial activity toward *Staphylococcus aureus*, *Bacillus cereus* and *Nocardia gardenen* with MIC 125 μg/ml [Ishiguro et al., 1993].

Dracorliodin

Dracorubin

5-Methoxy-7 –hydroxyflavan

Nordracorubin

The luridly named dragon's blood resin is principle derived from the scales of fruit belonging to *Daemonorops draco* Blume (Palmaceae). It has been used medicinally as a stimulant and astringent, especially in dentifrices and mouth washes. It has also found commercial use in varnishes and lacquers, imparting a mahogany stain to wood, and as a protectant for zinc in photoengraving and etching. These constituents showed activity against *Staphylococcus aureus* and *Mycobacterium smegmatis* [Rao et al., 1982].

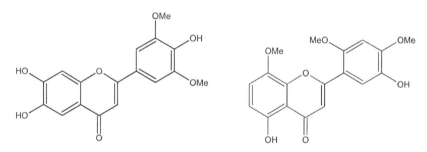

Euchrestaflavanone A	Bonannione A

Macarangaflavanone A	Macarangaflavanone B

From the dichloromethane extract of leaves of *Macaranga pleiostemona* (Euphorbiaceae) four antibacterial prenylated flavanones were isolated [Schutz et al., 1995]. Showed activity against *Escherichia coli* and *Micrococcus luteus* using a bioautographic method.

4′,6,7-Trihydroxy-3′,5′dimethoxyflavone	5,5′-Dihidroxy-2′,4′,8-trimethoxyflavone

These flavones showed antibiotic activity against *Staphylococcus aureus, Sarcina lutea, Escherichia coli,* and *Pseudomonas aeruginosa* [Zheng et al., 1996], were isolated from *Artemisia giraldii* Pam (Compositae) a species indigenous to north-weat China.

6-Prenylpinocembrin   2′,4′-Dihydroxy-5-(1′′-dimethylallyl)6- prenylpinocembrin

Found in Dalea elegans Hook (Fabaceae), exhibited activity against Bacillus subtilis, Staphylococcus aureus, Klebsiella pneumoniae, and Escherichia coli, [Ortega et al., 1996].

Isokaemferide   5,7,4'-Trihydroxy-3,8-dimethoxyflavone

5,7,4'-Trihydroxy-3,3'-dimethoxyflavone

From a hydrolysed methanolic extract from the *Psiadia trinervia* (Compositae) was isolated these flavonoids with antimicrobial activity against *C. cucumerinum* and Gram-positive bacterium *Bacillus cereus.* Ayanin and casticin at concentration of 20μg and 10 μg of chrysosplenol-D and 5,7,4'-Trihydroxy-3,8-dimethoxyflavone were sufficient to inhibit growth of *Cladosporium cucumerinum* .

Four of the isolates, 5,7,4'-Trihydroxy-3,3'-dimethoxyflavone, chrysosplenol-D, isokaemferide and 5,7,4'-Trihydroxy-3,8-dimethoxyflavone were active against *Bacillus cereus* (4 μg) [Wang et al., 1989].

Aurentiacin A   2′,4′-Dihydroxy-6′-methoxy-3′,5′-dimethylchalcone

2′,6′-Dihydroxy-4′-methoxy-3′,5′-dimethyldihydrochalcone

2'-Hydroxy-4',6'-dimethoxy-3'-methyldihydrochalcone

2',6'-Dihydroxy-4'-methoxy-3'-methyldihydrochalcone

Found in *Myrica serrata* Lamarck (Myricaceae), were actives against *Candida albicans, Cladosporium cucumerinum* and *Bacillus subtilis* [Gafner et al., 1996]. All compounds were devoid of growth inhibitory activity against *C. albicans*, chalcones 2',4'-Dihydroxy-6'-methoxy-3',5'-dimethylchalcone and aurentiacin A were active against *Cladosporium cucumerinum, Bacillus subtilis, and Escherichia coli* .

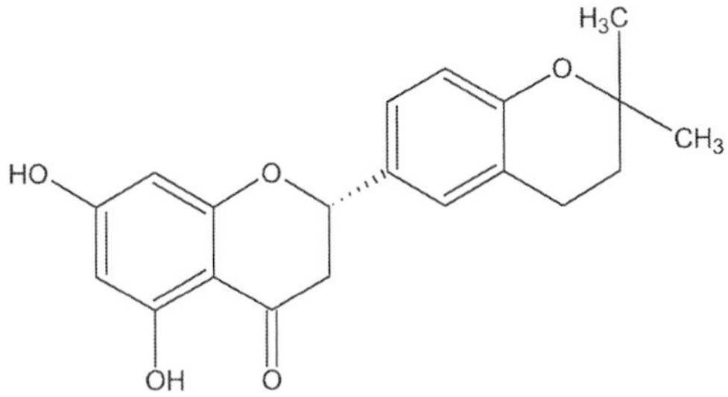

Cyclolicoflavanone

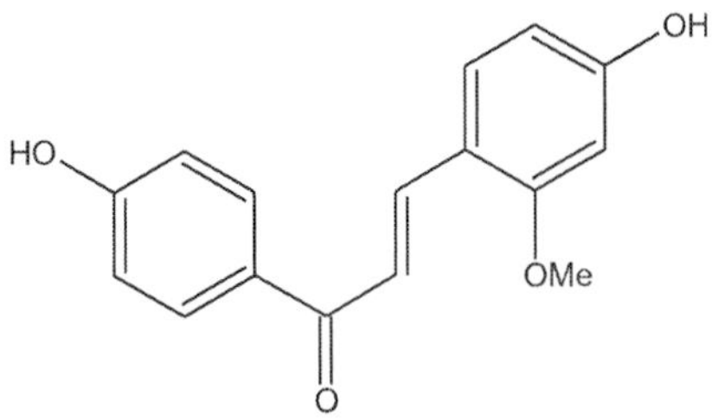

Echinatin

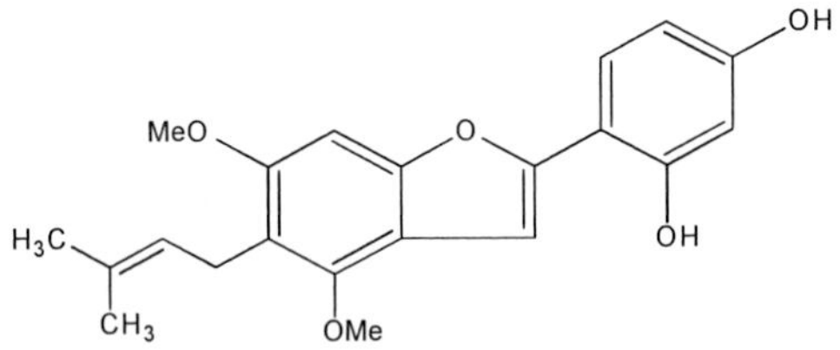

Gancaonin I

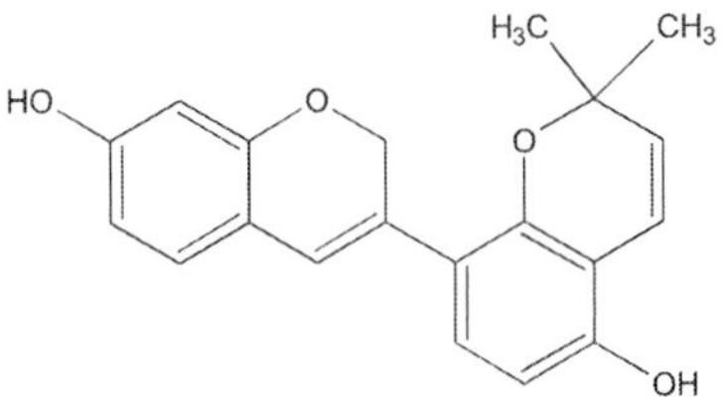

Glabrene

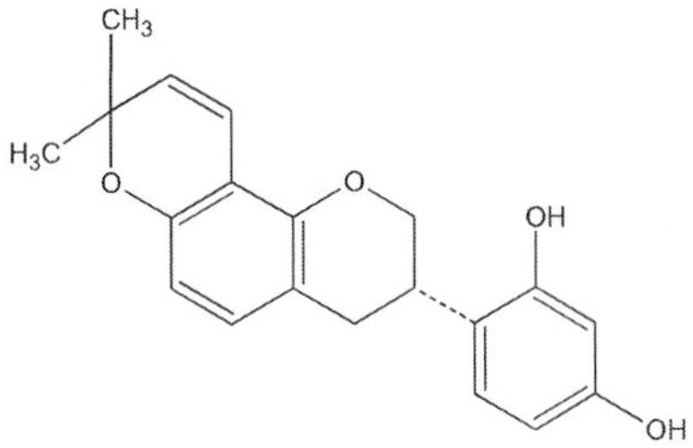

Glabridin

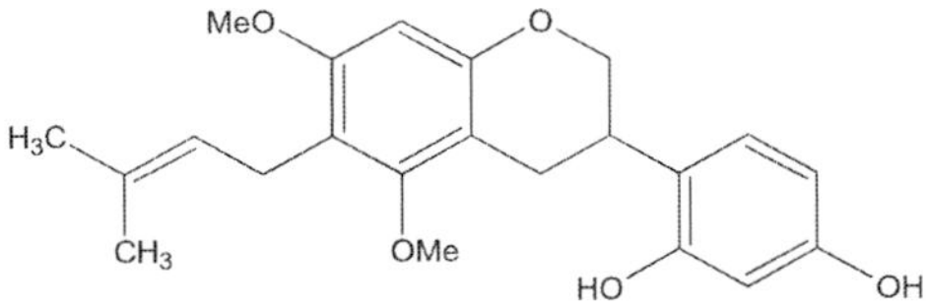

Glyasperin D

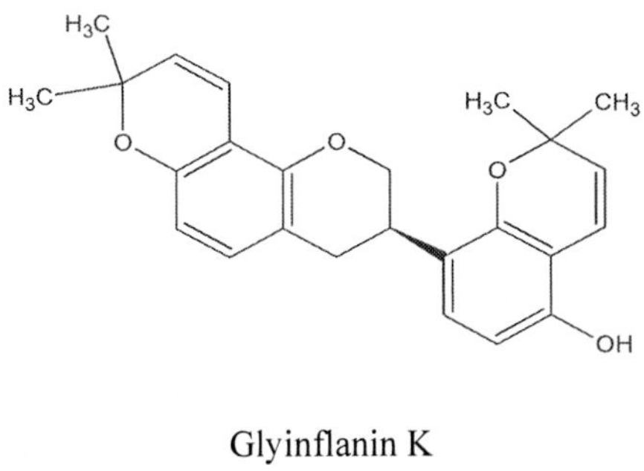

Glyinflanin K

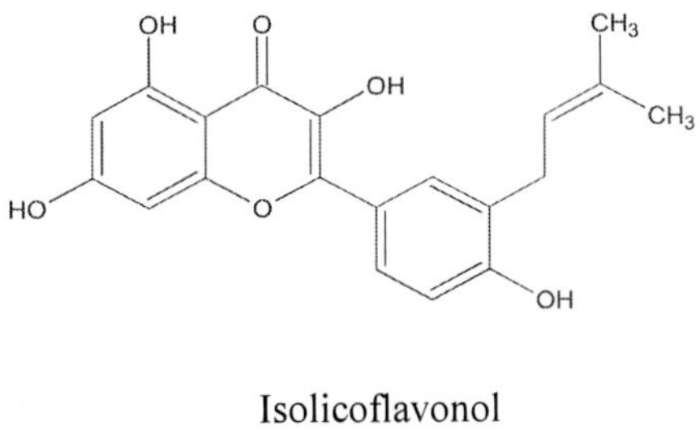

Isolicoflavonol

Lespedezaflavanone B

Licoagrodione

Licochalcone A

Licochalcone B

Licochalcone C

Licochalcone D

Licoflavanone

Licoricidin 4′-O-Methylglabridin Tenuifolin B

Glycyrrhiza species has been used by man for at least 4000 years. Partly because of its present commercial value and partly because of continuing interest in the anti-inflammatory activity of extracts known in commerce as Russian and Xinjiang licorices, constituted by *Glycyrrhiza glabra, G. inflate* and *G. lepidota* (Leguminosae) exhibited potent antimicrobial and antioxidant activity. All of these compounds inhibited the growth of gram-positive bacteria *Staphylococcus aureus* and *Bacillus subtilis*. In particular, the potencies of the antimicrobial activity of licochalcone A and glabridin were comparable to that of a well-known antibiotic, streptomycin [Okada et al., 1989]. Also possess activity against *Staphylococcus aureus, Mycobacterium smegmatis, Escherichia coli, Salmonella gallinarum, Kliebsiella pneumoniae* and *Candida albican* [Haraguchi et al., 1998, Mitscher et al., 1983].

These prenylated flavanone named licoflavanone were isolated from the leaves of the *Glycyrrhiza glabra* (Leguminosae) Shown to have activity against *Bacillus subtilis, Staphylococcus aureus* and *Candida albicans* [Fukui et al., 1988]. Licoflavanone is active against *Pseudomonas aeruginosa, Bacillus subtilis, Staphylococcus aureus Candida albicans, Trichophyton mentagrophytes, Aspergillus niger* and *Kliebsiella pneumoniae* [Li et al., 1998, Fukui et al., 1988].

Licochalcone A and B, and glyasperin D exhibited antimicrobial activity (MIC = 3.13-12.5 µg/ml) against *Staphylococcus aureus*. Glabrene, licoisoflavanone B, isolicoflavonol, and gancaonin I also showed the antibacterial activity against these strains (MIC = 1.56-25 µg/ml). These compounds exhibited antimicrobial activity against *Micrococcus luteus* and *Bacillus subtilis* (MIC=3.13-25 µg/ml) but not against *Klebsiella pneumoniae* and *Pseudomonas aeruginosa* [Fukai et al., 2002].

Licochalcone A has various uses in the food and pharmaceutical industries; The vegetative cell growth of *Bacillus subtilis* was inhibited with licochalcone A. Thus, licochalcone A could be a useful compound for the development of antibacterial agents for the preservation of foods containing high concentrations of salts and proteases, in which cationic peptides might be less effective [Tsukiyama et al., 2002].

Auriculatin

Bidwillon A

Bidwillon B

8-γ,γ-Dimethylallyldaidzein

Found in *Erythrina bidwilli* (Leguminosae) showed antimicrobial activity against *Fusobacterium nucleatum*, and *Prevotella intermedia* (Inuma et al., 1992). In a bioassay-guided fractionation using *Staphylococcus aureus*, the flavanones sigmoidin-B-4'-methylether and abyssinone V, the pterocarpans calopocarpin and neorautenol, and the isoflavanone bidwillon A were identified as the active components. Sigmoidin B 4' -methylether and calopocarpin were the most active principles of the stem bark of *Erythrina burttii* Ball. (Leguminosae) against the fungi *Trychophyton mentagrophyte* and *S. aureus*. All compounds were inactive against *E. coli*. The acetate derivatives la and 4a were inactive, and hence the presence of free phenolic group(s) appears to be important for antimicrobial activities of all compounds [Yenesewa et al., 2005].

Calopocarpin

Sigmoidin B-4'-methylether

Neorautenol

Found in the hard resins of hop, *Humulus lupulus* (Cannabidaceae). Showed a high antifungal activity against *Trichophyton mentagrophytes* and *T. rubrum* also showed slight activity against *Mucor* spp [Natarajan et al., 2008].

6-Isopentenyl-naringenin

Isoxanthohumol

Xanthohumol

Eriosemaone A

Eriosemaone B

Eriosemaone C

Eriosemaone D

Flemichin D

Found in the roots of *Eriosema tuberosum* (Leguminosae) exhibited antifungal activity against *Cladosporium cucumerinun* and *Candida albicans* at range of 5-10 µg/ml [Ma et al., 1995].

2,4,6-Trihydroxy-3(3-phenylpropionyl) benzaldehyde

2,4, 6-Trihydroxy-3methyl-5(3-phenyl propionyl)benzaldehyde

2,4,5, 6-Tetrahydroxy-3-(3-phenylpropionyl)benzaldehyde

3-Phenyl-1-(2,4,6-trihydroxyphenyl)-1-propanone

1-(2,4,6-Trihydroxy-3-methyl)-3-phenyl-1-propanone

Found in *Psidium actangulum* (Myrtaceae). Possesses antifungal, antifeedant and antibacterial activities. Showed activity against *Pseudoperonospora cubensis, Pseudo monas cubensis, Botrytis cinerea, Puccinia recondita* and *Phytophthora infestans* [Sato et al., 1995a].

Naringenin   Sakuranetin

The flavanones naringenin and sakuranetin were isolated from *Piper crassinervinum* (Piperaceae). Both compounds showed inhibition of fungal growth of *Cladosporium cladosporioides* and *Cladosporium sphaerospermum.* Sakuranetin was the most potent with activities comparable to the controls nystatin and Miconazole [Daneluttea et al., 2003].

Bolusanthin III

Bolusanthin IV

Isogancaonin C

Bolusanthus speciosus Harms (Fabaceae), otherwise called Tree Wisteria, is monotypic and endemic in subtropical South Africa, Botswana, Zimbabwe, Mozambique and Zambia. The dried inner bark is used to relieve abdominal pains, emetism and tuberculosis. From chloroform and ethyl acetate extract of the root wood was isolated three flavonoids (isogancaonin C, bolusanthin III and bolusanthin IV) whith strong antimicrobial activities against *Escherichia coli, Bacillus subtilis, Staphylococcus, aureus* and *Candida mycoderma.* The isolated compounds also showed moderate to strong radical scavenging properties against DPPH radical [Erasto et al., 2004].

Hesperetin

Naringin

Neohesperidin

Neoeriocitrin

Neohesperidin, hesperetin, neoeriocitrin, eriodictyol, naringin and naringenin isolated from ethanolic extract from *Citrus bergamia* Risso (Bergamot) were found to be active against (*Escherichia coli, Pseudomonas putida, Salmonella enterica*), Gram-negative bacteria (*Listeria innocua, Bacillus subtilis, Staphylococcus aureus, Lactococcus lactis*) and the yeast *Saccharomyces cerevisiae*) and their antimicrobial potency increased after enzymatic deglycosylation. The minimum inhibitory concentrations of flavonoids, were found to be in the range 200 to 800 μg ml^{-1} [Mandalari et al., 2007].

4-Hydroxylonchocarpin

Isobavachalcone

Kanzonol C

Stipulin

Extract of the twigs of Dorstenia barteri (Moraceae) contains isobavachalcone, 4-hydroxylonchocarpin and kanzonol C prevented the growth of Citrobacter freundii, Enterobacter aerogens, Proteus mirabilis, Proteus vulgaris, Bacillus megaterium, Bacillus stearothermophilus and Candida albicans at the lowest MIC value of 0.3 μg/ml. Isobavachalcone, which appeared as the most active compound [Mbaveng et al., 2008].

Albanol B   Kenusanone A   kuraridin

Kuwanon C   Mulberrofuran G   Papyriflavonol A

Sophoraflavanone D   Sophoraisoflavanone A

Prenylated flavonoids, papyriflavonol A, kuraridin, sophoraflavanone D and sophoraisoflavanone A exhibited a good antifungal activity against *Candida albicans*. Kuwanon C, mulberrofuran G, albanol B, and kenusanone A, showed strong antibacterial activity against *Escherichia coli, Salmonella typhimurium, Staphylococcus epidermis* and *S. aureus*. These compounds *were* purified from five different medicinal plants *Morus alba L., Morus mongolica* Schneider, *Broussnetia papyrifera* (L.) *Vent, Sophora flavescens Ait* and *Echinosophora koreensis* [Sohn et al., 2004].

Tangeritin

Nobiletin

Polymethoxylated flavonoids, were isolated and identified from peel extracts of *Citrus* spp. (Rutaceae), which presented antimicrobial activity especially against *Microsporum canis* and *Trichophyton mentagrophytes*. Tangeritin and nobiletin were isolated from *Citrus reticulata*; showed antimicrobial activity againts two opportunistic bacteria (*Escherichia coli* and *Staphylococcus aureus*) [Johann et al., 2007].

Apigenin

Genkwanin

5-Hydroxy-7,4'-dimethoxyflavone

Antibacterial flavonoids were isolated by bioassay-guided fractionation from *Combretum erythrophyllum* (Combretaceae) showed antimicrobial activity against Gram-positive and Gram-negative bacteria. All compounds had good activity against *Vibrio cholerae* and *Enterococcus faecalis*, with MIC values in the range of 25-50 µg/ml. Rhamnocitrin and quercetin-5,3'-dimethylether also inhibited *Micrococcus luteus* and *Shigella sonei* at 25 µg/ml. With the exception of 5-hydroxy-7,4'-dimethoxy-flavone the flavonoids were not toxic towards human lymphocytes. This compound is potentially toxic to human cells and exhibited the poorest antioxidant activity whereas rhamnocitrin and rhamnazin exhibited strong antioxidant activity. Genkwanin; rhamnocitrin; quercetin-5,3'-dimethylether; rhamnazin had a higher anti-inflammatory activity than the positive control mefenamic acid [Martini et al., 2004].

Quercetin-3,3'-dimethylether

Rhamnocitrin

Rhamnazin

2',6'-Dihydroxy-3'-methyl-4'-methoxy-dihydrochalcone

Eucalyptin

8-Desmethyl-eucalyptin

Extracts of Eucalyptus globulus, E. maculata and E. viminalis (Mirtaceae) significantly inhibited the growth of Gram-positive bacteria Staphylococcus aureus, Bacillus cereus, Enterococcus faecalis, Alicyclobacillus acidoterrestris and Propionibacterium acnes, and of a fungus Trichophyton mentagrophytes, but they did not show strong antibacterial activity against Gram-negative bacteria Escherichia coli, and Pseudomonas putida. 2',6'-dihydroxy-3'-methyl-4'-methoxy-dihydrochalcone, eucalyptin and 8-desmethyl-eucalyptin, isolated from E. maculata extracts, exhibited potent antimicrobial activities with MIC ranging from 1.0 to 31 μgml [Takahashi et al., 2004].

Wogonin

Oroxindin

The phytochemicals betulinic acid, wogonin and oroxindin isolated from the aerial parts of *Bacopa monnieri* (Scrophulariaceae) and *Holmskioldia sanguinea* (Verbenaceae) showed significant antifungal activity against the fungi *Alternaria alternata* and *Fusarium fusiformis*. Inhibition of root growth germination of wheat seeds was observed for all three compounds which showed 100% inhibition at 10 μg/mL. Wogonin showed potent inhibition of *Alternaria alternata* compared with oroxindin at a concentration of 4 μg/mL [Chaudhuri et al., 2004].

Apigenin-7-O-glucoside

Isoorientin

Luteolin

Orientin

Stems methanol extract from *Daphne gnidium* L. (Thymelaeaceae) exhibited antibacterial activity against *Bacillus lentus* and *Escherichia coli*, but was inactive against fungi. The most active compounds were daphnetin and genkwanin (Cottiglia et al., 2001).

Quercetin 3-O-α-arabinoside

Distichin

A prenylated coumarin Pavietin, has been isolated from the leaves of an *Aesculus pavia* together with quercitrin, quercetin 3-O-α-arabinoside, and distichin. Mixture of these flavonoids resulted in weak or no activity to inhibit mycelial growth [Curir et al., 2007].

Guaijaverin

Morin-3-O-α-L-lyxopyranoside

Morin-3-O-α-arabopyranoside

Antibacterial compounds were isolated from leaves of *Psidium guajava* L. (Myrtaceae). The flavonoid glycosides, morin-3-O-α-L-lyxopyranoside and morin-3-O-α-arabopyranoside showed minimum inhibition concentration of 200 ug/ml for each against *Salmonella enteritidis*, and 250 ug/ml and 300 ug/ml against *Bacillus cereus* respectively [Hidetoshi and Gen-ichi 2002]. Guaijaverin showed antimicrobial activity against *Streptococcus mutans* [Prabu et al., 2006]. In addition, galactose-specific lectin isolated from guava fruit ripe were shown to bind to *E-coli* (a common diarrhea-causing organism), preventing its adhesion to the intestinal wall and thus preventing infection resulting diarrhea [Coutiño et al., 2001].

Epigallocatechin-(4β→8)-gallocatechin-(4β→S) benzylthioether

Epigallocatechin-(4β→6)-epigallocatechin-(4β→S) benzylthioether

Epigallocatechin-(4β→8)-epigallocatechin-(4β→S) benzylthioether

Epicatechin-(4β→8)-epigal)-ocatechin-(4β→S) benzylthioether

Gallocatechin benzylthioether

Epigallocatechin benzylthioether

Catechin benzylthioether

Epicatechin benzylthioether

The proanthocyanidin from the leaves of the forage legume *Dorycnium rectum* (Leguminosae) differs from other temperate proanthocyanidin-containing forage legumes in that the range of polymers extends up to very high degrees of polymerisation. Epigallocatechin was the most abundant extension unit and the terminating flavan-3-ols comprised largely catechin and gallocatechin units in equal proportions. Formation of thiolyated dimmer products showed the interflavan-linkages of the lower molecular weight proanthocyanidins to be predominantly C4 →C8 with a small amount of C4→C6. Proanthocyanidins showed antibacterial activity at 100 µg/ml against pure cultures of microbes selected from the ruminal population *Clostridium aminophilum*, *Butyrivibrio fibrisolvens* and *Clostridium proteoclasticum* significantly dependent on their structure but not so against *Ruminococcus albus* and *Peptostreptococcus anaerobius* [Sivakumaran et al., 2004].

Agnuside

5'-Hydroxy-3',4', 3, 6, 7-pentamethoxyflavone

Iso-orientin

Luteolin

4',5,7-Trihydroxy-3'-O-β-D-glucuronic acid-6"-methylester

4',5,7-Trihydroxy-3'-O-β-D-glucuronic acid-6"-methylester showed promising activity against *T. mentagrophytes* and *C. neoformans* of MIC 6.25 μg/ml as compared to standard antifungal drug fluconazole, having MIC of 2 μg/ml against *T. mentagrophytes*. 5'-hydroxy-3',4',3,6,7-penta- methoxyflavone showed activity of MIC 12.5 μg/ml against *C. neoformans* whereas *Iso*-orientin showed activity against *T. mentagrophytes*. At similar concentration, luteolin showed moderate activity (25 μg/ml) against each test organism. 4',5,7-Trihydroxy-3'-O-β-D-glucuronic acid-6"-methylester was found to be most active at MIC 6.25 μg/ml among all the isolated compounds from *Vitex negundo* (Verbenaceae) [Sathiamoorthy et al., 2007].

Dalhorridin   Dalhorridinin

Oalspinin   Oalspinosin

Occurrs in *Dalbergia horrida* (Leguminosae). These flavonoids showed analgesic, anti-inflammatory, CNS depressant and mild anti-bacterial properties [Narayanan et al., 2007].

Diplacone

3'-O-Methyl-5'-hydroxydiplacone

3'-O-Methyl-5'-O-methyldiplacone

3'-O-Methyldiplacone

Mimulone

Tomentodiplacone

Tomentodiplacone B

C-6-geranylflavonoids were isolated from an ethanol extract of *Paulownia tomentosa* Steud (Scrophulariaceae) fruits. 3'-O-Methyl-5'-hydroxydiplacone, 3'-O-methyl-5'-O-methyldiplacone and 3'-O-methyldiplacol proved to be the most active of the compounds isolated. The 3'-methoxy-4',5'-dihydroxyphenyl ring B of 3'-O-methyl-5'-hydroxydiplacone and 3',5'-methoxy-4-hydroxy substitution seem to be important for the activity due to an increase in the planar character of the molecule. The OH-3 group of 3'-O-methyldiplacol also increases the activity of the compound in comparison with the corresponding flavanone 3'-O-methyldiplacone. Some studies have reported greater activity against Gram-positive bacteria than Gram-negative. This was demonstrated clearly with the C-geranyl flavonoids of *P. tomentosa*. None of the compounds tested showed activity *against E. coli, P. aeruginosa,* or *S. enteritidis*. This is probably due to the lipophilic character of the compounds tested caused by the presence of the geranyl side chain. Some of flavanones have been tested in a liposome membrane model, and it was shown that the presence of a lipophilic substituent on the flavonoid skeleton increased the alteration of membrane fluidity. The resistance of Gram-negative bacteria to the compounds isolated is probably caused by the more complex structure and hydrophilic nature of their cell walls [Smejkal et al., 2008].

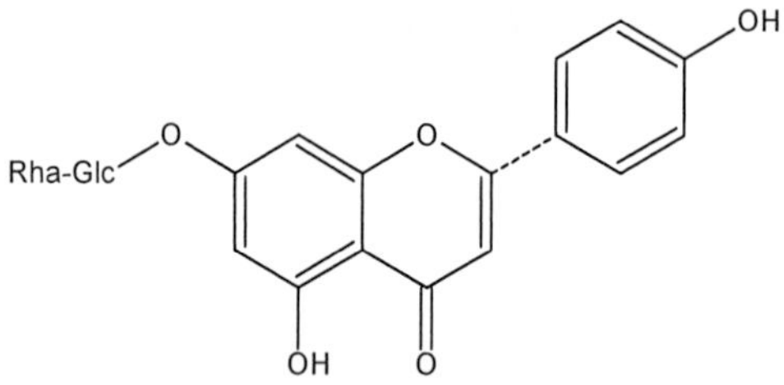

Apigenin-7-rutinoside

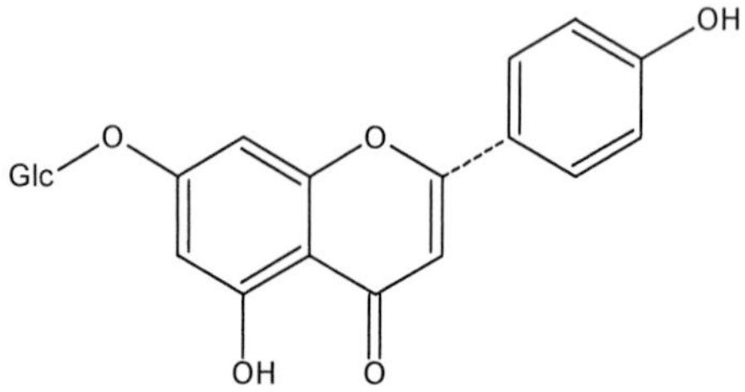

Apigenin-7-O-β-D-glucopyranoside

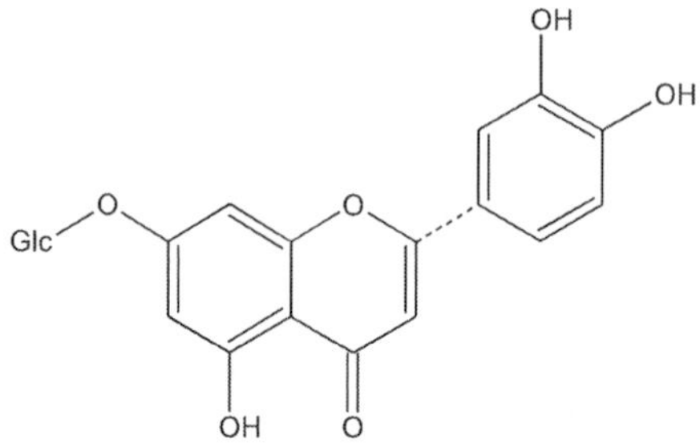

Cynaroside

Luteolin-7-rutinoside

Cynara scolymus L. (Cichorioideae) leaf extracts showed flavonoids with antimicrobial activities. Among them, chlorogenic acid, cynarin and luteolin-7-rutinoside, exhibited a relatively higher activity than other compounds; in addition, they were more effective against fungi than bacteria. The minimum inhibitory concentrations of these compounds were between 50 and 200 µg/ml [Zhu et al., 2004].

Scandenone

Tiliroside

The flavonoid derivatives, scandenone, tiliroside, quercetin-3,7-O-α-L-dirhamnoside and kaempferol-3,7- O-α-L-dirhamnoside, showed antibacterial and antifungal activities against *Escherichia coli, Pseudomonas aeruginosa, Proteus mirabilis, Klebsiella pneumoniae, Acinetobacter baumannii, Staphylococcus aureus, Bacillus subtilis,* and *Enterococcus faecalis,* as well as the *fungus Candida albicans* by a microdilution method. All of the compounds tested were found to be quite active against *S. aureus* and *E. faecalis* with MIC values of 0,5 µg/ml, followed by *E. coli* (2 µg/ml), K. pneumoniae (4 µg/ml), A. baumannii (8 µg/ml), and *B. subtilis* (8 µg/ml), while they inhibited *C. albicans* at 1 µg/ml as potent as ketoconazole [Ozcelik et al., 2006].

5,7-Dibenzyloxyflavanone

2'-Hydroxy-4',6'-dibenzyloxychalcone

5,7-Dibenzyloxyflavanone

2'-Hydroxy-4',6'-dibenzyloxychalcone

From the dichloromethane extract of the flowers of *Helichrysum gymnocomum* (Asteraceae) flavonoids, and acylphloroglucinol, were isolated. Compounds have MIC values below 64 μg/ml against a selection of pathogens, including *Staphylococcus aureus* (6.3 μg/ml) and methicillin and gentamycin resistant strain of *S. aureus* (7.8 μg/ml). With the exception of 5,7-dibenzyloxyflavanone, the other compounds had notable activity (45-63 μg/ml) towards *Pseudomonas aeruginosa*. Compounds having antimicrobial activities less than 64 μg/ml are accepted as having notable antimicrobial activity and those compounds exhibiting activity at concentrations below 10 μg/ml are considered "clinically significant". The isolated compounds from *H. gymnocomum* had MIC values below 64 μg/ml. Acylphloroglucinols are known to be microbio-logically active against anti-staphylococcal (16-32 μg/ml) [Drewes and van Vuuren, 2008].

Angusticomin B

Bartericin A

Gancaonin Q

Found in *Dorstenia angusticomis* Engl. (Moraceae).The interval of antimicrobial effect of 0.61-78.12 µg/ml was observed for gancaonin Q and stipulin against *Gram-negative bacteria: Citrobacter freundii, Enterobacter aerogens, Enterobacter cloacae, Escherichia coli, Klebsiella pneumoniae, Morganella morganii, Proteus mirabilis, Proteus vulgaris, Pseudomonas aeruginosa, Shigella dysenteriae, Shigella flexneri, Salmonella typhi, Salmonella typhymurium Gram-positive bacteria: Bacillus cereus, Bacillus megaterium, Bacillus stearothermophilus, Bacillus subtilis, Staphylococcus aureus, Streptococcus faecalis, Yeasts: Candida albicans, Candida krusei* and *Candida gabrata.* While values lower than 0.31 µg/ml and up to 39.06 µg/ml were obtained with bartericin A [Kuete et al., 2007]. Flavonoids are known to complex with cell wall components and adhesins to prevent the microbial growth [Rojas et al., 1992] and this can be the possible mechanism by which all compounds exhibit their actions.

Appollinine

Lanceolatin A

Pseudosemiglabrin

Semiglabrin

Tephrosia species (Leguminosae) used medicinally and as fish poison, are known to be a source of flavonoids. 7-oxygenated 8-prenyl flavones, semiglabrin, pseudosemiglabrin, appollinine and lanceolatin A, have been isolated from *Tephrosia nubica*. The four flavanoids exhibit an antifungal activity against *Aspergillus niger, Penicillium funiculosum, Fusarium moniliforum* and *Phoma* spp [Ammar and 1988]. Regarding the subsitution pattern within the tested compounds, the methoxy group at the 7 position in appollinine and lanceolatin A which possess a positive effect on fungal inhibition, the compounds semiglabrinand and pseudosemiglabrin, without a methoxy group at the 7 position shows also an activity against these fungi. It seems that the fungicidal property of the prenylated flavones is specific to individual fungi, substances and their concentration and no absolute generalization is possible in this context.

(2S)-3´,4´-Dihydroxy-7-methoxyflavan

(2S)-7,4´-Dihydroxy-3´-methoxyflavan

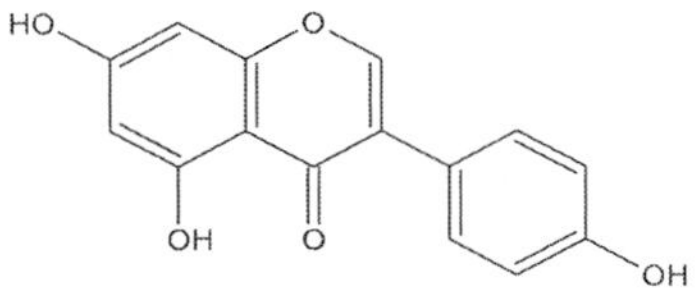

Genistein

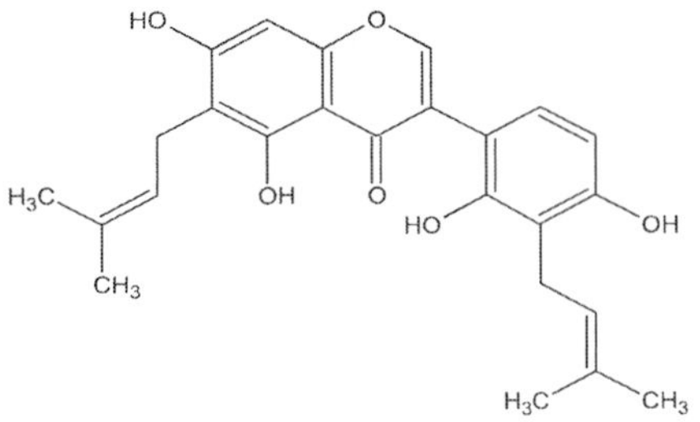

2′-Hydroxylupalbigenin

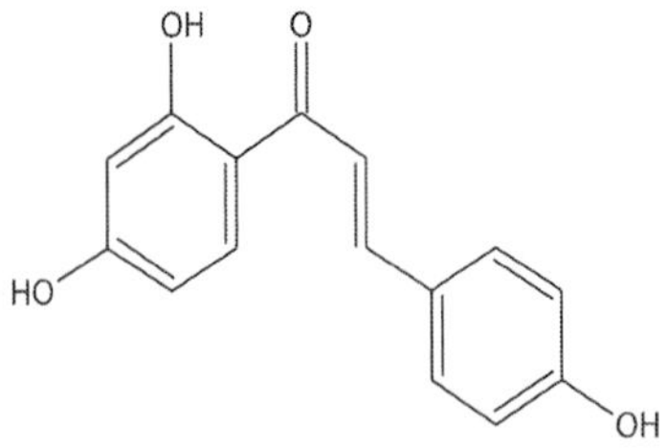

Isoliquiritigenin

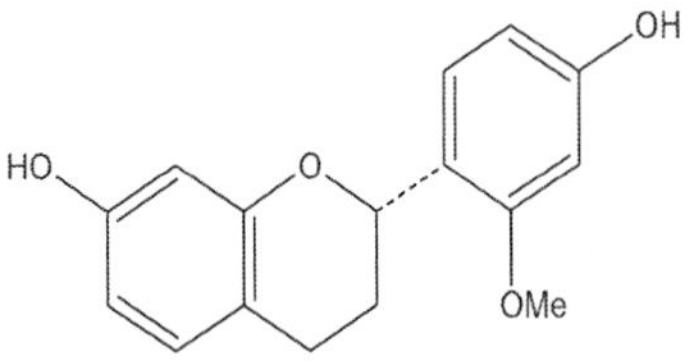

2′-Methyl ether (2S)-7,4′- dihydroxyflavan

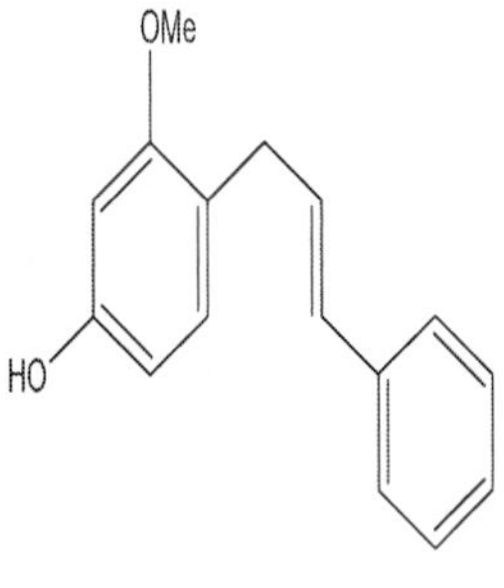

Obtustyrene

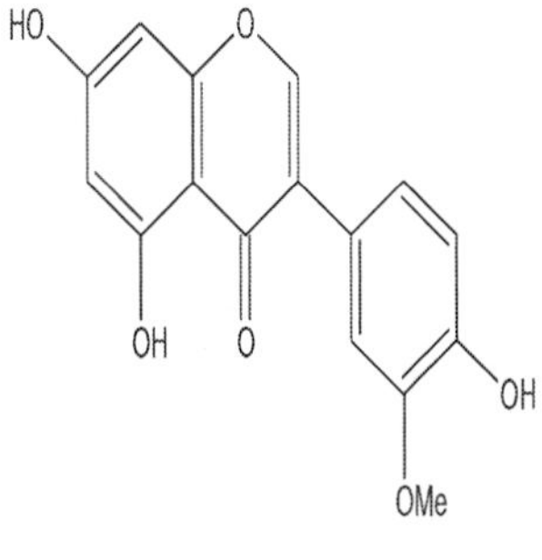

3′-O-Methylorobol

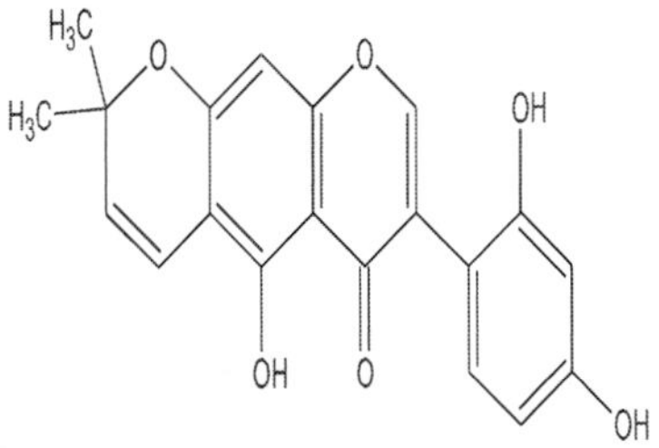

Parvisoflavone B

Found in *Bauhinia Manca* (Leguminosae), these compound together with Licoisoflavone B, lupinisoflavone A, lupinisoflavone B, lupinisoflavone C, lupinisoflavone D, lupisoflavone, lupalbigenin possess significant antifungal activity against *Botrytis cinerea, Claviceps viridis, Coprinus cinereus, Rhizoctonia solani* and *Saprolegnia asterophora* (Achenbach et al., 1988).

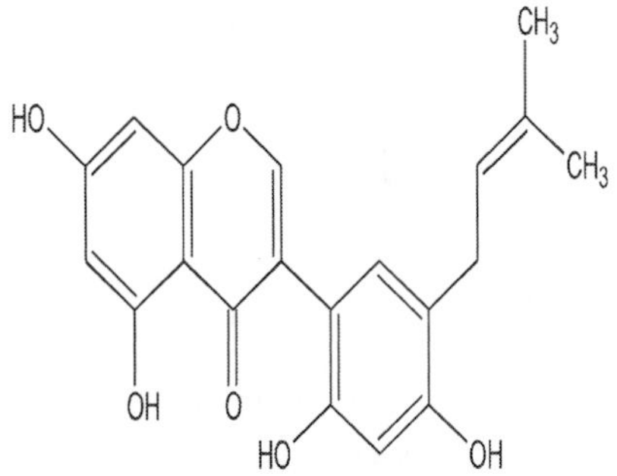

Allolicoisoflavone A

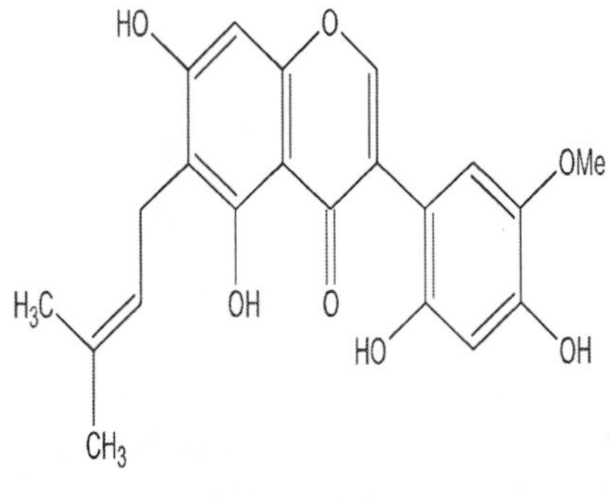

Isopiscerythrone

Piscisoflavone A   Piscisoflavone B

These isoflavones are constituents of *Piscidia erythrina* (Leguminosae) were found be strongly antifungal when applied at 50 and 100 μg/ml against *Cladosporium herbarum* [Moriyama et al., 1992].

Cyclokievitone   5-Deoxykievitone

Induced as a phytoalexin in *Phaseolus vulgaris* (Leguminosae). It has antifungal activity [Ingham, 1983[b]].

Dalbergioidin   Kievitone

Kievitone and dalbergioidin induced as aphytoalexin in many Leguminosae as *Dolichos biflorus,* have antibacterial activity against *Pseudomonas, Xanthomonas* and *Achromobacter* spp. It shows antifungal activity [Dewick, 1988, Harbone, 1989].

Dracorhodin

Dracorubin

5-Methoxy-7-hydroxyflavan

Nordracorubin

These constituents of *Daemonorops draco* Blume (Palmaceae) showed activity against *Staphylococcus aureus* and *Mycobacterium smegmatis* [Rao et al., 1982].

Chalconaringenin

3,5-Dihydroxy-6,7,8-trimethoxyflavone

Occurs in *Helichrysum odoratissimum* (Asteraceae), have activity against *Bacillus subtilis* and *Staphylococcus aureus* (Puyvelde et al., 1989).

Isokaempferide

5,7,4′-Trihydroxy-3,8-dimethoxyflavone

5,7,4′-Trihydroxy-3,8, 3′-trimethoxyflavone

From a hydrolysed methanolic extract from the *Psiadia trinervia* (Compositae) was isolated these flavonoids with antimicrobial activity against *C. cucumerinum* and Gram-positive bacterium *Bacillus cereus* [Wang et al., 1989].

Flemiflavanone D   5,7,4′-Trihydroxy-6,8-diprenylisoflavone

Eryvarigatin

Flemiflavanone D, was found in *Flemingia stricta* L. (Palmaceae) showed antimicrobial activity. The other diprenylisoflavone were isolated from *Erythrina fusca* (Leguminosae) roots [Harbone, 1989].

6,8-Dimethyl-3,7-dimethoxy- kaempferol   6,8-Dimethyl-3-methoxy- kaempferol

6,8-Dimethyl-3,7-dimethoxy- quercetin

6,8-Dimethyl-3-methoxy-quercetin

6-Methyl-3- methoxy-quercetin

6- Methyl-3,7,3′-trimethoxy-quercetin

6- Methyl-3,7-dimethoxy-quercetin

These C-methylflavonols were isolated from *Piliostigma thonningii* (Schum.) (Caesalpiniaceae). The structure-activity relationship observed for the C-methylflavonols that the 5,7-dihydroxylation is necessary for antibacterial activity and methoxylation at C-7 significantly reduces activity , the 3′-OH may not be essential for antibacterial activity. Thus, the most active of the isolated compounds is 6-C-methylquercetin-3-methyl ether against *Staphylococcus aureus* (MIC 1.125 mM) conforms with requisite structural features [Ibewuike et al., 1997].

References

Abd-El-Hady, F. K. & Ouf, S. A. (1993). Fungitoxic effect of different substances from *Solenostemma argel* (Del) Hayne on some shoot surface fungi. *Zentralblatt fur krobiologie*, *148*, 598-607.

Achenbach, H., Stocker, M. & Constela, M. A. (1988). Flavonoids and other constituents of Balhinia Manca. *Phytochemistry*, *27*, 1835-1841.

Ammar, N. M. & El-Diwany, A. I. (1988). Antimicrobial study of Tephosia nubica flavones. J. Islam. *Academic Sci.*, *1*, 72-73.

Awouafack, M. D., Kouam, S. F., Hussain, H., Ngamga, D., Tane, P., Schulz, B., Green, I. R. & Krohn, K. (2008). Antimicrobial Prenylated Dihydrochalcones from Eriosema glomerata. *Planta Med.*, *74*, 50-54.

Barberan, F. T., Sanmartin, E. I., Lorente, F. T. & Rumbero, A. (1990). Antimicrobial phenolic compounds from three Spanish *Helichrysum* species. *Phytochemistry*, *29*, 1093-1095.

Bernard, F. X., Sable, S. & Cameron, B. (1997). Glycosylated flavones as selective inhibitors of topoisomerase IV, *Antimicrob Agents Chemother*, *41*, 992-998.

Bhakuni, D. S. & Chaturvedi, R. (1984). Chemical constituents of Crotalaria madurensis. *J Natural Products*, *47*, 585-591.

Bloor, S. J. (1995). An antimicrobial kaemferol-diacyl-rhamnoside from Pentachondra pumila. *Phytochemistry*, *38*, 1033-1035.

Bojasel, G., Majindal, R. R. T., Gashe, B. A. & Wanjala, C. C. W. (2002). Antimicrobial Flavonoids from Bolusanthus speciosus. *Planta Med.*, *68*, 615-620.

Bremner, P. D. & Meyer, J. M. 1998. Pinocernbrin chalcone: an antibacterial compound from Helichrysum trilineatum. *Planta Med.*, *64*, 777.

Chaudhuri, P. K., Srivastava, R., Kumar, S. & Kumar, S. (2004). Phytotoxic and antimicrobial *constituents of Bacopa monnieri and Holmskioldia sanguinea. Phytother Res., 18, 114-117.*

Cottiglia, F., Loy, G., Garau, D., Floris, C., Casu, M., Pompei, R. & Bonsignore, L. (2001). Antimicrobial evaluation of coumarins and flavonoids from the stems of Daphne gnidium L. *Phytomedicine*, *8*, 302-305.

Coutiño, R. R., Hernández, C. P. & Giles, R. H. (2001). Lectins in fruits having gastrointestinal activity: their participation in the hemagglutinating property of *Escherichia coli* O157:H7. *Archives of Medical Research*, *32*, 251-257.

Curir, P., Galeotti, F., Marcello, D., Barile, E. & Lanzotti, V. (2007). Pavietin, a Coumarin from *Aesculus pavia* with Antifungal Activity. *J Nat Prod.*, *70*, 1668-1671.

Curir, P., Dolci, M., Lanzotti, V. & Taglialatela-Scafati, O. (2001). Kaempferide triglycoside: a posible factor of resistance of carnation (*Dianthus caryophyllus*) to *Fusarium oxysporum* f. Sp. Dianthi. *Phytochemistry*, *56*, 717-721.

Cushnie, T. P. & Lamb, A. J. (2005). Antimicrobial activity of flavonoids. *Int J Antimicrob Agents*, *26*, 343-356.

Cushnie, T. P., Hamilton, V. E., Chapman, D. G., Taylor, P. W. & Lamb, A. J. (2007). Aggregation of *Staphy- lococcus aureus* following treatment with the antibacterial flavonol galangin. dihydroxyflavone showed both good antimicrobial and antioxidative activities.: *J Appl Microbiol.*, *103*, 1562-1567.

Daneluttea, A. P., Henrique, J., Lago, M. C. M. & Massuo, J. K. (2003). Antifungal flavanones and prenylated hydroquines from *Piper crassinervium* Kunth. *Phytochemistry*, *64*, 555-559.

Deng, Y., Lee, J. P., Tianasoa-Ramamonjy, M., Snyder, J. K., Etages, S. A. D., Kanada, D., Snyder, M. P. & Turner, C. J. (2000). New antimicrobial flavanones from Physena madagascariensis. *J Nat Prod.*, *63*, 1082-1089.

Dewick, P. M. (1988). *The isoflavonoids.* In The flavonoids:Advances in research since 1980. Harbone J.B. London: Chapman, & Hall.

Donnelly, D. M. X. & Sheridan, M. G. (1988). The neoflavonoids. In the flavonoids: Advances in research since 1980 London: Chaprnand and Hall, 234.

Drewes, S. E. & van Vuuren, S. F. (2008). Antimicrobial acylphloroglucinols and dibenzyloxy flavonoids from flowers of Helichrysum gymnocomum. *Phytochemistry, 69,* 1745-1749.

Dubois, J. L. & Sneden, A. T. (1995). Dihydrolicoisoflavone, a new isoflavone from Swartzia polyphyllla. *J Nat Prod., 58,* 629-632.

Elsohlyl, H. N., Joshi, A. S., Nimrod, A. C., Walker, L. A. & Clark, A. M. (2001). Antifungal Chalcones from Maclura tinctoria. *Planta Med., 67,* 87-89.

Erasto, P., Bojase-Moleta, G. & Majinda, R. R. T. (2004). Antimicrobial and antioxidant flavonoids from the root wood of Bolusanthus speciosus. *Phytochemistry, 65,* 875-880.

Ferrari, F., Botta, B. & De Lima, R. A. (1983). Flavonoids and isoflavonoids from Zollernia paraensis. *Phytochemistry, 22,* 1663-1664.

Fukai, T., Marumo, A., Kaitou, K., Kanda, T., Terada, S. & Nomura, T. (2002). Antimicrobial activity of licorice flavonoids against methicillin-resistant Staphylococcus aureus. *Fitoterapia, 73,* 536-539.

Fukai, T., Oku, Y., Hano, Y. & Terada, S. (2004). Antimicrobial activities of hydrophobic 2-arylbenzofurans and an isoflavone against vancomycin-resistant Enterococci and methicillin- resistant Staphylococcus aureus. *Planta Med., 7,* 685-687.

Fukui, H., Goto, K. & Tabata, M. (1988). Two antimicrobial flavanones from the leaves of Glycyrrhiza glabra. *Chem Pharm Bull, 36,* 4174-4176.

Gafner, S., Wolfender, J., Mavi, S. & Hostettman, K. (1996). Antifungal and antibacterial chalcones from Myrica serrata. *Planta Med., 62,* 67-69.

Garo, E., Maillard, S. A., Mavi, S. & Hostettmann, K. (1996). Five flavansd from Mariscus psilostachys. *Phytochemistry, 43,* 1265-1269.

Ghazal, S. A., Abuzarqa, M. & Mahasneh, A. M. (2006). Antimicrobial activity of *Polygonum equisetiforme* extracts and flavonoids. *Phytother Res., 6,* 265-269.

Grosvenor, P. W. & Gray, D. O. (1998). Coluteol and Colutequinone B, more antifungal isoflavonoids from Colutea arborescens. *J Nat Prod., 61,* 99-101.

Gutkin, G., Norbedo, C., Mollerach, M., Ferraro, G. & Coussio, J. D. (1984). Antibacterial activity of Achyrocline flaccida. *J Ethnopharm, 10,* 319-321.

Haraguchi, H., Tanimoto, K., Tamura, Y., Mizutani, K. & Kinoshita, T. (1998). Mode of antibacterial action of retrochalcones from *Glycyrrhiza inflata, Phytochemistry, 48,* 125-129.

Harbone, J. B. (1988). The flavonoids : Advances in Research since 1980. London Chapman & Hall. 67.

Harbone, J. B. (1989). Phytochemical methods. Methods if, plant biochemistry. London Academia Press, 1, 56.

Harborne, J. B. & Baxter, H. (1999). *The handbook of natural flavonoids Vols 1 and 2,* John Wiley and Sons, Chichester, UK.

Harsh, M. L. & Nag, T. N. (1984). Antimicrobial principles from in vitro tissue culture of Peganum harmala. *J Nat Prod., 47,* 902-903.

Hidetoshi, A. & Gen-ichi, D. (2002). Isolation of Antimicrobial Compounds from Guava (*Psidium guajava* Lo) and their Structural Elucidation. *Biosci Biotechnol Biochem., 66,* 1727-1730.

Hilliard, J. J., Krause, H. M. & Bernstein, J. I. (1995). A comparison of active site binding of 4-quinolones and novel flavone gyrase inhibitors to DNA gyrase, *Adv Exp Med Biol., 390,* 59–69.

Hufford, C. H., Jia, Y., Cromm, E. M., Muhammed, I., Okunade, A. L. & Clark, A. M. (1993). Antimicrobial compounds from Petalostemum purpureum. *J Nat Prod.*, *56*, 1878-1889.

Hwang, B. Y., Roberts, S. K., Chaddwwick, L. R., Wu, C. D. & Kinghorn, A. D. (2003). Antimicrobial Constituents from Goldenseal: (the Rhizomes of *Hydrastis canadensis*) against selected oral pathogens. *Planta Med.*, *69*, 623-627.

Ibewuike, J. C., Ogungbamila, F. O., Ogundaini, A. O., Okeke, I. N. & Bohlin, L. (1997). Antiiinflammatory and antibacterial activities of C-methylflavonols from Piliostigma thonningii. *Phytother Res.*, *11*, 281-284.

Ikigai, H., Nakae, T., Hara, Y. & Shimamura, T. (1993). Bactericidal catechins damage the lipid bilayer, *Biochim Biophys Acta*, *1147*, 132-136.

Ingham, J. L. (1983a). *Phytoalexin from the Leguminosae*. In Phytoalexins (Bailey, J. A. I and Mansfield, J. W.) Glasgow: Blackie 25.

Ingham, J. L. (1976). Fungal modification of pterocarpans phytoalexins from Melilotus alba and Trifolium pretense. *Phytochemistry*, *15*, 1489-1495.

Ingham, J. L. (1983b). Natural occurring isoflavonoids. *Progress in the chemistry of organic natural products*, *43*, 1-266.

Inuma, M., Okawa, Y., Tanaka, T., Ho, F., Kobayashi, Y. & Miyauchi, K. (1994). Anti-oral microbial activity of isoflavonoids in roots bark of Ormosia monosperma. *Phytochemistry*, *37*, 889-891.

Ishiguro, K., Nagata, S., Fukumoto, H., Yamaki, M., Iso, K. & Oyama, Y. (1993). An isopentenylated flavonol from Hypericum japonicum. *Phytochemistry*, *32*, 1583-1585.

Jayasinghe, L., Balasooriya, B. A. I. S., Padmini, W. C., Hara, N. & Fujimoto, Y. (2004). Geranyl chalcone derivatives with antifungal and radical scavenging properties from the leaves of Artocarpus nobilis. *Phytochemistry*, *65*, 1287-1290.

Johann, S., Lopes de Oliveira, V., Pizzolatti, M. G., Schripsema, J., Braz-Filho, R., Branco, A. & Smânia, A. (2007). Antimicrobial activity of wax and hexane extracts from *Citrus* spp. peels. Antimicrobial activity of wax and hexane extracts from *Citrus* spp. peels. Mem. Inst. Oswaldo Cruz 102: 59-68

Kasai, S., Watanabe, S., Kawabata, J., Tahara, S. & Mizutani, J. (1992). Antimicrobial catechin derivativess of Agrimonia pilosa. *Phytochemistry*, *31*, 787 -789.

Kodama, O., Miyakawa, J., Akatsuka, T. & Kiyosawa, S. (1992). Sakuranetin a flavanone phytoalexin from ultavioleta-irradiated rice leaves. *Phytochemistry*, *31*, 3807-3809.

Kofinas, C., Chinou, I., Loukis, A., Harvala, C., Maillard, M. & Hostettmann. (1998). Flavonoids and bioactive coumarins of Tordylium apulum. *Phytochemistry*, *48*, 637-641.

Komatsu, M., Yokoe, I. & Shirataki, Y. (1978). Studies on the constituents of *Sophora* species. XI11.11 Constituents of the aerial parts of Sophora tomentosa L. *Chem Pharm Bull*, *26*, 3863-3870.

Krauze-Baranowskaa, M. & Wiwart, M. (2003). Antifungal Activity of Biflavones from Taxus baccata and Ginkgo biloba. *Z Naturforsch*, *58*, 65-69.

Kuete, V., Metuno, R., Ngameni, B., Tsafack, A. M., Ngandeu, F., Fotso, G. F., Bezabih, M., Etoa, F., Ngadjuib, B. T., Abegaz, B. M. & Benga, V. P. (2007). Antimicrobial activity of the methanolic extracts and compounds from Treculia obovoidea (Moraceae). *Journal of Ethnopharmacology*, *112*, 531-536.

Kuete, V., Simo, I. K., Ngameni, B., Bigoga, J. D., Watchueng, J., Kapguepa, R. N., Etoa, F., Tchaleu, B. N. & Benga, V. P. (2007a). Antimicrobial activity of the methanolic extract, fractions and four flavonoids from the twigs of *Dorstenia angusticomis* Engl. (Moraceae). *Journal of Ethnopharmacology, 112,* 271-277.

Kuroyanagi, M., Arakawa, T., Hirayama, Y. & Hayashi, T. (1999). Antibacterial and antiandrogen flavonoids from Sophora flavescens. *J Nat Prod., 62,* 1595-1599.

Lane, G. A., Sutherland, O. R. W. & Skipp, R. A. (1987). Isoflavonoids as insect feeding deterrents and antifungal components from root of Lupinus angustifolius. *J Chem Ecol., 13,* 771-783.

Lee, D. G., Kim, H. K., Park, Y., Park, S. C., Woo, E. R., Jeong, H. G. & Hahm, K. S. (2003). Gram-positive bacteria specific properties of silybin derived from Silybum marianum. *Arch Pharm Res., 26,* 597-600.

Li, W., Asada, Y. & Yoshikawa, T. (1998). Antimicrobial flavonoids from Glycyrrhiza glabra hairy root cultures. *Planta Med., 64,* 746-747.

Lin, R., Chin, Y. & Lee, M. (2005). Antimicrobial Activity of Antibiotics in Combination with Natural Flavonoids against Clinical Extended-Spectrum β-Lactamase (ESBL)-producing Klebsiella pneumoniae. *Phytother Res., 19,* 612-617.

Lopes, N. P., Kato, M. J. & Yoshoida, M. (1999). Antifungal constituents from roots of Virola surinamensis. *Phytochemistry, 51,* 29-39

Ma, W. G., Fuzzati, N., Li, Q. S., Yang, C. R., Stoeckli-Evans, H. & Hostettman, K. (1995). Polyphenols from Eriosema tuberosum. *Phytochemistry, 39,* 1049-1061.

Mahmoud, Z. Y. (1981). Antimicrobial components from Maclura pomifera. *Planta Med., 42,* 299-301.

Maillard, M., Gupta, M. P. & Hostettmann, K. (1987). A new antifungal prenylated flavanone from Erythrina berteroana. *Planta Med., 53,* 563-564.

Mandalari, G., Bennett, R. N., Bisignano, G., Trombetta, D., Saija, A., Faulds, C. B., Gasson, M. J. & Narbad, A. (2007). Antimicrobial activity of flavonoids extracted from bergamot (*Citrus bergamia* Risso) peel, a byproduct of the essential oil industry. *J Applied Microbiol., 103,* 2056-2064.

Martini, N. D., Katerere, D. R. & Eloff, J. N. (2004). Biological activity of five antibacterial flavonoids from Combretum erythrophyllum (Combretaceae). *J Ethnopharmacol, 93,* 207-212.

Mbaveng, A. T., Ngameni, B., Kuete, V., Simo, I. K., Ambassa, P., Roy, R., Bezabih, M., Etoa, F. X., Malterud, K. E., Bremnes, I. E., Faegri, A., Moe, I. & Dugstad, S. E. (1985). Flavonoids from the wood of Salix caprea as inhibitors of wood-destroying fungi. *J Nat Prod., 48,* 559-563.

Messana, I., Ferrari, F. & Carmo, M. M. (1987). A new isoprenylated Flavone from Brosimopsis oblongifolia. *Planta Med., 53,* 541-543.

Ming, D., Brian, A. L., Hillhouse, B. J., French, C. J., Hudson, J. B. & Towers, G. H. N. (2002). Bioactive Constituents from Iryanthera megistophylla. *J Nat Prod., 65,* 1412-1416.

Mirzoeva, O. K., Grishanin, R. N. & Calder, P. C. (1997). Antimicrobial action of propolis and some of its components: the effects on growth, membrane potential and motility of bacteria, *Microbiol Res., 152,* 239-246.

Mitscher, L. A., Rao, G. S. R., Khanna, I., Veysoglu, T. & Drake, S. (1983). Antimicrobial agents from higher plants: prenylated flavonoids and other phenol from Glycyrrhiza lepidota. *Phytochemistry, 22,* 573-576.

Mizobuchi, S. & Sato, Y. (1984). A New flavanone with antifungal activity isolated from Hopst. *Agric Biol Chem.*, *48*, 2771-2775.

Monache, G. D., Botta, B., Vinciguerra, V., Mello, J. F. & Chiappeta, A. A. (1996). Antimicrobial isoflavanones from Desmodium Canum. *Phytochemistry*, *41*, 537-544.

Mori, A., Nishiko, C., Enoki, N. & Tawata, S. (1987a). Antibacterial activity and mode of ction of plant flavonoids against Proteus vulgaris and Staphylococcus aureus. *Phytochemistry*, *26*, 2231-2234.

Mori, A., Nishino, C., Enoki, N. & Tawata, S. (1987). Antibacterial activity and mode of action of plant flavonoids against Proteus vulgaris and Staphylococcus aureus, *Phytochemistry*, *26*, 2231-2234.

Moriyama, M., Satoshi, T., Ingham, J. L. & Mizutani, J. (1992). Isoflavones from the root bark of Piscidia erythrina. *Phytochemistry*, *31*, 683-687.

Murillo, J. I., Encarnación-Dimayuga, R., Malmstromb, J., Christophersen, C. & Franzblau, S. G. (2003). Antimycobacterial flavones from Haplopappus Sonorensis. *Fitoterapia*, *74*, 226-230.

Nanayakkara, D., Burandt, C. L. & Jacob, M. (2002). Flavonoids with Activity against Methicillin-Resistant Staphylococcus aureus from Dalea scandens var. paucifolia. *Planta Med.*, *68*, 519-522.

Narayanan, M. C., Rao, P. R., Shanmugan, N., Gopalakrishnan, S. M. & Devi, K. (2007). Isolation and characterisation of bioactive isoflavonoids from the roots of Dalbergia horrida. *Natural Product Res.*, *21*, 903-909.

Natarajan, P., Katta, S., Andrei, I., Ambati, V. R. & Haas, L. G. J. (2008). Positive antibacterial co-action between hop (Humulus lupulus) constituents and selected antibiotics. *Phytomedicine*, *15*, 194-201.

Negrete, R. E., Backhouse, N., Bravo, B., Erazo, S., Garcia, R. & Avendafio, S. (1987). Some flavonoids of *Centaurea floccosa* Hook. *Plantes medicinales et Phytotherapie*, *21*, 168-172.

Ngadjui, B. T., Abegaz, B. M., Meyer, J. J., Lall, N. & Beng, V. P. (2008). Antimicrobial activity of the crude extracts and five flavonoids from the twigs of Dorstenia barteri (Moraceae). *J Ethnopharmacol.*, *116*, 483-489.

Nkengfack, A. E., Vardamides, J. C., Fomun, Z. T. & Meyer, M. (1995). Prenylated isoflavones from Erythrina eriotrichia. *Phytochemistry*, *40*, 1803-1808.

Nomura, T. (1988). Phenolic compounds of the mulberry tree and related plants. *Progr Chem Org Nat Prod.*, *53*, 87-201.

Normark, S., Boman, H. G. & Matsson, E. (1969). Mutant of Escherichia coli with anomalous cell division and ability to decrease episomally and chromosomally mediated resistance to ampicillin and several other antibiotics. *J Bacteriol.*, *97*, 1334-1342.

Odebiyi, O. O. & Sofowora, E. A. (1979). Antimicrobial alkaloids from Nigerian Chewing sticl (Fagara zanthoxyloides). *Planta Med.*, *36*, 204-207.

Ohemeng, K. A., Schwender, C. F., Fu, K. P. & Barrett, J. F. (1993). DNA gyrase inhibitory and antibacterial activity of some flavones. *Bioorg Med Chem Lett*, *3*, 225-230.

Okada, K., Tamura, Y., Yamamoto, M., Inoue, Y., Takagaki, R. & Takahashi, K. (1989). Identification of antimicrobial and antioxidant constituents from licorice of Russian, and Xinnng Origin. *Chem Pharm Bull*, *37*, 2528-2530.

Ortega, M. C., Scarafia, M. E. & Juliani, H. R. (1996). Antimicrobial agents in Dalea elegans. *Fitoterapia LXVII*, 81-86.

Osawa, K., Yasuda, H., Maruyama, T., Morita, H., Takeya, K. & Itokawa, H. (1992). Isoflavanones from the heartwood of *Swartzia polyphylla* and their antibacterial activity against cariogenic bacteria, *Chem Pharm Bull*, *40*, 2970-2974.

Ozcelik, B., Orhan, I. & Toker, G. (2006). Antiviral and Antimicrobial Assessment of Some Selected Flavonoids. *Z Naturforsch.*, *61c*, 632-638.

Pan, S., Bhattacharyya, A., Ghosh, P. & Thakur, S. (1983). Studies on the antifungal activity of some naturally occuring coumarins. *Zeitschrijt fur Pfanzenkankheiten und Pfanzenschutz*, *90*, 265-268.

Park, K. D., Park, Y. S., Cho, S. J., Sun., Kim, S. H., Jung. & Kim, J. H. (2004). Antimicrobial activity of 3-O-acyl-(-)-epicatechin and 3-O-acyl-(+)-catechin derivatives. *Planta Med.*, *70*, 272-276.

Pegnyemb, D. E., Mbing, J. N., Atchade, A. T., Tih, R. G., Sondengam, B. L., Blond, A. & Bodo (2005). Antimicrobial biflavonoids from the aerial parts of *Ouratea sulcata. Phytochemistry*, *66*, 1922-1926.

Pepeljnjak, S., Kalodera, Z. & Zovko, M. (2005). Antimicrobial activity of flavonoids from Pelargonium radula (Cav.) L Herit. *Acta Pharm.*, *55*, 431-435.

Perry, N. B. & Foster, L. M. (1994). Antiviral and antifungal flavonoids, plus a triterpene from Hebe cupressoides. *Planta Med.*, *60*, 491-492.

Plaper, A., Golob, M., Hafner, I., Oblak, M., Solmajer, T. & Jerala, R. (2003). Characterization of quercetin binding site on DNA gyrase, *Biochem Biophys Res Commun.*, *306*, 530-536.

Prabu, G. R., Gnanamani, A. & Sadulla, S. (2006). Guaijaverin a plant flavonoid as potential antiplaque agent against Streptococcus mutans. *Journal of applied Microbiology.*, *101*, 487-495.

Puupponen-Pimiä, R., Nohynek, L., Alakomi, H. L. & Oksman-Caldentey, K. M. (2005). The action of berry phenolics against human intestinal pathogens. *Biofactors*, *23*, 243-251.

Puyvelde, L., Van, K., Costa, N., Munyjiabo, V., Nyirankuliza, S., Hakizamungu, E. & Schamp, N. (1989). Isolation of flavonoids and a chalcone from Helichrysum odoratissimum. *J Nat Prod.*, *52*, 629-633.

Pizzolattia, M. G., Vensona, A. F., Junior, A. S, Smania, E. F. A. & Braz-Filho, R. (2002). Epimeric flavalignans from *Trichilia catigua* (Meliaceae) with Antimicrobial Activity. Z. *Naturforsch*, *57*, 483-486.

Rahalison, L., Benathan, M., Monod, M., Frenk, E., Gupta, M. P., Solis, P. N., Fuzzati, N. & Hostettman, K. (1995). Antifungal principles of Baccharis pedunculata. *Planta Med.*, *61*, 360-362.

Rahman, M. M. & Gray, A. I. (2002). Antimicrobial constituents from the stem bark of Feronia limonia. *Phytochemistry*, *59*, 73-77.

Rahman, M. M., Gibbons, S. & Graya, A. I. (2007). Isoflavanones from Uraria picta and their antimicrobial activity. *Phytochemistry*, *68*, 1692-1697.

Rao, G. S. R., Gerhart, M. A., Lee, R. T., Mitscher, L. A. & Drake, S. (1982). Antimicrobial agents from higher plants dragon's blood resin. *J Nat Prod.*, *45*, 646-648.

Rocha, L., Marston, A., Auxiliadora, M., Kaplan, C., Stoeckli, H., Thull, U., T Esta, B. & Hostettmann, K. (1994). An antifungal y-pyrone and xanthones with monoamine oxidase inhibitors activity from Hypericum brasiliense. *Phytochemistry*, *36*, 1381-1385.

Rojas, A., Hernandez, L., Perreda-Mirranda, R. & Matg, R. (1992). Screening for antimicrobial activity of crude drug extract and pure natura] products from Mexican medicinal plants. *Journal of Ethnopharmacology*, *35*, 275-283.

Rwangabo, P. C. Claeys, M., Pieters, L., Corthout, J., Berghe, D. A., Vanden, A. & Vlietinck, A. J. (1988). Umuhengerin, a new antimicrobial active flavonoid from Lantana trifolia. *J Nat Prod.*, *51*, 966-968.

Saini, K. S. & Ghosa, S. (1984). Naturally occurring flavans unsubstituted in the heterocyclic ring. *Phytochemistry*, *23*, 2415-2421.

Sathiamoorthy, B., Gupta, P., Kumar, M., Chaturvedi, A. K., Shukla, P. K. & Mauryaa, R. (2007). New antifungal flavonoid glycoside from Vitex negundo. *Bioorg Med Chem Lett*, *17*, 239-242.

Sato, M., Fujiwara, S. & Tsuchiya, H. (1996). Flavones with antibacterial activity against cariogenic bacteria, *J Ethnopharmacol*, *54*, 171-176.

Sato, M., Tsuchiya, H., Akagiri, M., Takagi, N. & Iinuma, M. (1997). Growth inhibition of oral bacteria related to denture stomatitis by anti-candidal chalcones. *Aust Dent J.*, *42*, 343-346.

Sato, M., Tsuchiya, H., Takase, I., Kureshiro, H., Tanigaki, S. & Linuma, M. (1995). Antibacterial Aactivity of flavanone isolated from *Sophora exigua* against methicillin-resistant Staphylococcus aureus and its combination with antibiotics. *Phytother Res.*, *9*, 509-512.

Sato, S., Obara, H., Takeuchi, H., Tawaraya, T., Endo, A. & Onodera, J. 1995a. Síntesis of 2,4, 6-Trihydroxy-3methyl- and 2,4,5, 6-Tetrahydroxy-substituted 3-(3-phenylpropionyl) benzaldehyde and their bactericidal activity. *Phtochemistry*, *18*, 491-493.

Satoa, M., Fujiwarab, S., Tsuchiya, H., Fujiib, T., Iinumad, M., Tosa, H. & Ohkawa, Y. (1996). Flavones with antibacterial activity against cariogenic bacteria. *J Ethnopharm*, *54*, 171-176.

Schutt, C. & Netzl,y, D. (1991). Effect of apiforol and apigeninidin on growth of selected fungi. *J. Chem Ecology*, *17*, 2261-2266.

Schutz, B., Wright, A. D., Rali, T. & Sticher, O. (1995). Prenylated flavanones from leaves of Macaranga pleiostemona. *Phytochemistry*, *40*, 1273-1277.

Sekine, T., Inagaki, M., Ikegami, F., Fujii, Y. & Ruangrungsi, N. (1999). Six diprenylisoflavones, derrisisoflavones A-F, from Derris scandens. *Phytochemistry*, *52*, 87-94.

Shung, T., Huang, S., long, T., Lai, J. & Kuoh, C. (1988). Coumarins, acridone alkaloids and a flavone from Citrus grandis. *Phytochemistry*, *27*, 585-587.

Singh, M. & Singh, I. (1985). Two flavonoids glycosides from Cassia occidentalis Pods. *Planta Med.*, 525-526.

Sivakumaran, S., Molan, A. L., Meagher, L. P., Kolb, B., Foo, L. Y., Lane, G. A., Attwood, G. A., Fraser, K. & Michael Tavendale (2004). Variation in antimicrobial action of proarithocyanidins from Dorycnium rectum against rumen bacteria. *Phytochemistry*, *65*, 2485-2497.

Skibola, C. F. & Smith, M. T. (2000). Potential health impacts of excessive flavonoid intake, *Free Radic Biol Med.*, *29*, 456-459.

Smejkal, K., Chudfk, S., Kloucek, P., Marek, R., Cvacka, J., Urbanova, M., Julinek, O., Kokoska, L., Slapetova, T., Holubova, P., Zima, A. & Dvorskat, M. (2008). Antibacterial C-Geranylflavonoids from Paulownia tomentosa Fruits. *Nat Prod.*, *71*, 706-709.

Sohn, H. Y., Son, K. H., Kwon, C. S., Kwon, G. S. & Kang, S. S. (2004). Antimicrobial and cytotoxic activity of 18 prenylated flavonoids isolated from medicinal plants: Morus alba L., Morus mongolica Schneider, Broussnetia papyrifera (L.) Vent, Sophora flavescens Ait and Echinosophora koreensis Nakai. *Phytomedicine, 11,* 666-672.

Srinivas, K. V. N. S., Rao, Y. K., Mahender, I., Das, B., Rama, K. V. S., Krishna, K., Kishore, H. & Murty, U. S. N. (2003). Flavanoids from Caesalpinia pulcherrima. *Phytochemistry, 63,* 789-793.

Stapleton, P. D., Shah, S. & Hamilton-Miller, J. M. T. (2004). Anti-Staphylococcus aureus activity and oxacillin resistance modulating capacity of 3-*O*-acyl-catechins. *Int J Antimicrob Agents, 24,* 374-380.

Tahara, S., Ingham, J. L., Ankara, S., Mizutani, J., Harbone, J. B. (1984). Fungitoxic dihydrofura- noisoflavones and related compounds in white lupin, Lupinus albus. *Phytochemistry, 23,* 1889-1900.

Takahashi, T., Kokubo, R. & Sakaino, M. (2004). Antimicrobial activities of eucalyptus leaf extracts and flavonoids from Eucalyptus maculata. *Lett Appl Microbiol., 39,* 60-64.

Tan, R. X., Lu, H., Wolfende, J. L., Yu, T. T., Zheng, W. F., Yang, L., Gafner, S. & Hostettmann, K. 1999. Mono-and sesquiterpenes and antifungal constituents from Artemisia Species. *Planta Med., 65,* 64-67.

Taniguchi, M. & Kubo, I. (1993). Ethnobotanical drug discovery based on medicine menstrial in the African savanna: screening of east African plants for antimicrobial activity II. *J Nat Prod., 56,* 1539-1546.

Tereschuk, M. L., Riera, M. V. Q., Castro, G. R. & Abdala, L. R. (1997). Antimicrobial activity of flavonoids from leaves of Tagetes minuta. *J Ethnopharm, 56,* 227-232.

Tomas-Lorente, F., Iniesta-Sanmartin, E. & Tomas-Barberan, E. A. (1991). Antimicrobial phenolics from Helichrysum picardii. *Fitoterapia LXII,* 521-523.

Tsuchiya, H. & Iinuma, M. (2000). Reduction of membrane fluidity by antibacterial sophoraflavanone G isolated from Sophora exigua, *Phytomedicine, 7,* 161-165.

Tsuchiya, H., Sato M. & Miyazaki, T. (1996). Comparative study on the antibacterial activity of phytochemical flavanones against methicillin-resistant Staphylococcus aureus. *J Ethnopharmacol, 50,* 27-34.

Tsukiyama, R., Katsura, H., Tokuriki, N. & Kobayashi, M. (2002). Antibacterial activity of licochalcone A against spore-forming bacteria. *Antimicrob Agents Chemother, 46,* 1226-1230.

Urzua, A. & Cuadra, P. (1990). Acylated flavonoids aglycones from Gnaphalium robustum. *Phytochemistry, 29,* 1342-1343.

VanWagenen, B., Huddleston, J. & Cardellina, J. H. (1988). Native American food medicinal plants. Water-soluble constituents of Lomatium dissectum. *J Nat Prod., 51,* 1436-141.

Veluri, R., Weir, T. L., Bais, H. P., Stermitz, F. R. & Vivanco, J. M. (2004). Phytotoxic and antimicrobial activities of catechin derivatives. *J Agric Food Chem., 52,* 1077-82.

Waage, K. S. & Hedin, P. A. (1984a). Biologically-active flavonoids from Gossypium arboretum. *Phytochemistry, 23,* 2509-2511.

Waage, S. K. & Hedin, P. A. (1985). Quercetin 3-*O*-galactosyl-(1-6)-glucoside, a compound from narrow leaf vetch with antibacterial activity. *Phytochemistry, 24,* 243-245.

Waage, S. K. & Hedin, P. A. (1985a). Biologically-active flavonoids in Heterotheca camporum. *J. Mississipi Academy Sciences, 30,* 55-58.

Waage, S. K., Hedin, P. A. & Grimley, E. (1984). A biologically-active procyanidin from Machaerium floribundum. *Phytochemistry*, *23*, 2785-2787.

Wachter, G. A., Hoffmann, J. J., Furbacher, T., Blake, M. E. & Timmermann, B. N. (1999). Antibacterial and antifungal flavanones from Eysenhardtia texana. *Phytochemistry*, *52*, 1469-1471.

Wang, Y., Hamburger, M., Gueho, J. & Hostettman, K. (1989). Antimicrobial flavonoids from Psiadia trinervia and their methylated and acetylated derivatives. *Phytochemistry*, *28*, 2323-2327

Ward, F. E., Garling, D. L., Buckler, R. T., Lawler, D. M. & Cummings, D. P. (1981) Antimicrobial 3-methyl- eneflavanones, *J Med Chem.*, *24*, 1073-1077.

Yamamoto, Y., Matsunaga, K. & Friedman, H. (2004). Protective effects of green tea catechins on alveolar macrophages against bacterial infections. *Biofactors*, *21*, 119-121.

Yanagawa, Y., Yamamoto, Y., Hara, Y. & Shimamura, T. (2003). A combination effect of epigallocatechin gallate, a major compound of green tea catechins, with antibiotics on Helicobacter pylori growth in vitro. *Curr Microbiol.*, *47*, 244-249.

Yenesewa, A., Derese, S., Midiwo, J. O., Bii, C. C., Heydenreich, M. & Peter, M. G. (2005). Antimicrobial flavonoids from the stem bark of Erythrina burttii. *Fitoterapia*, *76*, 469-472.

Zheng, W., Tan, R. X., Yang, L. & Liu, Z. (1996). Two flavones from Artemisia giraldii and their antimicrobial activity. *Planta Med.*, *62*, 160-162.

Zhu, X., Zhang, H. & Lo, R. (2004). Phenolic Compounds from the Leaf Extract of Artichoke (Cynara scolymus L.) and Their Antimicrobial Activities. *J Agric Food Chem.*, *52*, 7272-7278.

Index

B

C

G

J

K

L

M

N

P

S

T

U

V

W

X

Y

Z